Parkinson's Disease: Advanced Research and Clinical Care

Parkinson's Disease: Advanced Research and Clinical Care

Editor: Dustin Campbell

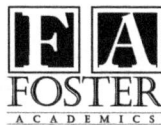

FA FOSTER
ACADEMICS

www.fosteracademics.com

www.fosteracademics.com

FA
FOSTER
ACADEMICS

Cataloging-in-Publication Data

Parkinson's disease : advanced research and clinical care / edited by Dustin Campbell.
     p. cm.
Includes bibliographical references and index.
ISBN 978-1-63242-732-8
1. Parkinson's disease. 2. Brain--Diseases. 3. Parkinson's disease--Research.
4. Parkinson's disease--Treatment. I. Campbell, Dustin.
RC382 .P37 2019
616.833--dc23

Foster Academics,
118-35 Queens Blvd., Suite 400,
Forest Hills, NY 11375, USA

ISBN 978-1-63242-732-8 (Hardback)

Contents

Preface...IX

Chapter 1 **Marijuana Compounds: A Nonconventional Approach to Parkinson's Disease Therapy** 1
Mariana Babayeva, Haregewein Assefa, Paramita Basu, Sanjeda Chumki and Zvi Loewy

Chapter 2 **Psychometric Evaluation of the Parkinson's Disease Activities of Daily Living Scale** 20
Stina B. Jonasson, Peter Hagell, Gun-Marie Hariz, Susanne Iwarsson and Maria H. Nilsson

Chapter 3 **A Meta-Analysis of *GBA*-Related Clinical Symptoms in Parkinson's Disease**......................................27
Yuan Zhang, Li Shu, Xun Zhou, Hongxu Pan, Qian Xu, Jifeng Guo, Beisha Tang and Qiying Sun

Chapter 4 **The Association between *LRRK2* G2385R and Phenotype of Parkinson's Disease in Asian Population** 34
Wei Di, Zhiyong Zeng, Jingyan Li, Xiaoling Liu, Minzhi Bo and Hua Lv

Chapter 5 **Diagnostic Validation for Participants in the Washington State Parkinson Disease Registry** 41
Hojoong M. Kim, James B. Leverenz, Daniel J. Burdick, Sindhu Srivatsal, Jennifer Pate, Shu-Ching Hu, Steven P. Millard, Marie Y. Davis, Ali Samii and Cyrus P. Zabetian

Chapter 6 **Sensitivity and Specificity of the ECAS in Parkinson's Disease and Progressive Supranuclear Palsy**..47
Jennifer A. Foley, Elaine H. Niven, Andrew Paget, Kailash P. Bhatia, Simon F. Farmer, Paul R. Jarman, Patricia Limousin, Thomas T. Warner, Huw R. Morris, Thomas H. Bak, Sharon Abrahams and Lisa Cipolotti

Chapter 7 **Insights into the Mechanisms Involved in Protective Effects of VEGF-B in Dopaminergic Neurons**...55
Beatrice Caballero, Scott J. Sherman and Torsten Falk

Chapter 8 **Correlation of Visuospatial Ability and EEG Slowing in Patients with Parkinson's Disease** 68
Dominique Eichelberger, Pasquale Calabrese, Antonia Meyer, Menorca Chaturvedi, Florian Hatz, Peter Fuhr and Ute Gschwandtner

Chapter 9 **Cognitive Function Characteristics of Parkinson's Disease with Sleep Disorders**............79
Jing Huang, Wenyan Zhuo, Yuhu Zhang, Hongchun Sun, Huan Chen, Peipei Zhu, Xiaobo Pan, Jianhao Yang and Lijuan Wang

Chapter 10   **Management of Psychosis in Parkinson's Disease: Emphasizing Clinical Subtypes and Pathophysiological Mechanisms of the Condition**................................85
Raquel N. Taddei, Seyda Cankaya, Sandeep Dhaliwal and K. Ray Chaudhuri

Chapter 11   **Event-Related Potentials in Parkinson's Disease Patients with Visual Hallucination**................................103
Yang-Pei Chang, Yuan-Han Yang, Chiou-Lian Lai and Li-Min Liou

Chapter 12   **Genetic Variants in SNCA and the Risk of Sporadic Parkinson's Disease and Clinical Outcomes**................................110
Clarissa Loureiro das Chagas Campêlo and Regina Helena Silva

Chapter 13   **Patterns and Predictors of Depression Treatment among Older Adults with Parkinson's Disease and Depression in Ambulatory Care Settings in the United States**................................121
Sandipan Bhattacharjee, Nina Vadiei, Lisa Goldstone, Ziyad Alrabiah and Scott J. Sherman

Chapter 14   **Programming for Stimulation-Induced Transient Nonmotor Psychiatric Symptoms after Bilateral Subthalamic Nucleus Deep Brain Stimulation for Parkinson's Disease**................................127
Xi Wu, Yiqing Qiu, Keith Simfukwe, Jiali Wang, Jianchun Chen and Xiaowu Hu

Chapter 15   **Genetic Variations and mRNA Expression of NRF2 in Parkinson's Disease**................................141
Caroline Ran, Karin Wirdefeldt, Lovisa Brodin, Mehrafarin Ramezani, Marie Westerlund, Fengqing Xiang, Anna Anvret, Thomas Willows, Olof Sydow, Anders Johansson, Dagmar Galter, Per Svenningsson and Andrea Carmine Belin

Chapter 16   **Crossing Virtual Doors: A New Method to Study Gait Impairments and Freezing of Gait in Parkinson's Disease**................................148
Luis I. Gómez-Jordana, James Stafford, C. (Lieke) E. Peper and Cathy M. Craig

Chapter 17   **Cognitive Training and Transcranial Direct Current Stimulation for Mild Cognitive Impairment in Parkinson's Disease**................................156
Blake J. Lawrence, Natalie Gasson, Andrew R. Johnson, Leon Booth and Andrea M. Loftus

Chapter 18   **Association between Objectively Measured Physical Activity and Gait Patterns in People with Parkinson's Disease: Results from a 3-Month Monitoring**................................168
Micaela Porta, Giuseppina Pilloni, Roberta Pili, Carlo Casula, Mauro Murgia, Giovanni Cossu and Massimiliano Pau

Chapter 19   **Predictors of Functional and Quality of Life Outcomes following Deep Brain Stimulation Surgery in Parkinson's Disease Patients: Disease, Patient and Surgical Factors**................................178
Hesham Abboud, Gencer Genc, Nicolas R. Thompson, Srivadee Oravivattanakul, Faisal Alsallom, Dennys Reyes, Kathy Wilson, Russell Cerejo, Xin Xin Yu, Darlene Floden, Anwar Ahmed, Michal Gostkowski, Ayman Ezzeldin, Hazem Marouf, Ossama Y. Mansou, Andre Machado and Hubert H. Fernandez

Chapter 20   **Should Skin Biopsies be Performed in Patients Suspected of Having Parkinson's Disease?**................................186
Timo Siepmann, Ana Isabel Penzlin, Ben Min-Woo Illigens and Heinz Reichmann

Chapter 21   **The Cognition of Maximal Reach Distance in Parkinson's Disease**..192
Satoru Otsuki and Masanori Nagaoka

Chapter 22   **Standardised Neuropsychological Assessment for the Selection of Patients
Undergoing DBS for Parkinson's Disease** 200
Jennifer A. Foley, Tom Foltynie, Patricia Limousin and Lisa Cipolotti

Chapter 23   **The Sources of Reactive Oxygen Species and its Possible Role in the
Pathogenesis of Parkinson's Disease** 213
Minrui Weng, Xiaoji Xie, Chao Liu, Kah-Leong Lim, Cheng-wu Zhang and Lin Li

Chapter 24   **Rivastigmine as a Symptomatic Treatment for Apathy in Parkinson's Dementia
Complex: New Aspects for this Riddle**...222
Rita Moretti, Paola Caruso and Matteo Dal Ben

Chapter 25   **Neuroprotective Effects of Salidroside in the MPTP Mouse Model of
Parkinson's Disease: Involvement of the PI3K/Akt/GSK3β Pathway**.......................................231
Wei Zhang, Hong He, Hujie Song, Junjie Zhao, Tao Li, Leitao Wu,
Xiaojun Zhang and Jianzong Chen

Chapter 26   **Antidyskinetic Treatment with MTEP Affects Multiple Molecular Pathways in
the Parkinsonian Striatum**..240
Jing-ya Lin, Zhen-guo Liu, Cheng-long Xie, Lu Song and Ai-juan Yan

Chapter 27   **Tremor Types in Parkinson Disease: A Descriptive Study using
a New Classification**..248
Alexandre Gironell, Berta Pascual-Sedano, Ignacio Aracil, Juan Marín-Lahoz,
Javier Pagonabarraga and Jaime Kulisevsky

Chapter 28   **Aerobic Exercise Preserves Olfaction Function in Individuals with
Parkinson's Disease** 253
Anson B. Rosenfeldt, Tanujit Dey and Jay L. Alberts

Chapter 29   **Identification of NURR1 (Exon 4) and FOXA1 (Exon 3) Haplotypes
Associated with mRNA Expression Levels in Peripheral Blood Lymphocytes of
Parkinson's Patients in Small Indian Population**..259
Jayakrishna Tippabathani, Jayshree Nellore, Vaishnavie Radhakrishnan,
Somashree Banik and Sonia Kapoor

Chapter 30   **The Importance of Connection to Others in QoL in MSA and PSP**.......................................267
Louise Wiblin, Rory Durcan, Mark Lee and Katie Brittain

Permissions

List of Contributors

Index

Preface

Parkinson's disease (PD) is a progressive disorder of the nervous system that affects the motor system. PD results in motor, neuropsychiatric, sensory and sleep diseases. Four cardinal motor symptoms in PD are tremor, postural instability, rigidity and slowness of movement. Neuropsychiatric disturbances such as disorders of mood, behavior, cognition and thought may also occur. An important underlying cause of Parkinson's disease is the death of cells in the substantia nigra, lower levels of dopamine in these regions and the build-up of proteins into Lewy bodies in the neurons. People exposed to certain pesticides and with head injuries in the past are at an increased risk of developing Parkinson's diseases. There is currently no cure for Parkinson's disease. The symptoms can be managed with the help of medications, rehabilitation, surgery and palliative care. This book discusses the fundamentals as well as modern approaches in the study of Parkinson's disease. It aims to shed light on some of the unexplored aspects of PD and the recent researches in this domain. It is a complete source of knowledge on the present status of this important disease.

This book has been the outcome of endless efforts put in by authors and researchers on various issues and topics within the field. The book is a comprehensive collection of significant researches that are addressed in a variety of chapters. It will surely enhance the knowledge of the field among readers across the globe.

It gives us an immense pleasure to thank our researchers and authors for their efforts to submit their piece of writing before the deadlines. Finally in the end, I would like to thank my family and colleagues who have been a great source of inspiration and support.

Editor

Marijuana Compounds: A Nonconventional Approach to Parkinson's Disease Therapy

Mariana Babayeva, Haregewein Assefa, Paramita Basu, Sanjeda Chumki, and Zvi Loewy

Touro College of Pharmacy, 230 West 125th Street, Room 530, New York, NY 10027, USA

Correspondence should be addressed to Mariana Babayeva; mariana.babayeva@touro.edu

Academic Editor: Jan Aasly

Parkinson's disease (PD), a neurodegenerative disorder, is the second most common neurological illness in United States. Neurologically, it is characterized by the selective degeneration of a unique population of cells, the nigrostriatal dopamine neurons. The current treatment is symptomatic and mainly involves replacement of dopamine deficiency. This therapy improves only motor symptoms of Parkinson's disease and is associated with a number of adverse effects including dyskinesia. Therefore, there is unmet need for more comprehensive approach in the management of PD. Cannabis and related compounds have created significant research interest as a promising therapy in neurodegenerative and movement disorders. In this review we examine the potential benefits of medical marijuana and related compounds in the treatment of both motor and nonmotor symptoms as well as in slowing the progression of the disease. The potential for cannabis to enhance the quality of life of Parkinson's patients is explored.

1. Introduction

Marijuana, the crude product (dried flowers, stems, seeds, and leaves) derived from the cannabis sativa plant, consists of more than 85 phytocannabinoids [1, 2]. The term phytocannabinoids is used to differentiate these plant-derived cannabinoids from the synthetic cannabinoids and the structurally different endogenous cannabinoids (endocannabinoids). Among the phytocannabinoids, Cannabidiol (CBD) and Δ9-Tetrahydrocannabinol (Δ9-THC, THC) are the major constituents of marijuana [3]. Δ9-THC is a psychoactive agent with analgesic and muscle relaxant property [3, 4]. While CBD is a nonpsychoactive compound and has been shown to have hypnotic, anxiolytic, antipsychotic, antioxidant, and neuroprotective effects [5], THC is a partial agonist at the cannabinoid receptor 1 (CB1) and receptor 2 (CB2). Unlike Δ9-THC, CBD has antagonistic/inverse agonistic property at CB1 receptor and appears to modulate Δ9-THC-associated side effects including anxiety, tachycardia, and hunger [3]. CBD also appears to potentiate the effect of endocannabinoids by inhibiting their inactivation, thereby alleviating psychotic symptom [6].

Despite the placement of marijuana in the schedule 1 category under the US Federal Controlled Substance Act [7] and the US Federal Government's continued opposition on its legalization, 24 states and Washington DC have enacted laws allowing marijuana to treat certain medical conditions [8]. The range and types of disease conditions for which medical marijuana have been approved vary from state to state. The most common disease conditions approved by the states include cancer, HIV/AIDS, glaucoma, chronic and/or severe pain, seizure/epilepsy, cachexia, and multiple sclerosis. Moreover, two cannabinoids (dronabinol and nabilone) have been approved by the FDA for clinical use. The synthetically produced Δ9-THC, dronabinol (Marinol®), is a schedule III drug, which is indicated in the treatment of chemotherapy-induced nausea and emesis as well as anorexia associated with weight loss in AIDS patients. A synthetic cannabinoid, nabilone (Cesamet®), is a schedule II drug that is indicated for the treatment of nausea and vomiting associated with cancer chemotherapy. Another cannabinoid, Cannabidiol (Epidiolex®), is in a clinical trial for the treatment of drug-resistant epilepsy in children [9]. A phytocannabinoid preparation, nabiximols (Sativex®), has been approved for the treatment of spasticity due to multiple sclerosis in a number of countries outside the United States. Nabiximols is an extract of *Cannabis sativa* L that consists of mainly THC and CBD [10, 11].

Although recent studies have provided strong evidence for the therapeutic benefit of medical marijuana [12–16], increasing access to cannabis and/or cannabinoids can result in side effects such as addiction, respiratory illness, and decline in cognitive processing. Cannabis use has been indicated as a potential cause, aggravator, or masker of major psychiatric symptoms, including psychotic, depressive, and anxiety disorders, particularly in young people [17–19]. Other negative effects include working memory deficits, reduced attention and processing speed, anhedonia, abnormal social behavior, and susceptibility to mood and anxiety disorders [20, 21]. While adult users seem comparatively resistant to cannabis-induced behavioral and brain morphologic changes, the individuals who start using cannabis during their early teens can have more severe and more long-lasting effects [22].

The target of medical marijuana and its constituents is the endocannabinoid system, which is involved in the modulation of a number of physiological functions. The endocannabinoid system includes the endocannabinoids, the cannabinoid receptors, and the enzymes involved in the biosynthesis and inactivation of the endocannabinoids [23] The cannabinoid receptors are mainly expressed in the central nervous system and the immune system, but they have also been identified in a number of other parts of the body including the cardiovascular system, the peripheral nervous system, the reproductive system, and the gastrointestinal tract. Due to its wide distribution and effects on a range of biological process, the cannabinoid system has become an attractive target for the development of drugs that can potentially be used for the treatment of a number of pathological conditions including mood disorders and movement disorders such as PD [24]. Components of the endocannabinoid system are abundant in the striatum and other parts of the basal ganglia and play a crucial role in modulating dopamine activity and motor functions [25–27].

Parkinson's disease (PD) is the second most common neurodegenerative disorder following Alzheimer's disease and the 14th leading cause of death in all age groups in the United States [28]. The prevalence of PD increases with age and is shown to be higher in males than females in some age groups [29]. The number of people with PD is projected at approximately 9 million by 2030 in the 15 most populous countries in the world [30, 31]. Neurologically PD is characterized by the destruction of dopaminergic cells in the pars compacta region of the substantia nigra in the midbrain, resulting in dopamine deficiency in the nerve terminals of the striatum in the forebrain [32]. These changes cause impairments not just to the motor system but also to the cognitive and neuropsychological systems [33]. The nigrostriatal pathway is one of the dopamine pathways in the brain that regulates movement. The exact cause for the loss of neuronal cells is unknown, and the trigger of dopaminergic degeneration seems to be multifactorial including environmental factors and genetic susceptibilities

[34–36]. Clinically, PD is characterized by resting tremor, muscle rigidity, bradykinesia, and postural instability [32, 34, 37, 38] and it is also associated with a number of nonmotor symptoms including depression, anxiety, constipation, orthostatic hypotension, fatigue, and sleep disorders, as well as, in advanced disease, dementia [39–44]. Although dopamine deficiency accounts for the major motor symptoms of the disease, loss of noradrenergic and serotoninergic nerve terminals in the limbic system may account for several of the nonmotor features seen in Parkinson's disease [45, 46].

Current therapy involves treatment of motor symptoms of PD through replacement of dopamine deficiency [47]. This includes (1) enhancement of the synthesis of brain dopamine by administration of levodopa, a dopamine precursor, (2) direct stimulation of dopamine receptors, (3) decreasing dopamine catabolism, and (4) stimulation of dopamine release and inhibition of dopamine reuptake from presynaptic sites. Another therapy involves restoring the normal balance of cholinergic and dopaminergic actions on the basal ganglia using anticholinergic drugs [47–49].

However these drugs treat only motor symptoms of Parkinson's disease and are associated with a number of adverse effects. Long-term use of levodopa, the mainstay therapy for PD, is associated with motor fluctuations [50] and levodopa-induced dyskinesia [51–53]. The monoamine oxidase B (MAO-B) inhibitors (selegiline and rasagiline) as well as inhibitors of catechol-o-methyltransferase, COMT (tolcapone and entacapone), are used mostly to reduce the motor fluctuations associated with levodopa therapy due to their levodopa-sparing effect [54–59]. Several dopamine agonists including pramipexole, ropinirole, rotigotine, and apomorphine are used as monotherapy in early stage of Parkinson disease or as adjunctive therapy with levodopa in patients with advanced PD in order to reduce motor fluctuations [56, 60–64]. In addition to their limited efficacy on motor symptoms and their adverse effects, drugs that are currently used for the treatment of PD do not have an effect on disease progression. Therefore, there is an urgent need for the development of safer drugs that treat both the motor and nonmotor symptoms of PD as well as drugs that slow the progression of the disease.

Medical marijuana has been demonstrated to improve motor symptoms including tremor, rigidity, and bradykinesia as well as nonmotor symptoms such as pain and sleep disorders of PD in observational studies [65]. Survey of PD patients in Colorado, USA, also indicated the beneficial effects of marijuana in alleviating nonmotor symptoms of PD [66]. Cannabidiol (CBD), one of the major constituents of marijuana, has been shown to be effective in the treatment of psychosis and sleep disorders in PD patients [67–69]. Another phytocannabinoid, Δ9-tetrahydrocannabivarin (Δ9-THCV, THCV), was studied in animal disease model of PD and found to have neuroprotective and symptom-relieving effects [70]. Therefore, marijuana may provide an alternative or add-on therapy for Parkinson's disease. In addition, Parkinson's disease has been listed as one of the disease conditions for which medical marijuana is allowed in Connecticut, Illinois, Massachusetts, New Hampshire, New

Mexico, and New York. However, it may also be covered under chronic illnesses in several other states.

In this review we seek to investigate any scientific evidence that indicates the potential use of marijuana and/or its components for the treatment of Parkinson's disease. The review aims to (i) examine briefly current treatment and the unmet need of PD therapy, (ii) assess the role of the cannabinoid system in the modulation of movement and neuroprotection, (iii) look at the mechanism of action of marihuana constituents in the modulation of movement and PD-associated disorders, (iv) assess other beneficial effects of marihuana that contribute to the amelioration of PD, and (v) gather scientific evidence on the clinical benefit of marijuana and/or its constituents in PD patients.

2. Marijuana and Its Influence on the Endocannabinoid System

Cannabis has been used to treat disease since ancient times. Marijuana is derived from the *Cannabis sativa L.* plant. Marijuana contains the active chemicals known as cannabinoids. At least 85 cannabinoids have been identified as unique compounds in *Cannabis* [1]. The therapeutic potential of many of these ligands still remains largely unexplored prompting a need for further research. The chemicals responsible for the medicinal effects of marijuana are D9-Tetrahydrocannabinol (THC) and Cannabidiol (CBD) [71, 72]. THC is the major psychoactive ingredient, acting primarily upon the central nervous system where it affects brain function. CBD is the major nonpsychoactive ingredient in cannabis and produces neuroprotective and anti-inflammatory effects [73]. Both compounds, TCH and CBD, have anticonvulsant properties [74]. Cannabinoids have also potential to alleviate motor disorders by reducing motor impairments and neuron degeneration [75]. In addition, cannabinoids have been shown to be effective in preclinical studies involving excitotoxicity, oxidative stress, neuroinflammation, and motor complications associated with PD [76].

Some cannabinoids (endocannabinoids or ECBs) are found in the body. Initially, ECBs were discovered in the brain and subsequently in the periphery in humans and animals. Endocannabinoids are produced by cultured neurons [77], microglia, and astrocytes [78]. ECBs interact with the endocannabinoid system and aid in regulation of memory, pleasure, concentration, thinking, movement and coordination, sensory and time perception, appetite, and pain [24, 79, 80]. The ECBs activate two guanine nucleotide-binding protein- (G-protein-) coupled cell membrane receptors, consequently named the cannabinoid type 1 (CB1) and type 2 (CB2) receptors [81]. CB1 receptors are located primarily in the central and peripheral neurons and CB2 receptors are predominantly found in immune cells [82]. CB1 receptors are important mediators in signaling pathways and have been identified on both glutamatergic and gamma-aminobutyric (GABA) neurons [83]. It is believed that one important role of the neuronal CB1 component is to modulate neurotransmitter release in a manner that maintains homeostasis by preventing the development of excessive neuronal activity in the central nervous system [82]. Animal models illustrate that activation of the CB1 receptor by their endogenous ligands can result in prominent neuroprotective effects and may prevent epileptic seizures [84]. Other studies suggest that activation of CB1 receptors offers neuroprotection against dopaminergic lesion and the development of L-DOPA-induced dyskinesias [85]. CB2 receptors are closely related to CB1 and are mainly expressed on T cells of the immune system, on macrophages and B cells, and in hematopoietic cells [86]. They are also expressed on peripheral nerve terminals where these receptors play a role in antinociception and the relief of pain [87]. In the brain, CB2 receptors are mainly expressed by microglial cells, where their role remains unclear [88].

The major identified ECBs are arachidonoyl ethanolamide (anandamide, AEA), 2-arachidonoyl glycerol (2-AG), O-arachidonoyl ethanolamine (virodhamine), and 2-arachidonoyl glyceryl ether (noladin ether) [89]. Both AEA and 2-AG are specific ligands of CB1 and CB2 receptors. Besides having activity on CB1 and CB2 receptors, AEA also has full agonistic activity at TRPV1 receptor [90]. AEA is localized in the brain and periphery [91]. In the brain AEA shows high distribution in the hippocampus, thalamus, striatum, and brainstem and to a lesser extent in the cerebral cortex and cerebellum [92]. Lower concentrations of AEA are found in human serum, plasma, and cerebrospinal fluid [93]. Similarly, 2-AG is observed in both the brain and periphery, although its concentration is almost 150 times higher in brain compared to that of AEA [92, 94, 95]. 2-AG has greater potency, stability, and agonistic activity at CB1 and CB2 receptors compared to that of AEA [96, 97]. Two prominent areas involved in the control of movement, such as the globus pallidus and the substantia nigra, contain not only the highest densities of CB1 receptors [88], but also the highest levels of ECBs, especially AEA [98, 99]. Tissue levels of AEA are regulated by fatty acid amide hydrolase (FAAH) [100]. It has also been shown that the basal ganglia contain the precursor of AEA [98, 99], supporting the theory of in situ synthesis for this compound. Studies have demonstrated that AEA synthesis is regulated by dopaminergic D2 receptors in the striatum, suggesting that the endocannabinoid system acts as an inhibitory feedback mechanism countering the dopamine-induced facilitation of motor activity [101].

Marijuana compound THC is CB_1 and CB_2 receptor partial agonist [82]. Due to the structural similarity of natural cannabinoid THC to the endogenous cannabinoid AEA, many therapeutic advantages of THC have been identified, such as lowering ocular pressure, inhibiting smooth muscle contractions, and increasing appetite [102]. When smoked, THC is rapidly absorbed from the lungs into the bloodstream and has an effect on the cannabinoid receptors. The central nervous system and specific areas of the brain contain the highest concentration of cannabinoid receptors. Therefore, cannabis or THC administration can create an overexcitation of the system that results in altered perceptions, pleasure, and mood [103].

Unlike THC, CBD has little affinity for CB1 and CB2 receptors but acts as an indirect antagonist of cannabinoid agonists. While this should cause CBD to reduce the effects of THC, it may potentiate THC's effects by increasing CB1 receptor density or through another CB1-related mechanism [73]. CBD is also an inverse agonist of CB2 receptors. CBD can counteract some of the functional consequences of CB1 activation in the brain, possibly by indirect enhancement of adenosine A1 receptors activity through equilibrative nucleoside transporter (ENT) inhibition [73]. CBD helps to augment some of THC's beneficial effects, as it reduces the psychoactivity of THC, enhances its tolerability, and widens THC's therapeutic window [104].

Other cannabinoids can also contribute to the cannabis medicinal effects. Studies in experimental models and humans have suggested anti-inflammatory, neuroprotective, anxiolytic, and antipsychotic properties of chemicals extracted from marijuana [6, 15, 82, 105, 106].

3. Cannabinoids and Parkinson's Disease

3.1. Changes in the Cannabinoid System in Parkinson's Disease. Recent data from several studies indicate the important role of the endocannabinoid system in Parkinson's disease. The components of the endocannabinoid system are highly expressed in the neural circuit of basal ganglia, which is part of a complex neuronal system. This neuronal system coordinates activities from different cortical regions that directly or indirectly participate in the control of movement [107, 108]. In the basal ganglia, the endocannabinoid system bidirectionally interacts with dopaminergic, glutamatergic, and GABAergic signaling systems [109]. Endocannabinoids play a dominant role in controlling transmission at synapses between cortical and striatal neurons, in mediating the induction of a particular form of synaptic plasticity, and in modulating basal ganglia activity and motor functions [110]. The progressive loss of dopaminergic neurons that occurs in PD leads to lower striatal levels of dopamine. These low levels of dopamine result in the alteration of the equilibrium between the direct and the indirect basal ganglia pathways and ECB signaling [111].

The cannabinoid signaling system mentioned above experiences a biphasic pattern of changes during the progression of PD [112]. Early and presymptomatic PD stages, characterized by neuronal malfunction with little evidence of neuronal death, are associated with desensitization/down-regulation of CB1 receptors and aggravation of various cytotoxic insults such as excitotoxicity, oxidative stress, and glial activation [113]. However, intermediate and advanced stages of PD, characterized by a deep nigral degeneration and manifestation of major Parkinsonian symptoms, are associated with upregulatory responses of CB1 receptors and the endocannabinoid ligands [113]. This could explain the potential of CB1 receptor ligands in alleviating common PD symptoms.

In the brain, CB1 receptors are expressed by GABAergic neurons innervating the external and internal segments of the globus pallidus and the substantia nigra [114–116]. CB1 receptors are also present in the corticostriatal glutamatergic terminals and in the excitatory projections from the subthalamic nucleus to the internal segment of the globus pallidus and the substantia nigra [114–116]. Within the striatum, CB1 receptors

are expressed in parvalbumin immune-reactive interneurons, cholinergic interneurons, and nitric oxide synthase-positive neurons [117, 118]. Animal models of Parkinson's disease show an increase in the density of CB1 receptors, levels of endogenous ligands, and CB1 receptor binding in the basal ganglia [119–122]. Endogenous cannabinoids activate CB1 receptors on presynaptic axons and reduce neurotransmitter and glutamate release, working as retrograde synaptic messengers released from postsynaptic neurons [123]. Similarly, activation of CB1 receptors inhibits both glutamate release from substantia nigra afferents and GABA release from striatal afferents. At the same time, activation of presynaptic CB1 receptors in the external segments of the globus pallidus can increase local GABA levels by reducing GABA reuptake from striatal afferents to the nucleus and decrease GABA release from striatal afferents of the substantia nigra [114, 116, 118]. Based on these evidences, it is thought that the function of the basal ganglia neuronal system is controlled by ECB. The presence of endocannabinoid systems in different neural structures and their interaction with dopaminergic, glutamatergic, and GABAergic neurotransmitter signaling systems make the components of endocannabinoid system ideal targets for a novel nondopaminergic treatment of PD.

Endocannabinoid signaling is also bidirectionally linked to dopaminergic signaling within the basal ganglia [118]. The CB1, D1, and D2 dopamine receptors are localized in the striatum [114, 115]. In animal models, CB1 and D2 dopamine receptors share a common pool of G proteins, suggesting the link of their signal transduction mechanisms [124, 125]. In addition, D2 receptor stimulation resulted in release of ECBs in the striatum [101]. However, stimulation of CB1 receptors completely inhibited D1-dopamine receptor mediated activation of adenylyl cyclase and decreased GABA release from striatal afferents of dopaminergic neurons of the substantia nigra resulting in an increased firing of these cells [114–116].

Another receptor involved in control of movement is transient receptor potential vanilloid type 1 (TRPV1), which is expressed in sensory neurons and basal ganglia circuitry of dopaminergic neurons [126, 127]. TRPV1 receptors are molecular integrators of nociceptive stimuli activated by endovanilloids [128]. TRPV1 also interacts with ECB. In particular, anandamide is one of the major endogenous activators of TRPV1 [129–131]. Studies have revealed that motor behavior can be suppressed by the activation of vanilloid receptors [98, 99], suggesting that TRPV1 receptors might play a role in the control of motor function.

3.2. Preclinical Data on the Endocannabinoid System as a Target for Parkinson's Disease Therapy. The association of cannabinoids with regulation of motor functions is well established [132–135]. The effect of the cannabinoids on motor activity depends on the impact of the endocannabinoid system on the dopaminergic, glutamatergic, and GABAergic signaling systems throughout the basal ganglia [112, 136]. The high density of cannabinoid, dopamine, and vanilloid-like receptors coupled with ECBs within the basal ganglia and cerebellum suggests a potential therapeutic role for the cannabinoids in the control of voluntary movement and in movement disorders such as Parkinson's disease [98, 99, 121, 137]. Additional indications of an important role of the endocannabinoid system in the control of movement involve an inhibitory action of cannabinoids through fine tuning of various classical neurotransmitters activity [138], prominent changes in transmission of ECBs in the basal ganglia [139], and alteration of the CB1 binding as well as CB1 availability in the substantia nigra [85, 112, 119, 120, 140, 141]. These data support the idea that cannabinoid- based compounds act on vital pathways of endocannabinoid transmission and therefore might be of therapeutic interest due to their potential to diminish motor symptoms in extrapyramidal disorders such as Parkinson's disease [27, 76, 142].

Research with cannabinoid agonists and antagonists demonstrates that the cannabinoids can modulate motor activity and produce alterations in corresponding molecular correlates [129, 143–145]. It has been widely reported that synthetic, plant-derived, or endogenous cannabinoid agonists exert a powerful motor inhibition in laboratory species [129, 144, 146–149]. This hypokinetic effect was shown to be mediated by the activation of CB1 receptors in neurons of the basal ganglia circuitry [88, 137, 141, 150–152]. Stimulation of the CB1 receptor by a synthetic cannabinoid HU-210 decreased spontaneous glutamatergic activity and reduced the rotations induced by levodopa/carbidopa by 34% in PD rats [153, 154]. Administration of CB1 receptor agonists THC and two synthetic cannabinoids WIN 55,212-2 and CP 55,940 increased extracellular dopamine concentrations in rats [152, 155, 156]. WIN 55,212-2 and CP 55,940 also weakened contralateral rotations induced by a selective D_1/D_5 receptor partial agonist SKF38393 without developing catalepsy in PD rats [148]. In a gender study THC produced an increase in tyrosine hydroxylase activity in parkin-null male mice (a model of early stages of PD) and caused a motor inhibition that was significantly greater compared to wild-type animals [122]. Treatment with THC inhibited motor activity and produced catalepsy in rats [109, 144, 146, 147] and caused antinociception and ring immobility in mice [157]. In other studies THC diminished the motor inhibition caused by 6-hydroxydopamine [70] and potentiated the hypokinetic effect of reserpine in rats more than 20-fold [135]. However, in a primate model of Parkinson's disease THC did not affect locomotor activity but increased bradykinesia [125].

Administration of WIN 55,212-2 increased stimulation of $GTP\gamma_S$ binding in the caudate nucleus, putamen, globus pallidus, and substantia nigra of marmosets, indicating an effective activation of CB1 signaling mechanisms [119, 120]. WIN 55,212-2 produced a dose-dependent reduction of the spontaneous motor activity and catalepsy in mutant Syrian hamsters, increased antidystonic efficacy of benzodiazepines [158], and significantly reduced the antikinetic effects of quinpirole in the reserpine-treated rats [159]. Treatment with WIN 55,212-2 also reduced levodopa-induced dyskinesias, attenuated axial, limb, and severe orolingual abnormal involuntary movements in 6-hyroxydopamine- (6-OHDA-) lesioned rats [160–163]. An endogenous cannabinoid agonist oleoylethanolamide (OAE) produced reduction in dyskinetic contralateral rotations correlated with reduction of molecular

associates of L-DOPA-induced dyskinesia: reduced FosB striatal overexpression and phosphoacetylation of hystone 3 [164]. Another synthetic agonist levonantradol decreased general and locomotor activity and increased bradykinesia in a primate model of Parkinson's disease [125]. Nabilone, a synthetic cannabinoid agonist, coadministered with levodopa significantly decreased total dyskinesia compared with levodopa alone treatment and increased the duration of antiparkinsonian action of levodopa by 76% in PD marmosets [165, 166].

Cannabinoid agonist anandamide (AEA) and its synthetic analog methanandamide increased the extracellular dopamine levels in the nucleus accumbens shell of rats by the activation of the mesolimbic dopaminergic system [167]. This dopamine increase was inhibited by the cannabinoid CB1 receptor antagonist rimonabant [167]. However, recent discoveries indicate that AEA is also able to activate vanilloid VR(1) receptors and that the activation of these receptors might also be responsible for changes in nigrostriatal dopaminergic activity and anandamide-induced hypokinesia [168–170]. AEA produced a tonic facilitation of glutamate release in the substantia nigra via stimulation of VR1 receptors, indicating the involvement of this receptor in motor and cognitive functions of the dopaminergic system [171]. Preclinical data have shown that AEA decreased the activity of nigrostriatal dopaminergic neurons and produced hypokinesia that was completely reversed by an antagonist of vanilloid-like receptors, capsazepine [129]. Additional studies have demonstrated that AEA inhibited ambulation and stereotypic behavior, increased inactivity, and occluded the effects of an agonist of vanilloid VR_1 receptors, livanil, on locomotion in mice, suggesting a common mechanism of action for the two compounds [170]. Treatment with anandamide lowered motor activity with the maximal inhibition by approximately 85% and produced hypothermia and analgesia in mice, increased the inactivity time, and markedly decreased the ambulation and the frequency of spontaneous non-ambulatory activities in rats [146, 147, 172, 173]. Moreover, AEA produced a decrease in spontaneous motor activity in laboratory animals similar to the reported actions of THC [129, 145, 153, 170]. The hypokinetic actions of AEA were boosted by coadministration with a selective inhibitor of endocannabinoid uptake N-(3-furylmethyl) eicosa-5,8,11,14-tetraenamide, UCM707 [174].

Tissue concentrations of endocannabinoids are important for producing motor effects. Levels and activities of AEA and 2-AG can be manipulated by inhibition of FAAH enzyme, the action of which is reduced in experimental models of PD [153, 175]. Animal studies have shown that the FAAH enzyme inhibitor [3-(3-carbamoylphenyl) phenyl] N-cyclohexylcarbamate (URB597) magnified and prolonged a rapid, brief dopamine increase that was produced by AEA [167]. Additional studies have confirmed that FAAH inhibition remarkably increases AEA tissue levels but reduces 2-AG levels [176, 177]. To determine whether FAAH inhibition has beneficial impact on PD symptoms the effect of the FAAH inhibitor, URB597, was studied in MPTP- lesioned marmosets. Treatment with URB597 increased plasma levels of AEA, did not modify the antiparkinsonian actions of L-DOPA, and reduced the magnitude of hyperactivity to levels equivalent to those seen in normal animals [178]. In PD mice URB597 prevented induced motor impairment [179]. Moreover, other FAAH inhibitors, JNJ1661010 and TCF2, also have anticataleptic properties [179]. These results reveal that FAAH inhibition may represent a new strategy for treatment of PD.

Overall, these results indicate that endogenous or exogenous cannabinoid agonists activate the dopaminergic system and play a very important role in modulation of motor behavior [180]. In addition to the effects on movement activity, cannabinoid agonists have demonstrated neuroprotective properties, suggesting that the cannabinoids have a promising pharmacological profile for not only improving Parkinsonian symptoms but also delaying PD progression [70, 85, 181–183].

The CB1 receptor antagonists can also influence movement syndromes of Parkinson's disease suggesting that modulation of the CB1 signaling system might be valuable in treatment of motor disorders. In a study with PD rats rimonabant (SR141716A), a selective antagonist of CB1 receptors has shown the potential to act as an antihypokinetic agent by enhancing glutamate release from excitatory afferents to the striatum [184]. Moreover, SR141716A prevented the effects of THC on dopamine release [156, 167] and also increased the locomotor activity in mice and rats preexposed to THC [170, 185]. SR141716A produced a 71% increase in motor activity in MPTP-lesioned marmosets with LID [136]. Coadministration of SR141716A with levodopa resulted in significantly less dyskinesia than administration of levodopa alone [136, 160]. SR141716A also reversed effect of the cannabinoid agonist WIN 55,212-2 and increased the locomotor activity in 6-OHDA-lesioned animals [159, 163]. Coadministration of SR141716A with a selective D_2/D_3 receptor agonist quinpirole reduced levels of AEA and 2AG by sevenfold in the globus pallidus, boosted the locomotive effects of quinpirole, and produced restoration of locomotion in animal models of Parkinson's disease [98, 99, 101, 136, 186]. In parkin-null mice SR141716A produced a decrease in tyrosine hydroxylase activity in the caudate–putamen and as result formed a hyperkinetic response [122]. However, SR141716A did not alleviate the motor deficits in a primate model of Parkinson's disease [125].

Another CB1 receptor antagonist AM251 and SR141716A produced antiparkinsonian effects in rats with very severe nigral degeneration (>95% cell loss) [187]. Local administration of these antagonists into denervated striatum, globus pallidus, and subthalamic nucleus reduced motor asymmetry in Parkinsonian rats [187, 188], which was inhibited by CB1 receptor agonist AM404 [187]. Another CB1 antagonist CE-178253 produced a 30% increase in motor behavior responses to L-DOPA in MPTP-treated rhesus monkeys but did not modify levodopa-induced dyskinesias [189]. THCV caused changes in glutamatergic transmission and attenuated the motor inhibition in PD rats [70]. Overall, these findings suggest that cannabinoid CB1 antagonists might be therapeutically effective in the control of Parkinson's disease and levodopa-induced dyskinesia [114, 190].

The activation of CB2 receptors might also contribute to some extent to the potential of cannabinoids in PD [191]. THCV, which is not only a CB1 antagonist but also a CB2 partial agonist, reduced the loss of tyrosine hydroxylase-positive neurons in the substantia nigra with preservation of these neurons in CB2 receptor-deficient mice [70]. CBD has also reduced the loss of tyrosine hydroxylase-positive neurons in the substantia nigra of PD rats. Both compounds, THCV and CBD, have acted via neuroprotective and antioxidant mechanisms [70, 182, 191]. CBD has also demonstrated significant effects in preclinical models of neurodegenerative disorders in combination with other cannabinoids [15, 70, 192]. CB2 receptor agonists display a promising pharmacological profile for delaying disease progression.

The cannabinoid pharmacologic manipulation represents a promising therapy to alleviate movement disorders and levodopa-induced dyskinesias. Thus, CB1 antagonists appear to have antiparkinsonian effects, while cannabinoid receptor agonists may be useful in the treatment of motor complications in Parkinson's disease.

3.3. Effect of Cannabinoids on Patients with Movement Disorders. Cannabis and related compounds have created significant research interest as a promising therapy in neurodegenerative and movement disorders. The successful use of tincture of *Cannabis indica* in treating PD was first described in Europe by Gowers [193]. Despite the lack of controlled studies, there is evidence that cannabinoids are of therapeutic value in the treatment of tics in Tourette syndrome, some forms of tremor and dystonia, chorea in Huntington's disease, the reduction of levodopa-induced dyskinesia in Parkinson's disease, and Parkinsonian syndromes [194–201].

A study with smoked cannabis queried 339 PD patients indicated that marijuana produced significant improvement of general PD symptoms in 46% of the patients; 31 % of them reported improvement in resting tremor, 38% reported relief from rigidity, 45% defined reduced bradykinesia, and 14% of the patients reported alleviated dyskinesias [202]. High urine concentration (>50 ng/ml) of the THC primary active metabolite, 11-HO-THC, was associated with relief from PD symptoms [202]. The dose and frequency of the cannabis administrations were important in relieving PD symptoms. Smoked cannabis also produced a statistically significant improvement in tremor, rigidity, and bradykinesia as well as improvement in sleep and pain scores in 22 PD patients [65]. In another study, smoked cannabis was responsible for a significant improvement in the mean total motor Unified Parkinson's Disease Rating Scale (UPDRS) score, tremor, rigidity, and bradykinesia in 17 patients with PD [203]. One dose of smoked marijuana provided symptoms relief for up to 3 hours [203]. Moreover, both studies reported significant improvement of nonmotor symptoms of PD, such as pain and sleep [65, 203]. However, smoked marijuana did not reduce Parkinsonian symptoms in 5 patients with idiopathic Parkinson's disease and severe tremor [204]. A clinical trial in 19 PD and 6 patients with levodopa-induced dyskinesia demonstrated that oral cannabis extract was ineffective for alleviating parkinsonism or dyskinesia [205].

Few studies have evaluated the effects of CBD on PD symptoms. In a pilot study CBD lowered total UPDRS scores and significantly reduced psychotic symptoms in 6 PD patients with psychosis [67]. In another study CBD administration produced no improvement in measures of motor and general symptoms in 21 PD patients [68, 69]. However, the group treated with CBD had significantly different mean total scores in the Parkinson's Disease Questionnaire, 39 compared to the placebo group [68, 69]. Oral CBD improved dyskinesia by up to 30% without a significant worsening of the parkinsonism in PD patients [206]. CBD withdrawal caused severe generalized dystonia [206].

Clinical studies have been conducted to evaluate the effect of a synthetic cannabinoid nabilone. Oral nabilone significantly reduced dyskinesia without aggravating parkinsonism in seven PD patients with severe L-DOPA-induced dyskinesia [207]. In another study, nabilone produced a 22% reduction in levodopa-induced dyskinesia in PD patients [208]. Nabilone showed efficacy not only against LID but also against bradykinesia in PD patients [209]. Some other cannabinoid related compounds such as CE178253, OEA, and HU-210 have also been reported to be efficacious against L-DOPA-induced dyskinesia and bradykinesia in PD [199, 209]. However, SR 141716 did not improve Parkinsonian motor disability in PD patients [210]. The American Academy of Neurology (AAN) review deemed marijuana "probably ineffective" for treating L-DOPA-induced dyskinesia [211]. These conflicting results indicate the need for more research in this area.

Several clinical studies have been performed to evaluate the effect of marijuana on dystonia. Inhaled cannabis has provided a marked reduction in dystonia and complete pain relief in patients with right hemiplegic painful dystonia. Moreover, the patients have been able to completely discontinue opioid use [212]. Smoked cannabis also improved idiopathic dystonia and generalized dystonia due to Wilson's disease [213, 214]. In a preliminary study, administration of CBD resulted in a 50% improvement in spasm severity and frequency in a patient with blepharospasm-oromandibular dystonia [215] and amelioration of the dystonic movements within 2-3 hours in patients with dystonic movement disorders [201]. CBD also improved dystonia by 20–50% in dystonic patients and stopped tremor and hypokinesia in 2 patients with Parkinson's disease [200]. Another cannabis compound, THC, produced a reduction of abnormal movement patterns in a 14-year-old girl with marked dystonia [216] and decreased intensity of myoclonic movements in a 13-year-old boy with athetosis and myoclonic movements [216]. In contrast to these findings, one study found no significant reduction in dystonia following treatment with nabilone [165, 166].

Studies have looked at the potential benefits of medical marijuana and cannabinoids for the treatment of Huntington's disease (HD). Nabilone versus placebo showed a treatment difference of 0.86 for total motor score; 1.68 for chorea; 3.57 for Unified Huntington's Disease Rating Scale (UHDRS) cognition; 4.01 for UHDRS behavior; and 6.43 for the neuropsychiatric inventory in HD patients [217]. However, in previous study nabilone was found to increase choreatic movements in patients with HD [197, 198]. AAN guideline examining the efficacy of marijuana for treating chorea in HD stated nabilone can be used for modest decreases in HD chorea [218]. Available data regarding the effect of CBD on HD symptoms are inconsistent. CBD produced improvement (20–40%) in the choreic movements in HD patients [219]. However, a latter study did not confirm the earlier finding [220]. A comparison of the effects of CBD and placebo on chorea severity in neuroleptic-free HD patients indicated no significant or clinically important differences [220].

Few studies have indicated that marijuana and THC can reduce tics and associated behavioral disorders in patients with Tourette's syndrome (TS) [221]. Cannabis inhalations produced a significant amelioration of TS symptoms [222]. Following marijuana administration 82% of TS patients ($N = 64$) reported a reduction, or complete remission of motor and vocal tics, and an amelioration of premonitory urges and obsessive-compulsive symptoms (OCB) [199]. Smoked marijuana also eliminated TS symptoms in one case study [223]. Administration of THC to a boy with TS improved tics and enhanced short-interval intracortical inhibition and the prolongation of the cortical silent period [224]. TCH significantly reduced tics and improve driving ability in a Tourette's patient [225]. Treatment with THC lowered the mean Cl specific over nonspecific binding ratio (V_3'') from 0.30 to 0.25 in six TS patients, although the difference was not significant. However V_3'' clearly declined in a patient with a marked clinical response [226]. To date, there have been only two controlled trials that investigated the effect of THC on TS [194], both of which reported a significant improvement of tics and OCB after THC administration [195, 196].

Considering the relevance of these data, the need for alternative treatments for PD motor and nonmotor symptoms, medical marijuana, or related compounds may provide a new approach to the treatment of Parkinson's disease.

4. Beneficial Effects of Cannabinoids in the Amelioration of Nonmotor Symptoms and Progression of Parkinson's Disease

4.1. Neuroprotective Actions of Cannabinoids. Cannabinoids have been shown to have neuroprotective effect due to their antioxidative, anti-inflammatory actions and their ability to suppress exitotoxicity. Plant-derived cannabinoids such as THC and CBD can provide neuroprotection against the in vivo and in vitro toxicity of 6-hydroxydopamine and this was thought to be due to their antioxidative property or modulation of glial cell function or a combination of both [182]. Studies found that CBD was able to recover 6-hydroxydopamine-induced dopamine depletion and also induced upregulation of Cu, Zn-superoxide dismutase, which is a key enzyme in endogenous defense against oxidative stress [70, 191, 227]. The reported data suggest that CBD also diminishes the increase in nicotinamide adenine dinucleotide phosphate (NADPH) oxidase expression and decreases the markers of oxidative stress, inflammation, and cell death in the kidneys [228]. Another study has also emphasized a role for superoxide anion produced by microglial NADPH oxidase in augmenting the demise of dopaminergic neurons in the PD brain [229]. The mechanism by which CBD acts to reduce NADPH oxidase expression and inhibit oxidative injury within the PD brain has yet to be confirmed but it seems to act through mechanisms independent of CB1 or CB2 receptors [76]. However, data obtained from recent studies have hinted towards a direct relationship between the CB1 receptor and mitochondrial functions in the brain [230]. The phenolic ring moieties in cannabinoids display antioxidant activity guarding against glutamate-induced neurotoxicity in a cellular model [231]. CBD produced reduction of hydroperoxide-induced oxidative damage and was more protective against glutamate neurotoxicity compared to ascorbate and a-tocopherol, indicating that CBD is a potent antioxidant [232]. Taken together, these discoveries support the hypothesis that treatment with cannabinoids having antioxidant effects may modulate mitochondrial reactive oxygen species production [233] in the PD brain.

Inflammation has been shown to be a crucial pathological factor responsible for the demise of dopaminergic neurons in PD [234–236]. Glial cells appear to play a key role in neuroinflammation, since higher levels of activated microglia are reported in the substantia nigra of patients with PD compared to brains of control subjects [237, 238]. Cannabinoids demonstrate anti-inflammatory activities by suppressing toxic cytokine release and microglia activation [181–183]. Increased CB2 receptor expression in nigral cells and stimulation of these receptors protect dopaminergic neurons from microglia-induced inflammation and regulate neuronal survival [70]. The cannabinoids are known to be able to activate the CB2 receptor, which mediate the anti-inflammatory effects of the compounds and preserve cells from excessive apoptosis. Recent evidence substantiates that some cannabinoids may attenuate the neuroinflammation associated with PD [191, 239–241]. Several studies showed that CBD has anti-inflammatory properties [242–246] and can produce beneficial effect in acute inflammation and chronic neuropathic states [5, 247, 248]. THC demonstrates anti-inflammatory effect via activation of the CB1 receptor [249–251]. In addition, cannabinoids provide anti-inflammation effect by reducing the vasoconstriction and restoring blood supply to the injured area [252]. All these data support that cannabinoids are potentially effective compounds for the treatment of neuroinflammatory conditions, including neurodegenerative diseases like PD.

Marijuana may prevent brain damage by protecting against neuronal injury. There are a few mechanisms by which cannabinoids provide neuroprotection. One of the mechanisms involves an induction/upregulation of cannabinoid CB2 receptors, mainly in reactive microglia, and regulates the influence of these glial cells on homeostasis of surrounding neurons [253]. In combination with the increased antitoxic effects observed in cell cultures containing glia, this suggests that immunomodulation produced by CB2 receptor activation may play a primary role in the neuroprotective properties of cannabinoids [182]. Another mechanism of neuroprotection is activation of CB1 receptors. Loss of dopaminergic neurons and greater degree of motor impairment in

CB1 knockout mice have been reported [85]. Cannabinoids activating the CB1 receptor are antiexcitotoxic due to suppression of glutamatergic activity with a subsequent decrease in calcium ion influx and eventual nitric oxide production [254–256]. Sativex-like combination of phytocannabinoids has been demonstrated to produce neuroprotective effect via interaction with both CB1 and CB2 receptors [134, 257]. In addition, THC reduced the loss of tyrosine hydroxylase-positive neurons in the substantia nigra [70] and exhibited neuroprotective effect by activation of the PPARγ receptors [258]. Overall, these data suggest that cannabinoids are neuroprotective in acute and chronic neurodegeneration and can delay or even stop progressive degeneration of brain dopaminergic system, a process that cannot be prevented currently.

4.2. Analgesic Effect of Cannabinoids. Pain is a relevant and often underestimated nonmotor symptom of PD [259, 260]. Pain affects more that 50% of people with this disorder and can cause extreme physical, psychological, and social disorders and worsen Parkinsonian disability [261, 262]. Different treatment options are used to treat PD pain [262–265]. However, these medications have significant side effects and do not provide universal efficacy [264, 265]. Cannabis is well known as a pain-relieving plant. The cannabinoid receptors in the central and peripheral nervous systems have been shown to modulate pain perception [266, 267].

Several clinical studies have been performed to investigate the effect of marijuana or cannabinoids on pain. Smoked cannabis significantly reduced neuropathic pain intensity as well as significantly improved mood disturbance, physical disability, and quality of life in HIV-patients [268]. Cannabis was effective at ameliorating neuropathic pain in patients with central and peripheral neuropathic pain [269]. Inhaled cannabis significantly reduced pain intensity (34%) compared to placebo in a clinical trial of painful distal symmetric polyneuropathy (DSPN) [270]. Whole plant extracts of *Cannabis sativa* produced statistically significant improvements on the mean pain severity score [271]. Cannabis-based medicine significantly decreased chronic pain intensity as well as sleep disturbance in multiple sclerosis patients [272, 273]. Oromucosal nabiximols (1 : 1 combination of the THC and CBD) produced a reduction in pain intensity scores in patients with neuropathic pain [274].

These findings are consistent with other discoveries supporting the efficacy of cannabis in relieving pain. The analgesic effect of cannabinoids has been reviewed [75, 211, 275–281]. The review of the literature suggests that marijuana and/or cannabinoids may be efficacious for pain relieving in various disease states including PD.

4.3. Antidepressant Effect of Cannabinoids. Depression is one of the common nonmotor symptoms of PD and the estimated rate varies widely, with an average prevalence of up to 50%. [282–284]. Despite its association with poor health outcomes and quality of life, depression in PD patients is underdiagnosed and undertreated [285–287]. Studies have indicated that the endocannabinoid system is involved in the regulation of mood and emotional behavior, and the loss or blockade of the endocannabinoid signaling system results in depressive symptoms [288]. For example, the CB1 receptor antagonist rimonabant has been shown to induce symptoms of anxiety and depression [289–291]. In addition, polymorphism of the gene that encodes the CB1 receptor has been associated with depression in PD [292]. In animal models, low level of THC produced antidepressant activity and increased serotogenic activity via activation of the CB1 receptor [293]. Animal studies have also shown that inhibition of hydrolysis of the endocannabinoid anandamide exerts antidepressive effect [294] and resulted in an increased serotonergic and noradrenergic neuronal activity in the midbrain. Currently available antidepressant drugs act via increasing serotonin and/or noradrenaline levels. These, and many other studies, indicate that the cannabinoid system is a potential target for the development of novel antidepressant drugs. Epidemiological studies have demonstrated that people who used cannabis daily or weekly exhibit less depressed mood and more positive effect than nonusers of cannabis [295]. Other studies have shown an association between heavy cannabis use and depressive symptoms. However, it is not clear whether the increased depressive symptoms are due to cannabis use or other factors that increased the risk of both depression and heavy use of cannabis [296]. Therefore, moderate use of cannabis in PD patients may help alleviate depressive symptoms and improve quality of life.

4.4. Effect of Cannabinoids on Sleep Disorders. Sleep disorders are common in PD patients and negatively affect the quality of life. The reported prevalence ranges from 25% to 98% and this wide variation could be due to differences in study design and diagnostic tools used [297]. The causes of the sleep disturbances in PD are multifactorial and include neurodegeneration and the medications used to treat motor symptoms of PD [298]. Various sleep disorders including rapid eye movement sleep behavior disorder, insomnia, sleep fragmentation, excessive daytime sleepiness, restless legs syndrome, and obstructive sleep apnea have been described in PD patients [299, 300]. Cannabidiol, the major nonpsychotic component of marijuana, has been reported to improve rapid eye movement sleep behavior disorder in PD patients [68, 69]. Marijuana has also been shown to improve nonmotor symptoms of PD including sleep [65]. In clinical trials involving 2000 patients with various pain conditions, nabiximols has been demonstrated to improve subjective sleep parameters [301]. Thus, marijuana could be used to enhance the quality of life of PD patients by alleviating sleep disorders and pain.

benefits of medical marijuana and cannabinoids in the treatment of both motor and nonmotor symptoms as well as in slowing the progression of the disease. We have looked into any scientific evidence that indicates the potential use of marijuana and/or related compounds for the treatment of PD. Current treatments of PD provide only relief of motor symptoms and are associated with adverse effects such as dyskinesia. In addition, these therapies do not slow the progression of the disease. Therefore, there is an urgent need for safer drugs that can treat both motor and nonmotor symptoms of PD as well as drugs that slow the progression of the disease.

In spite of the placement of marijuana in schedule 1 category under the US Federal Controlled Substance Act, 24 states and Washington DC have enacted laws allowing the use of marijuana to treat a range of medical conditions. Parkinson's disease has been listed as one of the disease conditions for which medical marijuana is allowed in a number of states. Research studies have provided evidence for the potential effectiveness of medical marijuana and its components in the treatment of PD as cannabinoids act on the same neurological pathway that is disrupted in Parkinson's disease. Involvement of the endocannabinoid system in the regulation of motor behavior, the localization of the cannabinoid receptors in areas that control movement, and the effect of cannabinoids on motor activity indicate that cannabinoids can be potentially used in the treatment of movement disorders. Cannabinoid agonists and antagonists have been shown to modulate the endocannabinoid system and modify motor activity. Cannabinoid receptor antagonists appear to produce antiparkinsonian effects while cannabinoid receptor agonists exert a powerful motor inhibition and may be useful in the treatment of motor complications. In addition, we have assessed the role of the cannabinoid system and marijuana constituents in neuroprotection as well as considered other beneficial effects of marijuana. Marijuana has been shown to improve nonmotor symptoms of PD such as depression, pain, sleep, and anxiety. Moreover, components of cannabis have been demonstrated to have neuroprotective effect due to their anti-inflammatory, antioxidative, and antiexcitotoxic properties. Due to combination of the above mentioned beneficial effects, cannabis may provide a viable alternative or addition to the current treatment of Parkinson's disease. However, there are concerns regarding the use of medical marijuana including lack of standardization and regulation, imprecise dosing, possible adverse effects, and medication interactions. Further studies are needed to provide more data on efficacy, safety, pharmacokinetics, and interactions of cannabinoids.

5. Summary

Cannabis and related compounds have recently been studied as promising therapeutic agents in treatment of neurodegenerative and movement disorders including Parkinson's disease. In this review we have examined the potential

References

[1] L. M. Borgelt, K. L. Franson, A. M. Nussbaum, and G. S. Wang, "The pharmacologic and clinical effects of medical cannabis," *Pharmacotherapy*, vol. 33, no. 2, pp. 195–209, 2013.

[2] M. A. ElSohly and D. Slade, "Chemical constituents of marijuana: the complex mixture of natural cannabinoids," *Life Sciences*, vol. 78, no. 5, pp. 539–548, 2005.

[3] E. B. Russo, "Taming THC: potential cannabis synergy and phytocannabinoid-terpenoid entourage effects," *British Journal of Pharmacology*, vol. 163, no. 7, pp. 1344–1364, 2011.

[4] E. J. Rahn and A. G. Hohmann, "Cannabinoids as Pharmacotherapies for neuropathic pain: from the bench to the bedside," *Neurotherapeutics*, vol. 6, no. 4, pp. 713–737, 2009.

[5] A. W. Zuardi, "Cannabidiol: from an inactive cannabinoid to a drug with wide spectrum of action," *Revista Brasileira de Psiquiatria*, vol. 30, no. 3, pp. 271–280, 2008.

[6] F. M. Leweke, D. Piomelli, F. Pahlisch et al., "Cannabidiol enhances anandamide signaling and alleviates psychotic symptoms of schizophrenia," *Translational Psychiatry*, vol. 2, no. 3, article e94, 2012.

[7] DEA (Drug Enforcement Administration), Drug Fact Sheet: Marijuana, http://www.dea.gov/druginfo/drug_data_sheets/Marijuana.pdf.

[8] ONDCP (Office of National Drug Control Policy), Marijuana Resource Center: State Laws Related to Marijuana, https://www.whitehouse.gov/ondcp/state-laws-related-to-marijuana.

[9] Y. Park, "Georgia Regents University. Epidiolex and Drug Resistant Epilepsy in Children (CBD)," In: ClinicalTrials.gov. Bethesda (MD): National Library of Medicine (US). NLM Identifier: NCT02397863, https://clinicaltrials.gov/ct2/show/NCT02397863.

[10] W. Notcutt, R. Langford, P. Davies, S. Ratcliffe, and R. Potts, "A placebo-controlled, parallel-group, randomized withdrawal study of subjects with symptoms of spasticity due to multiple sclerosis who are receiving long-term Sativex (nabiximols)," *Multiple Sclerosis Journal*, vol. 18, no. 2, pp. 219–228, 2012.

[11] A. Novotna, J. Mares, S. Ratcliffe et al., "A randomized, double-blind, placebo-controlled, parallel-group, enriched-design study of nabiximols* (Sativex®), as add-on therapy, in subjects with refractory spasticity caused by multiple sclerosis," *European Journal of Neurology*, vol. 18, no. 9, pp. 1122–1131, 2011.

[12] F. Grotenhermen and K. Müller-Vahl, "The therapeutic potential of cannabis and cannabinoids," *Deutsches Arzteblatt International*, vol. 109, no. 29-30, pp. 495–501, 2012.

[13] C. Scuderi, D. De Filippis, T. Iuvone, A. Blasio, A. Steardo, and G. Esposito, "Cannabidiol in medicine: a review of its therapeutic potential in CNS disorders," *Phytotherapy Research*, vol. 23, no. 5, pp. 597–602, 2009.

[14] T. Iuvone, G. Esposito, D. De Filippis, C. Scuderi, and L. Steardo, "Cannabidiol: a promising drug for neurodegenerative disorders?" *CNS Neuroscience and Therapeutics*, vol. 15, no. 1, pp. 65–75, 2009.

[15] A. J. Hill, C. M. Williams, B. J. Whalley, and G. J. Stephens, "Phytocannabinoids as novel therapeutic agents in CNS disorders," *Pharmacology and Therapeutics*, vol. 133, no. 1, pp. 79–97, 2012.

[16] P. Fusar-Poli, J. A. Crippa, S. Bhattacharyya et al., "Distinct effects of Δ9-tetrahydrocannabinol and cannabidiol on neural activation during emotional processing," *Archives of General Psychiatry Journal*, vol. 66, no. 1, pp. 95–105, 2009.

[17] D. T. Malone, M. N. Hill, and T. Rubino, "Adolescent cannabis use and psychosis: epidemiology and neurodevelopmental models," *British Journal of Pharmacology*, vol. 160, no. 3, pp. 511–522, 2010.

[18] G. Gerra, A. Zaimovic, M. L. Gerra et al., "Pharmacology and toxicology of cannabis derivatives and endocannabinoid agonists," *Recent Patents on CNS Drug Discovery*, vol. 5, no. 1, pp. 46–52, 2010.

[19] T. H. Moore, S. Zammit, A. Lingford-Hughes et al., "Cannabis use and risk of psychotic or affective mental health outcomes: a systematic review," *The Lancet*, vol. 370, no. 9584, pp. 319–328, 2007.

[20] M. G. Bossong and R. J. M. Niesink, "Adolescent brain maturation, the endogenous cannabinoid system and the neurobiology of cannabis-induced schizophrenia," *Progress in Neurobiology*, vol. 92, no. 3, pp. 370–385, 2010.

[21] M. Schneider, "Puberty as a highly vulnerable developmental period for the consequences of cannabis exposure," *Addiction Biology*, vol. 13, no. 2, pp. 253–263, 2008.

[22] F. Grotenhermen, "The toxicology of cannabis and cannabis prohibition," *Chemistry & Biodiversity*, vol. 4, no. 8, pp. 1744–1769, 2007.

[23] F. R. de Fonseca, I. del Arco, F. J. Bermudez-Silva, A. Bilbao, A. Cippitelli, and M. Navarro, "The endocannabinoid system: physiology and pharmacology," *Alcohol and Alcoholism*, vol. 40, no. 1, pp. 2–14, 2005.

[24] P. Pacher, S. Bátkai, and G. Kunos, "The endocannabinoid system as an emerging target of pharmacotherapy," *Pharmacological Reviews*, vol. 58, no. 3, pp. 389–462, 2006.

[25] T. Morera-Herreras, C. Miguelez, A. Aristieta, J. A. Ruiz-Ortega, and L. Ugedo, "Endocannabinoid modulation of dopaminergic motor circuits," *Frontiers in Pharmacology*, vol. 3, article 110, 2012.

[26] A. El Manira and A. Kyriakatos, "The role of endocannabinoid signaling in motor control," *Physiology*, vol. 25, no. 4, pp. 230–238, 2010.

[27] J. Fernández-Ruiz and S. González, "Cannabinoid control of motor function at the Basal Ganglia," *Handbook of Experimental Pharmacology*, vol. 168, pp. 479–507, 2005.

[28] J. Xu, K. D. Kochanek, and S. L. Murphy, "National vital statistics reports deaths: final data for 2007," *Statistics*, vol. 58, no. 3, p. 135, 2010.

[29] T. Pringsheim, N. Jette, A. Frolkis, and T. D. L. Steeves, "The prevalence of Parkinson's disease: a systematic review and meta-analysis," *Movement Disorders*, vol. 29, no. 13, pp. 1583–1590, 2014.

[30] E. R. Dorsey, R. Constantinescu, J. P. Thompson et al., "Projected number of people with Parkinson disease in the most populous nations, 2005 through 2030," *Neurology*, vol. 68, no. 5, pp. 384–386, 2007.

[31] L. C. S. Tan, "Epidemiology of parkinson's disease," *Neurology Asia*, vol. 18, no. 3, pp. 231–238, 2013.

[32] A. Galvan and T. Wichmann, "Pathophysiology of Parkinsonism," *Clinical Neurophysiology*, vol. 119, no. 7, pp. 1459–1474, 2008.

[33] L. C. Kwan and T. L. Whitehill, "Perception of speech by individuals with Parkinson's disease: a review," *Parkinson's Disease*, vol. 2011, Article ID 389767, 11 pages, 2011.

[34] B. Thomas and M. F. Beal, "Parkinson's disease," *Human Molecular Genetics*, vol. 16, no. 2, pp. R183–R194, 2007.

[35] G. E. Alexander, "Biology of Parkinson's disease: pathogenesis and pathophysiology of a multisystem neurodegenerative disorder," *Dialogues in Clinical Neuroscience*, vol. 6, no. 3, pp. 259–280, 2004.

[36] W. Dauer and S. Przedborski, "Parkinson's disease: mechanisms and models," *Neuron*, vol. 39, no. 6, pp. 889–909, 2003.

[37] M. C. Rodriguez-Oroz, M. Jahanshahi, P. Krack et al., "Initial clinical manifestations of Parkinson's disease: features and pathophysiological mechanisms," *The Lancet Neurology*, vol. 8, no. 12, pp. 1128–1139, 2009.

[38] T. Patel and F. Chang, "Parkinson's disease guidelines for pharmacists," *Canadian Pharmacists Journal*, vol. 147, no. 3, pp. 161–170, 2014.

[39] K. R. Chaudhuri, D. G. Healy, and A. H. V. Schapira, "Non-motor symptoms of Parkinson's disease: diagnosis and management," *The Lancet Neurology*, vol. 5, no. 3, pp. 235–245, 2006.

[40] B. Müller, J. Assmus, K. Herlofson, J. P. Larsen, and O.-B. Tysnes, "Importance of motor vs. non-motor symptoms for health-related quality of life in early Parkinson's disease," *Parkinsonism and Related Disorders*, vol. 19, no. 11, pp. 1027–1032, 2013.

[41] J. Latoo, M. Mistry, and F. J. Dunne, "Often overlooked neuropsychiatric syndromes in Parkinson's disease," *British Journal of Medical Practitioners*, vol. 6, no. 1, pp. 23–30, 2013.

[42] F. Stocchi, G. Abbruzzese, R. Ceravolo et al., "Prevalence of fatigue in Parkinson disease and its clinical correlates," *Neurology*, vol. 83, no. 3, pp. 215–220, 2014.

[43] D. C. Velseboer, R. J. de Haan, W. Wieling, D. S. Goldstein, and R. M. A. de Bie, "Prevalence of orthostatic hypotension in Parkinson's disease: a systematic review and meta-analysis," *Parkinsonism and Related Disorders*, vol. 17, no. 10, pp. 724–729, 2011.

[44] B. Connolly and S. H. Fox, "Treatment of cognitive, psychiatric, and affective disorders associated with Parkinson's disease," *Neurotherapeutics*, vol. 11, no. 1, pp. 78–91, 2014.

[45] P. Huot, S. H. Fox, and J. M. Brotchie, "Monoamine reuptake inhibitors in Parkinson's disease," *Parkinson's Disease*, vol. 2015, Article ID 609428, 71 pages, 2015.

[46] F. Gasparini, T. Di Paolo, and B. Gomez-Mancilla, "Metabotropic glutamate receptors for Parkinson's disease therapy," *Parkinson's Disease*, vol. 2013, Article ID 196028, 11 pages, 2013.

[47] C. G. Goetz and G. Pal, "Initial management of Parkinson's disease," *British Medical Journal*, vol. 349, Article ID 6258, 2014.

[48] A. Lees, "Alternatives to levodopa in the initial treatment of early Parkinson's disease," *Drugs and Aging*, vol. 22, no. 9, pp. 731–740, 2005.

[49] R. Katzenschlager, C. Sampaio, J. Costa, and A. Lees, "Anticholinergics for symptomatic management of Parkinson's disease," *Cochrane Database of Systematic Reviews*, no. 2, Article ID CD003735, 2003.

[50] S. Maranis, S. Tsouli, and S. Konitsiotis, "Treatment of motor symptoms in advanced Parkinson's disease: a practical approach," *Progress in Neuro-Psychopharmacology and Biological Psychiatry*, vol. 35, no. 8, pp. 1795–1807, 2011.

[51] R. Heumann, R. Moratalla, M. T. Herrero et al., "Dyskinesia in Parkinson's disease: mechanisms and current non-pharmacological interventions," *Journal of Neurochemistry*, vol. 130, no. 4, pp. 472–489, 2014.

[52] M. Politis, K. Wu, C. Loane et al., "Serotonergic mechanisms responsible for levodopa-induced dyskinesias in Parkinson's disease patients," *The Journal of Clinical Investigation*, vol. 124, no. 3, pp. 1340–1349, 2014.

[53] G. Porras, P. De Deurwaerdere, Q. Li et al., "L-dopa-induced dyskinesia: beyond an excessive dopamine tone in the striatum," *Scientific Reports*, vol. 4, article 3730, 2014.

[54] J. J. Chen, D. M. Swope, and K. Dashtipour, "Comprehensive review of rasagiline, a second-generation monoamine oxidase inhibitor, for the treatment of Parkinson's Disease," *Clinical Therapeutics*, vol. 29, no. 9, pp. 1825–1849, 2007.

[55] S. Lecht, S. Haroutiunian, A. Hoffman, and P. Lazarovici, "Rasagiline—a novel MAO B inhibitor in Parkinson's disease therapy," *Therapeutics and Clinical Risk Management*, vol. 3, no. 3, pp. 467–474, 2007.

[56] R. Pahwa, S. A. Factor, K. E. Lyons et al., "Practice parameter: Treatment of Parkinson disease with motor fluctuations and dyskinesia (an evidence-based review): report of the Quality Standards Subcommittee of the American Academy of Neurology," *Neurology*, vol. 66, no. 7, pp. 983–995, 2006.

[57] F. Stocchi and J. M. Rabey, "Effect of rasagiline as adjunct therapy to levodopa on severity of OFF in Parkinson's disease," *European Journal of Neurology*, vol. 18, no. 12, pp. 1373–1378, 2011.

[58] O. Rascol, D. J. Brooks, E. Melamed et al., "Rasagiline as an adjunct to levodopa in patients with Parkinson's disease and end-of-dose motor fluctuations: a randomised, double-blind, controlled trial," *The Lancet Neurology*, vol. 365, pp. 947–954, 2005.

[59] E. Tolosa and M. B. Stern, "Efficacy, safety and tolerability of rasagiline as adjunctive therapy in elderly patients with Parkinson's disease," *European Journal of Neurology*, vol. 19, no. 2, pp. 258–264, 2012.

[60] O. Rascol, D. J. Brooks, A. D. Korczyn, P. P. De Deyn, C. E. Clarke, and A. E. Lang, "A five-year study of the incidence of dyskinesia in patients with early Parkinson's disease who were treated with ropinirole or levodopa," *The New England Journal of Medicine*, vol. 342, no. 20, pp. 1484–1491, 2000.

[61] Parkinson Study Group, "Pramipexole vs levodopa as initial treatment for Parkinson disease: A randomized controlled trial. Parkinson Study Group," *The Journal of the American Medical Association*, vol. 284, no. 15, pp. 1931–1938, 2000.

[62] S. Perez-Lloret, M. V. Rey, P. L. Ratti, and O. Rascol, "Rotigotine transdermal patch for the treatment of Parkinson's disease," *Fundamental and Clinical Pharmacology*, vol. 27, no. 1, pp. 81–95, 2013.

[63] J.-P. Elshoff, W. Cawello, J.-O. Andreas, F.-X. Mathy, and M. Braun, "An update on pharmacological, pharmacokinetic properties and drug-drug interactions of rotigotine transdermal system in Parkinson's disease and restless legs syndrome," *Drugs*, vol. 75, no. 5, pp. 487–501, 2015.

[64] D. Deleu, Y. Hanssens, and M. G. Northway, "Subcutaneous apomorphine: an evidence-based review of its use in Parkinson's disease," *Drugs and Aging*, vol. 21, no. 11, pp. 687–709, 2004.

[65] I. Lotan, T. A. Treves, Y. Roditi, and R. Djaldetti, "Cannabis (medical marijuana) treatment for motor and non-motor symptoms of Parkinson disease," *Clinical Neuropharmacology*, vol. 37, no. 2, pp. 41–44, 2014.

[66] T. A. Finseth, J. L. Hedeman, R. P. Brown, K. I. Johnson, M. S. Binder, and B. M. Kluger, "Self-reported efficacy of cannabis and other complementary medicine modalities by Parkinson's disease patients in Colorado," *Evidence-Based Complementary and Alternative Medicine*, vol. 2015, Article ID 874849, 6 pages, 2015.

[67] A. W. Zuardi, J. A. S. Crippa, J. E. C. Hallak et al., "Cannabidiol for the treatment of psychosis in Parkinson's disease," *Journal of Psychopharmacology*, vol. 23, no. 8, pp. 979–983, 2009.

[68] M. H. N. Chagas, A. W. Zuardi, V. Tumas et al., "Effects of cannabidiol in the treatment of patients with Parkinson's disease: an exploratory double-blind trial," *Journal of Psychopharmacology*, vol. 28, no. 11, pp. 1088–1092, 2014.

[69] M. H. N. Chagas, A. L. Eckeli, A. W. Zuardi et al., "Cannabidiol can improve complex sleep-related behaviours associated with rapid eye movement sleep behaviour disorder in Parkinson's disease patients: a case series," *Journal of Clinical Pharmacy and Therapeutics*, vol. 39, no. 5, pp. 564–566, 2014.

[70] C. García, C. Palomo-Garo, M. García-Arencibia, J. A. Ramos, R. G. Pertwee, and J. Fernández-Ruiz, "Symptom-relieving and neuroprotective effects of the phytocannabinoid Δ^9-THCV in animal models of Parkinson's disease," *British Journal of Pharmacology*, vol. 163, no. 7, pp. 1495–1506, 2011.

[71] M. Shen and S. A. Thayer, "Δ^9-Tetrahydrocannabinol acts as a partial agonist to modulate glutamatergic synaptic transmission between rat hippocampal neurons in culture," *Molecular Pharmacology*, vol. 55, no. 1, pp. 8–13, 1999.

[72] R. Murase, R. Kawamura, E. Singer et al., "Targeting multiple cannabinoid anti-tumour pathways with a resorcinol derivative leads to inhibition of advanced stages of breast cancer," *British Journal of Pharmacology*, vol. 171, no. 19, pp. 4464–4477, 2014.

[73] O. Devinsky, M. R. Cilio, H. Cross et al., "Cannabidiol: pharmacology and potential therapeutic role in epilepsy and other neuropsychiatric disorders," *Epilepsia*, vol. 55, no. 6, pp. 791–802, 2014.

[74] M. Babayeva, M. Fuzailov, P. Rozenfeld, and P. Basu, "Marijuana compounds: a non-conventional therapeutic approach to epilepsy in children," *Journal of Addiction Neuropharmacology*, vol. 1, pp. 2–36, 2014.

[75] J. L. Croxford, "Therapeutic potential of cannabinoids in CNS disease," *CNS Drugs*, vol. 17, no. 3, pp. 179–202, 2003.

[76] J. Fernández-Ruiz, O. Sagredo, M. R. Pazos et al., "Cannabidiol for neurodegenerative disorders: important new clinical applications for this phytocannabinoid?" *British Journal of Clinical Pharmacology*, vol. 75, no. 2, pp. 323–333, 2013.

[77] Y. Hashimotodani, T. Ohno-Shosaku, M. Watanabe, and M. Kano, "Roles of phospholipase Cβ and NMDA receptor in activity-dependent endocannabinoid release," *The Journal of Physiology*, vol. 584, no. 2, pp. 373–380, 2007.

[78] Z. Hegyi, K. Holló, G. Kis, K. Mackie, and M. Antal, "Differential distribution of diacylglycerol lipase-alpha and N-acyl-phosphatidylethanolamine-specific phospholipase d immunoreactivity in the superficial spinal dorsal horn of rats," *Glia*, vol. 60, no. 9, pp. 1316–1329, 2012.

[79] P. G. Fine and M. J. Rosenfeld, "The endocannabinoid system, cannabinoids, and pain," *Rambam Maimonides Medical Journal*, vol. 4, no. 4, Article ID e0022, 2013.

[80] E. M. Marco, S. Y. Romero-Zerbo, M.-P. Viveros, and F. J. Bermudez-Silva, "The role of the endocannabinoid system in eating disorders: pharmacological implications," *Behavioural Pharmacology*, vol. 23, no. 5-6, pp. 526–536, 2012.

[81] C. R. Hiley, "Endocannabinoids and the heart," *Journal of Cardiovascular Pharmacology*, vol. 53, no. 4, pp. 267–276, 2009.

[82] R. G. Pertwee, "The diverse CB 1 and CB 2 receptor pharmacology of three plant cannabinoids: Δ 9-tetrahydrocannabinol, cannabidiol and Δ 9-tetrahydrocannabivarin," *British Journal of Pharmacology*, vol. 153, no. 2, pp. 199–215, 2008.

[83] J.-Y. Xu and C. Chen, "Endocannabinoids in synaptic plasticity and neuroprotection," *Neuroscientist*, vol. 21, no. 2, pp. 152–168, 2015.

[84] V. L. Hegde, M. Nagarkatti, and P. S. Nagarkatti, "Cannabinoid receptor activation leads to massive mobilization of myeloid-derived suppressor cells with potent immunosuppressive properties," *European Journal of Immunology*, vol. 40, no. 12, pp. 3358–3371, 2010.

[85] S. Pérez-Rial, M. S. García-Gutiérrez, J. A. Molina et al., "Increased vulnerability to 6-hydroxydopamine lesion and reduced development of dyskinesias in mice lacking CB1 cannabinoid receptors," *Neurobiology of Aging*, vol. 32, no. 4, pp. 631–645, 2011.

[86] D. Piomelli, "The molecular logic of endocannabinoid signalling," *Nature Reviews Neuroscience*, vol. 4, no. 11, pp. 873–884, 2003.

[87] L. A. Matsuda, S. J. Lolait, M. J. Brownstein, A. C. Young, and T. I. Bonner, "Structure of a cannabinoid receptor and functional expression of the cloned cDNA," *Nature*, vol. 346, no. 6284, pp. 561–564, 1990.

[88] M. Herkenham, A. B. Lynn, M. D. Little et al., "Cannabinoid receptor localization in brain," *Proceedings of the National Academy of Sciences of the United States of America*, vol. 87, no. 5, pp. 1932–1936, 1990.

[89] I. Ivanov, P. Borchert, and B. Hinz, "A simple method for simultaneous determination of N-arachidonoylethanolamine, N-oleoylethanolamine, N-palmitoylethanolamine and 2-arachidonoylglycerol in human cells," *Analytical and Bioanalytical Chemistry*, vol. 407, no. 6, pp. 1781–1787, 2015.

[90] R. G. Pertwee, A. C. Howlett, M. E. Abood et al., "International Union of Basic and Clinical Pharmacology. LXXIX. Cannabinoid receptors and their ligands: Beyond CB1 and CB2," *Pharmacological Reviews*, vol. 62, no. 4, pp. 588–631, 2010.

[91] N. T. Snider, V. J. Walker, and P. F. Hollenberg, "Oxidation of the endogenous cannabinoid arachidonoyl ethanolamide by the cytochrome P450 monooxygenases: physiological and pharmacological implications," *Pharmacological Reviews*, vol. 62, no. 1, pp. 136–154, 2010.

[92] M. W. Buczynski and L. H. Parsons, "Quantification of brain endocannabinoid levels: methods, interpretations and pitfalls," *British Journal of Pharmacology*, vol. 160, no. 3, pp. 423–442, 2010.

[93] C. C. Felder, A. Nielsen, E. M. Briley et al., "Isolation and measurement of the endogenous cannabinoid receptor agonist, anandamide, in brain and peripheral tissues of human and rat," *FEBS Letters*, vol. 393, no. 2-3, pp. 231–235, 1996.

[94] T. Sugiura, S. Kondo, S. Kishimoto et al., "Evidence that 2-arachidonoylglycerol but not N-palmitoylethanolamine or anandamide is the physiological ligand for the cannabinoid CB2 receptor. Comparison of the agonistic activities of various cannabinoid receptor ligands in HL-60 cells," *Journal of Biological Chemistry*, vol. 275, no. 1, pp. 605–612, 2000.

[95] T. Bisogno, F. Berrendero, G. Ambrosino et al., "Brain regional distribution of endocannabinoids: implications for their biosynthesis and biological function," *Biochemical and Biophysical Research Communications*, vol. 256, no. 2, pp. 377–380, 1999.

[96] R. Mechoulam, S. Ben-Shabat, L. Hanus et al., "Identification of an endogenous 2-monoglyceride, present in canine gut, that binds to cannabinoid receptors," *Biochemical Pharmacology*, vol. 50, no. 1, pp. 83–90, 1995.

[97] W. Gonsiorek, C. Lunn, X. Fan, S. Narula, D. Lundell, and R. W. Hipkin, "Endocannabinoid 2-arachidonyl glycerol is a full agonist through human type 2 cannabinoid receptor: antagonism by anandamide," *Molecular Pharmacology*, vol. 57, no. 5, pp. 1045–1050, 2000.

[98] V. Di Marzo, F. Berrendero, T. Bisogno et al., "Enhancement of anandamide formation in the limbic forebrain and reduction of endocannabinoid contents in the striatum of $\Delta9$-

tetrahydrocannabinol-tolerant rats," *Journal of Neurochemistry*, vol. 74, no. 4, pp. 1627–1635, 2000.

[99] V. Di Marzo, M. P. Hill, T. Bisogno, A. R. Crossman, and J. M. Brotchie, "Enhanced levels of endogenous cannabinoids in the globus pallidus are associated with a reduction in movement in an animal model of Parkinson's disease," *FASEB Journal*, vol. 14, no. 10, pp. 1432–1438, 2000.

[100] G. Palermo, I. Bauer, P. Campomanes et al., "Keys to lipid selection in fatty acid amide hydrolase catalysis: structural flexibility, gating residues and multiple binding pockets," *PLoS Computational Biology*, vol. 11, no. 6, article e1004231, 2015.

[101] A. Giuffrida, L. H. Parsons, T. M. Kerr, F. Rodríguez De Fonseca, M. Navarro, and D. Piomelli, "Dopamine activation of endogenous cannabinoid signaling in dorsal striatum," *Nature Neuroscience*, vol. 2, no. 4, pp. 358–363, 1999.

[102] L. De Petrocellis, M. G. Cascio, and V. Di Marzo, "The endocannabinoid system: a general view and latest additions," *British Journal of Pharmacology*, vol. 141, no. 5, pp. 765–774, 2004.

[103] B. S. Basavarajappa, "Neuropharmacology of the endocannabinoid signaling system-molecular mechanisms, biological actions and synaptic plasticity," *Current Neuropharmacology*, vol. 5, no. 2, pp. 81–97, 2007.

[104] I. G. Karniol and E. A. Carlini, "Pharmacological interaction between cannabidiol and δ9-tetrahydrocannabinol," *Psychopharmacologia*, vol. 33, no. 1, pp. 53–70, 1973.

[105] R. Mechoulam and Y. Shvo, "Hashish—I: the structure of cannabidiol," *Tetrahedron*, vol. 19, pp. 2073–2078, 1963.

[106] V. Di Marzo and A. Fontana, "Anandamide, an endogenous cannabinomimetic eicosanoid: 'killing two birds with one stone'," *Prostaglandins, Leukotrienes and Essential Fatty Acids*, vol. 53, no. 1, pp. 1–11, 1995.

[107] H. J. Groenewegen, "The basal ganglia and motor control," *Neural Plasticity*, vol. 10, no. 1-2, pp. 107–120, 2003.

[108] P. Calabresi, B. Picconi, A. Tozzi, V. Ghiglieri, and M. Di Filippo, "Direct and indirect pathways of basal ganglia: a critical reappraisal," *Nature Neuroscience*, vol. 17, no. 8, pp. 1022–1030, 2014.

[109] J. Fernández-Ruiz, "The endocannabinoid system as a target for the treatment of motor dysfunction," *British Journal of Pharmacology*, vol. 156, no. 7, pp. 1029–1040, 2009.

[110] B. D. Heifets and P. E. Castillo, "Endocannabinoid signaling and long-term synaptic plasticity," *Annual Review of Physiology*, vol. 71, pp. 283–306, 2009.

[111] E. Bezard, J. M. Brotchie, and C. E. Gross, "Pathophysiology of levodopa-induced dyskinesia: potential for new therapies," *Nature Reviews Neuroscience*, vol. 2, no. 8, pp. 577–588, 2001.

[112] S. V. More and D.-K. Choi, "Promising cannabinoid-based therapies for Parkinson's disease: motor symptoms to neuroprotection," *Molecular Neurodegeneration*, vol. 10, no. 1, article 17, 2015.

[113] M. García-Arencibia, C. García, and J. Fernández-Ruiz, "Cannabinoids and Parkinson's disease," *CNS and Neurological Disorders—Drug Targets*, vol. 8, no. 6, pp. 432–439, 2009.

[114] J. M. Brotchie, "CB1 cannabinoid receptor signalling in Parkinson's disease," *Current Opinion in Pharmacology*, vol. 3, no. 1, pp. 54–61, 2003.

[115] M. van der Stelt and V. Di Marzo, "The endocannabinoid system in the basal ganglia and in the mesolimbic reward system: implications for neurological and psychiatric disorders," *European Journal of Pharmacology*, vol. 480, no. 1–3, pp. 133–150, 2003.

[116] E. Benarroch, "Endocannabinoids in basal ganglia circuits: implications for Parkinson disease," *Neurology*, vol. 69, no. 3, pp. 306–309, 2007.

[117] F. R. Fusco, A. Martorana, C. Giampà et al., "Immunolocalization of CB1 receptor in rat striatal neurons: A Confocal Microscopy Study," *Synapse*, vol. 53, no. 3, pp. 159–167, 2004.

[118] M. Di Filippo, B. Picconi, A. Tozzi, V. Ghiglieri, A. Rossi, and P. Calabresi, "The endocannabinoid system in Pakinson's disease," *Current Pharmaceutical Design*, vol. 14, no. 23, pp. 2337–2346, 2008.

[119] I. Lastres-Becker, M. Cebeira, M. L. De Ceballos et al., "Increased cannabinoid CB1 receptor binding and activation of GTP-binding proteins in the basal ganglia of patients with Parkinson's syndrome and of MPTP-treated marmosets," *European Journal of Neuroscience*, vol. 14, no. 11, pp. 1827–1832, 2001.

[120] I. Lastres-Becker, F. Fezza, M. Cebeira et al., "Changes in endocannabinoid transmission in the basal ganglia in a rat model of Huntington's disease," *NeuroReport*, vol. 12, no. 10, pp. 2125–2129, 2001.

[121] T. M. Dawson and V. L. Dawson, "Rare genetic mutations shed light on the pathogenesis of Parkinson disease," *The Journal of Clinical Investigation*, vol. 111, no. 2, pp. 145–151, 2003.

[122] S. González, M. A. Mena, I. Lastres-Becker et al., "Cannabinoid CB_1 receptors in the basal ganglia and motor response to activation or blockade of these receptors in parkin-null mice," *Brain Research*, vol. 1046, no. 1-2, pp. 195–206, 2005.

[123] R. I. Wilson and R. A. Nicoll, "Endocannabinoid signaling in the brain," *Science*, vol. 296, no. 5568, pp. 678–682, 2002.

[124] J. P. Meschler, T. J. Conley, and A. C. Howlett, "Cannabinoid and dopamine interaction in rodent brain: effects on locomotor activity," *Pharmacology Biochemistry and Behavior*, vol. 67, no. 3, pp. 567–573, 2000.

[125] J. P. Meschler, A. C. Howlett, and B. K. Madras, "Cannabinoid receptor agonist and antagonist effects on motor function in normal and 1-methyl-4-phenyl-1,2,5,6-tetrahydropyridine (MPTP)-treated non-human primates," *Psychopharmacology*, vol. 156, no. 1, pp. 79–85, 2001.

[126] L. A. Batista, P. H. Gobira, T. G. Viana, D. C. Aguiar, and F. A. Moreira, "Inhibition of endocannabinoid neuronal uptake and hydrolysis as strategies for developing anxiolytic drugs," *Behavioural Pharmacology*, vol. 25, no. 5-6, pp. 425–433, 2014.

[127] É. Mezey, Z. E. Tóth, D. N. Cortright et al., "Distribution of mRNA for vanilloid receptor subtype 1 (VR1), and VR1- like immunoreactivity, in the central nervous system of the rat and human," *Proceedings of the National Academy of Sciences of the United States of America*, vol. 97, no. 7, pp. 3655–3660, 2000.

[128] E. Palazzo, F. Rossi, and S. Maione, "Role of TRPV1 receptors in descending modulation of pain," *Molecular and Cellular Endocrinology*, vol. 286, no. 1-2, supplement 1, pp. S79–S83, 2008.

[129] E. de Lago, R. de Miguel, I. Lastres-Becker, J. A. Ramos, and J. Fernández-Ruiz, "Involvement of vanilloid-like receptors in the effects of anandamide on motor behavior and nigrostriatal dopaminergic activity: in vivo and in vitro evidence," *Brain Research*, vol. 1007, no. 1-2, pp. 152–159, 2004.

[130] T. dos Anjos-Garcia, F. Ullah, L. L. Falconi-Sobrinho, and N. C. Coimbra, "CB1 cannabinoid receptor-mediated anandamide signalling reduces the defensive behaviour evoked through GABAA receptor blockade in the dorsomedial division of the ventromedial hypothalamus," *Neuropharmacology*, vol. 113, pp. 156–166, 2016.

[131] E. Lizanecz, Z. Bagi, E. T. Pásztor et al., "Phosphorylation-dependent desensitization by anandamide of vanilloid receptor-1 (TRPV1) function in rat skeletal muscle arterioles and in Chinese hamster ovary cells expressing TRPV1," *Molecular Pharmacology*, vol. 69, no. 3, pp. 1015–1023, 2006.

[132] A. V. Kravitz, B. S. Freeze, P. R. L. Parker et al., "Regulation of parkinsonian motor behaviours by optogenetic control of basal ganglia circuitry," *Nature*, vol. 466, no. 7306, pp. 622–626, 2010.

[133] A. C. Kreitzer and R. C. Malenka, "Endocannabinoid-mediated rescue of striatal LTD and motor deficits in Parkinson's disease models," *Nature*, vol. 445, no. 7128, pp. 643–647, 2007.

[134] O. Sagredo, M. R. Pazos, V. Satta, J. A. Ramos, R. G. Pertwee, and J. Fernández-Ruiz, "Neuroprotective effects of phytocannabinoid-based medicines in experimental models of Huntington's disease," *Journal of Neuroscience Research*, vol. 89, no. 9, pp. 1509–1518, 2011.

[135] D. E. Moss, S. B. McMaster, and J. Rogers, "Tetrahydrocannabinol potentiates reserpine-induced hypokinesia," *Pharmacology, Biochemistry and Behavior*, vol. 15, no. 5, pp. 779–783, 1981.

[136] M. Van Der Stelt, S. H. Fox, M. Hill et al., "A role for endocannabinoids in the generation of parkinsonism and levodopa-induced dyskinesia in MPTP-lesioned non-human primate models of Parkinson's disease," *FASEB Journal*, vol. 19, no. 9, pp. 1140–1142, 2005.

[137] T. Bisogno, F. Berrendero, G. Ambrosino et al., "Brain regional distribution of endocannabinoids: implications for their biosynthesis and biological function," *Biochemical and Biophysical Research Communications*, vol. 256, no. 2, pp. 377–380, 1999.

[138] M. C. Sañudo-Peña, K. Tsou, and J. M. Walker, "Motor actions of cannabinoids in the basal ganglia output nuclei," *Life Sciences*, vol. 65, no. 6-7, pp. 703–713, 1999.

[139] I. Lastres-Becker, H. H. Hansen, F. Berrendero et al., "Alleviation of motor hyperactivity and neurochemical deficits by endocannabinoid uptake inhibition in a rat model of Huntington's disease," *Synapse*, vol. 44, no. 1, pp. 23–35, 2002.

[140] M. Glass, M. Dragunow, and R. L. Faull, "The pattern of neurodegeneration in Huntington's disease: a comparative study of cannabinoid, dopamine, adenosine and GABA$_A$ receptor alterations in the human basal ganglia in Huntington's disease," *Neuroscience*, vol. 97, no. 3, pp. 505–519, 2000.

[141] K. Van Laere, C. Casteels, S. Lunskens et al., "Regional changes in type 1 cannabinoid receptor availability in Parkinson's disease in vivo," *Neurobiology of Aging*, vol. 33, no. 3, pp. 620.e1–620.e8, 2012.

[142] E. M. Romero, B. Fernández, O. Sagredo et al., "Antinociceptive, behavioural and neuroendocrine effects of CP 55,940 in young rats," *Developmental Brain Research*, vol. 136, no. 2, pp. 85–92, 2002.

[143] L. E. Long, R. Chesworth, X.-F. Huang, I. S. McGregor, J. C. Arnold, and T. Karl, "A behavioural comparison of acute and chronic 9- tetrahydrocannabinol and cannabidiol in C57BL/6JArc mice," *International Journal of Neuropsychopharmacology*, vol. 13, no. 7, pp. 861–876, 2010.

[144] W. R. Prescott, L. H. Gold, and B. R. Martin, "Evidence for separate neuronal mechanisms for the discriminative stimulus and catalepsy induced by Δ^9-THC in the rat," *Psychopharmacology*, vol. 107, no. 1, pp. 117–124, 1992.

[145] J. N. Crawley, R. L. Corwin, J. K. Robinson, C. C. Felder, W. A. Devane, and J. Axelrod, "Anandamide, an endogenous ligand of the cannabinoid receptor, induces hypomotility and hypothermia in vivo in rodents," *Pharmacology, Biochemistry and Behavior*, vol. 46, no. 4, pp. 967–972, 1993.

[146] J. Romero, R. de Miguel, E. García-Palomero, J. J. Fernández-Ruiz, and J. A. Ramos, "Time-course of the effects of anandamide, the putative endogenous cannabinoid receptor ligand, on extrapyramidal function," *Brain Research*, vol. 694, no. 1-2, pp. 223–232, 1995.

[147] J. Romero, L. Garcia, M. Cebeira, D. Zadrozny, J. J. Fernández-Ruiz, and J. A. Ramos, "The endogenous cannabinoid receptor ligand, anandamide, inhibits the motor behavior: role of nigrostriatal dopaminergic neurons," *Life Sciences*, vol. 56, no. 23-24, pp. 2033–2040, 1995.

[148] L. A. Anderson, J. J. Anderson, T. N. Chase, and J. R. Walters, "The cannabinoid agonists WIN 55,212-2 and CP 55,940 attenuate rotational behavior induced by a dopamine D1 but not a D2 agonist in rats with unilateral lesions of the nigrostriatal pathway," *Brain Research*, vol. 691, no. 1-2, pp. 106–114, 1995.

[149] J. Fernández-Ruiz, I. Lastres-Becker, A. Cabranes, S. González, and J. A. Ramos, "Endocannabinoids and basal ganglia functionality," *Prostaglandins Leukotrienes and Essential Fatty Acids*, vol. 66, no. 2-3, pp. 257–267, 2002.

[150] M. Herkenham, A. B. Lynn, M. Ross Johnson, L. S. Melvin, B. R. De Costa, and K. C. Rice, "Characterization and localization of cannabinoid receptors in rat brain: a quantitative in vitro autoradiographic study," *Journal of Neuroscience*, vol. 11, no. 2, pp. 563–583, 1991.

[151] A. G. Hohmann and M. Herkenham, "Localization of cannabinoid CB1 receptor mRNA in neuronal subpopulations of rat striatum: a double-label in situ hybridization study," *Synapse*, vol. 37, no. 1, pp. 71–80, 2000.

[152] J. Romero, I. Lastres-Becker, R. de Miguel, F. Berrendero, J. A. Ramos, and J. Fernández-Ruiz, "The endogenous cannabinoid system and the basal ganglia: biochemical, pharmacological, and therapeutic aspects," *Pharmacology and Therapeutics*, vol. 95, no. 2, pp. 137–152, 2002.

[153] P. Gubellini, B. Picconi, M. Bari et al., "Experimental parkinsonism alters endocannabinoid degradation: implications for striatal glutamatergic transmission," *The Journal of Neuroscience*, vol. 22, no. 16, pp. 6900–6907, 2002.

[154] Y. Gilgun-Sherki, E. Melamed, R. Mechoulam, and D. Offen, "The CB1 cannabinoid receptor agonist, HU-210, reduces levodopa-induced rotations in 6-hydroxydopamine-lesioned rats," *Pharmacology and Toxicology*, vol. 93, no. 2, pp. 66–70, 2003.

[155] D. T. Malone and D. A. Taylor, "Modulation by fluoxetine of striatal dopamine release following Δ^9-tetrahydrocannabinol: a microdialysis study in conscious rats," *British Journal of Pharmacology*, vol. 128, no. 1, pp. 21–26, 1999.

[156] G. Tanda, F. E. Pontieri, and G. Di Chiara, "Cannabinoid and heroin activation of mesolimbic dopamine transmission by a common $\mu 1$ opioid receptor mechanism," *Science*, vol. 276, no. 5321, pp. 2048–2050, 1997.

[157] R. G. Pertwee, A. Thomas, L. A. Stevenson et al., "The psychoactive plant cannabinoid, Δ 9- tetrahydrocannabinol, is antagonized by Δ 8- and Δ 9-tetrahydrocannabivarin in mice in vivo," *British Journal of Pharmacology*, vol. 150, no. 5, pp. 586–594, 2007.

[158] A. Richter and W. Löscher, "(+)-WIN 55,212-2, a novel cannabinoid receptor agonist, exerts antidystonic effects in mutant dystonic hamsters," *European Journal of Pharmacology*, vol. 264, no. 3, pp. 371–377, 1994.

[159] Y. P. Maneuf, A. R. Crossman, and J. M. Brotchie, "The cannabinoid receptor agonist WIN 55,212-2 reduces D_2, but not D_1, dopamine receptor-mediated alleviation of akinesia

in the reserpine-treated rat model of Parkinson's disease," *Experimental Neurology*, vol. 148, no. 1, pp. 265–270, 1997.

[160] G. Segovia, F. Mora, A. R. Crossman, and J. M. Brotchie, "Effects of CB1 cannabinoid receptor modulating compounds on the hyperkinesia induced by high-dose levodopa in the reserpine-treated rat model of Parkinson's disease," *Movement Disorders*, vol. 18, no. 2, pp. 138–149, 2003.

[161] M. G. Morgese, T. Cassano, V. Cuomo, and A. Giuffrida, "Antidyskinetic effects of cannabinoids in a rat model of Parkinson's disease: role of CB_1 and TRPV1 receptors," *Experimental Neurology*, vol. 208, no. 1, pp. 110–119, 2007.

[162] M. G. Morgese, T. Cassano, S. Gaetani et al., "Neurochemical changes in the striatum of dyskinetic rats after administration of the cannabinoid agonist WIN55,212-2," *Neurochemistry International*, vol. 54, no. 1, pp. 56–64, 2009.

[163] B. Ferrer, N. Asbrock, S. Kathuria, D. Piomelli, and A. Giuffrida, "Effects of levodopa on endocannabinoid levels in rat basal ganglia: implications for the treatment of levodopa-induced dyskinesias," *European Journal of Neuroscience*, vol. 18, no. 6, pp. 1607–1614, 2003.

[164] R. González-Aparicio and R. Moratalla, "Oleoylethanolamide reduces L-DOPA-induced dyskinesia via TRPV1 receptor in a mouse model of Parkinson's disease," *Neurobiology of Disease*, vol. 62, pp. 416–425, 2014.

[165] S. H. Fox, B. Henry, M. Hill, A. Crossman, and J. M. Brotchie, "Stimulation of Cannabinoid receptors reduces levodopa-induced dyskinesia in the MPTP-lesioned nonhuman primate model of Parkinson's disease," *Movement Disorders*, vol. 17, no. 6, pp. 1180–1187, 2002.

[166] S. H. Fox, M. Kellett, A. P. Moore, A. R. Crossman, and J. M. Brotchie, "Randomised, double-blind, placebo-controlled trial to assess the potential of cannabinoid receptor stimulation in the treatment of dystonia," *Movement Disorders*, vol. 17, no. 1, pp. 145–149, 2002.

[167] M. Solinas, Z. Justinova, S. R. Goldberg, and G. Tanda, "Anandamide administration alone and after inhibition of fatty acid amide hydrolase (FAAH) increases dopamine levels in the nucleus accumbens shell in rats," *Journal of Neurochemistry*, vol. 98, no. 2, pp. 408–419, 2006.

[168] P. M. Zygmunt, J. Petersson, D. A. Andersson et al., "Vanilloid receptors on sensory nerves mediate the vasodilator action of anandamide," *Nature*, vol. 400, no. 6743, pp. 452–457, 1999.

[169] D. Smart, M. J. Gunthorpe, J. C. Jerman et al., "The endogenous lipid anandamide is a full agonist at the human vanilloid receptor (hVR1)," *British Journal of Pharmacology*, vol. 129, no. 2, pp. 227–230, 2000.

[170] V. Di Marzo, I. Lastres-Becker, T. Bisogno et al., "Hypolocomotor effects in rats of capsaicin and two long chain capsaicin homologues," *European Journal of Pharmacology*, vol. 420, no. 2-3, pp. 123–131, 2001.

[171] S. Marinelli, V. Di Marzo, N. Berretta et al., "Presynaptic facilitation of glutamatergic synapses to dopaminergic neurons of the rat substantia nigra by endogenous stimulation of vanilloid receptors," *The Journal of Neuroscience*, vol. 23, no. 8, pp. 3136–3144, 2003.

[172] P. B. Smith, D. R. Compton, S. P. Welch, R. K. Razdan, R. Mechoulam, and B. R. Martin, "The pharmacological activity of anandamide, a putative endogenous cannabinoid, in mice," *Journal of Pharmacology and Experimental Therapeutics*, vol. 270, no. 1, pp. 219–227, 1994.

[173] E. Fride and R. Mechoulam, "Pharmacological activity of the cannabinoid receptor agonist, anandamide, a brain constituent," *European Journal of Pharmacology*, vol. 231, no. 2, pp. 313–314, 1993.

[174] E. De Lago, J. Fernández-Ruiz, S. Ortega-Gutiérrez, A. Viso, M. L. López-Rodríguez, and J. A. Ramos, "UCM707, a potent and selective inhibitor of endocannabinoid uptake, potentiates hypokinetic and antinociceptive effects of anandamide," *European Journal of Pharmacology*, vol. 449, no. 1-2, pp. 99–103, 2002.

[175] N. Ueda, R. A. Puffenbarger, S. Yamamoto, and D. G. Deutsch, "The fatty acid amide hydrolase (FAAH)," *Chemistry and Physics of Lipids*, vol. 108, no. 1-2, pp. 107–121, 2000.

[176] M. Maccarrone, "Fatty acid amide hydrolase: a potential target for next generation therapeutics," *Current Pharmaceutical Design*, vol. 12, no. 6, pp. 759–772, 2006.

[177] V. Di Marzo and M. Maccarrone, "FAAH and anandamide: is 2-AG really the odd one out?" *Trends in Pharmacological Sciences*, vol. 29, no. 5, pp. 229–233, 2008.

[178] T. H. Johnston, P. Huot, S. H. Fox et al., "Fatty Acid Amide Hydrolase (FAAH) inhibition reduces L-3,4- dihydroxyphenylalanine-induced hyperactivity in the 1-methyl-4-phenyl-1,2,3,6-tetrahydropyridine-lesioned non-human primate model of Parkinson's disease," *Journal of Pharmacology and Experimental Therapeutics*, vol. 336, no. 2, pp. 423–430, 2011.

[179] M. Celorrio, D. Fernández-Suáreza, E. Rojo-Bustamantea et al., "Fatty acid amide hydrolase inhibition for the symptomatic relief of Parkinson's disease," *Brain, Behavior, and Immunity*, vol. 57, pp. 94–105, 2016.

[180] M. Hodaie, J. S. Neimat, and A. M. Lozano, "The dopaminergic nigrostriatal system and Parkinson's disease: molecular events in development, disease, and cell death, and new therapeutic strategies," *Neurosurgery*, vol. 60, no. 1, pp. 17–28, 2007.

[181] A. Sayd, M. Antón, F. Alén et al., "Systemic administration of oleoylethanolamide protects from neuroinflammation and anhedonia induced by LPS in rats," *International Journal of Neuropsychopharmacology*, vol. 18, no. 6, pp. 1–14, 2015.

[182] I. Lastres-Becker, F. Molina-Holgado, J. A. Ramos, R. Mechoulam, and J. Fernández-Ruiz, "Cannabinoids provide neuroprotection against 6-hydroxydopamine toxicity in vivo and in vitro: relevance to Parkinson's disease," *Neurobiology of Disease*, vol. 19, no. 1-2, pp. 96–107, 2005.

[183] S. V. More, H. Kumar, I. S. Kim, S.-Y. Song, and D.-K. Choi, "Cellular and molecular mediators of neuroinflammation in the pathogenesis of Parkinson's disease," *Mediators of Inflammation*, vol. 2013, Article ID 952375, 12 pages, 2013.

[184] M. García-Arencibia, L. Ferraro, S. Tanganelli, and J. Fernández-Ruiz, "Enhanced striatal glutamate release after the administration of rimonabant to 6-hydroxydopamine-lesioned rats," *Neuroscience Letters*, vol. 438, no. 1, pp. 10–13, 2008.

[185] P. Huang, L.-Y. Liu-Chen, E. M. Unterwald, and A. Cowan, "Hyperlocomotion and paw tremors are two highly quantifiable signs of SR141716-precipitated withdrawal from delta9-tetrahydrocannabinol in C57BL/6 mice," *Neuroscience Letters*, vol. 465, no. 1, pp. 66–70, 2009.

[186] S. González, C. Scorticati, M. García-Arencibia, R. de Miguel, J. A. Ramos, and J. Fernández-Ruiz, "Effects of rimonabant, a selective cannabinoid CB1 receptor antagonist, in a rat model of Parkinson's disease," *Brain Research*, vol. 1073-1074, no. 1, pp. 209–219, 2006.

[187] E. Fernandez-Espejo, I. Caraballo, F. R. de Fonseca et al., "Cannabinoid CB1 antagonists possess antiparkinsonian efficacy only in rats with very severe nigral lesion in experimental parkinsonism," *Neurobiology of Disease*, vol. 18, no. 3, pp. 591–601, 2005.

[188] F. El Banoua, I. Caraballo, J. A. Flores, B. Galan-Rodriguez, and E. Fernandez-Espejo, "Effects on turning of microinjections into basal ganglia of D1 and D2 dopamine receptors agonists and the cannabinoid CB1 antagonist SR141716A in a rat Parkinson's model," *Neurobiology of Disease*, vol. 16, no. 2, pp. 377–385, 2004.

[189] X. Cao, L. Liang, J. R. Hadcock et al., "Blockade of cannabinoid type 1 receptors augments the antiparkinsonian action of levodopa without affecting dyskinesias in 1-methyl-4-phenyl-1,2,3,6- tetrahydropyridine-treated rhesus monkeys," *Journal of Pharmacology and Experimental Therapeutics*, vol. 323, no. 1, pp. 318–326, 2007.

[190] S. M. Papa, "The cannabinoid system in Parkinson's disease: multiple targets to motor effects," *Experimental Neurology*, vol. 211, no. 2, pp. 334–338, 2008.

[191] M. García-Arencibia, S. González, E. de Lago, J. A. Ramos, R. Mechoulam, and J. Fernández-Ruiz, "Evaluation of the neuroprotective effect of cannabinoids in a rat model of Parkinson's disease: importance of antioxidant and cannabinoid receptor-independent properties," *Brain Research*, vol. 1134, no. 1, pp. 162–170, 2007.

[192] J. Fernández-Ruiz, M. Moreno-Martet, C. Rodríguez-Cueto et al., "Prospects for cannabinoid therapies in basal ganglia disorders," *British Journal of Pharmacology*, vol. 163, no. 7, pp. 1365–1378, 2011.

[193] W. Gowers, *A Manual of Diseases of the Nervous System*, P. Blakiston's Son & Co, Philadelphia, Pa, USA, 1888.

[194] K. R. Müller-Vahl, "Treatment of Tourette syndrome with cannabinoids," *Behavioural Neurology*, vol. 27, no. 1, pp. 119–124, 2013.

[195] K. R. Müller-Vahl, U. Schneider, H. Prevedel et al., "Δ9-tetrahydrocannabinol (THC) is effective in the treatment of tics in Tourette syndrome: a 6-week randomized trial," *Journal of Clinical Psychiatry*, vol. 64, no. 4, pp. 459–465, 2003.

[196] K. R. Müller-Vahl, U. Schneider, A. Koblenz et al., "Treatment of Tourette's syndrome with Δ^9-tetrahydrocannabinol (THC): a randomized crossover trial," *Pharmacopsychiatry*, vol. 35, no. 2, pp. 57–61, 2002.

[197] K. R. Muller-Vahl, H. Kolbe, U. Schneider, and H. M. Emrich, "Cannabis in movement disorders," *Forschende Komplementarmedizin*, vol. 6, no. 3, pp. 23–27, 1999.

[198] K. R. Müller-Vahl, U. Schneider, and H. M. Emrich, "Nabilone increases choreatic movements in Huntington's disease," *Movement Disorders*, vol. 14, no. 6, pp. 1038–1040, 1999.

[199] K. R. Müller-Vahl, H. Kolbe, U. Schneider, and H. M. Emrich, "Cannabinoids: possible role in patho-physiology and therapy of Gilles de la Tourette syndrome," *Acta Psychiatrica Scandinavica*, vol. 98, no. 6, pp. 502–506, 1998.

[200] P. Consroe, R. Sandyk, and S. R. Snider, "Open label evaluation of cannabidiol in dystonic movement disorders," *International Journal of Neuroscience*, vol. 30, no. 4, pp. 277–282, 1986.

[201] R. Sandyk, S. R. Snider, P. Consroe, and S. M. Elias, "Cannabidiol in dystonic movement disorders," *Psychiatry Research*, vol. 18, no. 3, p. 291, 1986.

[202] K. Venderova, E. Ruzicka, V. Vorisek, and P. Visnovsky, "Survey on cannabis use in Parkinson's disease: subjective improvement of motor symptoms," *Movement Disorders*, vol. 19, no. 9, pp. 1102–1106, 2004.

[203] I. Lotan, T. Treves, Y. Roditi, and R. Djaldetti, "Medical marijuana (cannabis) treatment for motor and non-motor symptoms in Parkinson's disease. An open-label observational study," *Movement Disorders*, vol. 28, no. 1, p. 448, 2013.

[204] J. P. Frankel, A. Hughes, A. A. J. Lees, and G. M. Stern, "Marijuana for parkinsonian tremor," *Journal of Neurology, Neurosurgery & Psychiatry*, vol. 53, no. 5, p. 436, 1990.

[205] C. B. Carroll, P. G. Bain, L. Teare, X. Liu, C. Joint, and C. Wroath, "Cannabis for dyskinesia in Parkinson disease: a randomized double-blind crossover study," *Neurology*, vol. 63, pp. 1245–1250, 2004.

[206] S. R. Snider and P. Consroe, "Beneficial and adverse effects of cannabidiol in a Parkinson patient with sinemet-induced dystonic dyskinesia," *Neurology*, vol. 35, article 201, 1985.

[207] K. A. Sieradzan, S. H. Fox, J. Dick, and J. M. Brotchie, "The effects of the cannabinoid receptor agonist nabilone on L-DOPA induced dyskinesia in patients with idiopathic Parkinson's disease," *Movement Disorders*, vol. 13, supplement 2, p. 29, 1998.

[208] K. A. Sieradzan, S. H. Fox, M. Hill, J. P. R. Dick, A. R. Crossman, and J. M. Brotchie, "Cannabinoids reduce levodopa-induced dyskinesia in Parkinson's disease: A Pilot Study," *Neurology*, vol. 57, no. 11, pp. 2108–2111, 2001.

[209] P. Consroe, "Brain cannabinoid systems as targets for the therapy of neurological disorders," *Neurobiology of Disease*, vol. 5, no. 6, pp. 534–551, 1998.

[210] V. Mesnage, J. L. Houeto, A. M. Bonnet et al., "Neurokinin B, neurotensin, and cannabinoid receptor antagonists and Parkinson disease," *Clinical Neuropharmacology*, vol. 27, no. 3, pp. 108–110, 2004.

[211] B. S. Koppel, J. C. M. Brust, T. Fife et al., "Systematic review: efficacy and safety of medical marijuana in selected neurologic disorders: report of the Guideline Development Subcommittee of the American Academy of Neurology," *Neurology*, vol. 82, no. 17, pp. 1556–1563, 2014.

[212] A. Chatterjee, A. Almahrezi, M. Ware, and M. A. Fitzcharles, "A dramatic response to inhaled cannabis in a woman with central thalamic pain and dystonia," *Journal of Pain and Symptom Management*, vol. 24, no. 1, pp. 4–6, 2002.

[213] C. D. Marsden, "Treatment of torsion dystonia," in *Disorders of Movement, Current Status of Modern Therapy*, A. Barbeau, Ed., vol. 8, pp. 81–104, Lippincott Williams & Wilkins, Philadelphia, Pa, USA, 1981.

[214] M. C. Uribe Roca, F. Micheli, and R. Viotti, "Cannabis sativa and dystonia secondary to Wilson's disease," *Movement Disorders*, vol. 20, no. 1, pp. 113–115, 2005.

[215] S. R. Snider and P. Consroe, "Treatment of Meige's syndrome with cannabidiol," *Neurology*, vol. 34, article 147, 1984.

[216] R. Lorenz, "On the application of cannabis in paediatrics and epileptology," *Neuroendocrinology Letters*, vol. 25, no. 1-2, pp. 40–44, 2004.

[217] A. Curtis, I. Mitchell, S. Patel, N. Ives, and H. Rickards, "A pilot study using nabilone for symptomatic treatment in Huntington's disease," *Movement Disorders*, vol. 24, no. 15, pp. 2254–2259, 2009.

[218] M. J. Armstrong and J. M. Miyasaki, "Evidence-based guideline: pharmacologic treatment of chorea in Huntington disease: report of the guideline development subcommittee of the American Academy of Neurology," *Neurology*, vol. 79, no. 6, pp. 597–603, 2012.

[219] R. Sandyk, P. Consroe, L. Stern, S. R. Snider, and D. Bliklen, "Preliminary trial of cannabidiol in Huntington's disease," in *Marijuana: An International Research Report*, G. Chesher, P. Consroe, and R. Musty, Eds., Australian Government Publishing Service, Canberra, Australia, 1988.

[220] P. Consroe, J. Laguna, J. Allender et al., "Controlled clinical trial of cannabidiol in Huntington's disease," *Pharmacology, Biochemistry and Behavior*, vol. 40, no. 3, pp. 701–708, 1991.

[221] N. M. Kogan and R. Mechoulam, "Cannabinoids in health and disease," *Dialogues in Clinical Neuroscience*, vol. 9, no. 4, pp. 413–430, 2007.

[222] R. Sandyk and G. Awerbuch, "Marijuana and tourette's syndrome," *Journal of Clinical Psychopharmacology*, vol. 8, no. 6, pp. 444–445, 1988.

[223] M. Hemming and P. M. Yellowlees, "Effective treatment of Tourette's syndrome with marijuana," *Journal of Psychopharmacology*, vol. 7, no. 4, pp. 389–391, 1993.

[224] A. Hasan, A. Rothenberger, A. Münchau, T. Wobrock, P. Falkai, and V. Roessner, "Oral Δ9-tetrahydrocannabinol improved refractory Gilles de la Tourette syndrome in an adolescent by increasing intracortical inhibition: a case report," *Journal of Clinical Psychopharmacology*, vol. 30, no. 2, pp. 190–192, 2010.

[225] A. Brunnauer, F. M. Segmiller, T. Volkamer, G. Laux, N. Müller, and S. Dehning, "Cannabinoids improve driving ability in a Tourette's patient," *Psychiatry Research*, vol. 190, no. 2-3, p. 382, 2011.

[226] G. Berding, K. Müller-Vahl, U. Schneider et al., "[^{123}I]AM281 single-photon emission computed tomography imaging of central cannabinoid CB1 receptors before and after Δ9-tetrahydrocannabinol therapy and whole-body scanning for assessment of radiation dose in Tourette patients," *Biological Psychiatry*, vol. 55, no. 9, pp. 904–915, 2004.

[227] J. Ševčík and K. Mašek, "Potential role of cannabinoids in Parkinson's disease," *Drugs and Aging*, vol. 16, no. 6, pp. 391–395, 2000.

[228] H. Pan, P. Mukhopadhyay, M. Rajesh et al., "Cannabidiol attenuates cisplatin-Lnduced nephrotoxicity by decreasing oxidative/nitrosative stress, inflammation, and cell death," *Journal of Pharmacology and Experimental Therapeutics*, vol. 328, no. 3, pp. 708–714, 2009.

[229] M. S. Hernandes, C. C. Café-Mendes, and L. R. G. Britto, "NADPH oxidase and the degeneration of dopaminergic neurons in Parkinsonian mice," *Oxidative Medicine and Cellular Longevity*, vol. 2013, Article ID 157857, 13 pages, 2013.

[230] E. Hebert-Chatelain, L. Reguero, N. Puente et al., "Cannabinoid control of brain bioenergetics: exploring the subcellular localization of the CB1 receptor," *Molecular Metabolism*, vol. 3, no. 4, pp. 495–504, 2014.

[231] S. Yamaori, J. Ebisawa, Y. Okushima, I. Yamamoto, and K. Watanabe, "Potent inhibition of human cytochrome P450 3A isoforms by cannabidiol: role of phenolic hydroxyl groups in the resorcinol moiety," *Life Sciences*, vol. 88, no. 15-16, pp. 730–736, 2011.

[232] A. J. Hampson, M. Grimaldi, J. Axelrod, and D. Wink, "Cannabidiol and (−)Δ9-tetrahydrocannabinol are neuroprotective antioxidants," *Proceedings of the National Academy of Sciences of the United States of America*, vol. 95, no. 14, pp. 8268–8273, 1998.

[233] G. Bénard, F. Massa, N. Puente et al., "Mitochondrial CB1 receptors regulate neuronal energy metabolism," *Nature Neuroscience*, vol. 15, no. 4, pp. 558–564, 2012.

[234] S. Amor, F. Puentes, D. Baker, and P. Van Der Valk, "Inflammation in neurodegenerative diseases," *Immunology*, vol. 129, no. 2, pp. 154–169, 2010.

[235] S. Amor, L. A. N. Peferoen, D. Y. S. Vogel et al., "Inflammation in neurodegenerative diseases—an update," *Immunology*, vol. 142, no. 2, pp. 151–166, 2014.

[236] L. F. Clark and T. Kodadek, "The immune system and neuroinflammation as potential sources of blood-based biomarkers for Alzheimer's disease, Parkinson's disease, and huntington's disease," *ACS Chemical Neuroscience*, vol. 7, no. 5, pp. 520–527, 2016.

[237] M. A. Mena and J. García De Yébenes, "Glial cells as players in parkinsonism: the 'good,' the 'bad,' and the 'mysterious' glia," *Neuroscientist*, vol. 14, no. 6, pp. 544–560, 2008.

[238] P. L. McGeer and E. G. McGeer, "Glial reactions in Parkinson's disease," *Movement Disorders*, vol. 23, no. 4, pp. 474–483, 2008.

[239] N. Stella, "Cannabinoid and cannabinoid-like receptors in microglia, astrocytes, and astrocytomas," *Glia*, vol. 58, no. 9, pp. 1017–1030, 2010.

[240] A. Klegeris, C. J. Bissonnette, and P. L. McGeer, "Reduction of human monocytic cell neurotoxicity and cytokine secretion by ligands of the cannabinoid-type CB2 receptor," *British Journal of Pharmacology*, vol. 139, no. 4, pp. 775–786, 2003.

[241] G. Esposito, C. Scuderi, C. Savani et al., "Cannabidiol in vivo blunts β-amyloid induced neuroinflammation by suppressing IL-1β and iNOS expression," *British Journal of Pharmacology*, vol. 151, no. 8, pp. 1272–1279, 2007.

[242] B. Watzl, P. Scuderi, and R. R. Watson, "Influence of marijuana components (THC and CBD) on human mononuclear cell cytokine secretion in vitro," *Advances in Experimental Medicine and Biology*, vol. 288, pp. 63–70, 1991.

[243] M. D. Srivastava, B. I. S. Srivastava, and B. Brouhard, "Δ9 Tetrahydrocannabinol and cannabidiol alter cytokine production by human immune cells," *Immunopharmacology*, vol. 40, no. 3, pp. 179–185, 1998.

[244] A. M. Malfait, R. Gallily, P. F. Sumariwalla et al., "The nonpsychoactive cannabis constituent cannabidiol is an oral anti-arthritic therapeutic in murine collagen-induced arthritis," *Proceedings of the National Academy of Sciences of the United States of America*, vol. 97, no. 17, pp. 9561–9566, 2000.

[245] R. Mechoulam, L. A. Parker, and R. Gallily, "Cannabidiol: an overview of some pharmacological aspects," *Journal of Clinical Pharmacology*, vol. 42, no. 11, pp. 11S–19S, 2002.

[246] R. Mechoulam, M. Peters, E. Murillo-Rodriguez, and L. O. Hanuš, "Cannabidiol—recent advances," *Chemistry and Biodiversity*, vol. 4, no. 8, pp. 1678–1692, 2007.

[247] B. Costa, M. Colleoni, S. Conti et al., "Oral anti-inflammatory activity of cannabidiol, a non-psychoactive constituent of cannabis, in acute carrageenan-induced inflammation in the rat paw," *Naunyn-Schmiedeberg's Archives of Pharmacology*, vol. 369, no. 3, pp. 294–299, 2004.

[248] B. Costa, A. E. Trovato, F. Comelli, G. Giagnoni, and M. Colleoni, "The non-psychoactive cannabis constituent cannabidiol is an orally effective therapeutic agent in rat chronic inflammatory and neuropathic pain," *European Journal of Pharmacology*, vol. 556, no. 1–3, pp. 75–83, 2007.

[249] F. Assaf, M. Fishbein, M. Gafni, O. Keren, and Y. Sarne, "Pre- and post-conditioning treatment with an ultra-low dose of Δ9-tetrahydrocannabinol (THC) protects against pentylenetetrazole (PTZ)-induced cognitive damage," *Behavioural Brain Research*, vol. 220, no. 1, pp. 194–201, 2011.

[250] P. E. Szmitko and S. Verma, "Does cannabis hold the key to treating cardiometabolic disease?" *Nature Clinical Practice Cardiovascular Medicine*, vol. 3, no. 3, pp. 116–117, 2006.

[251] M. Fishbein-Kaminietsky, M. Gafni, and Y. Sarne, "Ultralow doses of cannabinoid drugs protect the mouse brain from inflammation-induced cognitive damage," *Journal of Neuroscience Research*, vol. 92, no. 12, pp. 1669–1677, 2014.

[252] O. Sagredo, M. García-Arencibia, E. de Lago, S. Finetti, A. Decio, and J. Fernández-Ruiz, "Cannabinoids and neuroprotection in basal ganglia disorders," *Molecular Neurobiology*, vol. 36, no. 1, pp. 82–91, 2007.

[253] D. A. Price, A. A. Martinez, A. Seillier et al., "WIN55,212-2, a cannabinoid receptor agonist, protects against nigrostriatal cell loss in the 1-methyl-4-phenyl-1,2,3,6-tetrahydropyridine mouse model of Parkinson's disease," *European Journal of Neuroscience*, vol. 29, no. 11, pp. 2177–2186, 2009.

[254] J. Martínez-Orgado, D. Fernández-López, I. Lizasoain, and J. Romero, "The seek of neuroprotection: introducing cannabinoids," *Recent Patents on CNS Drug Discovery*, vol. 2, no. 2, pp. 131–139, 2007.

[255] J. Romero and J. Martínez-Orgado, "Cannabinoids and neurodegenerative diseases," *CNS and Neurological Disorders—Drug Targets*, vol. 8, no. 6, pp. 440–450, 2009.

[256] M. F. Beal, "Excitotoxicity and nitric oxide in Parkinson's disease pathogenesis," *Annals of Neurology*, vol. 44, no. 3, pp. S110–S114, 1998.

[257] S. Valdeolivas, V. Satta, R. G. Pertwee, J. Fernández-Ruiz, and O. Sagredo, "Sativex-like combination of phytocannabinoids is neuroprotective in malonate-lesioned rats, an inflammatory model of Huntington's disease: role of CB1 and CB2 receptors," *ACS Chemical Neuroscience*, vol. 3, no. 5, pp. 400–406, 2012.

[258] M. Zeissler, C. Hanemann, J. Zajicek, and C. Carroll, "FAAH inhibition is protective in a cell culture model of Parkinson's disease," *Journal of Neurology, Neurosurgery & Psychiatry*, vol. 83, supplement 2, p. A15, 2012.

[259] M. Sophie and B. Ford, "Management of pain in Parkinson's disease," *CNS Drugs*, vol. 26, no. 11, pp. 937–948, 2012.

[260] E. G. Silva, M. A. Viana, and E. M. Quagliato, "Diagnostic of parkinsonian syndrome in a Brazilian movement disorders clinic," *Revista Neurociências*, vol. 13, no. 4, pp. 173–177, 2005.

[261] M. Tinazzi, C. Del Vesco, E. Fincati et al., "Pain and motor complications in Parkinson's disease," *Journal of Neurology, Neurosurgery and Psychiatry*, vol. 77, no. 7, pp. 822–825, 2006.

[262] J. I. Sage, "Pain in Parkinson's disease," *Current Treatment Options in Neurology*, vol. 6, no. 3, pp. 191–200, 2004.

[263] R. H. Dworkin, E. M. Nagasako, B. S. Galer, R. D. Hetzel, and J. T. Farrar, "Assessment of pain and pain-related quality of life in clinical trials," in *Handbook of Pain Assessment*, D. C. Turk and R. Melzack, Eds., pp. 519–548, Guilford, New York, NY, USA, 2nd edition, 2001.

[264] R. H. Dworkin, M. Backonja, M. C. Rowbotham et al., "Advances in neuropathic pain: diagnosis, mechanisms, and treatment recommendations," *Archives of Neurology*, vol. 60, no. 11, pp. 1524–1534, 2003.

[265] R. H. Dworkin, A. E. Corbin, J. P. Young Jr. et al., "Pregabalin for the treatment of postherpetic neuralgia: a randomized, placebo-controlled trial," *Neurology*, vol. 60, no. 8, pp. 1274–1283, 2003.

[266] L. Greenbaum, I. Tegeder, Y. Barhum, E. Melamed, Y. Roditi, and R. Djaldetti, "Contribution of genetic variants to pain susceptibility in Parkinson disease," *European Journal of Pain*, vol. 16, no. 9, pp. 1243–1250, 2012.

[267] A. Calignano, G. La Rana, A. Giuffrida, and D. Piomelli, "Control of pain initiation by endogenous cannabinoids," *Nature*, vol. 394, no. 6690, pp. 277–281, 1998.

[268] R. J. Ellis, W. Toperoff, F. Vaida et al., "Smoked medicinal cannabis for neuropathic pain in HIV: a randomized, crossover clinical trial," *Neuropsychopharmacology*, vol. 34, no. 3, pp. 672–680, 2009.

[269] B. Wilsey, T. Marcotte, A. Tsodikov et al., "A randomized, placebo-controlled, crossover trial of cannabis cigarettes in neuropathic pain," *Journal of Pain*, vol. 9, no. 6, pp. 506–521, 2008.

[270] D. I. Abrams, C. A. Jay, S. B. Shade et al., "Cannabis in painful HIV-associated sensory neuropathy: a randomized placebo-controlled trial," *Neurology*, vol. 68, no. 7, pp. 515–521, 2007.

[271] J. S. Berman, C. Symonds, and R. Birch, "Efficacy of two cannabis based medicinal extracts for relief of central neuropathic pain from brachial plexus avulsion: results of a randomised controlled trial," *Pain*, vol. 112, no. 3, pp. 299–306, 2004.

[272] K. B. Svendsen, T. S. Jensen, and F. W. Bach, "Does the cannabinoid dronabinol reduce central pain in multiple sclerosis? Randomised double blind placebo controlled crossover trial," *British Medical Journal*, vol. 329, no. 7460, pp. 253–257, 2004.

[273] D. J. Rog, T. J. Nurmikko, T. Friede, and C. A. Young, "Randomized, controlled trial of cannabis-based medicine in central pain in multiple sclerosis," *Neurology*, vol. 65, no. 6, pp. 812–819, 2005.

[274] T. J. Nurmikko, M. G. Serpell, B. Hoggart, P. J. Toomey, B. J. Morlion, and D. Haines, "Sativex successfully treats neuropathic pain characterised by allodynia: a randomised, double-blind, placebo-controlled clinical trial," *Pain*, vol. 133, no. 1–3, pp. 210–220, 2007.

[275] K. P. Hill, "Medical marijuana for treatment of chronic pain and other medical and psychiatric problems: a clinical review," *The Journal of the American Medical Association*, vol. 313, no. 24, pp. 2474–2483, 2015.

[276] M. E. Lynch and F. Campbell, "Cannabinoids for treatment of chronic non-cancer pain; a systematic review of randomized trials," *British Journal of Clinical Pharmacology*, vol. 72, no. 5, pp. 735–744, 2011.

[277] M. I. Martín Fontelles and C. Goicoechea García, "Role of cannabinoids in the management of neuropathic pain," *CNS Drugs*, vol. 22, no. 8, pp. 645–653, 2008.

[278] M. Iskedjian, B. Bereza, A. Gordon, C. Piwko, and T. R. Einarson, "Meta-analysis of cannabis based treatments for neuropathic and multiple sclerosis-related pain," *Current Medical Research and Opinion*, vol. 23, no. 1, pp. 17–24, 2007.

[279] S. Corey, "Recent developments in the therapeutic potential of cannabinoids," *Puerto Rico Health Sciences Journal*, vol. 24, no. 1, pp. 19–26, 2005.

[280] P. F. Smith, "Cannabinoids in the treatment of pain and spasticity in multiple sclerosis," *Current Opinion in Investigational Drugs*, vol. 3, no. 6, pp. 859–864, 2002.

[281] F. A. Campbell, M. R. Tramèr, D. Carroll, D. J. M. Reynolds, R. A. Moore, and H. J. McQuay, "Are cannabinoids an effective and safe treatment option in the management of pain? A qualitative systematic review," *British Medical Journal*, vol. 323, no. 7303, pp. 13–16, 2001.

[282] W. J. G. Hoogendijk, I. E. C. Sommer, G. Tissingh, D. J. H. Deeg, and E. C. Wolters, "Depression in Parkinson's disease: the impact of symptom overlap on prevalence," *Psychosomatics*, vol. 39, no. 5, pp. 416–421, 1998.

[283] M. Yamamoto, "Depression in Parkinson's disease: its prevalence, diagnosis, and neurochemical background," *Journal of Neurology*, vol. 248, no. 3, pp. III5–11, 2001.

[284] J. S. A. M. Reijnders, U. Ehrt, W. E. J. Weber, D. Aarsland, and A. F. G. Leentjens, "A systematic review of prevalence studies of depression in Parkinson's disease," *Movement Disorders*, vol. 23, no. 2, pp. 183–189, 2008.

[285] A. Schrag, A. Hovris, D. Morley, N. Quinn, and M. Jahanshahi, "Caregiver-burden in parkinson's disease is closely associated with psychiatric symptoms, falls, and disability," *Parkinsonism & Related Disorders*, vol. 12, no. 1, pp. 35–41, 2006.

[286] A. Schrag, "Quality of life and depression in Parkinson's disease," *Journal of the Neurological Sciences*, vol. 248, no. 1-2, pp. 151–157, 2006.

[287] H. Reichmann, C. Schneider, and M. Löhle, "Non-motor features of Parkinson's disease: depression and dementia," *Parkinsonism and Related Disorders*, vol. 15, no. 3, pp. S87–S92, 2009.

[288] B. B. Gorzalka and M. N. Hill, "Putative role of endocannabinoid signaling in the etiology of depression and actions of antidepressants," *Progress in Neuro-Psychopharmacology and Biological Psychiatry*, vol. 35, no. 7, pp. 1575–1585, 2011.

[289] M. Navarro, E. Hernández, R. M. Muñoz et al., "Acute administration of the CB1 cannabinoid receptor antagonist SR 141716A induces anxiety-like responses in the rat," *NeuroReport*, vol. 8, no. 2, pp. 491–496, 1997.

[290] F. A. Moreira and B. Lutz, "The endocannabinoid system: emotion, learning and addiction," *Addiction Biology*, vol. 13, no. 2, pp. 196–212, 2008.

[291] F. A. Moreira and J. A. S. Crippa, "The psychiatric side-effects of rimonabant," *Revista Brasileira de Psiquiatria*, vol. 31, no. 2, pp. 145–153, 2009.

[292] F. J. Barrero, I. Ampuero, B. Morales et al., "Depression in Parkinson's disease is related to a genetic polymorphism of the cannabinoid receptor gene (CNR1)," *The Pharmacogenomics Journal*, vol. 5, no. 2, pp. 135–141, 2005.

[293] F. R. Bambico, P. R. Hattan, J. P. Garant, and G. Gobbi, "Effect of delta-9-tetrahydrocannabinol on behavioral despair and on pre- and postsynaptic serotonergic transmission," *Progress in Neuro-Psychopharmacology & Biological Psychiatry*, vol. 38, no. 1, pp. 88–96, 2012.

[294] G. Gobbi, F. R. Bambico, R. Mangieri et al., "Antidepressant-like activity and modulation of brain monoaminergic transmission by blockade of anandamide hydrolysis," *Proceedings of the National Academy of Sciences of the United States of America*, vol. 102, no. 51, pp. 18620–18625, 2005.

[295] T. F. Denson and M. Earleywine, "Decreased depression in marijuana users," *Addictive Behaviors*, vol. 31, no. 4, pp. 738–742, 2006.

[296] L. Degenhardt, W. Hall, and M. Lynskey, "Exploring the association between cannabis use and depression," *Addiction*, vol. 98, no. 11, pp. 1493–1504, 2003.

[297] B. Porter, R. MacFarlane, and R. Walker, "The frequency and nature of sleep disorders in a community-based population of patients with Parkinson's disease," *European Journal of Neurology*, vol. 15, no. 1, pp. 46–50, 2008.

[298] A. Videnovic and D. Golombek, "Circadian and sleep disorders in Parkinson's disease," *Experimental Neurology*, vol. 243, pp. 45–56, 2013.

[299] L. M. Trotti and D. L. Bliwise, "Treatment of the sleep disorders associated with Parkinson's disease," *Neurotherapeutics*, vol. 11, no. 1, pp. 68–77, 2014.

[300] M. Stacy, "Sleep disorders in Parkinson's disease: epidemiology and management," *Drugs and Aging*, vol. 19, no. 10, pp. 733–739, 2002.

[301] E. B. Russo, G. W. Guy, and P. J. Robson, "Cannabis, pain, and sleep: lessons from therapeutic clinical trials of sativex, a cannabis-based medicine," *Chemistry & Biodiversity*, vol. 4, no. 8, pp. 1729–1743, 2007.

Psychometric Evaluation of the Parkinson's Disease Activities of Daily Living Scale

Stina B. Jonasson,[1,2] Peter Hagell,[3] Gun-Marie Hariz,[4] Susanne Iwarsson,[1] and Maria H. Nilsson[1,5]

[1]Department of Health Sciences, Faculty of Medicine, Lund University, Lund, Sweden
[2]Department of Neurology and Rehabilitation, Skåne University Hospital, Lund, Sweden
[3]The PRO-CARE Group, School of Health and Society, Kristianstad University, Kristianstad, Sweden
[4]Department of Community Medicine and Rehabilitation, Occupational Therapy, Umeå University, Umeå, Sweden
[5]Memory Clinic, Skåne University Hospital, Malmö, Sweden

Correspondence should be addressed to Stina B. Jonasson; stina.jonasson@med.lu.se

Academic Editor: Hélio Teive

Objective. To evaluate a set of psychometric properties (i.e., data completeness, targeting, and external construct validity) of the Parkinson's disease Activities of Daily Living Scale (PADLS) in people with Parkinson's disease (PD). Specific attention was paid to the association between PADLS and PD severity, according to the Hoehn & Yahr (H&Y) staging. *Methods.* The sample included 251 persons with PD (mean age 70 [SD 9] years). Data collection comprised a self-administered postal survey, structured interviews, and clinical assessments at home visits. *Results.* Data completeness was 99.6% and the mean PADLS score was 2.1. Floor and ceiling effects were 22% and 2%, respectively. PADLS scores were more strongly associated ($r_s > 0.5$) with perceived functional independence, ADL dependency, walking difficulties, and self-rated PD severity than with variables such as PD duration and cognitive function ($r_s < 0.5$). PADLS scores differed across H&Y stages (Kruskal-Wallis test, $p < 0.001$). Those in H&Y stages IV-V had more ADL disability than those in stage III (Mann–Whitney U test, $p < 0.001$), whereas there were no significant differences between the other stages. *Conclusion.* PADLS revealed excellent data completeness, acceptable targeting, and external construct validity. It seems to be well suited as a rough estimate of ADL disability in people with PD.

1. Introduction

The ability to perform activities of daily living (ADL) is essential for independent living. ADL includes activities such as feeding, dressing, bathing, cooking, cleaning, and shopping. People with Parkinson's disease (PD) often experience ADL limitations already early during the disease course [1]. Poor ADL performance may result in dependence and is negatively associated with health-related quality of life [2]. Thus, adequate assessments of ADL are important to be able to monitor ADL performance throughout the course of disease in order to provide optimal treatment, care, and rehabilitation for people with PD.

There are various ways of assessing ADL. The assessment can be based on observations of actual ADL performance, interviews, or self-ratings. Assessments can address difficulties in performing ADL, dependence on assistance from others and from assistive devices, or a combination of both [3]. Several ADL rating scales have been psychometrically tested and recommended for use with people with PD [3]. These rating scales typically include around ten items and have been shown to be highly associated with walking difficulties (r_s 0.74–0.86) [4] and physical functioning (r 0.63–0.77) [5, 6]. Lower associations have been reported between ADL disability and depressive symptoms (r_s 0.45–0.61) [7, 8], general health (r 0.42–0.47) [5], PD duration (r_s 0.40) [7], cognitive function (r_s 0.18–0.23) [8], and age (r_s 0.16) [7], respectively. The association between ADL disability and PD motor symptoms has shown large variations among studies (r 0.37–0.68; r_s 0.52–0.87) [5–7, 9]. Large variations apply also for the association between ADL disability and PD severity (r 0.54–0.59; r_s 0.36–0.83) [5–9].

The Parkinson's disease Activities of Daily Living Scale (PADLS) is a single-item self-reported rating scale targeting ADL in people with PD [10]. Since its development in 2001, the PADLS has been used in various PD studies; see, for example, [11–15]. To the best of our knowledge, its psychometric properties have only been reported in the original publication [10] and in a conference abstract [16]. These studies [10, 16] reported test-retest reliability (weighted Kappa 0.70; r 0.89) and external construct validity in terms of associations with, for example, motor symptoms (r 0.65; r_s 0.55), complications of PD therapy (r_s 0.56), depressive symptoms (r 0.43), PD duration (r 0.39; r_s 0.32), and frequency of social activities (r 0.02–0.44). A recent review listed PADLS as a "suggested" rating scale for assessment of ADL in people with PD, and it was argued that more psychometric studies are needed before PADLS can be classified as "recommended" [3]. The review also noted a lack of studies regarding the association between PADLS and the Hoehn & Yahr staging (H&Y, i.e., a classification of PD severity [17]) and the Unified Parkinson's Disease Rating Scale (UPDRS, which assesses PD signs and symptoms [18]).

Thus, this study aimed to evaluate a set of psychometric properties (i.e., data completeness, targeting, and external construct validity) of PADLS scores in people with PD. Specific attention was paid to the association between PADLS and PD severity according to H&Y.

2. Materials and Methods

We utilized cross-sectional baseline data of the project "Home and Health in People Ageing with PD." Details regarding the project design and methods have been published elsewhere [19]. The project was conducted in accordance with the Helsinki Declaration and was approved by the Regional Ethical Review Board in Lund, Sweden (number 2012/558). All participants gave their written informed consent.

2.1. Participants and Recruitment. Participants were recruited from three hospitals in Skåne County, Sweden. A detailed flow chart of the recruitment procedure has been published [20]. A total of 653 persons met the inclusion criterion of a PD diagnosis (ICD-10: G20.9) since at least one year. Of those, 158 were excluded due to difficulties in understanding or speaking Swedish (n = 10), severe cognitive difficulties (n = 91), or other reasons that made them unable to give informed consent or take part in the majority of the data collection (e.g., hallucinations or a recent stroke, n = 57). Fifty-eight persons were excluded since they lived outside Skåne County. The remaining 437 persons were invited to participate, but 22 of those were unreachable and two had a revised diagnosis. Out of the remaining 413 participants, 157 (38%) declined. Another five persons were excluded since they had not responded to the PADLS by themselves or not responded within two months from the home visit (part of the data collection) or due to extensive missing data. This resulted

in a final study sample of 251 participants (mean age 70 [SD 9] years; 39% women). Further participant characteristics are presented in Table 1.

2.2. Data Collection. The data collection is comprised of a self-administered postal survey and a subsequent home visit, which included interview-administered questionnaires and questions as well as clinical assessments. The home visits were conducted by two registered occupational therapists who had undergone project-specific training. More details regarding the procedure have been described elsewhere [19].

The self-administered postal survey included the PADLS, a single-item self-reported rating scale that addresses perceived ADL difficulties and dependence on others as well as on assistive devices during various ADL [10]. Respondents are instructed to rate how their PD has affected their day-to-day activities during the past month according to five response categories ranging from 1 (no difficulties with day-to-day activities) to 5 (extreme difficulties with day-to-day activities), but each response option also has a more detailed description. For example, "2: mild difficulties" includes the following description: "Slowness with some aspects of house-work, gardening or shopping. Able to dress and manage personal hygiene completely independently but rate is slower." PADLS scores have also been dichotomized into "not needing help from others in daily activities" versus "needing help" (PADLS 1-2 versus 3–5) [21].

In addition, the postal survey included a question on self-rated general health (possible item score 1–5, higher = worse) [22] and the Generic Walk-12 (Walk-12G), which assesses perceived walking difficulties in everyday life (possible total score 0–42, higher = worse) [23].

The structured interview during the home visit included a question on PD duration and three study-specific questions targeting social activities. The latter were self-rated by asking about the frequency of visiting/receiving visits from friends/family (almost never; once or twice a year, once or twice a month, once or twice a week, or every day; scored 1–5, resp.). Moreover, depressive symptoms were self-rated using the Geriatric Depression Scale (GDS-15; possible total score 0–15, higher = worse) [24]. Perceived functional independence was assessed according to an item from the Neuropsychological Aging Inventory (possible item score 0–10, higher = better) [25]. Finally, ADL dependency was assessed using the ADL Staircase [26]. Based on the internationally well-known and widely used Katz' ADL Index [27], the ADL Staircase is a conceptually and theoretically sound instrument supported by research demonstrating reliability and validity [28, 29] as well as methodological considerations for use in different populations [30, 31]. Dependence in nine ADL items is rated based on a combination of interview and observation (possible total score 0–9, higher = worse) [26].

Motor symptoms were clinically assessed according to the UPDRS part III (possible total score 0–108, higher = worse), whereas complications of PD therapy were assessed according to the UPDRS part IV (possible total score 0–23, higher = worse) [18]. Cognitive function was assessed by using the Montreal Cognitive Assessment (MoCA; possible total score 0–30, higher = better) [32]. PD severity was

TABLE 1: Participants' characteristics ($n = 243$–251, depending on missing data).

Characteristics	Median (first-third quartile) unless otherwise stated
Sex (women), n (%)	99 (39)
Age (years), mean (SD), min–max	70 (9), 45–93
Parkinson duration (years)	8 (5–13)
Parkinson severity (Hoehn & Yahr)[1]	3 (2-3)
Parkinson severity (self-rated), n (%)	
Mild	85 (34)
Moderate	116 (46)
Severe	49 (20)
Motor symptoms (UPDRS part III)[2]	30 (22–39)
Complications of therapy (UPDRS part IV)[3]	4 (2–7)
Self-rated general health (RAND-36)[1]	3 (3-4)
ADL dependency (ADL staircase)[4]	1 (0–3)
Perceived functional independence[5]	9 (7–10)
Walking difficulties in daily life (Generic Walk-12)[6]	14 (7–24)
Depressive symptoms (Geriatric Depression Scale)[7]	2 (1–4)
Cognitive function (Montreal Cognitive Assessment)[8]	26 (22–28)

UPDRS = Unified Parkinson's Disease Rating Scale; ADL = activities of daily living; possible score ranges and directions: [1]1–5, higher = worse; [2]0–108, higher = worse; [3]0–23, higher = worse; [4]0–9, higher = worse; [5]0–10, higher = better; [6]0–42, higher = worse; [7]0–15, higher = worse; [8]0–30, higher = better.

assessed using the H&Y (stages I–V, higher = worse) [17]. In addition, the participants rated their overall PD severity as either mild, moderate, or severe (scored 1–3, resp.). Assessments at the home visits were conducted at a time point when the participant reported feeling at their best.

2.3. Data Analyses. Statistical analyses were performed in IBM SPSS Statistics, version 24. Analyses included data completeness, targeting, and external construct validity of the PADLS. Two-tailed p values were used and the level of statistical significance was set to $p < 0.05$.

2.3.1. Data Completeness. Data completeness refers to the degree to which a rating scale is completed [33, 34] and was calculated as the percentage of participants who responded to the PADLS. A maximum of 10% missing data has been suggested as a limit for acceptable data completeness [35].

2.3.2. Targeting. Targeting refers to the scale's ability to mirror the levels of the targeted variable (e.g., ADL disability) in the study sample [33]. The mean score of a well-targeted rating scale should be close to the scale's midpoint and scores should range the full span of possible scale scores [34]. Skewness should be less than ±1 [34] and floor and ceiling effects should not exceed 15–20% [33, 34, 36]. That is, less than 15–20% of the study sample should score 1 or 5 on the PADLS, respectively.

2.3.3. External Construct Validity. External construct validity of a rating scale is supported when scores are more strongly associated with related constructs and more weakly associated with nonrelated constructs [37]. In this study, associations between PADLS and other scores were explored by Spearman's correlation coefficients (r_s). The hypotheses were based on clinical reasoning and previous studies regarding associations between ADL and other variables [4–10, 16]. The associations (r_s) between PADLS and walking difficulties in daily life, perceived functional independence, self-rated PD severity, ADL dependency, motor symptoms, and complications of PD therapy were anticipated to be >0.5 [4–7, 9, 10, 16]. The associations between PADLS and depressive symptoms as well as general health were anticipated to be around 0.5 [5, 7, 8, 10]. The associations between PADLS and PD duration, age, cognitive function, and frequency of social activities were anticipated to be <0.5 [5, 7, 8, 10, 16].

Kruskal-Wallis and Mann–Whitney U tests were used to explore whether PADLS scores differed between H&Y stages. H&Y stages IV and V were merged due to few participants in H&Y stage V ($n = 6$).

3. Results

All but one participant responded to the PADLS, resulting in 99.6% data completeness. The score distribution is presented in Table 2. The mean score was 2.1 and scale scores ranged the full span (i.e., 1–5). Fifty-four participants chose the lowest ("best") response option (22% floor effect) whereas six participants chose the highest ("worst") response option (2% ceiling effect).

PADLS scores correlated >0.5 with walking difficulties in daily life, perceived functional independence, self-rated PD severity, and ADL dependency. The associations between PADLS scores and other studied variables were weaker (Table 3). The Kruskal-Wallis test showed that PADLS scores differed across H&Y stages ($p < 0.001$). Specifically, those in H&Y stages IV and V had higher PADLS scores than those in H&Y stage III (Mann–Whitney U test, $p < 0.001$), whereas there were no significant differences between the other H&Y stages (Table 4).

TABLE 2: Score distribution of the Parkinson's disease Activities of Daily Living Scale (PADLS).

PADLS response options (abbreviated)	n (%)[1]
(1) No difficulties with day-to-day activities	54 (22)
(2) Mild difficulties with day-to-day activities	130 (52)
(3) Moderate difficulties with day-to-day activities	49 (20)
(4) High levels of difficulties with day-to-day activities	11 (4)
(5) Extreme difficulties with day-to-day activities	6 (2)
Mean score (SD)	2.1 (0.9)
Median (first-third quartile)	2 (2-3)
Skewness (SE)	0.94 (0.15)
Floor/ceiling effect	21.6%/2.4%

[1] One person did not respond to the PADLS, resulting in $n = 250$.

4. Discussion

This study confirmed that the PADLS has satisfactory psychometric properties for use in the PD population. The PADLS revealed excellent data completeness; only one participant left the form blank. This indicates that the scale is easy to understand and perceived as relevant [38] by people with PD. The finding probably reflects the single-item nature of the scale, which might favor data completeness. Targeting was generally acceptable, with small ceiling effects. However, floor effects were above the recommended level [33, 34, 36]. Small floor and ceiling effects are desirable in order to enable separation of people and detect changes [33]. More than one-fifth scored the lowest possible and reported no difficulties with day-to-day activities. This floor effect may purely mirror the PD severity of the present sample. That is, 85 participants self-rated their PD as mild and 50 were classified as H&Y stage I. With such a high prevalence of mild PD severity it is not surprising that also ADL disabilities were rated as low or nonexisting. On the other hand, a previous study [1] reported that restrictions in ADL are often seen early during the disease. Already at their first visit to a neurological centre, those later diagnosed with PD had more ADL disabilities than healthy age-matched controls [1]. Although the PADLS showed generally satisfactory psychometric properties, its single-item nature makes it a coarse indicator unsuitable as an outcome measure due to the uncertainty associated with such scores. Notably, floor effects indicate that it is especially important to complement this scale with a more detailed ADL assessment for people with mild PD-symptoms.

External construct validity of the PADLS was generally supported by largely expected associations with other variables. However, the associations with motor symptoms and complications of PD therapy were lower than expected. In comparison to the present sample, the participant characteristics in previous studies [5, 6, 9, 10, 16] show no clear patterns that could explain our relatively weak association between, for example, ADL disability and motor symptoms. However, previous studies have shown large variations in association between motor symptoms and ADL disability, and our findings are within the range of previous studies [5–7, 9, 10, 16].

Indeed, varying results in previous studies imply a challenge when stating a priori hypotheses, which is essential for the exploration of a scale's external construct validity [37]. We do find our hypothesis of the association between ADL disabilities and motor symptoms reasonable, as several items in UPDRS part III (i.e., motor symptoms) do capture disabilities. It should be kept in mind that ADL is a complex phenomenon, affected by environmental characteristics and prerequisites as well as by the use of various assistive devices. Moreover, existing ADL assessments cover different activities, and the majority do not take individual or subgroup specific activity preferences and patterns into consideration. All considered, ADL rating scales take different aspects into account and include different activities, making the definition of a priori hypotheses a delicate matter.

Although PADLS scores increased with increasing H&Y stages, the differences across these stages were small. The finding that PADLS scores differed only between H&Y stage III versus stages IV and V is not surprising. That is, the definition of H&Y stage III states that "patients are still physically capable of leading independent lives" whereas stages IV-V define a "severely disabling" PD [17].

4.1. Limitations. Data completeness might have been affected by the study design. That is, our data collectors were instructed to screen all self-administered ratings at the subsequent home visit. In case of missing values, the data collectors were instructed to ask the participants to add responses. However, another psychometric study based on the same data collection did report missing values that were close to those collected in another sample not using the same procedure [39].

One could argue that using polychoric and polyserial correlation coefficients would have been a theoretically better choice than r_s when studying the external construct validity of the PADLS. This is since r_s and r tend to attenuate estimated correlations between ordinal data [40, 41], such as the PADLS. Since previous studies did not use polychoric or polyserial correlations [4–10, 16], we used methods similar to those used before in order to enhance comparability with previous studies. However, reanalyses using polychoric correlations yielded generally somewhat stronger coefficients, as expected (data available on request). In addition, this study does not cover all psychometric aspects. For example, test-retest reliability was not evaluated.

Our decision to use the ADL Staircase [26] and not the UPDRS part II [18] to study external construct validity in terms of ADL deserves a comment since the latter is commonly used in PD research. Given the complexity of the phenomenon at target (i.e., ADL), our ambition was to use data collected with an ADL rating scale based on conceptual and theoretical underpinnings. As such, ADL is not disease specific but a generic human phenomenon. Although UPDRS part II is recommended as a disability instrument [3], it contains items that are not conceptually related to the ADL construct [42]. Recently the Movement Disorder Society task force documented this as a major drawback as "the 13 items of the UPDRS-ADL do not all assess disability,

TABLE 3: Spearman correlations (r_s) between Parkinson's disease Activities of Daily Living Scale (PADLS) scores and other variables.

Variable	r_s	p value
Walking difficulties in daily life (Generic Walk-12)	0.66	<0.001
Perceived functional independence	−0.62	<0.001
Parkinson severity (self-rated)	0.59	<0.001
ADL dependency (ADL staircase)	0.54	<0.001
Depressive symptoms (Geriatric Depression Scale)	0.40	<0.001
Motor symptoms (UPDRS part III)	0.39	<0.001
Self-rated general health (RAND-36)	0.38	<0.001
Parkinson duration	0.33	<0.001
Complications of therapy (UPDRS part IV)	0.29	<0.001
Age	0.23	<0.001
Cognitive function (Montreal Cognitive Assessment)	−0.19	0.002
Frequency of social activities: visits family	−0.10	0.104
Frequency of social activities: visits friends	−0.06	0.332
Frequency of social activities: receives visits from family or friends	0.02	0.774

Higher scores are worse for all variables, except for perceived functional independence and cognitive function (higher = better) and frequency of social activities (higher = more social activities). This implies that more, for example, walking difficulties and less, for example, functional independence are associated with more ADL disability (positive and negative correlation coefficients, resp.); ADL = activities of daily living; UPDRS = Unified Parkinson's Disease Rating Scale; n = 243–250, depending on missing data.

TABLE 4: Descriptive data of Parkinson's disease Activities of Daily Living Scale (PADLS) scores across Hoehn & Yahr stages.

Hoehn & Yahr		PADLS, median (first-third quartile)	Need help from others in daily activities, n (%)[1]
Stage	n (%)		
I	50 (20)	2 (1-2)	5 (10%)
II	72 (29)	2 (1-2)	11 (15%)
III	67 (27)	2 (2-2)	12 (18%)
IV-V	61 (24)	3 (2–3.5)	38 (62%)

[1]PADLS dichotomized: those who scored >2 were classified as needing help from others.

with 7 of 13 assessing impairments, not functional status (speech, salivation, swallowing, falling, freezing, tremor, and sensory complaints)" [3]. While we consider choosing the ADL Staircase a methodological strength, it should be kept in mind that the comparability with PD studies that used UPDRS part II is limited.

It needs to be emphasized that the PADLS is a single-item rating scale and as such, it only gives a rough, global estimate of a person's ADL disabilities. Still, it should be noted that although the abbreviated response categories are phrased, for example, "mild difficulties in day-to-day activities," the PADLS captures both perceived difficulties, dependence on others and on assistive devices during ADL performance. Moreover, it includes both personal and instrumental ADL. As such, the PADLS can be useful in clinical practice as well as in research for purposes of providing a crude categorization of levels of ADL disabilities. However, a more comprehensive rating scale is needed if a more thorough ADL assessment is warranted, and especially so for those with less severe ADL

disabilities. This is in agreement with recommendations from the developers of the PADLS, who stated that the scale is not suitable for use in isolation but should be considered a complement to existing scales [10].

5. Conclusions

We found the self-reported, single-item rating scale PADLS to yield scores with excellent data completeness, acceptable targeting, and external construct validity. The PADLS seems to be well suited for providing a rough indicator of ADL disability in people with PD. As psychometric testing is a continuous process, further studies focusing on additional aspects, such as responsiveness, minimal important difference, and response category functioning, are warranted.

Acknowledgments

The authors thank the participants for their cooperation, registered nurses Jan Reimer, Susanne Lindskov, and Eva Aronsson for selection of participants, and registered occupational therapists Maya Kylén and Malin Mejstad for data collection. The "Home and Health in People Ageing with PD" project was funded by numerous sources in Sweden: the Strategic Research Area in Neuroscience at Lund University (MultiPark), the Swedish Research Council, the Ribbingska Foundation, the Greta and Johan Kock Foundation, the Swedish Association of Persons with Neurological Disabilities (NHR), the Norrbacka-Eugenia Foundation, NEURO Sweden, and the Swedish Parkinson Foundation. The study was conducted within the context of Centre for Ageing and

Supportive Environments (CASE) at Lund University, Sweden, financed by the Swedish Research Council for Health, Working Life and Welfare (Forte). Peter Hagell was supported by Kristianstad University, Kristianstad, Sweden.

References

[1] G.-M. Hariz and L. Forsgren, "Activities of daily living and quality of life in persons with newly diagnosed Parkinson's disease according to subtype of disease, and in comparison to healthy controls," *Acta Neurologica Scandinavica*, vol. 123, no. 1, pp. 20–27, 2011.

[2] B. J. Lawrence, N. Gasson, R. Kane, R. S. Bucks, and A. M. Loftus, "Activities of daily living, depression, and quality of life in Parkinson's disease," *PLoS ONE*, vol. 9, no. 7, Article ID e102294, 2014.

[3] L. M. Shulman, M. Armstrong, T. Ellis et al., "Disability Rating Scales in Parkinson's Disease: Critique and Recommendations," *Movement Disorders*, vol. 31, no. 10, pp. 1455–1465, 2016.

[4] P. Martinez-Martin et al., "A new clinical tool for gait evaluation in Parkinson's disease," *Clinical Neuropharmacology*, vol. 20, no. 3, pp. 183–194, 1997.

[5] L. M. Rubenstein et al., "The usefulness of the functional status questionnaire and medical outcomes study short form in parkinson's disease research," *Quality of Life Research*, vol. 7, no. 4, pp. 279–290, 1998.

[6] N. Weisscher, B. Post, R. J. De Haan, C. A. W. Glas, J. D. Speelman, and M. Vermeulen, "The AMC Linear Disability Score in patients with newly diagnosed Parkinson disease," *Neurology*, vol. 69, no. 23, pp. 2155–2161, 2007.

[7] T. Gazibara, I. Stankovic, A. Tomic et al., "Validation and cross-cultural adaptation of the Self-Assessment Disability Scale in patients with Parkinson's disease in Serbia," *Journal of Neurology*, vol. 260, no. 8, pp. 1970–1977, 2013.

[8] A. E. Lang, S. Eberly, C. G. Goetz et al., "Movement disorder society unified Parkinson disease rating scale experiences in daily living: Longitudinal changes and correlation with other assessments," *Movement Disorders*, vol. 28, no. 14, pp. 1980–1986, 2013.

[9] E. Martignoni, F. Franchignoni, C. Pasetti, G. Ferriero, and D. Picco, "Psychometric properties of the Unified Parkinson's Disease Rating Scale and of the Short Parkinson's Evaluation Scale," *Neurological Sciences*, vol. 24, no. 3, pp. 190-191, 2003.

[10] J. P. Hobson, N. I. Edwards, and R. J. Meara, "The Parkinson's Disease Activities of Daily Living Scale: a new simple and brief subjective measure of disability in Parkinson's disease," *Clinical Rehabilitation*, vol. 15, no. 3, pp. 241–246, 2001.

[11] K. Rosqvist, P. Hagell, P. Odin, H. Ekström, S. Iwarsson, and M. H. Nilsson, "Factors associated with life satisfaction in Parkinson's disease," *Acta Neurologica Scandinavica*, vol. 136, no. 1, pp. 64–71, 2017.

[12] C. A. Brown, E. M. Cheng, R. D. Hays, S. D. Vassar, and B. G. Vickrey, "SF-36 includes less Parkinson Disease (PD)-targeted content but is more responsive to change than two PD-targeted health-related quality of life measures," *Quality of Life Research*, vol. 18, no. 9, pp. 1219–1237, 2009.

[13] S. B. Jonasson, M. H. Nilsson, and J. Lexell, "Psychometric properties of four fear of falling rating scales in people with Parkinson's disease," *BMC Geriatrics*, vol. 14, no. 1, article no. 66, 2014.

[14] Y. Olsson, L. Clarén, A. Alvariza, K. Årestedt, and P. Hagell, "Health and social service access among family caregivers of people with Parkinson's disease," *Journal of Parkinson's Disease*, vol. 6, no. 3, pp. 581–587, 2016.

[15] B. Lindholm, P. Hagell, O. Hansson, and M. H. Nilsson, "Prediction of falls and/or near falls in people with mild Parkinson's disease," *PLoS ONE*, vol. 10, no. 1, Article ID e0117018, 2015.

[16] P. Hagell, G. M. Hariz, and M. H. Nilsson, "P1.131 The Parkinson's disease activities of daily living scale (PADLS) revisited," *Parkinsonism & Related Disorders*, vol. 15, p. S62, 2009.

[17] M. M. Hoehn and M. D. Yahr, "Parkinsonism: onset, progression and mortality.," *Neurology*, vol. 17, no. 5, pp. 427–442, 1967.

[18] S. Fahn, R. L. Elton, and Members of the UPDRS Development Committee, "Unified Parkinson's Disease Rating Scale," in *Recent developments in Parkinson's disease*, S. Fahn, Ed., vol. 2, pp. 153–163, MacMillan Healthcare Information, Florham Park, NJ, USA, 293-304, 1987.

[19] M. H. Nilsson and S. Iwarsson, "Home and health in people ageing with Parkinson's disease: Study protocol for a prospective longitudinal cohort survey study," *BMC Neurology*, vol. 13, article no. 142, 2013.

[20] M. Kader, S. Ullén, S. Iwarsson, P. Odin, and M. H. Nilsson, "Factors contributing to perceived walking difficulties in people with Parkinson's disease," *Journal of Parkinson's Disease*, vol. 7, no. 2, pp. 397–407, 2017.

[21] B. Lindholm, P. Hagell, O. Hansson, and M. H. Nilsson, "Factors associated with fear of falling in people with Parkinson's disease," *BMC Neurology*, vol. 14, no. 1, article no. 19, 2014.

[22] R. D. Hays, C. D. Sherbourne, and R. M. Mazel, "The RAND 36-Item Health Survey 1.0," *Health Economics*, vol. 2, no. 3, pp. 217–227, 1993.

[23] S. Bladh, M. H. Nilsson, G.-M. Hariz, A. Westergren, J. Hobart, and P. Hagell, "Psychometric performance of a generic walking scale (Walk-12G) in multiple sclerosis and Parkinson's disease," *Journal of Neurology*, vol. 259, no. 4, pp. 729–738, 2012.

[24] J. I. Sheikh and J. A. Yesavage, "Geriatric Depression Scale (GDS): recent evidence and development of a shorter version," *Clinical Gerontologist*, vol. 5, no. 1-2, pp. 165–173, 1986.

[25] W. Oswald, *Neuropsychological Aging Inventory (NAI) manual*, Hogrefe & Huber Publishing, Toronto, Canada, 2005.

[26] U. Sonn and K. Hulter Asberg, "Assessment of activities of daily living in the elderly. A study of a population of 76-year-olds in Gothenburg, Sweden," *Scandinavian Journal of Rehabilitation Medicine*, vol. 23, no. 4, pp. 193–202, 1991.

[27] S. Katz, A. B. Ford, R. W. Moskowitz, B. A. Jackson, and M. W. Jaffe, "Studies of illness in the aged. the index of adl: a standardized measure of biological and psychosocial function," *Journal of the American Medical Association*, vol. 185, pp. 914–919, 1963.

[28] W. D. Spector, S. Katz, J. B. Murphy, and J. P. Fulton, "The hierarchical relationship between activities of daily living and instrumental activities of daily living," *Journal of Chronic Diseases*, vol. 40, no. 6, pp. 481–489, 1987.

[29] U. Jakobsson, "The ADL-staircase: Further validation," *International Journal of Rehabilitation Research*, vol. 31, no. 1, pp. 85–88, 2008.

[30] S. Iwarsson, "Environmental influences on the cumulative structure of instrumental ADL: An example in osteoporosis patients in a Swedish rural district," *Clinical Rehabilitation*, vol. 12, no. 3, pp. 221–227, 1998.

[31] S. Iwarsson, V. Horstmann, F. Oswald, and H.-W. Wahl, "Socio-cultural care, service context, and IADL dependence among very old European women," *Topics in Geriatric Rehabilitation*, vol. 26, no. 1, pp. 32–45, 2010.

[32] Z. S. Nasreddine, N. A. Phillips, V. Bédirian et al., "The Montreal Cognitive Assessment, MoCA: a brief screening tool for mild cognitive impairment," *Journal of the American Geriatrics Society*, vol. 53, no. 4, pp. 695–699, 2005.

[33] J. Hobart and S. Cano, "Improving the evaluation of therapeutic interventions in multiple sclerosis: The role of new psychometric methods," *Health Technology Assessment*, vol. 13, no. 12, 2009.

[34] J. Hobart, A. Riazi, D. Lamping, R. Fitzpatrick, and A. Thompson, "Improving the evaluation of therapeutic interventions in multiple sclerosis: development of a patient-based measure of outcome," *Health Technology Assessment*, vol. 8, no. 9, 2004.

[35] R. N. Saris-Baglama et al., *SF Health Outcomes Scoring Software User's Guide*, Quality Metric Inc, 2004.

[36] C. A. McHorney and A. R. Tarlov, "Individual-patient monitoring in clinical practice: are available health status surveys adequate?" *Quality of Life Research*, vol. 4, no. 4, pp. 293–307, 1995.

[37] D. L. Streiner, G. R. Norman, and J. Cairney, *Health Measurement Scales. A Practical Guide to Their Development and Use*, Oxford University Press, New York, NY, USA, 5th edition, 2015.

[38] H. C. W. de Vet, "Measurement in medicine : a practical guide," in *Practical guides to biostatistics and epidemiology*, p. 338, Cambridge University Press, Cambridge, UK, 2011.

[39] M. H. Nilsson, P. Hagell, and S. Iwarsson, "Psychometric properties of the General Self-Efficacy Scale in Parkinson's disease," *Acta Neurologica Scandinavica*, vol. 132, no. 2, pp. 89–96, 2015.

[40] E. Babakus and C. E. Ferguson, "On choosing the appropriate measure of association when analyzing rating scale data," *Journal of the Academy of Marketing Science*, vol. 16, no. 1, pp. 95–102, 1988.

[41] J. B. Carroll, "The nature of the data, or how to choose a correlation coefficient," *Psychometrika*, vol. 26, no. 4, pp. 347–372, 1961.

[42] G.-M. Hariz, M. Lindberg, M. I. Hariz, and A. T. Bergenheim, "Does the ADL part of the Unified Parkinson's Disease Rating Scale measure ADL? An evaluation in patients after pallidotomy and thalamic deep brain stimulation," *Movement Disorders*, vol. 18, no. 4, pp. 373–381, 2003.

3

A Meta-Analysis of *GBA*-Related Clinical Symptoms in Parkinson's Disease

Yuan Zhang,[1] Li Shu,[1] Xun Zhou,[1] Hongxu Pan,[1] Qian Xu,[1,2,3] Jifeng Guo,[1,2,3,4,5,6] Beisha Tang,[1,2,3,4,5,6,7,8] and Qiying Sun[2,3,7]

[1]Department of Neurology, Xiangya Hospital, Central South University, Changsha, Hunan 410008, China
[2]National Clinical Research Center for Geriatric Disorders, Changsha, Hunan 410078, China
[3]Key Laboratory of Hunan Province in Neurodegenerative Disorders, Central South University, Changsha, Hunan 410008, China
[4]Parkinson's Disease Center of Beijing Institute for Brain Disorders, Beijing 100069, China
[5]Collaborative Innovation Center for Brain Science, Shanghai 200032, China
[6]Collaborative Innovation Center for Genetics and Development, Shanghai 200438, China
[7]Department of Geriatrics, Xiangya Hospital, Central South University, Changsha, Hunan 410008, China
[8]Center for Medical Genetics, School of Life Sciences, Central South University, Changsha, Hunan 410008, China

Correspondence should be addressed to Qiying Sun; sunqiying2015@163.com

Academic Editor: Jan Aasly

Background. GBA gene had been proved to be a crucial gene to the risk of PD. Numerous studies had discussed about the unique clinical characteristics of PD patients with *GBA* carriers (*GBA* + PD). However, there was lack of updated comprehensive analysis on the topic. In order to clarify the association between *GBA* variants and the clinical phenotypes of PD, we conducted this comprehensive meta-analysis. *Method.* Medline, Embase, and Cochrane were used to perform the searching. Strict selection criteria were followed in screening for new published articles or data. Revman 5.3 software was applied to perform the total statistical analysis, and funnel plots in the software were used to assess the publication biases. *Results.* A total of 26 articles including 931 *GBA* + PD and 14861 *GBA* noncarriers of PD (*GBA* − PD) were involved in the final meta-analysis, and 14 of them were either newly added publications or related data newly analyzed compared with the version published in 2015. Then, a series of symptoms containing depression, orthostatic hypotension, motor fluctuation, wearing-off, and freezing were newly analyzed due to more articles eligible. Besides, clinical features like family history, AAO, UPDRS-III, H-Y, and dementia previously analyzed were updated with new data added. Significant statistical differences were found in wearing-off, family history, AAO, UPDRS-III, and dementia (OR: 1.14, 1.65; MD: −3.61, 2.17; OR: 2.44; *p*: 0.03, <0.00001, <0.00001, 0.003, and <0.00001). Depression was slightly associated with *GBA* + PD (OR: 1.47; *p*: 0.04). Clinical symptoms such as H-Y, orthostatic hypotension, motor fluctuation, and freezing did not feature *GBA* + PD. *Conclusion.* Our results demonstrated that there were unique clinical features in *GBA* + PD which can help the management of the whole duration of PD patients.

1. Introduction

Parkinson's disease (PD), a common neurodegenerative disease, was featured by motor symptoms containing bradykinesia, resting tremor, rigidity, and postural instability. Nonmotor symptoms (NMS) such as cognitive impairment, olfactory dysfunction, and depression were also common in PD patients. Nowadays, the pathogenesis of PD remains elusive. Genetic factors have been demonstrated to cause PD and, to some extent, participate in modifying the phenotypes of PD [1–3].

GBA gene, encoding the lysosomal enzyme glucocerebrosidase (GCase), is the causative gene of Gaucher's disease (GD) [4]. *GBA* variants can increase the risk of PD up to 10 times, which was the strongest genetic factor contributing to the risk of PD [5, 6]. Nowadays, more than 300 mutations in *GBA* were reported [7–9]. The latest comprehensive meta-analysis had proved the importance of *GBA* variants such as

L444P, N370S, R120W, IVS2 + 1G > A, H255Q, D409H, RecNciI, E326K, and T369M to PD risks [10].

In addition to the contribution of *GBA* to the development of PD, studies have reported PD patients with *GBA* carriers (*GBA* + PD) manifested special clinical features compared to idiopathic PD. In the year of 2015, our group conducted a study combining the results of our new original research and meta-analysis on the association between *GBA* variants and the clinical features of PD [11]. The data indicated that *GBA* + PD are more inclined to onset at early age, initially with bradykinesia, have family history and develop to dementia when compared with *GBA* noncarriers of PD patients (*GBA* − PD). However, with more published articles, there were new clinical features such as depression, motor complications, and freezing gaits focused by researchers which will help draw a full picture of clinical features of *GBA* + PD or *GBA* − PD with complete motor symptoms (MSs) and NMSs [12–14]. Combined with newly published articles and newly involved data of previous articles, we performed a comprehensive analysis on clinical features of *GBA* + PD.

2. Methods

2.1. Selection Criteria. We conducted this meta-analysis based on PICOS (participants, interventions, controls, outcomes, and studies) rules.

2.1.1. Participants. All PD patients being diagnosed with widely accepted diagnostic criteria [15].

2.1.2. Interventions. DNAs were expanded by PCR-based methods or other accepted methods and analyzed by Sanger sequencing or other regular methods.

2.1.3. Controls. Controls were PD patients without carrying *GBA* variants.

2.1.4. Outcomes. A specific clinical feature of *GBA* carriers and noncarriers in PD patients were reported.

2.1.5. Study Types. Original studies such as case-only study, cohort study, or case-control study were conducted.

2.2. Literature Search. We searched articles in English using Medline database in Pubmed, Embase database in Ovid, and the Cochrane database. Key words were "GBA," "gluco-cerebrosidase," "Parkinso*" and "PD." The latest search was done on March 1, 2018. Overlapping articles from different databases were excluded. Two researchers (Yuan Zhang and Li Shu) performed the search independently. In case of disagreements, a third researcher (Qiying Sun) was consulted to arrive at a consensus.

2.3. Data Extraction. Comprehensive data were retrieved including the following items: publication year, first author,

ethnicity, country, number of *GBA* + PD and *GBA* − PD, and corresponding clinical information. Two researchers did the extraction independently. Another author was asked to participate in the process when confronted with problems. The quality of all case-control studies were assessed according to the Newcastle-Ottawa Scale (NOS) [16].

2.4. Statistical Analysis. The total statistical analysis was performed in Revman 5.3 software. The final results were demonstrated by pooled odds ratio (OR) or mean difference (MD) and 95% CI (confidence interval). When the data were dichotomous variables, pooled odds ratio (OR) was calculated, otherwise when the data were continuous outcomes, pooled mean difference (MD) was expressed. Heterogeneity was reflected by Q statistic (p value) and I^2 statistic. $p > 0.1$, $I^2 \leq 50\%$ indicated that the heterogeneity was not significant and suggested a fixed model (FM) be applied. Otherwise, a random model (RM) was used. The shape of funnel plot was used to reflect publication biases. Sensitivity analysis was performed by removing each original study sequentially to test the stability of the results.

3. Results

The complete information of searching process is shown in the flowchart (Figure 1), and the information of all included studies is demonstrated in Table 1. A total of 26 articles including 931 *GBA* + PD and 14861 *GBA* − PD were involved in the final meta-analysis, and 14 of them, which contained 582 *GBA* + PD and 8217 *GBA* − PD, were either newly added publications or related data newly analyzed compared with the version published in 2015 [11]. Then, a series of symptoms containing depression, orthostatic hypotension, motor fluctuation, wearing-off, and freezing were newly analyzed due to more articles eligible. Besides, clinical features like family history, age at onset (AAO), Unified Parkinson's Disease Rating Scale Part III (UPDRS-III), Hoehn–Yahr (H-Y), and dementia previously analyzed were updated with new data added. Due to the importance of disease duration in clinical characteristics of disease, we first conducted comparison of disease duration between *GBA* + PD and *GBA* − PD. We found that there was no statistical difference between the two groups (MD: 0.17, p: 0.47) (Supplementary Table 1; Supplementary Figure 1).

For the five (depression, orthostatic hypotension, motor fluctuation, wearing-off, and freezing) newly involved clinical characteristics in this meta-analysis (Table 2, Supplementary Figure 1), they belonged to NMS and motor complications. As can be seen from Table 2, significant statistical difference was found in wearing-off (OR: 1.14; p: 0.03). Slightly statistical significance was found in depression of *GBA* + PD (OR: 1.47; p: 0.04). Clinical symptoms such as orthostatic hypotension, motor fluctuation, and freezing did not feature *GBA* + PD in this meta-analysis.

As to the five updated clinical features of *GBA* + PD with newly involved data (Table 2, Supplementary Figure 1), they were family history, AAO, UPDRS-III, H-Y, and dementia. From the tables, significant statistical differences were found

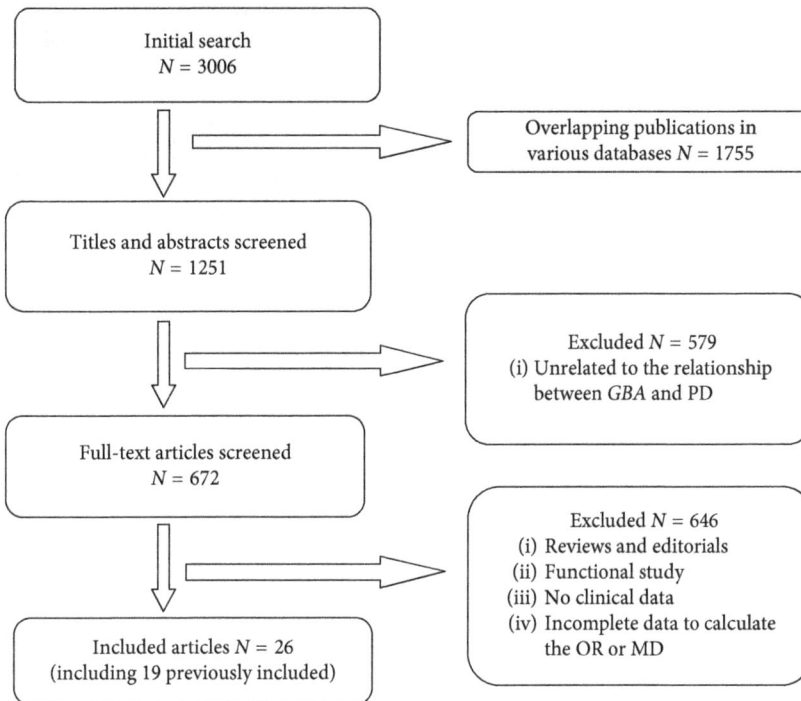

FIGURE 1: Flowchart illustrating the literature screening process.

in family history, AAO, UPDRS-III, and dementia (OR: 1.65; MD: −3.61, 2.17; OR: 2.44; *p*: <0.00001, <0.00001, 0.003, and <0.00001). We found a change in statistical differences in UPDRS-III scores from previous negative results, while we almost reached the same conclusion in analyzing family history, AAO, H-Y, and dementia.

All publications included were of high quality with the NOS scores above 7. According to the funnel plots (Supplementary Figure 2), the biases were rare. By removing articles one after another, the results of the remainder did not change significantly indicating that the results of our meta-analysis were stable.

4. Discussion

In our meta-analysis, we analyzed five new clinical features (depression, orthostatic hypotension, motor fluctuation, wearing-off, and freezing) and updated data of five previous analyzed clinical features (family history, AAO, UPDRS-III, H-Y, and dementia). We made the conclusion that GBA + PD patients had unique clinical features such as were more likely to have family history, earlier onset age, higher UPDRS-III scores, and develop dementia, depression, and wearing-off phenomena after adjusting disease duration.

Our meta-analysis about the demographic information of GBA + PD suggested that the carriers were more likely to have earlier age at onset with a mean of 3.6 years. Previous studies have shown that GBA + PD developed PD 1.7–6.0 years earlier than GBA − PD which were similar to our analysis [17]. Additionally, GBA + PD were more likely to have family history. These basic features of GBA carriers

will contribute to the targeted screening of the gene in researches.

As to other clinical features such as MSs and NMSs, our analysis demonstrated severe MSs reflected by higher UPDRS-III scores accompanied by motor complications like wearing-off phenomena and high possibilities to develop NMSs such as dementia and depression. Previous studies [18–20] have suggested deteriorative manifestations of GBA + PD such as higher UPDRS-III scores, easily presenting dementia, and motor complications. Since separating different subcategories of PD is crucial to better understand disease mechanisms, predict disease progression, or design clinical researches, recently, Fereshtehnejad et al. [21] reported that important clinical features and scales such as UPDRS I-III scores, NMSs-related scales such as Montreal Cognitive Assessment (MoCA) evaluating cognitive functions, and Epworth Sleepiness Scale (ESS) evaluation sleep disturbances were key factors defining clinical subtypes of PD. Our analysis found unique clinical features of GBA + PD which almost matched a diffuse malignant subtype in PD in the previous classifications which needed a more active treatment strategy for the deleterious prognosis.

The mechanism underlying GBA + PD prominent clinical features remains elusive. Some studies suggested that GBA mutations can cause dysfunctional GCase which finally led to α-synuclein aggregations in PD brains and in dopaminergic neurons [22]. As α-synuclein was vital pathological feature in PD brains, the promotion of GBA mutations to α-synuclein aggregations may explain the deleterious clinical features of GBA + PD. The dysfunctions in pathways outside classic basal ganglia may explain the NMS features of GBA + PD. The cortex dysfunction caused

TABLE 1: The characteristics of the related phenotypes data updated in all publications included.

Year, first author	NOS	Country	Groups	n	Family history	AAO	UPDRS-III	H-Y	Dementia	Depression	Orthostatic hypotension	Wearing-off	Motor fluctuation	Freezing
2017, Cilia et al. [25]*	8	Italy	GBA+PD	123	38	52.4 ± 10.2	33.5 ± 14.2	—	25 (93)	—	12 (65)	—	48 (82)	28 (92)
			GBA−PD	2641	446	57.4 ± 10.6	30.4 ± 13.7	—	240 (1254)	—	89 (840)	—	726 (168)	332 (1210)
2017, Davis et al. [26]*	7	American	GBA+PD	27	—	62.0 ± 9.0	31.8 ± 10.6	—	9	—	—	—	—	—
			GBA−PD	675	—	68.4 ± 8.6	27.5 ± 12.9	—	58	—	—	—	—	—
2016, Thaler et al. [27]*	7	Israel	GBA+PD	12	—	51.4 ± 10.7	28.8 ± 9.6	2.9 ± 0.6	—	—	—	—	—	—
			GBA−PD	12	—	58.7 ± 5.7	21.7 ± 6.5	2.1 ± 0.7	—	—	—	—	—	—
2016, Swan et al. [28]*	7	Israel	GBA+PD	31	—	57.0 ± 12.7	16.7 ± 8.7	2.3 ± 1.1	—	10	—	—	—	—
			GBA−PD	55	—	59.7 ± 11.4	20.4 ± 13.2	2.2 ± 0.9	—	7	—	—	—	—
2016, Dan et al. [29]*	8	China	GBA+PD	40	—	—	—	—	—	16	—	—	—	—
			GBA−PD	1007	—	—	—	—	—	191	—	—	—	—
2015, Gan-Or et al. [24]*	7	Israel	GBA+PD	19	—	—	—	—	—	—	—	—	—	—
			GBA−PD	101	—	—	—	—	—	—	—	—	—	—
2014, Brockmann et al. [22]*	7	Germany	GBA+PD	33	—	—	—	2.7 ± 0.7	—	—	—	—	—	—
			GBA−PD	26	—	—	—	2.5 ± 0.7	—	—	—	—	—	—
2014, Wang et al. [30]#	8	China	GBA+PD	49	—	—	—	—	—	28 (49)	9 (34)	11 (37)	5 (37)	—
			GBA−PD	1366	—	—	—	—	—	583 (1366)	221 (843)	169 (922)	90 (924)	—
2014, Malec-Litwinowicz et al. [31]#	7	Poland	GBA+PD	5	—	—	—	—	—	4	1	—	—	—
			GBA−PD	117	—	—	—	—	—	43	21	—	—	—
2014, Li et al. [32]#	7	Japan	GBA+PD	34	—	—	—	—	—	—	5	20	—	—
			GBA−PD	113	—	—	—	—	—	—	21	49	—	—
2014, Pulkes et al. [33]#	7	China, Thailand	GBA+PD	17	—	—	—	—	—	—	—	8	—	2
			GBA−PD	191	—	—	—	—	—	—	—	82	—	21
2013, Kumar et al. [34]#	7	Serbia	GBA+PD	21	—	—	—	—	—	—	—	—	—	0 (19)
			GBA−PD	339	—	—	—	—	—	—	—	—	—	8 (287)
2011, Lesage et al. [35]#	8	Europeans	GBA+PD	100	—	—	—	—	—	—	—	—	47 (76)	—
			GBA−PD	1291	—	—	—	—	—	—	—	—	532 (902)	—
2008, Gan-Or et al. [36]#	7	Israel	GBA+PD	71	—	—	—	—	—	6	—	—	—	—
			GBA−PD	283	—	—	—	—	—	28 (280)	—	—	—	—

Abbreviations: *publications newly updated; #publications previously included, and this table only exhibits the updated clinical data in the previous publications included; other clinical features were shown in the published manuscript [11]. PD, Parkinson's disease; GBA + PD, PD with GBA mutations; GBA − PD, PD without GBA mutations; AAO, age at onset; UPSRS-III, the Part III of Unified Parkinson Disease Rating Scale; H-Y, Hoehn–Yahr Rating Scale. AAO, UPDRS-III, and H-Y were presented as mean and standard deviation; others were shown as count data. n, total number of patients whose clinical information was available in each group.

TABLE 2: *GBA*-related phenotypes updated to our previous meta-analysis.

Phenotypes	Number of articles (total/updated)	Total number of GBA + PD	Total number of GBA − PD	OR or MD (95% CI) updated	p value	Previous OR or MD (95% CI)
Family history[*][a]	11/1	558	9330	**1.65 (1.34, 2.02)**	**<0.00001**	**1.5 (1.18, 1.91)**
AAO[*][b]	17/4	622	11079	**−3.61 (−5.04, −2.17)**	**<0.00001**	**−3.10 (−4.88, −1.32)**
UPDRS-III[*][b]	9/4	335	6100	**2.17 (0.72, 3.62)**	**0.003**	1.61 (−0.65, 3.87)
H-Y[*][b]	11/3	275	3863	**0.18 (0.00, 0.35)**	**0.05**	0.06 (−0.06, 0.17)
Dementia[*][a]	8/2	224	2696	**2.44 (1.79, 3.33)**	**<0.00001**	**3.21 (1.97, 5.24)**
Depression[#][a]	5	196	2825	**1.47 (1.02, 2.13)**	**0.04**	—
Orthostatic hypotension[#][a]	4	138	1913	1.24 (0.79, 1.94)	0.35	—
Motor fluctuation[#][a]	3	195	2894	0.9 (0.66, 1.24)	0.53	—
Wearing-off[#][a]	3	88	1226	**1.68 (1.05, 2.69)**	**0.03**	—
Freezing[#][a]	3	128	1688	1.14 (0.74, 1.77)	0.55	—

Abbreviations: [*]phenotypes updated new publications; [#]phenotypes newly analyzed. PD, Parkinson's disease; GBA + PD, PD with GBA mutations; GBA - PD, PD without GBA mutations; AAO, age at onset; UPSRS-III, the Part III of Unified Parkinson Disease Rating Scale; OR, odds ratio; MD, mean deviation; CI, confidence interval. Bold OR or MD, 95% CI, and p values reflected statistically significance results; a, dichotomous variables reflected by OR (95% CI); b, continuous outcomes reflected by MD (95% CI).

by global brain degeneration can damage functions of specific areas of brains and cause dementia or depression [23]. However, the number of researches was limited, and more mechanism studies were needed in the future.

Previously, our comprehensive meta-analysis in *GBA* variants had proved the importance of *GBA* mutations to PD risks [10]. To clarify the role of *GBA* in PD clinical features more clearly, we did this meta-analysis. Our results demonstrated a clear phenotype-genotype correlation in *GBA* + PD. Knowing the unique features of *GBA* carriers will contribute to predicting the clinical course of *GBA* + PD and be benefit for the symptomatic treatments. The results of this meta-analysis can do a contribution to the precise treatments based on genetic screening and help delay the progression of the disease with more active and effective therapeutic strategies.

To evaluate the meta-analysis more objectively, there were some limitations which cannot be ignored. First, possible biases were inevitable because the included original studies were cross-sectional and possible biases existed in pooled analyses of these studies such as age, gender, or other correlated clinical phenotypes. Further longitudinal designed studies will be needed to confirm these results. Second, because most of these researches included mixed different specific variants together as *GBA* + PD or *GBA* − PD (Supplementary Table 1), we could not separate each variant with corresponding phenotype data and were not able to conduct pooled analysis based on specific variants of *GBA*. With more original articles conducted based on specific variants of *GBA* and phenotype, we may be able to do a more accurate analysis to help understand the relationship between the genotype and phenotype better. Third, although our updated meta-analysis was a comprehensive pooled analysis of *GBA*-associated clinical presentations, for the limited articles, we failed to prove the relationship of other clinical features such as rapid eye movement sleep behavior disorder (RBD) or freezing

which were demonstrated to be associated with *GBA* previously [24].

5. Conclusion

Our meta-analysis suggested an increased risk of having family history, dementia, depression, wearing-off, earlier onset age, and higher UPDRS-III scores with *GBA* + PD. However, variants in *GBA* had no relationship with H-Y, orthostatic hypotension, motor fluctuations, and freezing in PD. More data were needed to do complete analysis on different variants and different ethnics of *GBA*, and the corresponding clinical manifestations which can help the management of the whole duration of PD patients.

Authors' Contributions

YZ and LS have contributed equally to this work and are co-first authors. YZ, LS, and QS chose the topic and designed the experiments. YZ, LS, and QS performed the analysis. YZ, LS, QS, and BT analyzed the data. YZ, LS, and QS wrote the manuscript. XZ, HP, QX, and JG performed data management and figure modification.

Acknowledgments

This work was supported by grants from the National Natural Science Foundation of China (Nos. 81430023 and 81401059), the National Key Plan for Scientific Research and Development of China (Nos. 2016YFC1306000 and 2017YFC0909100), and Hunan Provincial Innovation Foundation for Postgraduate (No. CX2017B066).

Supplementary Materials

Supplementary Figure 1: forest plots of the association between phenotypes and PD risks in total. (A)–(J) respond to the phenotypes of family history, age at onset, UPDRS-III, H-Y, dementia, depression, orthostatic hypotension, motor fluctuation, wearing-off, and freezing individually. Supplementary Figure 2: funnel plots of the association between phenotypes and PD risks in total. (A)–(J) respond to the phenotypes of family history, age at onset, UPDRS-III, H-Y, dementia, depression, orthostatic hypotension, motor fluctuation, wearing-off, and freezing individually. Supplementary Table 1: the GBA variants reported in included articles. Abbreviations: C, carriers of GBA variants; NC, noncarriers of GBA variants; NA, not available. (*Supplementary Materials*)

References

[1] L. V. Kalia and A. E. Lang, "Parkinson's disease," *The Lancet*, vol. 386, no. 9996, pp. 896–912, 2015.

[2] Y. Zhang, Q. Y. Sun, R. H. Yu, J.-f. Guo, B.-S. Tang, and X.-X. Yan, "The contribution of GIGYF2 to Parkinson's disease: a meta-analysis," *Neurological Sciences*, vol. 36, no. 11, pp. 2073–2079, 2015.

[3] K. Li, B. S. Tang, Z. H. Liu et al., "LRRK2 A419V variant is a risk factor for Parkinson's disease in Asian population," *Neurobiology of Aging*, vol. 36, no. 10, pp. 2908.e11–2908.e15, 2015.

[4] G. A. Grabowski, "Gaucher disease. enzymology, genetics, and treatment," *Advances in Human Genetics 21*, pp. 377–441, Springer Nature, Basel, Switzerland, 1993.

[5] Z. Yu, T. Wang, J. Xu et al., "Mutations in the glucocerebrosidase gene are responsible for Chinese patients with Parkinson's disease," *Journal of Human Genetics*, vol. 60, no. 2, pp. 85–90, 2015.

[6] A. Lwin, E. Orvisky, O. Goker-Alpan, M. E. LaMarca, and E. Sidransky, "Glucocerebrosidase mutations in subjects with parkinsonism," *Molecular Genetics and Metabolism*, vol. 81, no. 1, pp. 70–73, 2004.

[7] G. O'Regan, R. M. deSouza, R. Balestrino, and A. H. Schapira, "Glucocerebrosidase mutations in Parkinson disease," *Journal of Parkinson's Disease*, vol. 7, no. 3, pp. 411–422, 2017.

[8] K. Fan, B. S. Tang, Y. Q. Wang et al., "The GBA, DYRK1A and MS4A6A polymorphisms influence the age at onset of Chinese Parkinson patients," *Neuroscience Letters*, vol. 621, pp. 133–136, 2016.

[9] J. F. Guo, K. Li, R. L. Yu et al., "Polygenic determinants of Parkinson's disease in a Chinese population," *Neurobiology of Aging*, vol. 36, no. 4, pp. 1765.e1–1765.e6, 2015.

[10] Y. Zhang, L. Shu, Q. Sun et al., "Integrated genetic analysis of racial differences of common GBA variants in Parkinson's disease: a meta-analysis," *Frontiers in Molecular Neuroscience*, vol. 11, 2018.

[11] Y. Zhang, Q. Y. Sun, Y. W. Zhao et al., "Effect of GBA mutations on phenotype of Parkinson's disease: a study on Chinese population and a meta-analysis," *Parkinson's Disease*, vol. 2015, article 916971, 10 pages, 2015.

[12] J. Aharon-Peretz, H. Rosenbaum, and R. Gershoni-Baruch, "Mutations in the glucocerebrosidase gene and Parkinson's disease in Ashkenazi Jews," *New England Journal of Medicine*, vol. 351, no. 19, pp. 1972–1977, 2004.

[13] C. P. da Silva, M. A. G. de, P. H. Cabello Acero et al., "Clinical profiles associated with LRRK2 and GBA mutations in Brazilians with Parkinson's disease," *Journal of the Neurological Sciences*, vol. 381, pp. 160–164, 2017.

[14] R. Torok, D. Zadori, N. Torok et al., "An assessment of the frequency of mutations in the GBA and VPS35 genes in Hungarian patients with sporadic Parkinson's disease," *Neuroscience Letters*, vol. 610, pp. 135–138, 2016.

[15] A. J. Hughes, S. E. Daniel, L. Kilford, and A. J. Lees, "Accuracy of clinical diagnosis of idiopathic Parkinson's disease: a clinico-pathological study of 100 cases," *Journal of Neurology, Neurosurgery & Psychiatry*, vol. 55, no. 3, pp. 181–184, 1992.

[16] A. Stang, "Critical evaluation of the Newcastle-Ottawa scale for the assessment of the quality of nonrandomized studies in meta-analyses," *European Journal of Epidemiology*, vol. 25, no. 9, pp. 603–605, 2010.

[17] R. Asselta, V. Rimoldi, C. Siri et al., "Glucocerebrosidase mutations in primary parkinsonism," *Parkinsonism & Related Disorders*, vol. 20, no. 11, pp. 1215–1220, 2014.

[18] M. Beavan, A. McNeill, C. Proukakis et al., "Evolution of prodromal clinical markers of Parkinson disease in a GBA mutation-positive cohort," *JAMA Neurology*, vol. 72, no. 2, pp. 201–208, 2015.

[19] T. Oeda, A. Umemura, Y. Mori et al., "Impact of glucocerebrosidase mutations on motor and nonmotor complications in Parkinson's disease," *Neurobiology of Aging*, vol. 36, no. 12, pp. 3306–3313, 2015.

[20] B. Creese, E. Bell, I. Johar, P. Francis, C. Ballard, and D. Aarsland, "Glucocerebrosidase mutations and neuropsychiatric phenotypes in Parkinson's disease and lewy body dementias: review and meta-analyses," *American Journal of Medical Genetics Part B: Neuropsychiatric Genetics*, vol. 177, no. 2, pp. 232–241, 2018.

[21] S. M. Fereshtehnejad, Y. Zeighami, A. Dagher, and R. B. Postuma, "Clinical criteria for subtyping Parkinson's disease: biomarkers and longitudinal progression," *Brain*, vol. 140, no. 7, pp. 1959–1976, 2017.

[22] K. Brockmann, K. Srulijes, S. Pflederer et al., "GBA-associated Parkinson's disease: reduced survival and more rapid progression in a prospective longitudinal study," *Movement Disorders*, vol. 30, no. 3, pp. 407–411, 2015.

[23] M. Beavan and A. H. Schapira, "Glucocerebrosidase gene mutation and preclinical markers of Parkinson disease-reply," *JAMA Neurology*, vol. 72, no. 6, p. 724, 2015.

[24] Z. Gan-Or, A. Mirelman, R. B. Postuma et al., "GBA mutations are associated with rapid eye movement sleep behavior disorder," *Annals of Clinical and Translational Neurology*, vol. 2, no. 9, pp. 941–945, 2015.

[25] R. Cilia, S. Tunesi, G. Marotta et al., "Survival and dementia in GBA-associated Parkinson's disease: the mutation matters," *Annals of Neurology*, vol. 80, no. 5, pp. 662–673, 2016.

[26] M. Y. Davis, C. O. Johnson, J. B. Leverenz et al., "Association of GBA mutations and the E326K polymorphism with motor and cognitive progression in Parkinson disease," *JAMA Neurology*, vol. 73, no. 10, pp. 1217–1224, 2016.

[27] A. Thaler, T. Gurevich, A. Bar Shira et al., "A "dose" effect of mutations in the GBA gene on Parkinson's disease phenotype," *Parkinsonism & Related Disorders*, vol. 36, pp. 47–51, 2017.

[28] M. Swan, N. Doan, R. A. Ortega et al., "Neuropsychiatric characteristics of GBA-associated Parkinson disease," *Journal of the Neurological Sciences*, vol. 370, pp. 63–69, 2016.

[29] X. Dan, C. Wang, J. Zhang et al., "Association between common genetic risk variants and depression in Parkinson's

disease: A dPD study in Chinese," *Parkinsonism & Related Disorders*, vol. 33, pp. 122–126, 2016.

[30] C. Wang, Y. Cai, Z. Gu et al., "Clinical profiles of Parkinson's disease associated with common leucine-rich repeat kinase 2 and glucocerebrosidase genetic variants in Chinese individuals," *Neurobiology of Aging*, vol. 35, no. 3, pp. 725.e1–725.e6, 2014.

[31] M. Malec-Litwinowicz, M. Rudzinska, M. Szubiga, M. Michalski, T. Tomaszewski, and A. Szczudlik, "Cognitive impairment in carriers of glucocerebrosidase gene mutation in Parkinson disease patients," *Neurologia i Neurochirurgia Polska*, vol. 48, no. 4, pp. 258–261, 2014.

[32] Y. Li, T. Sekine, M. Funayama et al., "Clinicogenetic study of GBA mutations in patients with familial Parkinson's disease," *Neurobiology of Aging*, vol. 35, no. 4, pp. 935.e3–935.e8, 2014.

[33] T. Pulkes, L. Choubtum, S. Chitphuk et al., "Glucocerebrosidase mutations in Thai patients with Parkinson's dis-ease," *Parkinsonism & Related Disorders*, vol. 20, no. 9, pp. 986–991, 2014.

[34] K. R. Kumar, A. Ramirez, A. Gobel et al., "Glucocerebrosidase mutations in a Serbian Parkinson's disease population," *European Journal of Neurology*, vol. 20, no. 2, pp. 402–405, 2013.

[35] S. Lesage, M. Anheim, C. Condroyer et al., "Large-scale screening of the Gaucher's disease-related glucocerebrosidase gene in Europeans with Parkinson's disease," *Human Molecular Genetics*, vol. 20, no. 1, pp. 202–210, 2011.

[36] Z. Gan-Or, N. Giladi, U. Rozovski et al., "Genotype-phenotype correlations between GBA mutations and Parkinson disease risk and onset," *Neurology*, vol. 70, no. 24, pp. 2277–2283, 2008.

4

The Association between *LRRK2* G2385R and Phenotype of Parkinson's Disease in Asian Population: A Meta-Analysis of Comparative Studies

Wei Di[ID],[1,2] Zhiyong Zeng,[3] Jingyan Li,[2] Xiaoling Liu,[2] Minzhi Bo,[4] and Hua Lv[ID][2]

[1]Department of Neurology, Xiangya Hospital, Central South University, Changsha, Hunan 410008, China
[2]Department of Neurology, Shaanxi Provincial People's Hospital, Third Affiliated Hospital of Medical College, Xi'an Jiaotong University, Xi'an, Shaanxi 710068, China
[3]Pediatric Department, The Second People's Hospital of Longgang District, Shenzhen, Guangdong 518112, China
[4]Xi'an Medical College, Xi'an, Shaanxi 710068, China

Correspondence should be addressed to Hua Lv; lvh2113@126.com

Academic Editor: Cristine Alves da Costa

Numerous studies have investigated the relationship between the *LRRK2* G2385R variant and clinical characteristics in Parkinson's disease (PD), but the results have been inconsistent. This study investigated whether the *LRRK2* G2385R variant was associated with a unique clinical phenotype of PD in the Asian population, using a meta-analysis. The PubMed, Web of Science, EMBASE, CNKI, and WANFANG databases were searched until September 2017. The strict selection criteria and exclusion criteria were determined, and mean differences (MD) or odds ratios (OR) with 95% confidence intervals (CI) were used to assess the strength of associations. Statistical analyses and graphics were performed using Review Manager 5.3. Sixteen related case-control studies were included in the meta-analysis. The *LRRK2* G2385R carriers significantly more often presented a family history (OR: 1.98; 95% CI: 1.16–3.39; $P = 0.01$) and had a longer disease duration (MD = 0.47, 95% CI: 0.01–0.93, $P = 0.04$) and a higher MMSE score (MD = 1.02, 95% CI: 0.43–1.62 $P = 0.0007$) than *LRRK2* G2385R noncarriers. There were no significant differences in sex distribution, age at onset, initial symptoms, motor symptoms, depression, levodopa-equivalent dose, and related complications between *LRRK2* G2385R-carrier and *LRRK2* G2385R-noncarrier PD patients. Our results suggested that most of the clinical characteristics of PD patients with *LRRK2* G2385R mutations are similar to those of *LRRK2* G2385R noncarriers among Asian PD patients, except for the more common family history, relatively longer disease duration, and higher MMSE scores in the former group.

1. Introduction

Parkinson's disease (PD) is the second most common neurodegenerative disorder. PD is defined by the presence of bradykinesia and at least one of the following symptoms: muscular rigidity, rest tremor, or postural instability. It is characterized by the cardinal motor symptoms of resting tremor, rigidity, bradykinesia, and postural instability, and a variety of nonmotor symptoms, such as olfactory dysfunction, psychiatric disorders, autonomic disturbances, and cognitive decline, among others. Although the etiology of PD has not been fully elucidated, it is thought to be the result of the interaction between genetic and environmental factors [1].

A number of candidate genes involved in PD etiology have been identified. Among them, mutations in the leucine-rich repeat kinase 2 gene (*LRRK2*) have been consistently reported to be the most frequent known cause of both sporadic and familial PD [2]. In particular, the G2385R polymorphism in *LRRK2* is an important genetic risk factor for PD in Asian individuals, as evidenced by various independent studies.

In recent years, genotype-phenotype correlation studies have suggested that PD patients with the *LRRK2* G2385R variant may exhibit some unique clinical characteristics, although some results were contradictory. Available studies have found that *LRRK2* G2385R carriers had a higher frequency of family history [3], longer disease duration [4], a lower age at onset [5], a higher proportion of postural instability and gait disorder (PIGD) phenotype [6], and a higher Mini-Mental State Examination (MMSE) score than PD patients who do not carry the *LRRK2* G2385R [6]. Moreover, a higher levodopa-equivalent dose (LED) and a higher proportion of levodopa-induced complications, including motor fluctuations and dyskinesia, were also observed in PD patients with the *LRRK2* G2385R variant in some studies [6, 7]. However, several other findings indicated that neither demographic data nor clinical presentation differed significantly between *LRRK2* G2385R carriers and noncarriers [8–10].

Taken together, there is no consensus about the relationship between *LRRK2* G2385R and clinical manifestations of PD patients. Here, we performed a meta-analysis to investigate whether *LRRK2* G2385R was associated with the clinical presentation of PD.

2. Methods

The literature search strategies, inclusion and exclusion criteria, outcome measurements, and methods of statistical analysis were completed according to the Preferred Reporting Items for Systematic Reviews and Meta-analysis and Meta-analysis of Observational Studies in Epidemiology recommendations for study reporting [11–13]. All analyses were based on previously published studies; thus, ethical approval and patient consent were not required.

2.1. Literature Search Strategy. A literature search was performed for publications up to September 2017 without restriction to regions, publication types, or languages. The primary sources were the electronic databases of PubMed, Web of Science, EMBASE, CNKI, and WANFANG. The following terms and their combinations were searched in [All Fields]: Parkinson disease, Parkinson's disease, Parkinson*, LRRK2 G2385R, LRRK2 Gly2385Arg, LRRK2 c.7153G>A. The reference lists of the included studies were screened to find further relevant studies.

2.2. Inclusion and Exclusion Criteria. Studies were selected when they met all the following criteria and the following studies were included if they met any of the following criteria: (1) observational studies, such as case-control studies and cohort studies; (2) comparative studies, which had to include an *LRRK2* G2385R-carrier PD group and an *LRRK2* G2385R-noncarrier PD group; (3) studies of association between specific clinical features (motor symptoms and nonmotor symptoms) and the *LRRK2* G2385R mutation; and (4) the diagnosis of PD had to be made according to the United Kingdom Parkinson Disease Society Brain Bank criteria. The following studies were excluded: (1) review articles, case reports, editorials; (2) duplicated reports (when multiple reports studying the same participants were published, the latest or most complete report was included); (3) studies with incomplete data, which included studies that did not compare *LRRK2* G2385R-carrier and *LRRK2*

G2385R-noncarrier PD patients; and (4) functional studies, such as animal experiments and cell experiments studies.

2.3. Data Extraction and Outcomes of Interest. Data from the included studies were extracted and summarized independently by two authors (Wei Di and Zhi-yong Zeng). Any disagreements were resolved by the senior authors (Jing-yan Li and Hua Lv). The primary outcomes were the comparison of clinical characteristics including motor symptoms and nonmotor symptoms in the two study groups (*LRRK2* G2385R carriers and noncarriers).

2.4. Quality Assessment and Statistical Analysis. The quality of selected studies was evaluated using the Newcastle–Ottawa Quality Assessment Scale (NOS) [14], which included three factors: patient selection, comparability of the study groups, and assessment of outcome. A score of 0–9 was allocated to each study. Studies that achieved six or more points were considered to be of high quality. The assessments were conducted by two authors (Wei Di and Zhi-yong Zeng).

All statistical analyses and graphics were generated using Review Manager 5.3 (Cochrane Collaboration, Oxford, England). The weighted mean difference (MD) and odds ratios (OR) were used to compare continuous and dichotomous variables, respectively. All results were reported with 95% confidence intervals (CIs). Statistical heterogeneity between studies was assessed using the chi-square test with significance set at $P \leq 0.10$, and heterogeneity was quantified using the I^2 statistic. The random effect model was used if there was heterogeneity between studies; alternatively, the fixed effect model was used [15]. Z tests were conducted to assess the association between the *LRRK2* G2385R variant and clinical characteristics. *P* values < 0.05 indicated statistically significant differences. Sensitivity analysis was performed in each comparison. Funnel plot analyses were used to screen for potential publication bias.

3. Results

3.1. Characteristics of Eligible Studies. A total of 359 studies were identified by searching in PubMed, Web of Science, EMBASE, CNKI, and WANFANG electronic databases. Sixteen eligible studies were included in the final statistical analysis [3–10, 16–23]. The detailed flow chart of study selection and reasons for exclusion are shown in Figure 1. All publications were full-text articles. Agreement between the two reviewers was 97% for study selection and 94% for quality assessment of trials. The detailed characteristics of all included studies are summarized in Table 1. All studies were performed on Asian individuals. The NOS score of all the included studies were no less than 6, indicating that none of the included studies were of low quality.

3.2. Meta-Analysis Results

3.2.1. Family History. PD patients with family history are defined as having at least one first- or second-degree relative

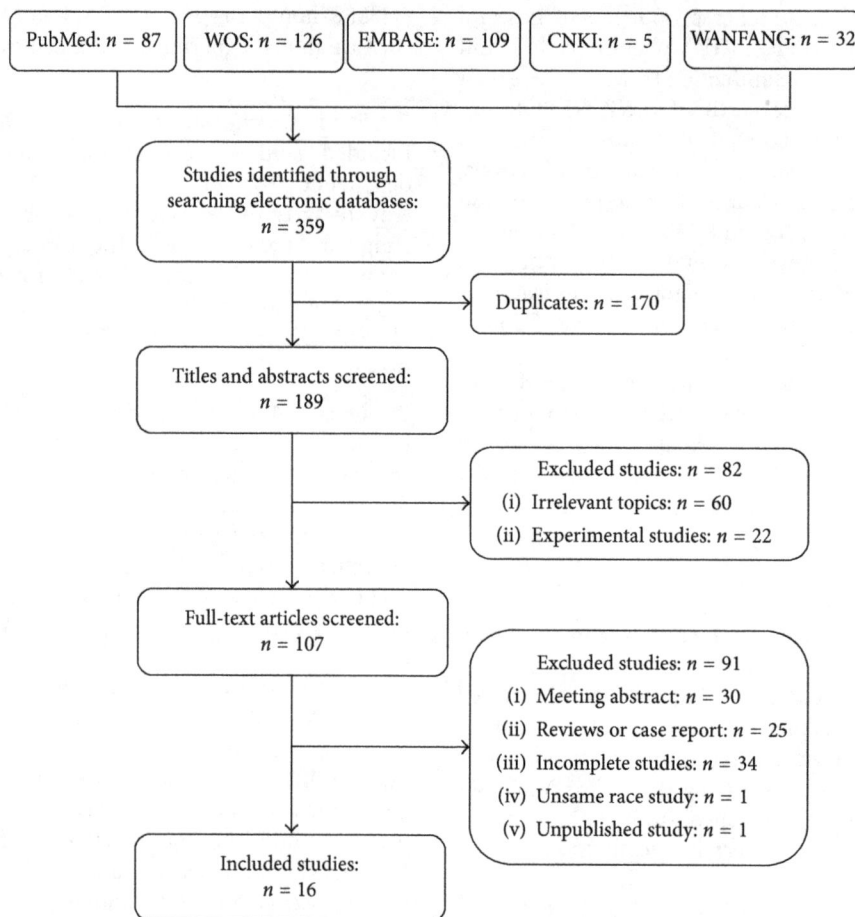

FIGURE 1: Flow diagram of studies included publication.

with a diagnosis of PD. Five studies assessed the relationship between *LRRK2* G2385R status and family history of PD, and the data showed that a family history of PD was significantly more common in the *LRRK2* G2385R carriers than in the *LRRK2* G2385R noncarriers (OR: 1.98; 95% CI: 1.16–3.39; $P = 0.01$) (Supplementary Figure 1).

3.2.2. Sex Distribution. Twelve studies included a sex distribution analysis between *LRRK2* G2385R-carrier PD group and *LRRK2* G2385R-noncarrier PD group. There was no significant association between males and *LRRK2* G2385R carrier status (OR = 0.85, 95% CI: 0.70–1.02, $P = 0.08$, Supplementary Figure 2).

3.2.3. Disease Duration. There were seven studies that mentioned the difference in disease duration between *LRRK2* G2385R-carrier PD patients and *LRRK2* G2385R-noncarrier PD patients. The average disease duration in carriers of the *LRRK2* G2385R was slightly longer than that in noncarriers (MD = 0.47, 95% CI: 0.01–0.93, $P = 0.04$, Supplementary Figure 3).

3.2.4. Age at Onset. Twelve studies assessed the relationship between *LRRK2* G2385R status and age at onset (AAO) of

PD patients. Four studies referred to AAO in early-onset PD patients. Another four studies were concerned with late-onset PD patients. No statistically significant differences were recorded between *LRRK2* G2385R-carrier PD group and *LRRK2* G2385R-noncarrier PD group (mean AAO: MD = −0.06, 95% CI: −0.15 to 0.03, $P = 0.19$, Supplementary Figure 4A; AAO in early-onset PD: MD = −2.43, 95% CI: −0.55 to 5.42, $P = 0.11$, Supplementary Figure 4B; AAO in late-onset PD: MD = −1.54, 95% CI: −3.38 to 0.30, $P = 0.10$, Supplementary Figure 4C).

3.2.5. Initial Symptoms. Four common initial symptoms, including tremor, rigidity, bradykinesia, and postural instability, were compared between *LRRK2* G2385R-carrier PD group and *LRRK2* G2385R-noncarrier PD group. No significant differences were observed (tremor: OR = 1.05, 95% CI: 0.76–1.45, $P = 0.76$, Supplementary Figure 5A; rigidity: OR = 1.14, 95% CI: 0.70–1.86, $P = 0.60$, Supplementary Figure 5B; bradykinesia: OR = 1.17, 95% CI: 0.76–1.79, $P = 0.48$, Supplementary Figure 5C; postural instability: OR = 0.97, 95% CI: 0.39–2.39, $P = 0.94$, Supplementary Figure 5D).

3.2.6. Disease Severity. The H-Y and UPDRS-III were commonly used to evaluate disease severity. Six studies

TABLE 1: Characteristics of included publication.

Article	Country	LRRK2 G2385R	Number	Family history	Sex (male)	Disease duration	AAO (n)	AAO (EOPD)	AAO (LOPD) (n)	Initial Tremor	Initial Bradykinesia	Initial PI	Initial Rigidity	H-Y	UPDRS-III	Motor Tremor	Motor Rigidity	Motor Bradykinesia	Motor PIGD	MMSE	Depression	LED (mg)	Motor fluctuation	Dyskinesia	NOS score
An et al. [5]	China	Carriers	71	—	40	—	52.75±9.84	42.96±7.23	58.40±5.93	37	—	—	—	2.16±0.91	—	—	—	—	—	—	—	—	—	—	8
		noncarriers	529	—	314	—	56.32±11.26	40.81±7.35	61.07±7.27	263	—	—	—	2.33±0.98	—	—	—	—	—	—	—	—	—	—	
Cai et al. [10]	China	Carriers	49	—	28	5.18±2.58	56.8±10.7	41.6±5.91	61.3±7.04	34	24	0	18	2.47±0.89	21.4±8.78	—	—	—	—	—	—	—	—	—	8
		noncarriers	461	—	275	4.92±3.36	58.6±11.0	42.9±5.5	63.2±7.33	299	224	9	168	2.57±0.93	22.1±8.35	—	—	—	—	—	—	—	—	—	
Cao et al. [7]	China	Carriers	14	0	5	8.57±8.71	57.1±11.0	—	—	8	7	5	7	1.7±0.4	19.6±5.1	—	—	—	—	—	—	—	—	3	7
		noncarriers	221	13	128	5.52±4.81	54.4±13.4	—	—	134	102	64	83	2.0±0.8	20.5±7.3	—	—	—	—	—	—	—	—	57	
Cao et al. [16]	China	Carriers	25	—	16	—	—	—	—	—	—	—	—	2.2±0.8	—	—	—	—	—	—	—	—	—	—	5
		noncarriers	43	—	28	—	—	—	—	—	—	—	—	2.4±0.74	—	—	—	—	—	—	—	—	—	—	
Chan et al. [17]	Hong Kong	Carriers	—	—	—	—	—	42.7±2.3 (3)	74.3±4.9 (4)	—	—	—	—	—	—	—	—	—	—	—	—	—	—	—	6
	China	noncarriers	—	—	—	—	—	38.3±6.6 (34)	69.2±10.7 (44)	—	—	—	—	—	—	—	—	—	—	—	—	—	—	—	
Di Fonzo et al. [18]	Taiwan	Carriers	61	—	34	13.4±6.2	53.2±12.5	—	—	—	—	—	—	—	—	—	—	—	—	—	—	—	—	—	8
	China	noncarriers	547	—	328	11.2±6.0	55.0±11.9	—	—	—	—	—	—	—	—	—	—	—	—	—	—	—	—	—	
Farrer et al. [3]	Taiwan	Carriers	34	6	18	7.3±5.4	54.9±11.8	—	—	—	—	—	—	—	—	24	32	30	12	—	—	457.6±246.6	12	13	8
	China	noncarriers	376	20	214	7.2±4.6	58.0±11.7	—	—	—	—	—	—	—	—	258	343	365	150	—	—	444.6±270.9	122	117	
Funayama et al. [20]	Japan	Carriers	—	—	—	—	54.0±10.6 (50)	42.5±5.8 (17)	59.9±7.0 (33)	—	—	—	—	—	—	—	—	—	—	—	—	—	—	—	7
		noncarriers	—	—	—	—	50.3±14.9 (389)	37.1±9.4 (180)	61.6±7.8 (209)	—	—	—	—	—	—	—	—	—	—	—	—	—	—	—	
Fung et al. [22]	Taiwan	Carriers	27	—	—	—	61.5±11.3	—	—	—	—	—	—	—	—	26	26	27	—	—	—	—	—	—	7
	China	noncarriers	278	—	—	—	61.9±10.5	—	—	—	—	—	—	—	—	252	261	269	—	—	—	—	—	—	
Fu et al. [19]	China	Carriers	37	8	21	—	55±11.7	—	—	21	11	1	3	—	—	—	—	—	—	—	—	—	—	—	7
		noncarriers	365	51	201	—	55.0±11.0	—	—	220	81	16	26	—	—	—	—	—	—	—	—	—	—	—	
Gao et al. [7]	China	Carriers	36	2	21	4.1±2.7	60.5±10.4	—	—	—	—	—	—	—	—	16	—	—	16	27.2±3.4	—	—	13	6	6
		noncarriers	139	10	73	3.8±3.2	58.2±8.8	—	—	—	—	—	—	—	—	55	—	—	73	25.3±4.0	—	—	15	6	
Hong et al. [21]	Korean	Carriers	23	—	7	3.8±3.1	—	—	—	—	—	—	—	—	19.8±11.2	—	—	—	—	25.6±4.4	5	—	—	—	7
		noncarriers	276	—	136	4.2±3.3	—	—	—	—	—	—	—	—	23.6±8.7	—	—	—	—	25.0±4.0	56	—	—	—	
Kim et al. [9]	Korean	Carriers	82	—	35	—	55.3±11.5	—	—	—	—	—	—	2.15±0.83	—	—	—	—	—	—	—	—	—	—	9
		noncarriers	841	—	373	—	54.7±10.8	—	—	—	—	—	—	2.08±0.81	—	—	—	—	—	—	—	—	—	—	
Sun et al. [6]	China	Carriers	76	—	37	6.57±4.21	55.57±8.78	—	—	—	—	—	—	—	24.55±12.08	29	—	—	43	27.78±2.68	27	553.67±329.84	27	4	7
		noncarriers	225	—	125	5.73±3.55	57.05±8.92	—	—	—	—	—	—	—	26.52±12.64	140	—	—	69	26.96±2.92	58	467.71±286.34	50	8	
Tan et al. [8]	Singapore	Carriers	33	5	16	—	59.0±11.0	—	—	—	—	—	—	—	26.0±11.0	—	—	—	—	—	—	467.0±275.0	—	7	5
		noncarriers	29	0	18	—	59.0±10.0	—	—	—	—	—	—	—	27.0±11.0	—	—	—	—	—	—	537.0±287.0	—	11	
Zhou et al. [23]	China	Carriers	26	—	—	—	—	—	—	—	—	—	—	1.82±0.58	—	—	—	—	—	—	—	—	—	—	7
		noncarriers	176	—	—	—	—	—	—	—	—	—	—	1.76±0.76	—	—	—	—	—	—	—	—	—	—	

TABLE 2: Summarized results of the meta-analysis.

Subjects	Effect model	MD/OR (95% CI)	P value	Study heterogeneity			
				Chi^2	df	I^2 (%)	P value
Family history	Fixed	1.98 [1.16–3.39]	0.01	5.42	4	26	0.25
Gender (male)	Fixed	0.85 [0.70–1.02]	0.08	6.09	11	0	0.87
Disease duration	Fixed	0.47 [0.01–0.93]	0.04	8.16	6	27	0.23
AAO	Fixed	−0.06 [−0.15 to 0.03]	0.19	16.32	11	33	0.13
AAO (early-onset)	Random	2.43 [−0.55 to 5.42]	0.11	19.47	3	85	0.0002
AAO (late-onset)	Random	−1.54 [−3.38 to 0.30]	0.10	6.67	3	55	0.08
Initial symptoms—tremor	Fixed	1.05 [0.76–1.45]	0.76	0.70	3	0	0.87
Initial symptoms—rigidity	Fixed	1.14 [0.70–1.86]	0.60	0.61	2	0	0.74
Initial symptoms—bradykinesia	Fixed	1.17 [0.76–1.79]	0.48	0.61	2	0	0.74
Initial symptoms—PI	Fixed	0.97 [0.39–2.39]	0.94	0.78	2	0	0.68
H-Y	Fixed	−0.09 [−0.20 to 0.01]	0.07	7.39	5	32	0.19
UPDRS-III	Fixed	−1.35 [−2.82 to 0.11]	0.07	1.56	4	0	0.82
Motor symptoms—tremor	Random	0.88 [0.40–1.91]	0.74	10.41	3	71	0.02
Motor symptoms—rigidity	Fixed	1.59 [0.48–5.27]	0.45	0.01	1	0	0.94
Motor symptoms—bradykinesia	Fixed	0.43 [0.15–1.24]	0.12	1.90	1	47	0.17
Motor symptoms—PIGD	Random	1.24 [0.48–3.23]	0.66	12.47	2	84	0.002
MMSE	Fixed	1.02 [0.43–1.62]	0.0007	2.27	2	12	0.32
Depression	Fixed	1.46 [0.90–2.37]	0.13	0.39	1	0	0.53
LED	Fixed	0.14 [−0.06 to 0.33]	0.17	3.78	2	47	0.15
Motor fluctuation	Random	1.73 [0.99–3.01]	0.05	7.52	2	73	0.02
Dyskinesia	Random	1.26 [0.63–2.54]	0.52	8.26	4	52	0.08

involved H-Y analysis, and five studies involved UPDRS-III analysis in *LRRK2* G2385R-carrier PD and *LRRK2* G2385R-noncarrier PD patients. No significant differences were discovered (H-Y: MD = −0.09, 95% CI: −0.20 to 0.01, P = 0.07, Supplementary Figure 6A; UPDRS-III: MD = −1.35, 95% CI: −2.82 to 0.11, P = 0.07, Supplementary Figure 6B).

3.2.7. Motor Symptoms. Tremor, rigidity, bradykinesia, PIGD are the main motor manifestations of PD patients. Four studies assessed the relationship between *LRRK2* G2385R status and the tremor phenotype of PD patients. Three studies focused on the PIGD phenotype, and two studies analyzed rigidity and bradykinesia phenotype. The meta-analysis results of these studies showed that there were no significant differences in the above motor phenotypes in the *LRRK2* G2385R-carrier PD group compared to *LRRK2* G2385R-noncarrier PD group (tremor: OR = 0.88, 95% CI: 0.40–1.91, P = 0.74, Supplementary Figure 7A; rigidity: OR = 1.59, 95% CI: 0.48–5.27, P = 0.45, Supplementary Figure 7B; bradykinesia: OR = 0.43, 95% CI: 0.15–1.24, P = 0.12, Supplementary Figure 7C; PIGD: OR = 1.24, 95% CI: 0.48–3.23, P = 0.66, Supplementary Figure 7D).

3.2.8. Nonmotor Symptoms. Only MMSE scores and the proportion of patients with depression were assessed owing to incomplete data about other nonmotor symptoms. Three studies included an MMSE score analysis in both groups and showed a significantly higher MMSE score in the *LRRK2* G2385R-carrier PD group than in the *LRRK2* G2385R-noncarrier PD group (MD = 1.02, 95% CI: 0.43–1.62, P = 0.0007, Supplementary Figure 8A). Two studies included a depression analysis, but there was no significant association between depression and *LRRK2* G2385R status (OR = 1.46, 95% CI: 0.90–2.37, P = 0.13, Supplementary Figure 8B).

3.2.9. Levodopa Therapy and Related Complications. There were some studies that mentioned the LED and related complications, including motor fluctuation and dyskinesia. The meta-analysis results of these studies showed no significant differences for LED, motor fluctuation, or dyskinesia between the *LRRK2* G2385R-carrier PD group and the *LRRK2* G2385R-noncarrier PD group (LED: MD = 0.14, 95% CI: −0.06 to 0.33, P = 0.17, Supplementary Figure 9A; motor fluctuation: OR = 1.73, 95% CI: 0.99–3.01, P = 0.05, Supplementary Figure 9B; dyskinesia: OR = 1.26, 95% CI: 0.63–2.54, P = 0.52, Supplementary Figure 9C).

Taken together, the *LRRK2* G2385R-carrier PD group more often presented a family history of PD and had a longer disease duration and a higher MMSE score than the *LRRK2* G2385R-noncarrier PD group. However, *LRRK2* G2385R carriers showed no significant differences in sex distribution, AAO, initial symptoms, motor symptoms and grade of severity, depression, or LED and levodopa-related complications compared to *LRRK2* G2385R noncarriers. The results of the meta-analysis are summarized in Table 2.

3.3. Sensitivity Analysis and Publication Bias. A sensitivity analysis was made in comparison with significant heterogeneity among the studies. When the heterogeneity among the studies was significant, we performed sensitivity analyses by excluding the relatively low-quality studies; the same results were obtained. Therefore, we can conclude that the sensitivity is low and that the results are reliable. As there were fewer than 10 high-quality studies in most comparisons in our meta-analysis, an accurate publication bias assessment could not be performed. However, we completed a funnel plot to estimate publication bias. There were no asymmetries in the funnel plot and no significant publication biases of the meta-analysis.

4. Discussion

In this meta-analysis, we extensively analyzed the relationship between *LRRK2* G2385R carrier status and clinical manifestations of PD in an Asian population. The *LRRK2* G2385R-carrier PD group significantly more often had a family history of PD than did the *LRRK2* G2385R-noncarrier PD group. The average disease duration in the *LRRK2* G2385R-carrier PD group was slightly longer than that in the *LRRK2* G2385R-noncarrier PD group. The mean MMSE score was significantly lower in the *LRRK2* G2385R-noncarrier PD group than in the *LRRK2* G2385R-carrier PD group.

Additionally, we observed that there were no significant differences in most of the clinical characteristics, including sex distribution, AAO, initial symptoms, motor symptoms and grade of severity, depression, and LED and levodopa-related complications between *LRRK2* G2385R-carrier and *LRRK2* G2385R-noncarrier PD patients. These results indicated that PD patients carrying a *LRRK2* G2385R mutation is associated with a significantly overlapping phenotype when compared with idiopathic PD. This finding is in line with those of previous studies reporting that G2019S carrier patients exhibit clinical features quite similar to those of noncarriers, with some mild differences [24–26]. One possible reason for this was that a broad spectrum of clinical characteristics may be caused by gene-gene interaction or gene-environment interactions, affecting the genotype and progression of the disease.

Nonmotor symptoms in PD are quite common and contribute to the patient's disability [27]. Associations between the genotype and nonmotor symptoms in PD patients have attracted research attention in recent years. To date, a few studies have focused mainly on several specific nonmotor symptoms, rather than on the general nonmotor symptom profile. Therefore, we failed to find sufficient data to assess the nonmotor symptoms of PD patients in the context of *LRRK2* G2385R status. For MMSE scores, given that only three published papers were included in the meta-analysis, a publication bias is likely to be present. A detailed clinical characterization of PD patients carrying *LRRK2* variants is warranted.

The NOS scores of all included publications were rated from 6 points to 9 points, providing a reliable bottom for the current analysis. No statistically significant publication bias or heterogeneity between different studies was detected in our meta-analysis. However, several limitations may have influenced the precision of our results. First, given that the number of included studies was limited, publication bias could potentially occur, even though we used various searching approaches and statistical analyses to minimize the publication bias. Second, although this meta-analysis included all the published case-control cohorts, some unpublished results may have been neglected.

5. Conclusion

In conclusion, our study suggested that most of the clinical characteristics of PD patients with the *LRRK2* G2385R mutation were similar to those of *LRRK2* G2385R noncarriers among Asian individuals, except for a more common family history, relatively longer disease duration, and higher MMSE scores in the *LRRK2* G2385R carriers. These findings strengthen our understanding of the clinical and genetic heterogeneity of PD and may have implications for diagnosis and therapy of PD. However, further larger samples and multicenter cooperative studies in different populations are warranted to clarify the relevance between the *LRRK2* G2385R genotype and clinical phenotype of PD.

Acknowledgments

This work was supported by grants from the China Postdoctoral Science Foundation (2016M600638), National Natural Science Foundation of China (81500965), and Shaanxi Provincial Natural Science Foundation (2017 JM8042).

References

[1] C. M. Tolleson and J. Y. Fang, "Advances in the mechanisms of Parkinson's disease," *Discovery Medicine*, vol. 15, pp. 61–66, 2013.

[2] D. G. Healy, M. Falchi, S. S. O'Sullivan et al., "Phenotype, genotype, and worldwide genetic penetrance of LRRK2-associated Parkinson's disease: a case-control study," *Lancet Neurology*, vol. 7, no. 7, pp. 583–590, 2008.

[3] M. J. Farrer, J. T. Stone, C. H. Lin et al., "Lrrk2 G2385R is an ancestral risk factor for Parkinson's disease in Asia," *Parkinsonism and Related Disorders*, vol. 13, no. 2, pp. 89–92, 2007.

[4] L. Cao, T. Zhang, Q. Xiao et al., "The prevalence of LRRK2 Gly2385Arg variant in Chinese Han population with Parkinson's disease," *Movement Disorders*, vol. 22, no. 16, pp. 2439–2443, 2007.

[5] X. K. An, R. Peng, T. Li et al., "LRRK2 Gly2385Arg variant is a risk factor of Parkinson's disease among Han-Chinese from mainland China," *European Journal of Neurology*, vol. 15, pp. 301–305, 2008.

[6] Q. Sun, T. Wang, T. F. Jiang et al., "Effect of a leucine-rich repeat kinase 2 variant on motor and non-motor symptoms in Chinese Parkinson's disease patients," *Aging and Disease*, vol. 7, pp. 230–236, 2016.

[7] C. Gao, H. Pang, X. G. Luo, Y. Ren, H. Shang, and Z. Y. He, "LRRK2 G2385R variant carriers of female Parkinson's disease are more susceptible to motor fluctuation," *Journal of Neurology*, vol. 260, no. 11, pp. 2884–2889, 2013.

[8] E. K. Tan, S. Fook-Chong, and Z. Yi, "Comparing LRRK2 Gly2385Arg carriers with noncarriers," *Movement Disorders*, vol. 22, no. 5, pp. 749-750, 2007.

[9] J. M. Kim, J. Y. Lee, H. J. Kim et al., "The LRRK2 G2385R variant is a risk factor for sporadic Parkinson's disease in the Korean population," *Parkinsonism and Related Disorders*, vol. 16, no. 2, pp. 85–88, 2010.

[10] J. Cai, J. Lin, W. Chen et al., "Association between G2385R and R1628P polymorphism of LRRK2 gene and sporadic Parkinson's disease in a Han-Chinese population in southeastern China," *Neurological Sciences*, vol. 34, pp. 2001–2006, 2013.

[11] D. F. Stroup, J. A. Berlin, S. C. Morton et al., "Meta-analysis of observational studies in epidemiology: a proposal for reporting. Meta-analysis of Observational Studies in Epidemiology (MOOSE) group," *JAMA*, vol. 283, no. 15, pp. 2008–2012, 2000.

[12] A. Liberati, D. G. Altman, J. Tetzlaff et al., "The PRISMA statement for reporting systematic reviews and meta-analyses of studies that evaluate health care interventions: explanation and elaboration," *Journal of Clinical Epidemiology*, vol. 62, no. 10, pp. e1–34, 2009.

[13] X. Fan, T. Lin, K. Xu et al., "Laparoendoscopic single-site nephrectomy compared with conventional laparoscopic nephrectomy: a systematic review and meta-analysis of comparative studies," *European Urology*, vol. 62, no. 4, pp. 601–612, 2012.

[14] G. A. S. B. Wells, D. O'Connell, J. Peterson, V. Welch, and M. T. P. Losos, *The Newcastle-Ottawa Scale (NOS) for Assessing the Quality of Nonrandomised Studies in Meta-Analyses*, July 2015, http://www.ohri.ca/programs/clinical pidemiology/oxford.asp.

[15] J. P. T. Higgins and S. Green, *Cochrane Handbook for Systematic Reviews of Interventions. Cochrane Collaboration*, John Wiley and Sons, New York, NY, USA, 2008.

[16] M. Cao, Z. Q. Gu, Y. Li et al., "Olfactory dysfunction in Parkinson's disease patients with the LRRK2 G2385R variant," *Neuroscience Bulletin*, vol. 32, no. 6, pp. 572–576, 2016.

[17] D. K. Chan, P. W. Ng, V. Mok et al., "LRRK2 Gly2385Arg mutation and clinical features in a Chinese population with early-onset Parkinson's disease compared to late-onset patients," *Journal of Neural Transmission*, vol. 115, pp. 1275–1277, 2008.

[18] A. Di Fonzo, Y. H. Wu-Chou, C. S. Lu et al., "A common missense variant in the LRRK2 gene, Gly2385Arg, associated with Parkinson's disease risk in Taiwan," *Neurogenetics*, vol. 7, no. 3, pp. 133–138, 2006.

[19] X. Fu, Y. Zheng, H. Hong et al., "LRRK2 G2385R and LRRK2 R1628P increase risk of Parkinson's disease in a Han Chinese population from Southern Mainland China," *Parkinsonism and Related Disorders*, vol. 19, no. 3, pp. 397-398, 2013.

[20] M. Funayama, Y. Li, H. Tomiyama et al., "Leucine-rich repeat kinase 2 G2385R variant is a risk factor for Parkinson disease in Asian population," *Neuroreport*, vol. 18, no. 3, pp. 273–275, 2007.

[21] J. H. Hong, Y. K. Kim, J. S. Park et al., "Lack of association between LRRK2 G2385R and cognitive dysfunction in Korean patients with Parkinson's disease," *Journal of Clinical Neuroscience*, vol. 36, pp. 108–113, 2017.

[22] H. C. Fung, C. M. Chen, J. Hardy, A. B. Singleton, and Y. R. Wu, "A common genetic factor for Parkinson disease in ethnic Chinese population in Taiwan," *BMC Neurology*, vol. 6, no. 1, p. 47, 2006.

[23] Y. Zhou, X. Luo, F. Li et al., "Association of Parkinson's disease with six single nucleotide polymorphisms located in four PARK genes in the northern Han Chinese population," *Journal of Clinical Neuroscience*, vol. 19, no. 7, pp. 1011–1015, 2012.

[24] A. Bouhouche, H. Tibar, R. Ben El Haj et al., "LRRK2 G2019S mutation: prevalence and clinical features in Moroccans with Parkinson's disease," *Parkinson's Disease*, vol. 2017, Article ID 2412486, 2017.

[25] R. N. Alcalay, A. Mirelman, R. Saunders-Pullman et al., "Parkinson disease phenotype in Ashkenazi Jews with and without LRRK2 G2019S mutations," *Movement Disorders*, vol. 28, no. 14, pp. 1966–1971, 2013.

[26] D. W. Li, Z. Gu, C. Wang et al., "Non-motor symptoms in Chinese Parkinson's disease patients with and without LRRK2 G2385R and R1628P variants," *Journal of Neural Transmission*, vol. 122, no. 5, pp. 661–667, 2015.

[27] S. Bostantjopoulou, Z. Katsarou, C. Karakasis, E. Peitsidou, D. Milioni, and N. Rossopoulos, "Evaluation of non-motor symptoms in Parkinson's Disease: an underestimated necessity," *Hippokratia*, vol. 17, pp. 214–219, 2013.

5

Diagnostic Validation for Participants in the Washington State Parkinson Disease Registry

Hojoong M. Kim [ID],[1,2] James B. Leverenz,[3] Daniel J. Burdick,[4] Sindhu Srivatsal,[5] Jennifer Pate,[1] Shu-Ching Hu,[1,2] Steven P. Millard,[1] Marie Y. Davis,[1,2] Ali Samii,[1,2] and Cyrus P. Zabetian [ID][1,2]

[1]Veterans Affairs Puget Sound Health Care System, Seattle, WA, USA
[2]Department of Neurology, University of Washington School of Medicine, Seattle, WA, USA
[3]Lou Ruvo Center for Brain Health, Cleveland Clinic, Cleveland, OH, USA
[4]Booth Gardner Parkinson's Care Center, EvergreenHealth Medical Center, Kirkland, WA, USA
[5]Virginia Mason Medical Center, Seattle, WA, USA

Correspondence should be addressed to Hojoong M. Kim; kimhoj@uw.edu

Academic Editor: Hélio Teive

Background. The Washington State Parkinson Disease Registry (WPDR) was created to facilitate recruitment for Parkinson's disease (PD) research studies conducted in the Pacific Northwest. The success of registries that rely on self-report is dependent on the accuracy of the information provided by participants, particularly diagnosis. *Objective and Methods.* Our goal was to assess diagnostic accuracy within the WPDR cohort. We randomly selected and attempted to contact 168 of the 1,278 actively enrolled WPDR participants. Those who responded were invited to undergo an interview and neurological examination performed by a PD specialist. If an in-person assessment was not possible, we sought information collected during participation in prior research studies or from review of medical records. A diagnosis was considered "validated" if the individual met UK Parkinson's Disease Society Brain Bank (UKBB) clinical diagnostic criteria for PD. *Results.* Data were ascertained for 106 participants; 77 underwent an in-person assessment, 21 had data available from a prior research study, and 8 provided access to medical records. Diagnostic accuracy within the overall sample was 93.4% (95% confidence interval (86.4%, 97.1%)). Seven patients did not fulfill UKBB criteria for the following reasons: early severe autonomic involvement ($n = 3$), history of neuroleptic treatment ($n = 1$), presence of the Babinski sign ($n = 1$), or insufficient supportive criteria ($n = 2$). *Conclusions.* Our results indicate that studies which use the WPDR for recruitment will rarely encounter patients who are misdiagnosed. This further supports the utility of the WPDR as an effective recruitment tool for PD research in the Pacific Northwest.

1. Introduction

2017 marked the 200th anniversary of James Parkinson's *Essay on the Shaking Palsy*, describing a neurodegenerative disorder that is known today as Parkinson's disease (PD) [1]. PD is the second most common neurodegenerative disorder, and it is estimated that the number of cases in the most populous nations will double to as much as 9.3 million by 2030 [2].

Neuroprotective therapy that delays progression has remained elusive despite advances in symptomatic treatment and an improved understanding of the genetics and pathophysiology of the disease. The average time from FDA application to approval of drugs is 12 years [3], and the time spent on patient recruitment and enrollment is a major limiting factor in this process [4]. Reducing the time required for these activities could substantially accelerate drug development. Well-characterized disease registries are one tool that can provide researchers with immediate access to a pool of prescreened individuals who are willing to participate in clinical studies [5].

To date, there are several PD registries in the US established to serve different functions. The Nebraska [6] and

California PD registries [7] were established primarily as epidemiologic tools to study the incidence and prevalence of the disease and to identify potential demographic and environmental risk factors. In contrast, the PD Registry of the Muhammad Ali Parkinson Center [8] and Fox Trial Finder [9] were created to facilitate enrollment in PD-related research on a national or international scale. We established the Washington State Parkinson Disease Registry (WPDR) in 2007 with a similar intent but with a focus on patients and research studies in the Pacific Northwest [10]. Diagnostic accuracy is a challenge for any disease registry in which diagnosis is by self-report, and the lower the accuracy, the lower the overall utility of both epidemiologic and research registries. In this study, we sought to validate the accuracy of self-reported PD diagnosis among participants in the WPDR.

2. Methods

2.1. WPDR Overview. The WPDR became operational and began enrollment in 2007. All prospective participants are first screened in-person, by telephone, or with an online questionnaire to determine if they have received a diagnosis of PD from a clinician (regardless of specialty). Those who self-report a diagnosis of PD are then invited to enroll; the informed consent process is completed in-person or by telephone. At the time of enrollment, information on demographics and disease characteristics is obtained. These data include initial and current motor symptoms, age at onset and diagnosis, PD-related medication and neurosurgical history, complications of treatment, nonmotor symptoms, and family history of PD. A subset of these data is updated annually using a questionnaire that is sent and returned by mail. The WPDR database and research staff are housed at the VA Puget Sound Health Care System (VAPSHCS) in Seattle. Researchers who wish to use the WPDR for recruitment submit an application which is reviewed by a committee of five investigators. Data collected in some studies that use the WPDR for recruitment are subsequently deposited back into the WPDR database to improve the depth and quality of information available for future use.

As of April 30, 2018, 2,130 PD patients have enrolled in the WPDR and after removing participants who are now deceased or have withdrawn, 1,521 are considered "active." Sixty-two studies have previously used or are currently using the WPDR for assistance with recruitment.

2.2. Validation Study: Subject Selection and Data Acquisition. The goal of this project was to estimate the proportion of patients enrolled in the WPDR who met the UK Parkinson's Disease Society Brain Bank (UKBB) clinical diagnostic criteria for PD [11] based on data obtained from a randomly selected subset of the cohort. We estimated that a sample size of between 100 and 125 was sufficient for this purpose. For these estimates, we used misdiagnosis rates of 5%, 10%, and 20% to span the positive predictive values (PPV) of the UKBB criteria reported in two clinicopathologic validation studies [12, 13]. For these misdiagnosis rates, the margin of error (half-width of the 95% confidence interval) was ±5%, ±6%, and ±8% for $n = 100$, and ±4%, ±6%, and ±7% for $n = 125$.

The validation study began on January 31, 2011, and at that time, a total of 1,354 patients had enrolled in the WPDR. Of those patients, we were notified of 76 deaths or withdrawals since initial entry, resulting in 1,278 active enrollments. We randomly ranked the entire active cohort from 1 to 1,278 using the sample function in the R software package and attempted to contact subjects in rank order [14]. See Figure 1 for details of the study progression. If a subject was successfully contacted, we sought permission to perform a study assessment which included a detailed neurological examination and interview. If the patient declined, we sought permission to obtain medical records from their current and/or prior neurologist(s). For the groups who were not assessed in-person, did not provide access to medical records, and could not be contacted, we searched the WPDR database to determine if they had participated in a previous study that provided suitable data back to us. Such data, if available, were used in the validation process. All study procedures were approved by the VAPSHCS Institutional Review Board, and all participants provided informed consent.

2.3. Validation Study: In-Person Assessments. Validation study visits were performed by a PD specialist (DJB, MYD, SCH, HMK, JBL, AS, SS, and CPZ) at our research clinic at the VAPSHCS or at the participant's place of residence. The assessment included an interview focused on PD symptoms and medications, a general neurologic examination, and the Movement Disorder Society-sponsored version of the Unified Parkinson Disease Rating Scale (MDS-UPDRS) Part III. The following information was obtained: past medical, surgical, and social history; age at onset; motor symptoms present at onset; and characteristics of tremor, rigidity, bradykinesia, and balance/gait difficulties. The general neurologic examination focused on ocular movements, sensory function, cerebellar function, general gait testing, and deep tendon reflexes.

2.4. Validation Study: Consensus Conferences. A core group of three PD specialists (HMK, JBL, and CPZ) attended every consensus conference, and others (DJB, MYD, SCH, AS, and SS) attended on an ad hoc basis. For each participant, a single specialist presented data available from the validation study assessment, previous studies that used the WPDR, or records from the treating neurologist. After review and discussion of the data, a consensus was reached as to whether each subject met UKBB criteria for PD. All data acquisition procedures, medical record reviews, and consensus conferences were conducted between January 31, 2011 and October 7, 2013.

3. Results

We initially attempted to contact the first 125 WPDR participants on the rank list and invite them to undergo an

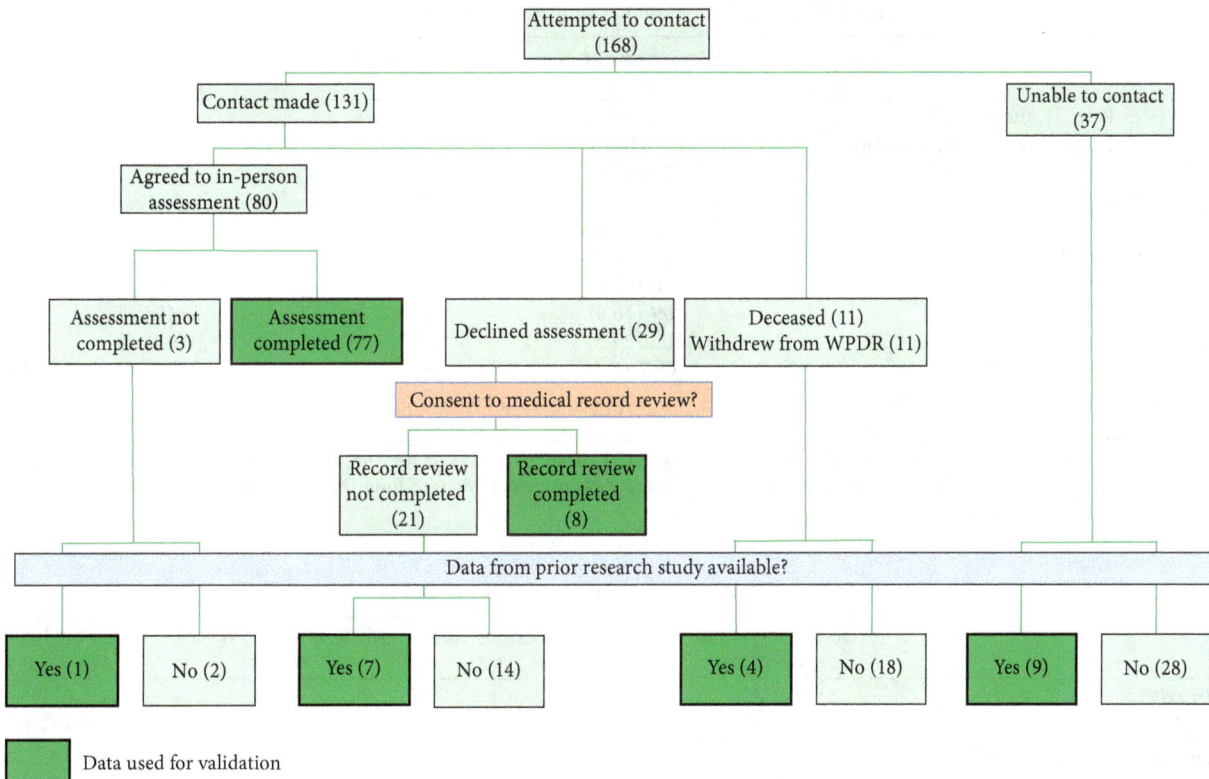

FIGURE 1: Data used for validation.

in-person assessment. Some patients could not be contacted, declined an assessment, or did not have data available from medical records or other studies. We then sought to contact an additional 43 participants in rank order until the minimum sample size was attained. In total, data from 106 patients were included in the final validation analysis (Figure 1). Of these participants, 77 were assessed in-person, 8 provided access to records from their treating neurologist (who were all movement disorder specialists), and 21 had data available from a prior research study that utilized the WPDR. This last source of data was a study on PD genetics in which a movement disorder specialist interviewed and examined each participant and based on this information determined whether the individual met UKBB criteria. We were able to reach a consensus (unanimous) decision on fulfillment of UKBB criteria for all 106 patients.

The clinical and demographic characteristics of the patients who were assessed in-person and not assessed in-person (i.e., data derived from a previous study or by medical record review) are presented in Table 1. Postural instability was more frequent in the patients who were not assessed in-person (65.5% vs. 39.0%, $p = 0.02$), but otherwise there were no significant differences between the two groups.

Of the patients with data available, 99/106 (93.4%, 95% confidence interval (86.4%, 96.1%)) fulfilled UKBB criteria at consensus conference (Table 2). The reasons for not fulfilling UKBB criteria were as follows: five participants had an exclusion criterion on Step 2 (neuroleptic treatment at onset

of symptoms, $n = 1$; presence of the Babinski sign, $n = 1$; early severe autonomic involvement, $n = 3$), and two individuals had less than three supportive prospective positive criteria on Step 3. The subject with neuroleptic exposure had been diagnosed with schizophrenia over 30 years prior to the onset of asymmetric left-sided resting tremor. This individual was also judged to have excellent levodopa responsiveness. The subject with the Babinski sign had examination findings and a history that were otherwise consistent with a clinical diagnosis of PD including a longstanding response to levodopa, medication-related wearing off, and peak dose dyskinesias. Of the three subjects with early severe autonomic involvement, two were thought to meet criteria for multiple system atrophy-parkinsonism (MSA-P). Both subjects who failed UKBB Step 3 had features atypical for PD including early postural instability, only a modest response to levodopa, and in one instance, symmetric parkinsonism.

4. Discussion

The success of disease registries that rely on self-report is highly dependent on the accuracy of the information provided by participants, most importantly diagnosis. Using data collected from a prospective in-person assessment, supplemented with information from prior research participation and medical records, we found that a large proportion of the WPDR participants sampled (93.4%) fulfilled UKBB criteria for PD. This suggests that studies which utilize

TABLE 1: Clinical and demographic characteristics of the study cohort.

	Assessed in-person (n = 77)	Not assessed in-person (n = 29)	Combined cohort (n = 106)	p value[a]
MDS-UPDRS Part III, mean (SD)	37.0 (18.0)	N/A	N/A	N/A
Hoehn and Yahr scale score median (range)	2 (1–5)	N/A	N/A	N/A
Mean (SD)	2.5 (0.9)			
Bradykinesia, n (%)	77 (100)	29 (100)	106 (100)	1.0[b]
Rigidity, n (%)	73 (94.8)	29 (100)	102 (96.2)	0.57[b]
Resting tremor, n (%)	51 (66.2)	24 (82.8)	75 (70.8)	0.15[b]
Postural instability, n (%)	30 (39.0)	19 (65.5)	49 (46.2)	0.02[b]
Male, n (%)	59 (76.6)	20 (69.0)	79 (74.5)	0.46[b]
Disease duration, mean (SD)	11.0 (7.5)	10.7 (7.3)	10.9 (7.4)	0.89[c]
Age at assessment, mean (SD)	69.7 (8.4)	66.6 (12.3)	68.8 (9.6)	0.15[c]
Duration between enrollment and assessment (years), Mean (SD)[d]	2.7 (1.0)	N/A	N/A	N/A

[a]Comparing patients in the "assessed in-person" and "not assessed in-person" groups; [b]Fisher's exact test; [c]unpaired t-test; [d]calculated only for "assessed in-person" group since data ascertained for the "not assessed in-person" group was sometimes derived from clinical or research visits that occurred before enrollment in the WPDR validation study.

TABLE 2: Reasons why diagnoses failed to validate.

	Assessed in-person (n = 77)	Data from previous study (n = 21)	Medical record review (n = 8)	Combined cohort (n = 106)
UKBB criteria				
Fulfilled, n (%)	71 (92.2)	20 (95.2)	8 (100)	99 (93.4)
Reasons for not fulfilling UKBB criteria				
Early severe autonomic involvement	2[a]	1	0	3[a]
Neuroleptic treatment at onset	1	0	0	1
Babinski sign	1	0	0	1
<3 Step III supportive criteria	2	0	0	2

[a]Two of these patients met criteria for MSA-P.

the WPDR for recruitment will only rarely encounter patients who are misdiagnosed.

We believe that there are two major factors that contributed to the high validation rate observed in our study. First, movement disorder specialists, who render PD diagnoses with greater accuracy than other practitioners [15], have cared for a greater proportion of WPDR participants than is typical for the US PD population. For example, 83.0% (88/106) of the WPDR patients successfully sampled, and 72.1% (922/1278) of the entire cohort reported that they were diagnosed or received care from a movement disorder specialist. In contrast, a recent nationwide poll conducted on behalf of the Michael J Fox Foundation found that only 45% of patient respondents had ever seen a movement disorder specialist [16]. Second, relatively few of the WPDR participants sampled were in an early stage of disease; only 24.5% (26/106) were within five years of symptom onset at the last data collection time point. Diagnostic accuracy is lowest in the early stages of PD since the assessment of some characteristics (e.g., motor progression and response to dopaminergic therapy) requires longitudinal information and features of atypical parkinsonism often emerge later in the course of the disease [17].

Of the four other large US-based PD registries of which we are aware, two (the Nebraska PD Registry [18] and the Fox Trial Finder (FTF) [19]) have performed validation studies. In the FTF study, over ten thousand members were invited to participate and 166 ultimately completed a virtual research visit via video conferencing with a neurologist specializing in PD. Though specific clinical diagnostic criteria were not used, the neurologists judged PD as the most likely diagnosis for 97% of the individuals. The Nebraska study attempted to contact 1,402 registrants and eventually interviewed and then either performed a medical record review (n = 172) or an in-person examination (n = 40) on a subset of patients. A movement disorder specialist used the available data to assign a "percentage probability of PD" based on global impression, and a diagnosis was considered confirmed if the probability was >50%. A PD diagnosis was validated for 82% of the patients who underwent medical record review and 77.5% of the patients who were directly examined. Comparisons between these validation efforts and ours are limited by important differences in methodology. Unlike the FTF and Nebraska studies, we examined the majority of participants in-person and used the most widely accepted clinical diagnostic criteria [11] rather than relying on a clinician's overall impression to render a diagnosis. Also, we were able to assess the validity of the diagnoses for the majority (106/168; 63.1%) of individuals who were initially targeted for recruitment in our validation study. In contrast, a much lower proportion of the target sample participated in the FTF (~2%) and Nebraska (~15%) studies, and thus these two studies were more susceptible to participation bias. However, it is not surprising that the validation rate of the FTF was similar to the WPDR. Both are self-selected research registries, and the participants sampled in the two studies had a similar disease duration at assessment (WPDR, 10.9 years; FTF, 8.0 years) and most had received care from a PD specialist (WPDR, 83.0%; FTF, 67.1%). The lower validation rate observed in the Nebraska study is expected since participants entered the registry as newly diagnosed cases and many of the initial diagnoses were rendered by nonneurologists.

Our study had several limitations. We were not able to perform an in-person assessment or obtain data for 36.9% (62/168) of the subjects targeted for validation for a variety of reasons (Figure 1). It is possible that the accuracy of the PD diagnosis was lower in these individuals than in those who were successfully sampled, which would bias our results. For a subset of subjects who could not be examined in-person, we used data from a prior research study to validate diagnosis. Such individuals might be more likely to have an accurate diagnosis by virtue of the fact that they previously participated in PD research. Finally, the definition of a validated case was based on clinical (UKBB) criteria alone. We selected the UKBB criteria because at the time we conducted our study, they were by far the most widely used clinical diagnostic criteria in research settings. Furthermore, the UKBB criteria have been validated in two clinicopathologic studies and were found to have PPVs of 82% [13] and 92% [12]. However, since the participants in our study did not undergo autopsy confirmation, a small proportion of the "validated" cases might have been misdiagnosed.

5. Conclusion

In a recent viewpoint, Dorsey and Bloem highlighted the global burden that PD poses in the coming decades, calling this the "Parkinson Pandemic" [20]. In order to meet this challenge, recruitment for clinical research must become more efficient to reduce delays in study completion. Research registries have great promise to assist in this endeavor, and since the establishment of the WPDR in 2007, sixty-two studies in the Pacific Northwest have utilized the WPDR for assistance with recruitment. Registries that rely on self-reported diagnosis of PD are limited if the diagnostic accuracy is low. Here, we have provided evidence that the vast majority of participants in the WPDR have been accurately diagnosed with PD. This underscores the value of the WPDR as an impactful resource for use by PD research studies in the Pacific Northwest.

Disclosure

The content is the responsibility of the authors alone and does not necessarily reflect the views or policies of the Department of Veterans Affairs or the United States Government.

Acknowledgments

This work was funded by grants from the APDA, Northwest Collaborative Care, Northwest Parkinson's Foundation, and Washington State Department of Health. During the conduct of this work, Daniel Burdick, Sindhu Srivatsal, and Marie Davis were supported by the VA Advanced Fellowship Program in Parkinson's Disease. This material is the result of work supported with resources and the use of facilities at the VA Puget Sound Health Care System.

References

[1] P. A. Kempster, B. Hurwitz, and A. J. Lees, "A new look at James Parkinson's Essay on the Shaking Palsy," *Neurology*, vol. 69, no. 5, pp. 482–485, 2007.

[2] E. R. Dorsey, R. Constantinescu, J. P. Thompson et al., "Projected number of people with Parkinson disease in the most populous nations, 2005 through 2030," *Neurology*, vol. 68, no. 5, pp. 384–386, 2007.

[3] G. A. Van Norman, "Drugs, devices, and the FDA: part 1: an overview of approval processes for drugs," *JACC: Basic to Translational Science*, vol. 1, no. 3, pp. 170–179, 2016.

[4] T. J. Scott, A. C. O'Connor, A. N. Link, and T. J. Beaulieu, "Economic analysis of opportunities to accelerate Alzheimer's disease research and development," *Annals of the New York Academy of Sciences*, vol. 1313, no. 1, pp. 17–34, 2014.

[5] J. Cummings, P. S. Aisen, B. DuBois et al., "Drug development in Alzheimer's disease: the path to 2025," *Alzheimer's Research and Therapy*, vol. 8, no. 1, p. 39, 2016.

[6] D. Strickland and J. M. Bertoni, "Parkinson's prevalence estimated by a state registry," *Movement Disorders*, vol. 19, no. 3, pp. 318–323, 2004.

[7] T. Hampton, "Parkinson disease registry launched," *JAMA*, vol. 293, no. 2, p. 149, 2005.

[8] ClinicalTrials.gov, *Parkinson's Disease Registry of the Muhammad Ali Parkinson Center*, National Library of Medicine (US), https://clinicaltrials.gov/ct2/show/NCT00217321, 2018.

[9] Michaeljfox.org, "Fox trial finder," https://foxtrialfinder.michaeljfox.org, 2017.

[10] H. M. Kim, A. Samii, E. Martinez, G. Richards, C. Zabetian, and J. B. Leverenz, "The Washington Parkinson disease registry (WPDR): a state-wide research registry," *Movement Disorders*, vol. 22, p. IX, 2007.

[11] W. R. Gibb and A. J. Lees, "The relevance of the Lewy body to the pathogenesis of idiopathic Parkinson's disease," *Journal of Neurology, Neurosurgery and Psychiatry*, vol. 51, no. 6, pp. 745–752, 1988.

[12] A. J. Hughes, S. E. Daniel, and A. J. Lees, "Improved accuracy of clinical diagnosis of Lewy body Parkinson's disease," *Neurology*, vol. 57, no. 8, pp. 1497–1499, 2001.

[13] A. J. Hughes, S. E. Daniel, L. Kilford, and A. J. Lees, "Accuracy of clinical diagnosis of idiopathic Parkinson's disease: a clinico-pathological study of 100 cases," *Journal of Neurology, Neurosurgery and Psychiatry*, vol. 55, no. 3, pp. 181–184, 1992.

[14] R Development Core Team, *R: A Language and Environment for Statistical Computing*, R Foundation for Statistical Computing, Vienna, Austria, 2008, http://www.R-project.org.

[15] A. J. Hughes, S. E. Daniel, Y. Ben-Shlomo, and A. J. Lees, "The accuracy of diagnosis of parkinsonian syndromes in a specialist movement disorder service," *Brain*, vol. 125, no. 4, pp. 861–870, 2002.

[16] Partnersinparkinsons.org, "Partners in Parkinson's Harris Poll: topline results," https://www.partnersinparkinsons.org/partners-in-parkinsons-news/partners-in-parkinsons-harris-poll-Topline-results, 2018.

[17] G. Rizzo, M. Copetti, S. Arcuti, D. Martino, A. Fontana, and G. Logroscino, "Accuracy of clinical diagnosis of Parkinson disease: a systematic review and meta-analysis," *Neurology*, vol. 86, no. 6, pp. 566–576, 2016.

[18] J. M. Bertoni, P. M. Sprenkle, D. Strickland, and N. Noedel, "Evaluation of Parkinson's disease in entrants on the Nebraska State Parkinson's Disease Registry," *Movement Disorders*, vol. 21, no. 10, pp. 1623–1626, 2006.

[19] E. R. Dorsey, J. D. Wagner, M. T. Bull et al., "Feasibility of virtual research visits in fox trial finder," *Journal of Parkinson's Disease*, vol. 5, no. 3, pp. 505–515, 2015.

[20] E. R. Dorsey and B. R. Bloem, "The Parkinson pandemic-A call to action," *JAMA Neurology*, vol. 75, no. 1, pp. 9-10, 2018.

Sensitivity and Specificity of the ECAS in Parkinson's Disease and Progressive Supranuclear Palsy

Jennifer A. Foley[ID],[1,2] Elaine H. Niven,[3] Andrew Paget,[1] Kailash P. Bhatia,[1,2]
Simon F. Farmer,[1,2] Paul R. Jarman,[1,2] Patricia Limousin,[1,2] Thomas T. Warner,[1,4]
Huw R. Morris[ID],[1,5] Thomas H. Bak[ID],[6,7,8] Sharon Abrahams,[6,7,8] and Lisa Cipolotti[ID][1,2,9]

[1]National Hospital for Neurology and Neurosurgery, Queen Square, London, UK
[2]UCL Institute of Neurology, Queen Square, London, UK
[3]School of Social Sciences (Psychology), University of Dundee, Dundee, UK
[4]Reta Lila Weston Institute of Neurological Studies, UCL Institute of Neurology, Queen Square, London, UK
[5]Department of Clinical Neuroscience, UCL Institute of Neurology, Queen Square, London, UK
[6]Human Cognitive Neuroscience–PPLS, University of Edinburgh, Edinburgh, UK
[7]Centre for Cognitive Ageing and Cognitive Epidemiology, University of Edinburgh, Edinburgh, UK
[8]Anne Rowling Regenerative Neurology Clinic, University of Edinburgh, Edinburgh, UK
[9]Dipartimento di Scienze Psicologiche, Pedagogiche e della Formazione, Università degli Studi di Palermo, Palermo, Italy

Correspondence should be addressed to Lisa Cipolotti; l.cipolotti@ucl.ac.uk

Academic Editor: Xiao-Ping Wang

Disentangling Parkinson's disease (PD) and progressive supranuclear palsy (PSP) may be a diagnostic challenge. Cognitive signs may be useful, but existing screens are often insufficiently sensitive or unsuitable for assessing people with motor disorders. We investigated whether the newly developed ECAS, designed to be used with people with even severe motor disability, was sensitive to the cognitive impairment seen in PD and PSP and able to distinguish between these two disorders. Thirty patients with PD, 11 patients with PSP, and 40 healthy controls were assessed using the ECAS, as well as an extensive neuropsychological assessment. The ECAS detected cognitive impairment in 30% of the PD patients, all of whom fulfilled the diagnostic criteria for mild cognitive impairment. The ECAS was also able to detect cognitive impairment in PSP patients, with 81.8% of patients performing in the impaired range. The ECAS total score distinguished between the patients with PSP and healthy controls with high sensitivity (91.0) and specificity (86.8). Importantly, the ECAS was also able to distinguish between the two syndromes, with the measures of verbal fluency offering high sensitivity (82.0) and specificity (80.0). In sum, the ECAS is a quick, simple, and inexpensive test that can be used to support the differential diagnosis of PSP.

1. Introduction

It has now been over 50 years since progressive supranuclear palsy (PSP) was first described as a progressive neurological disorder with motor, ocular, and cognitive features [1]. Clinically, it remains difficult to distinguish from Parkinson's disease (PD) [2, 3], particularly in the early stages [4]. Even when using agreed criteria, the accuracy of diagnosis is not 100% [5]. As it has a significantly worse prognosis than PD, with a more rapid progression [6], early detection is crucial for enabling access to appropriate interventions and

support, as well as identifying patients suitable for clinical trials. In the absence of any disease-specific biomarkers, there is a need for a quick, simple, and inexpensive test that can be used for the differential diagnosis of PSP.

Both PSP and PD are characterised by extrapyramidal syndromes, each of which can comprise symptoms of bradykinesia, rigidity, and/or postural instability [7]. Both disorders can feature eye movement abnormalities, and although the presence of the supranuclear vertical gaze palsy in PSP is diagnostically helpful, it is not universal [8, 9] and may be absent until quite late in the disease [10]. Although both disorders are thought to feature some similar cognitive signs, there is evidence to suggest that the specific cognitive profile may be a useful distinguishing feature [11].

Early cognitive impairment is a feature of PSP, which may precede the motor or ocular signs [12]. The profile is mainly that of executive dysfunction [13] and cognitive slowing [14], with markedly reduced verbal fluency [15, 16]. Deficits in other domains, including memory [17], language [18–20], visuospatial [16, 18], and social cognition [21–23], have also been reported.

In contrast, early stages of PD are characterised by only mild deficits in executive functions [24–27], but with illness progression, there is evolution from a mild cognitive impairment (MCI) to dementia, with greater involvement of posterior-based visual functions [28–30].

Existing screens of cognitive functioning can be criticised for being insufficiently sensitive to the cognitive profile of both PD and PSP. For example, the most widely used cognitive screen, the MMSE [31], has no measure of verbal fluency. Both the MMSE and the Addenbrooke's Cognitive Examination [32] have inadequate assessment of executive function. Their ensuing ceiling effects give them a low detection rate for cognitive impairment in Parkinsonian syndromes [33–35]. The Frontal Assessment Battery [36] does assess verbal fluency and executive function but has no measure of memory, language, or visuospatial function. Similarly, the Dementia Rating Scale (DRS) [37] has no measure of language or visuospatial function. This reliance upon the executive functions reduces its ability to discriminate PSP from PD [38] or frontotemporal syndromes [39]. The DRS also has a lengthy administration time and requires specialised testing materials, impractical for routine bedside use. The Montreal Cognitive Assessment [40] does have a measure of verbal fluency but does not accommodate for physical disability. Indeed, none of the existing assessments were designed specifically for people with movement disorders, such as Parkinsonian syndromes. Tasks involving speaking, writing, or drawing can be influenced by motor symptoms such as tremor, rigidity, bradykinesia, apraxia, or dysarthria; thus, a genuine cognitive impairment might be sometimes difficult to distinguish from motor dysfunction and performance decrements exaggerated by physical disability.

The ECAS [41] was recently developed as a brief assessment for the identification of cognitive and behavioural changes in disorders characterised by prominent motor symptoms, such as amyotrophic lateral sclerosis (ALS). It was developed to be used with patients with even severe physical disability and thus may be suitable for detecting cognitive impairment in all motor disorders. Many of the subtests can be performed either orally or manually, with some measures corrected for motor speed, reducing the impact that physical disability may have upon performance on cognitive tests [42]. It also allows the clinician to track cognitive impairment throughout the disease course, crucial for any longitudinal studies.

The ECAS has been standardised using a sample of healthy controls, providing normative data for clinical use [41]. It has also been validated against other screening tools

[43, 44] and extensive neuropsychological assessment [45]. It is available in English [41], German [46], Swiss German [46], Italian [44], and Chinese [47]. However, it remains untested whether the ECAS is also sensitive to the cognitive impairment observed in other progressive movement disorders. Thus, the aims of the present study were to determine firstly whether the ECAS is sensitive to the cognitive impairment seen in PD and PSP and secondly whether it is able to distinguish between these disorders, in order to support the differential diagnosis of PSP.

2. Methods

2.1. Participants. All patients were recruited from the National Hospital for Neurology and Neurosurgery, Queen Square, London. PSP patients (9 males and 2 females) were diagnosed using the NINDS-SPSP criteria [48] and had a mean illness duration of 3.73 years (range 1–11 years). PD patients (24 males and 6 females) fulfilled the Queen Square Brain Bank criteria for PD and had a mean illness duration of 5.67 years (range 0–14 years). All patients with PD-MCI were identified using the Movement Disorder Society Task Force guidelines [49], in which impairment (<2 SD) is present on at least two tests of cognitive functioning, either within or across different cognitive domains.

The healthy controls were those reported by Niven et al. [45]. They (26 males and 14 females) were recruited through the Psychology Department of the University of Edinburgh. No participant had significant neurological or psychiatric history.

The research was done in accordance with the Declaration of Helsinki and approved by the NRES Committee London-Queen Square and the University of Edinburgh's Department of Psychology Ethics Committee.

2.2. Measures. The ECAS is a 15–20-minute screen that includes assessment of the following domains: (1) fluency (free: words beginning with "S" and fixed: words beginning with "T" but with only four letters); (2) executive functions, separate from verbal fluency (Reverse Digit Span, Alternation, Inhibitory Sentence Completion, and Social Cognition); (3) language (Naming, Comprehension, and Spelling); (4) memory (Immediate Recall, Delayed Percentage Retention, and Delayed Recognition); and (5) visuospatial (Dot Counting, Cube Counting, and Number Location). Verbal fluency measures take into account the slowing of motor responses, by generating a verbal fluency index corrected for motor speed. Previously published ECAS normative data [41] were used to classify the abnormality of performance on each domain and calculate the total score out of a maximum of 136 (lower score indicating worse performance), with any scores <2 SD considered to be impaired.

Extensive neuropsychological testing was administered to assess the same domains (fluency, executive functions, language, memory, and visuospatial; Table 1). Mood was assessed using the Hospital Anxiety and Depression Scale [50], and patients were also assessed using the Apathy Scale [51].

Scores for the neuropsychological assessments were compared with published normative data. For each measure,

TABLE 1: Neuropsychological assessment.

Domain	Subdomain	Measures
Fluency		Phonemic verbal fluency index [42] (VFi): words beginning with "P" and "R"
Executive functions	Inhibition	Hayling Sentence Completion Test [52]: total unconnected errors (converted but not scaled); latency score (time taken to complete unconnected sentences minus time taken for connected sentences)
	Shifting and rule detection	Brixton Spatial Anticipation Test [52]: total number of errors
	Social	Reading the Mind in the Eyes–Revised [53]: total number of correct ones
Language	Naming	Graded Naming Test [54]
	Spelling	Graded Difficulty Spelling Test [55]
Memory		Adult Memory and Information Processing Battery [56]: immediate story recall; delayed story recall
Visuospatial		The Visual Object and Space Perception Battery [57]: cube analysis; number location

TABLE 2: Demographics of the participants.

	PSP patients		PD patients		Controls	
	Mean (SD)	Range	Mean (SD)	Range	Mean (SD)	Range
Age	66.82 (7.08)	53–77	63.33 (7.89)	50–80	62.70 (10.48)	39–88
Duration of symptoms (years)	3.73 (3.20)	1–11	5.67 (3.47)	0–14	—	—
Gender (female)	2	—	6	—	14	—
Education, mean years (SD)	15.27 (4.98)	10–26	14.33 (3.22)	9–23	12.25 (3.39)	9–25
HADS Depression	8.50 (5.50)	1–15	6.77 (4.39)	0–16	2.40 (1.81)	0–6
HADS Anxiety	8.50 (5.79)	2–17	9.17 (4.13)	3–18	4.83 (2.75)	0–11
Apathy	17.67 (12.04)	4–34	15.90 (10.26)	4–42	—	—

HADS: Hospital Anxiety and Depression Scale.

patients were judged to be impaired if scores were ≤ 2 SD. In the case where multiple measures were used, performance was classified as impaired when ≤ 2 SD on one of the two or two of the three measures was used.

2.3. Statistical Analyses. Data were analysed using SPSS v.19. Between-group comparisons were made using analyses of variance, and Pearson's and Spearman's correlations were used to detail the relationships between measures. Receiver operating characteristic (ROC) curve analyses were used to determine the relative sensitivity and specificity of the ECAS for the two patient groups.

3. Results

3.1. Demographics. Demographic details are given in Table 2. There were no significant group differences in age or education, and patients did not differ in symptom duration. There were significant group effects found for both HADS Anxiety (F (2, 75) = 13.04; $p < 0.001$) and Depression (F (2, 77) = 19.03; $p < 0.001$), with post hoc analysis revealing that patients had significantly higher burden of symptoms than healthy controls but no significant group difference between patient groups. There was no significant group difference in apathy scores between patient groups.

3.2. Performance on the ECAS. There was a significant effect of diagnosis on ECAS performance (Table 3). PSP patients had significantly lower total scores than PD patients and healthy controls, and PD patients had significantly lower

total scores than healthy controls (all $p < 0.017$). There was a significant effect of diagnosis on all domains, except visuospatial. PSP patients performed worse than PD patients and healthy controls on fluency, language, executive function, and memory (all $p < 0.017$). PD patients performed worse than healthy controls on executive function only ($p < 0.017$).

When compared to published normative data, 81.8% ($n = 9$) of the PSP patients and 30.0% of the PD patients ($n = 9$) were impaired on the ECAS. PSP patients demonstrated most frequent impairments in fluency, language, and memory (each $n = 7$; 63.6%) and then executive function ($n = 6$; 54.5%) and visuospatial ($n = 3$; 27.3%). PD patients demonstrated most frequent impairments in language ($n = 9$; 30.0%), executive function and memory (each $n = 8$; 26.7%), and then fluency and visuospatial (each $n = 5$; 16.7%). There were no significant correlations between duration of symptoms and ECAS scores in either patient groups.

In order to investigate the specific nature of the impairment in both patient groups, individual domains were further investigated. In fluency, post hoc comparisons revealed a significant effect of diagnosis on both free fluency (F (2, 23.16) = 15.19; $p < 0.017$) and fixed fluency (F (2, 21.63) = 8.30; $p < 0.017$), with PSP patients performing worse than PD patients and healthy controls (all $p < 0.017$), but with no significant differences between PD patients and healthy controls. In language, there was a significant group effect on spelling (F (2, 76) = 10.58; $p < 0.017$), with PSP patients performing worse than PD

TABLE 3: ECAS scores of the participants.

	PSP patients		PD patients		Controls		F (df)	p
	Mean (SD)	Range	Mean (SD)	Range	Mean (SD)	Range		
Total (max. 136)	85.09 (24.46)	54–126	109.87 (13.52)	78–126	120.61 (7.06)	100–132	17.44 (2, 22.09)[a]	<0.001
Executive function (max. 48)	29.27 (13.27)	9–46	36.93 (6.05)	19–44	42.11 (3.49)	33–48	12.56 (2, 22.22)[a]	<0.001
Language (max. 28)	23.18 (5.06)	15–28	26.67 (2.11)	19–28	27.50 (0.80)	25–28	5.76 (2, 21.01)[a]	<0.001
Fluency (max. 24)	8.18 (8.74)	0–22	18.73 (4.83)	6–24	20.74 (2.39)	12–24	12.37 (2, 21.91)[a]	<0.001
Memory (max. 24)	10.27 (6.90)	0–20	15.67 (4.25)	3–22	18.39 (2.53)	13–23	10.85 (2, 22.76)[a]	<0.001
Visuospatial (max. 12)	11.09 (1.87)	6–12	11.47 (1.04)	8–12	11.87 (0.67)	8–12	2.33 (2, 22.86)[a]	0.066

[a]Welch's adjusted F ratio.

TABLE 4: Neuropsychological assessment performance of participants.

		PSP patients		PD patients		Healthy controls		F (df)	p	Post hoc
		Mean (SD)	Range	Mean (SD)	Range	Mean (SD)	Range			
Fluency	"P" VFi	10.90 (6.30)	2.37–19.67	4.13 (2.98)	0.96–14.50	3.68 (1.96)	1.52–9.33	22.65 (2.78)	<0.001	PSP < PD
	"R" VFi	14.16 (13.16)	2.50–41.00	4.12 (2.11)	2.00–9.50	3.65 (1.73)	1.72–9.33	22.37 (2.76)	<0.001	PSP < PD
Executive function	Hayling: B–A time	69.14 (86.55)	5–251	33.00 (28.04)	−3 to 126	34.88 (28.96)	−5 to 121	2.88 (2.73)	0.06	
	Hayling: errors	6.57 (5.56)	0–14	5.17 (5.89)	0–29	8.75 (9.17)	0–32	1.80 (2.73)	0.17	
	Brixton	38.43 (3.21)	35–43	34.54 (9.71)	16–50	35.08 (8.23)	15–47	0.59 (2.70)	0.56	
	Reading the Mind in the Eyes	20.50 (5.43)	14–29	23.93 (5.06)	13–35	26.35 (3.81)	17–34	5.72 (2.71)	<0.01	PSP < HC
Language	Graded Naming Test	20.64 (5.85)	9–26	23.20 (3.61)	13–29	24.15 (6.64)	14–57	1.71 (2.78)	0.19	
	Graded Difficulty Spelling Test	19.64 (8.44)	2–29	22.29 (6.01)	7–30	22.53 (4.50)	12–29	1.15 (2.76)	0.32	
Memory	Immediate Story Recall	24.45 (14.20)	0–41	27.04 (9.73)	7–49					
	Delayed Story Recall	23.64 (15.54)	0–40	25.46 (9.61)	7–46					
	Retention	80.16 (32.96)	0–111.11	93.92 (14.75)	62.50–136.00	94.49 (12.74)	58.82–12.27	3.12 (2.77)	0.05	
Visuospatial	Cube Analysis	8.91 (1.58)	6–10	8.83 (1.62)	5–10	9.63 (0.87)	5–10	23.61 (2.78)	<0.05	PSP < HC
	Number Location	8.45 (2.46)	2–10	9.20 (1.00)	7–10	9.43 (0.71)	7–10	2.90 (2.78)	0.06	

VFi: Verbal Fluency Index.

patients and healthy controls (both $p < 0.017$), but with no significant difference between PD patients and healthy controls. In memory, there was a significant group effect on immediate recall (F (2, 24.04) = 11.47; $p < 0.017$) and retention (F (2, 20.69) = 8.92; $p < 0.017$), but not recognition. PSP patients performed significantly worse than PD patients and healthy controls on both of these (both $p < 0.017$), but with no significant difference between PD patients and healthy controls. In executive functions, there were significant group effects on reverse digit span (F (2, 25.96) = 7.60; $p < 0.017$), alternation (F (2, 22.92) = 5.66; $p < 0.017$), and social cognition (F (2, 20.42) = 9.49; $p < 0.017$). Both PSP and PD patients performed significantly worse than healthy controls on reverse digit span and social cognition (all $p < 0.017$), but with no significant differences between patient

groups. PSP patients performed significantly worse than PD patients and healthy controls on alternation ($p < 0.017$), but with no significant difference between PD patients and healthy controls.

3.3. Performance on Full Neuropsychological Assessment. Upon full neuropsychological assessment, there was a significant effect of diagnosis on fluency, executive function, and visuospatial domains (Table 4). Specifically, there were significant group differences on both measures of fluency, with PSP patients performing worse than PD patients and healthy controls. There were no significant differences between PD patients and healthy controls. In addition, PSP patients performed worse than healthy controls on the

Reading the Mind in the Eyes Test and Cube Analysis, but with no significant differences between PSP and PD patients, or between PD patients and healthy controls.

When scores on each of the neuropsychological assessments were compared with published normative data, there was a significant group difference in incidence of impairment in one domain only: fluency (χ^2 (1) = 7.61; $p < 0.001$). Nine of the 11 PSP patients (81.8%) were classified as impaired on at least one measure of verbal fluency, in comparison with only 33.3% ($n = 10$) of the 30 PD patients.

3.4. Diagnostic Accuracy of the ECAS for Cognitive Impairment in PD. Within the PD patients, a total of 17 (56.67%) met the criteria for PD-MCI. When PD and PD-MCI groups were compared, there were no significant differences in age, education, or symptom duration. However, on the ECAS, the PD-MCI group had significantly lower total scores (t (20.25) = 5.14; $p < 0.001$) and performed worse on executive function (t (23.83) = 3.02; $p < 0.01$), verbal fluency (t (22.52) = 3.26; $p < 0.01$), memory (t (28) = 3.09; $p < 0.01$), and visuospatial subscales (t (16.00) = 3.11; $p < 0.01$). On full neuropsychological assessment, the PD-MCI group also performed significantly worse on the Brixton Test (t (24) = 3.81; $p < 0.001$), Reading the Mind in the Eyes Test (t (26) = 2.75; $p < 0.05$), Graded Naming Test (t (28) = 4.32; $p < 0.001$), and Cube Analysis (t (20.69) = 2.801; $p < 0.05$).

ROC curve analysis revealed that the total score of the ECAS is able to discriminate between PD and PD-MCI with high sensitivity (88.2%) and 100% specificity, when using a threshold score of 112.50/136. The AUC is 0.93 (SE = 0.06; $p < 0.001$). Confidence intervals are 0.81 (lower bound) and 1.00 (upper bound). Indeed, all PD patients who performed in the impaired range on the ECAS fulfilled the diagnostic criteria for PD-MCI.

3.5. Diagnostic Accuracy of the ECAS for PSP. ROC curve analysis also revealed that the ECAS is highly specific (86.8%) and sensitive (91.0%) when discriminating PSP patients from healthy controls using a threshold score of 113.50/136. The AUC is 0.91 (SE = 0.67; $p < 0.001$). Confidence intervals are 0.79 (lower bound) and 1.00 (upper bound). All PSP patients who performed in the impaired range on the ECAS demonstrated impairment upon full neuropsychological testing, including impairment on at least one measure of verbal fluency.

3.6. Diagnostic Accuracy of the ECAS for Distinguishing between PD and PSP. The second aim of the study was to determine whether the ECAS is able to distinguish between PD and PSP, in order to support the early and accurate diagnosis of PSP. ROC curve analysis showed that the measure is able to discriminate between PD and PSP (when comparing all patients, irrespective of cognitive performance), with high specificity (76.7%) and sensitivity (72.7%), using a threshold score of 103.50/136 (Figure 1). The AUC is 0.80 (SE = 0.09; $p < 0.01$). Confidence intervals are 0.62 (lower bound) and 0.98 (upper bound). This

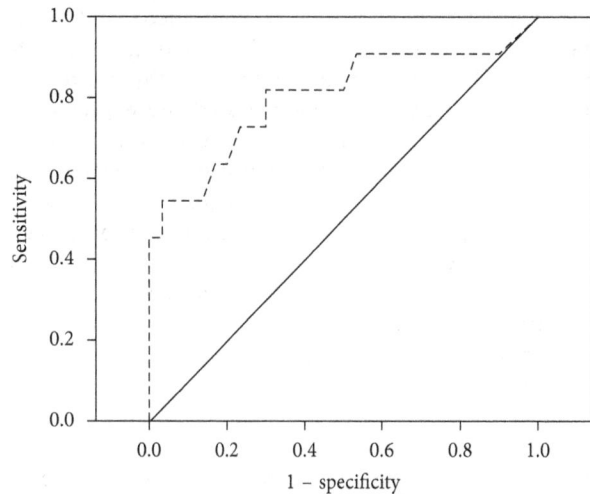

FIGURE 1: ROC curve depicting sensitivity and specificity of the ECAS, when comparing the PD and PSP patients (higher sensitivity scores indicate lower performance).

generated three false negatives and seven false positives. The false positives were all patients who fulfilled the criteria for PD-MCI.

Within the ECAS, fluency was the best predictor of PSP, with high specificity (80.0%) and sensitivity (82.0%) using a threshold score of 17/24. The AUC is 0.84 (SE = 0.08; $p < 0.01$). Confidence intervals are 0.69 (lower bound) and 1.00 (upper bound). This generated two false negatives and six false positives (five PD-MCI and one PD). This is in contrast to when using the raw number of words generated in the two fluency tasks as a predictor, which has lower sensitivity (77.8%) and specificity (79.2%) when using a threshold score of 17.5.

4. Discussion

Our study has shown that the ECAS is sensitive to the cognitive impairment seen in PD. We found that 30% of PD patients were impaired on the ECAS, all of whom also demonstrated impairments upon full neuropsychological testing and fulfilled the criteria for PD-MCI. Indeed, ROC curve analyses revealed that the ECAS has excellent sensitivity and complete specificity for detection of PD-MCI. On the ECAS, PD patients demonstrated impairments in a number of domains but performed significantly worse than healthy controls on one domain only: executive function. PD-MCI patients also demonstrated deficits in language and visuospatial functioning. These findings confirm the greater involvement of posterior functions with more advanced Parkinson's disease [30] but also suggest that the pattern of impairment can be fairly heterogeneous, even involving language. This is in accordance with the findings of the MDS Task Force [49], who also report impairments in a range of cognitive domains, including language.

Our data also show that the ECAS is sensitive to the cognitive impairment in PSP. We found that 81.8% of PSP patients were impaired on both the ECAS and full neuropsychological testing, including at least one measure of fluency. Again, ROC curve analyses confirmed that the ECAS total score gave excellent sensitivity and specificity for detection of PSP when compared with healthy controls. On the ECAS, PSP patients demonstrated the expected impairment in fluency, but also executive function, memory, and language. On extensive neuropsychological testing, PSP patients demonstrated impairments in fluency as well as executive function and visuospatial. The prominence of fluency and executive impairment on both the ECAS and full neuropsychological testing is in accordance with previous descriptions [13, 15, 16, 28], confirming that the ECAS is sensitive to the typical profile of cognitive impairment in PSP.

Importantly, we also found that the ECAS was able to distinguish between PD and PSP. ROC curve analysis revealed that the ECAS total score was sensitive and specific to PSP, with verbal fluency being the best discriminator. The ECAS was able to identify all PSP cases demonstrating cognitive impairment upon full testing. The few false positives mostly reflected PD patients with advanced cognitive impairment.

The strikingly reduced verbal fluency found on the ECAS and full testing confirms this as the cognitive hallmark of PSP. Importantly, the ECAS revealed this marked deficit even after accounting for the slowed motor speed. This contrasts with impairments in other cognitive domains, such as memory, which can improve by up to 50% given sufficient extra time [58, 59]. This impoverished verbal fluency, alongside the frequent family reports of reduced spontaneous speech and conversation initiation, likely reflects a cognitive adynamia beyond that of simple bradyphrenia but rather a more significant impairment in the generation of a "fluent sequence of novel thought" [19, 60]. This may reflect a deficit in novel thought generation and/or its appropriate sequencing [61]. Indeed, it has been argued that the akinesia in motor abilities, reduction of verbal fluency in cognition, and apathy in behaviour are all different manifestations of the same underlying disorder [62].

PSP patients also demonstrated impairments in other domains, which supports the findings of previous studies. In accordance with previous reports of poor delayed recall [17], our PSP patients displayed impaired verbal recall on the ECAS, with three of the seven PSP patients impaired on both the ECAS and full testing. Our patients also demonstrated language impairment, reflecting spelling difficulties, in accordance with previous studies [20, 63, 64]. Spelling was more impaired on the ECAS, perhaps because its spelling test comprises nouns, verbs, and compounds of low-to-medium frequency, with a longer mean length. In contrast, the spelling test used upon full testing contained mostly nouns of high-to-low frequency, with a shorter mean length. Our patients also demonstrated impaired visuospatial function, which supports previous findings [16, 18]. Nearly a third of PSP patients were impaired on the ECAS, with all of these also impaired upon full testing.

The PD and PSP patients both performed poorly on measures of social cognition. These findings echo previous reports of impaired performance on tests of theory of mind and social norms [22, 44, 65–67].

5. Conclusions

The ECAS captures the core cognitive deficit of reduced verbal fluency, as well as the wider cognitive profile of PSP. This may allow longitudinal testing to track progression as verbal fluency reaches floor. It was possible to use the ECAS with all the patients who took part in this study, despite often severe motor symptoms, indicating that it would be well tolerated in those with advanced disease. This suggests that the ECAS is suited for bedside use for detecting cognitive impairment in Parkinsonian syndromes and for distinguishing different cognitive profiles within these, in order to support differential diagnosis. Full neuropsychological assessment can then be used to further elucidate the specific clinical profile of each patient. Future research should examine its sensitivity for detecting cognitive impairment in other progressive movement disorders.

Acknowledgments

The authors thank Dr. Francisco Musich for his assistance with data collection. Part of this research was supported by an award from the Motor Neurone Disease Association (Sharon Abrahams/Apr11/6070). The study sponsor funded the testing of the control participants, as part of a larger study investigating the use of the ECAS in ALS.

References

[1] J. C. Steele, J. C. Richardson, and J. Olszewski, "Progressive supranuclear palsy," *Archives of Neurology*, vol. 10, no. 4, pp. 333–359, 1964.

[2] T. H. Bak and J. R. Hodges, "The neuropsychology of progressive supranuclear palsy," *Neurocase*, vol. 4, no. 2, pp. 89–94, 1998.

[3] I. Litvan, Y. Agid, J. Jankovic et al., "Accuracy of clinical criteria for the diagnosis of progressive supranuclear palsy (Steele-Richardson-Olszewski syndrome)," *Neurology*, vol. 46, no. 4, pp. 922–930, 1996.

[4] R. George, V. Krishnan, B. Mohan, and P. Maniyar, "Parkinson's disease and early stages of progressive supranuclear palsy: a neurological mimicry," *Journal of Case Reports*, vol. 5, pp. 377–381, 2015.

[5] A. J. Hughes, S. E. Daniel, Y. Ben-Shlomo, and A. J. Lees, "The accuracy of diagnosis of parkinsonian syndromes in a specialist movement disorder service," *Brain*, vol. 125, no. 4, pp. 861–870, 2002.

[6] S. S. O'Sullivan, L. A. Massey, D. R. Williams et al., "Clinical outcomes of progressive supranculear palsy and multiple system atrophy," *Brain*, vol. 131, no. 5, pp. 1362–1372, 2008.

[7] D. R. Willams and A. J. Lees, "Progressive supranuclear palsy: clinicopathological concepts and diagnostic challenges," *Lancet Neurology*, vol. 8, no. 3, pp. 270–279, 2010.

[8] I. Litvan, D. A. Grimes, A. E. Lang et al., "Clinical features differentiating patients with post-mortem confirmed progressive supranuclear palsy and corticobasal degeneration," *Journal of Neurology*, vol. 246, pp. II1–II5, 1999.

[9] E. H. Pinkhardt, R. Jurgens, W. Becker, F. Valdarno, A. C. Ludolph, and J. Kassubek, "Differential diagnostic value of eye movement recording in PSP-parkinsonism, Richardson's syndrome, and idiopathic Parkinson's disease," *Journal of Neurology*, vol. 255, no. 12, pp. 1916–1925, 2008.

[10] D. R. Williams, R. de Silva, D. C. Paviour et al., "Characteristics of two distinct clinical phenotypes in pathologically proven progressive supranuclear palsy: Richardson's syndrome and PSP-parkinsonism," *Brain*, vol. 128, no. 6, pp. 1247–1258, 2005.

[11] R. G. Brown, L. Lacomblez, B. G. Landwehrmeyer et al., "Cognitive impairment in patients with multiple system atrophy and progressive supranuclear palsy," *Brain*, vol. 133, no. 8, pp. 2382–2393, 2010.

[12] L. Donker Kaat, A. J. W. Boon, W. Kamphorst, R. Ravid, H. J. Duivenvoorden, and J. C. van Swieten, "Frontal presentation in progressive supranuclear palsy," *Neurology*, vol. 69, no. 8, pp. 723–729, 2007.

[13] B. Pillon, B. Dubois, A. Ploska, and Y. Agid, "Severity and specificity of cognitive impairment in Alzheimer's, Huntington's and Parkinson's diseases and progressive supranuclear palsy," *Neurology*, vol. 41, no. 5, pp. 634–643, 1991.

[14] B. Dubois, B. Pillon, F. Legault, Y. Agid, and F. Lhermitte, "Slowing of cognitive processing in progressive supranuclear palsy: a comparison with Parkinson's disease," *Archives of Neurology*, vol. 45, no. 11, pp. 1194–1199, 1998.

[15] T. H. Bak, L. M. Crawford, V. C. Hearn, P. S. Mathuranath, and J. R. Hodges, "Subcortical dementia revisited: similarities and differences in cognitive function between progressive supranuclear palsy (PSP), corticobasal degeneration (CBD) and multiple system atrophy (MSA)," *Neurocase*, vol. 11, no. 4, pp. 268–273, 2005.

[16] T. Rittman, B. C. Ghosh, P. McColgan et al., "The Addenbrooke's Cognitive Examination for the differential diagnosis and longitudinal assessment of patients with parkinsonian disorders," *Journal of Neurology, Neurosurgery, and Psychiatry*, vol. 84, no. 5, pp. 544–551, 2013.

[17] M. Zarei, H. R. Pouretemad, T. Bak, and J. R. Hodges, "Autobiographical memory in progressive supranuclear palsy," *European Journal of Neurology*, vol. 17, no. 2, pp. 238–241, 2010.

[18] T. H. Bak, D. Caine, V. C. Hearn, and J. R. Hodges, "Visuospatial functions in atypical parkinsonian syndromes," *Journal of Neurology, Neurosurgery, and Psychiatry*, vol. 77, no. 4, pp. 454–456, 2006.

[19] G. Robinson, T. Shallice, and L. Cipolotti, "Dynamic aphasia in progressive supranuclear palsy: a deficit in generating a fluent sequence of novel thought," *Neuropsychologia*, vol. 44, no. 8, pp. 1344–1360, 2006.

[20] J. D. Rohrer, D. Paviour, A. M. Bronstein, S. S. O'Sullivan, A. Lees, and J. D. Warren, "Progressive supranuclear palsy syndrome presenting as progressive nonfluent aphasia: a neuropsychological and neuroimaging analysis," *Movement Disorders*, vol. 25, no. 2, pp. 179–188, 2010.

[21] B. C. P. Ghosh, J. B. Rowe, A. J. Calder, J. R. Hodges, and T. H. Bak, "Emotion recognition in progressive supranuclear palsy," *Journal of Neurology, Neurosurgery, and Psychiatry*, vol. 80, no. 10, pp. 1143–1145, 2009.

[22] B. C. P. Ghosh, A. J. Calder, P. V. Peers et al., "Social cognitive deficits and their neural correlates in progressive supranuclear palsy," *Brain*, vol. 135, no. 7, pp. 2089–2102, 2012.

[23] F. M. O'Keefe, B. Murray, R. F. Coen et al., "Loss of insight in frontotemporal dementia, corticobasal degeneration and progressive supranuclear palsy," *Brain*, vol. 130, no. 3, pp. 753–764, 2007.

[24] R. Cools, E. Stefanova, R. A. Barker, T. W. Robbins, and A. M. Owen, "Dopaminergic modulation of high-level cognition in Parkinson's disease: the role of the prefrontal cortex revealed by PET," *Brain*, vol. 125, no. 3, pp. 584–594, 2002.

[25] J. D. E. Gabrieli, J. Singh, G. T. Stebbins, and C. G. Goetz, "Reduced working memory span in Parkinson's disease: evidence for the role of frontostriatal system in working and strategic memory," *Neuropsychology*, vol. 10, no. 3, pp. 322–332, 1996.

[26] A. McKinlay, R. C. Grace, J. C. Dalrymple-Alford, and D. Roger, "Characteristics of executive function impairment in Parkinson's disease patients without dementia," *Journal of the International Neuropsychological Society*, vol. 16, no. 2, pp. 268–277, 2010.

[27] J. Uekermann, I. Daum, M. Bielawski et al., "Differential executive control impairments in early Parkinson's disease," in *Journal of Neural Transmission. Supplementa*, T. Müller and P. Riederer, Eds., pp. 39–51, Springer, Berlin, Germany, 2004.

[28] R. Brown and C. D. Marsden, "Visuospatial function in Parkinson's disease," *Brain*, vol. 109, no. 5, pp. 987–1002, 1986.

[29] R. S. Weil, A. E. Schrag, J. D. Warren, S. J. Crutch, A. J. Lees, and H. R. Morris, "Visual dysfunction in Parkinson's disease," *Brain*, vol. 139, no. 11, pp. 2827–2843, 2016.

[30] C. H. Williams-Gray, T. Foltynie, C. E. G. Brayne, T. W. Robbins, and R. A. Barker, "Evolution of cognitive dysfunction in an incident Parkinson's disease cohort," *Brain*, vol. 130, no. 7, pp. 1787–1798, 2007.

[31] M. F. Folstein, S. E. Folstein, and P. R. McHugh, ""Mini-mental state": a practical method for grading the cognitive state of patients for the clinician," *Journal of Psychiatric Research*, vol. 12, no. 3, pp. 189–198, 1975.

[32] E. Mioshi, K. Dawson, J. Mitchell, R. Arnold, and J. R. Hodges, "The Addenbrooke's Cognitive Examination Revised (ACE-R): a brief cognitive test battery for dementia screening," *International Journal of Geriatric Psychiatry*, vol. 21, no. 11, pp. 1078–1085, 2006.

[33] T. H. Bak, T. T. Rogers, L. M. Crawford, V. C. Hearn, P. S. Mathuranath, and J. R. Hodges, "Cognitive bedside assessment in atypical parkinsonian syndromes," *Journal of Neurology, Neurosurgery, and Psychiatry*, vol. 76, no. 3, pp. 420–422, 2005.

[34] E. Fiorenzato, L. Weis, C. Falup-Pecurariu et al., "Montreal Cognitive Assessment (MoCA) and Mini-Mental State Examination (MMSE) performance in progressive supranuclear palsy and multiple system atrophy," *Journal of Neural Transmission*, vol. 123, no. 12, pp. 1435–1442, 2016.

[35] T. H. Bak and E. Mioshi, "A cognitive bedside assessment beyond the MMSE: the Addenbrooke's Cognitive Examination," *Practical Neurology*, vol. 7, pp. 245–249, 2007.

[36] B. Dubois, A. Slachevsky, I. Litvan, and B. Pillon, "The FAB: a Frontal Assessment Battery at bedside," *Neurology*, vol. 55, no. 11, pp. 1621–1626, 2000.

[37] S. Mattis, *Dementia Rating Scale (DRS)*, Psychological Assessment Resources, Lutz, FL, USA, 1998.

[38] J. Kulisevsky and J. Pagonabarraga, "Cognitive impairment in Parkinson's disease: tools for diagnosis and assessment," *Movement Disorders*, vol. 24, no. 8, pp. 1103–1110, 2009.

[39] M. Stamelou, J. Diehl-Schmid, A. Hapfelmeier et al., "The frontal assessment battery is not useful to discriminate progressive supranuclear palsy from frontotemporal dementias," *Parkinsonism and Related Disorders*, vol. 21, no. 10, pp. 1264–1268, 2015.

[40] Z. S. Nasreddine, N. A. Phillips, V. Bedirian et al., "The Montreal Cognitive Assessment, MoCA: a brief screening tool

for mild cognitive impairment," *Journal of the American Geriatrics Society*, vol. 53, no. 4, pp. 696–699, 2005.

[41] S. Abrahams, J. Newton, E. Niven, J. Foley, and T. H. Bak, "Screening for cognition and behaviour changes in ALS," *Amyotrophic Lateral Sclerosis and Frontotemporal Degeneration*, vol. 15, no. 1-2, pp. 9–14, 2014.

[42] S. Abrahams, P. N. Leigh, A. Harvey, G. N. Vythelingum, D. Grise, and L. H. Goldstein, "Verbal fluency and executive dysfunction in amyotrophic lateral sclerosis (ALS)," *Neuropsychologia*, vol. 38, no. 6, pp. 734–747, 2000.

[43] D. Lulé, C. Burkhardt, S. Abdulla et al., "The Edinburgh Cognitive and Behavioural Amyotrophic Lateral Sclerosis Screen: a cross-sectional comparison of established screening tools in a German-Swiss population," *Amyotrophic Lateral Sclerosis and Frontotemporal Degeneration*, vol. 16, no. 1-2, pp. 16–23, 2015.

[44] B. Poletti, F. Solca, L. Carelli et al., "The validation of the Italian Edinburgh Cognitive and Behavioural ALS Screen (ECAS)," *Amyotrophic Lateral Sclerosis and Frontotemporal Degeneration*, vol. 17, no. 7-8, pp. 489–498, 2016.

[45] E. Niven, J. Newton, J. Foley et al., "Validation of the Edinburgh Cognitive and Behavioural Amyotrophic Lateral Sclerosis Screen (ECAS): a cognitive tool for motor disorders," *Amyotrophic Lateral Sclerosis and Frontotemporal Degeneration*, vol. 16, no. 3-4, pp. 172–179, 2015.

[46] M. Loose, C. Burkhardt, H. Aho-Özhan et al., "Age and education-matched cut-off scores for the revised German/Swiss-German version of ECAS," *Amyotrophic Lateral Sclerosis and Frontotemporal Degeneration*, vol. 17, no. 5-6, pp. 374–376, 2016.

[47] S. Ye, Y. Ji, C. Li, J. He, X. Liu, and F. Dongsheng, "The Edinburgh Cognitive and Behavioural ALS Screen in a Chinese amyotrophic lateral sclerosis population," *PLoS One*, vol. 11, no. 5, article e0155496, 2016.

[48] I. Litvan, Y. Agid, and D. Calne, "Clinical research criteria for the diagnosis of progressive supranuclear palsy (Steele-Richardson-Olszewski syndrome): Report of the NINDS-SPSP International Workshop," *Neurology*, vol. 47, no. 1, pp. 1–9, 1996.

[49] I. Litvan, J. G. Goldman, A. I. Tröster et al., "Diagnostic criteria for mild cognitive impairment in Parkinson's disease: Movement Disorder Society Task Force guidelines," *Movement Disorders*, vol. 27, no. 3, pp. 349–356, 2012.

[50] A. S. Zigmond and R. P. Snaith, "The hospital anxiety and depression scale," *Acta Psychiatrica Scandinavica*, vol. 67, no. 6, pp. 361–370, 1983.

[51] R. S. Marin, R. C. Biedrzycki, and S. Firinciogullari, "Reliability and validity of the apathy evaluation scale," *Psychiatry Research*, vol. 38, no. 2, pp. 143–162, 1991.

[52] P. W. Burgess and T. Shallice, *The Hayling and Brixton Tests*, Thames Valley Test Company, Bury St Edmunds, UK, 1997.

[53] S. Baron-Cohen, S. Wheelwright, J. Hill, Y. Raste, and I. Plumb, "The "Reading the Mind in the Eyes" Test Revised Version: a study with normal adults, and adults with Asperger syndrome or high-functioning autism," *Journal of Child Psychology and Psychiatry*, vol. 42, no. 2, pp. 241–251, 2001.

[54] P. McKenna and E. K. Warrington, *Graded Naming Test*, NFER-Nelson, London, UK, 1983.

[55] D. M. Baxter and E. K. Warrington, "Measuring dysgraphia: a graded-difficulty spelling test," *Behavioural Neurology*, vol. 7, no. 3-4, pp. 107–116, 1994.

[56] A. K. Coughlan and S. E. Hollows, *The Adult's Memory and Information Processing Battery*, St James' University Hospital, Leeds, UK, 1985.

[57] E. K. Warrington and M. James, *The Visual Object and Space Perception Battery*, Thames Valley Test Company, Bury St Edmunds, UK, 1991.

[58] M. L. Albert, R. G. Feldman, and A. L. Willis, "The subcortical dementia of progressive supranuclear palsy," *Journal of Neurology, Neurosurgery, and Psychiatry*, vol. 37, no. 2, pp. 121–130, 1974.

[59] A. Kertesz and P. McMonagle, "Behavior and cognition in corticobasal degeneration and progressive supranuclear palsy," *Journal of the Neurological Sciences*, vol. 289, no. 1-2, pp. 138–143, 2010.

[60] G. A. Robinson, D. Spooner, and W. J. Harrison, "Frontal dynamic aphasia in progressive supranuclear palsy: distinguishing between generation and fluent sequencing of novel thoughts," *Neuropsychologia*, vol. 77, pp. 62–75, 2015.

[61] G. A. Robinson, "Primary progressive dynamic aphasia and Parkinsonism: generation, selection and sequencing deficits," *Neuropsychologia*, vol. 51, no. 13, pp. 2534–2547, 2013.

[62] T. H. Bak, "Movement disorders: why movement and cognition belong together," *Nature Reviews Neurology*, vol. 7, no. 1, pp. 10–12, 2011.

[63] B. Boeve, D. Dickson, J. Duffy, J. Bartleson, M. Trenerry, and R. Petersen, "Progressive nonfluent aphasia and subsequent aphasic dementia associated with atypical progressive supranuclear palsy pathology," *European Neurology*, vol. 49, no. 2, pp. 72–78, 2003.

[64] K. A. Josephs and J. R. Duffy, "Apraxia of speech and non-fluent aphasia: a new clinical marker for corticobasal degeneration and progressive supranuclear palsy," *Current Opinion in Neurology*, vol. 21, no. 6, pp. 688–692, 2008.

[65] M. E. Bodden, R. Dodel, and E. Kalbe, "Theory of mind in Parkinson's disease and related basal ganglia disorders: a systematic review," *Movement Disorders*, vol. 25, no. 1, pp. 13–27, 2010.

[66] A. Halpin, K. Rascovsky, L. Massimo, D. Irwin, C. McMillan, and M. Grossman, "Evidence of social norm deficits in progressive supranuclear palsy," *Neurology*, vol. 86, no. 16, pp. P5–194, 2016.

[67] M. Roca, T. Torralva, E. Gleichgerrcht et al., "Impairments in social cognition in early medicated and unmedicated Parkinson disease," *Cognitive and Behavioural Neurology*, vol. 23, no. 3, pp. 152–158, 2010.

7

Insights into the Mechanisms Involved in Protective Effects of VEGF-B in Dopaminergic Neurons

Beatrice Caballero,[1,2] Scott J. Sherman,[1] and Torsten Falk[1,3]

[1]*Department of Neurology, College of Medicine, University of Arizona, Tucson, AZ 85724, USA*
[2]*Department of Cellular and Molecular Medicine, College of Medicine, University of Arizona, Tucson, AZ 85724, USA*
[3]*Department of Pharmacology, College of Medicine, University of Arizona, Tucson, AZ 85724, USA*

Correspondence should be addressed to Torsten Falk; tfalk@u.arizona.edu

Academic Editor: Antonio Pisani

Vascular endothelial growth factor-B (VEGF-B), when initially discovered, was thought to be an angiogenic factor, due to its intimate sequence homology and receptor binding similarity to the prototype angiogenic factor, vascular endothelial growth factor-A (VEGF-A). Studies demonstrated that VEGF-B, unlike VEGF-A, did not play a significant role in angiogenesis or vascular permeability and has become an active area of interest because of its role as a survival factor in pathological processes in a multitude of systems, including the brain. By characterization of important downstream targets of VEGF-B that regulate different cellular processes in the nervous system and cardiovascular system, it may be possible to develop more effective clinical interventions in diseases such as Parkinson's disease (PD), Amyotrophic Lateral Sclerosis (ALS), and ischemic heart disease, which all share mitochondrial dysfunction as part of the disease. Here we summarize what is currently known about the mechanism of action of VEGF-B in pathological processes. We explore its potential as a homeostatic protective factor that improves mitochondrial function in the setting of cardiovascular and neurological disease, with a specific focus on dopaminergic neurons in Parkinson's disease.

1. Introduction

Parkinson's disease (PD) is a progressive neurodegenerative disease affecting approximately 1.5 million people in the United States. This disease involves the loss of neurons of the substantia nigra pars compacta (SNpc), as well as the loss of dopaminergic nerve terminals in its target area, the striatum. Lewy bodies, abnormal aggregates of protein, are the pathological hallmark of PD. The diminishing number of dopaminergic neurons ultimately leads to the depletion of dopamine content in the striatum [1] and results in a variety of motor and nonmotor deficits [2]. There are several theories behind the pathogenesis of PD but all hold in common a central idea of mitochondrial dysfunction among both sporadic and familial forms of the disease. Mitochondrial dysfunction may be the result of bioenergetics defects, mitochondrial DNA mutations, alteration in mitochondrial dynamics, and presence of mutated proteins associated with mitochondria [3]. Defects in mitochondrial respiration are

involved in human PD, as demonstrated in a study reporting accidental infusions of the toxin 1-methyl-4-phenyl-1,2,3, 6-tetrahydropyridine (MPTP), which selectively inhibits a component of the electron transport chain, mitochondrial complex 1 [4, 5]. This toxin is selectively taken up by dopaminergic neurons, leading to cell loss in the SNpc and a Parkinsonian state. Other toxins, such as the pesticide rotenone, also inhibit complex 1, inducing dopaminergic degeneration in humans and rodents, supporting the idea that mitochondrial dysfunction plays a central role in the pathogenesis of PD [6]. The "multiple hit" hypothesis of the pathogenesis of PD suggests that multiple insults have to come together to cause PD [7]. Calcium-induced toxicity may be one of the "hits" contributing to the selective vulnerability of dopaminergic neurons in PD. It has been observed that engagement of L-type calcium channels during autonomous pacemaking increases the sensitivity of SNpc dopaminergic neurons to mitochondrial toxins in animal models of PD. Human epidemiological data also supports a linkage between

L-type calcium channels and the risk of developing PD [8]. There are also implications of genetic mutations in mitochondrial dysfunction. DJ-1, encoded by the *PARK7* gene, protects neurons against oxidative stress and cell death. Deletion of DJ-1 exacerbated elevated mitochondrial oxidant stress due to calcium entry, demonstrating that neurodegenerative changes in PD may be driven by metabolic stress created by calcium entry, particularly in the face of genetic factors that compromise defense mechanisms [8]. The first gene to be linked to familial PD was *SNCA*, which encodes the protein α-synuclein, and since α-synuclein is also a main contributor to Lewy bodies in idiopathic PD it is of special importance for PD. Both monomeric and oligomeric forms of α-synuclein have differential effects on mitochondria, including increasing calcium, inhibitory effects on complex I activity, and inducing reactive oxygen species (ROS), as reviewed in [9]. Another familial form of early-onset PD can be caused by mutations in PTEN-induced kinase 1 (PINK1), where PINK1 mutations or knockdown of PINK1 results in an increase of α-synuclein aggregates in cell-culture PD models, decrease in mitochondrial respiration, and a decrease in ATP synthesis [3]. Functionally, PINK1 is a kinase and phosphorylates parkin and ubiquitin to regulate mitophagy *(vide infra)*. And finally, the *Parkin* gene, the causative gene for an autosomal recessive form of PD, has been shown to be necessary for autophagy of mitochondria. The connection between PD and mitochondria suggests that malfunction in the mitochondrial quality control process can lead to an accumulation of defective mitochondria and cell death [10].

Properties maintaining mitochondrial homeostasis are collectively known as mitochondrial dynamics and these processes, such as mitochondrial fission, fusion, and transport, interact to maintain the electron transport chain function, prevent buildup of damaged proteins, control mitochondrial turnover, and regulate cell death processes. Defects in any of these processes may be involved in PD pathogenesis [11]. With regard to PD, a significant amount of evidence supports the role of mitochondrial dysregulation in the pathophysiology of this disease. The high vulnerability of dopaminergic neurons to metabolic dysfunction may be due to their elevated bioenergetic requirements and particular morphological characteristics of these neurons such as a high density of axonal mitochondria and complex axonal arborizations [12].

Current treatments such as L-dihydroxyphenylalanine (L-DOPA) and deep brain stimulation, while effective, do not address the underlying issue of neurodegeneration involved in PD and serve to provide only symptomatic relief. Because these methods do not address the core cause of PD nor halt disease progression, there is need for improved therapeutic options aimed at identifying the cause of dopaminergic cell loss.

Similarities may exist among signaling pathways during pathological states involving the nervous system and cardiovascular system, and reviewing the role of VEGF-B can provide new perspectives for medically important diseases. The role of VEGF-B remains ambiguous compared to VEGF-A, which is the archetypal angiogenic factor and the most extensively studied among the VEGF family [13]. VEGF-B has

the potential to protect both cardiomyocytes from ischemic injury and neurons from degeneration. It is important to identify the similarities and differences between VEGF-B actions in these processes in order to determine areas of further research.

2. Vascular Endothelial Grown Factor Family

Vascular endothelial growth factor (VEGF) was first isolated in 1983 by Senger and colleagues and identified as vascular permeability factor (VPF) due to its ability to stimulate vascular permeability [14]. However, in 1989 Napoleone Ferrara and colleagues purified the same protein, which was distinguished for its role as a potent endothelial mitogen. It was then renamed "vascular endothelial growth factor" (VEGF). The protein purified by Ferrara and colleagues was the most biologically active isoform of the VEGF family, VEGF-A [15]. Although VEGF-A is the most studied isoform, there are 4 other identified members that make up the VEGF family, VEGF-B, VEGF-C, VEGF-D, and PlGF (placental growth factor) [16]. The VEGF family is known to bind to three receptor tyrosine kinases, known as vascular endothelial growth factor receptor-1, -2, and -3 (VEGFR-1–3; sometimes also referred to as flt-1, flk-1, and flt-4), activating several signaling cascades which regulate a multitude of cellular functions [17]. VEGFRs have an approximately 750-amino-acid residue extracellular domain organized into seven immunoglobulin-like folds as well as a single transmembrane region and an intracellular tyrosine kinase domain interrupted by a kinase-insert domain [16]. The VEGF ligands bind to these three main receptors with differing specificities. VEGFs are dimeric glycoproteins of approximately 40 kDa that bind the RTKs and cross-link them as dimers. As a result, the RTK's cytoplasmic tyrosine kinase domains autophosphorylate, which then triggers an intracellular signaling cascade that transduces the signal initiated by VEGF-binding into the cell [17]. This paper will focus on VEGFR-1 and VEGFR-2 regulators and their interactions with VEGF ligands. Both VEGFR-1 and VEGFR-2 are high affinity receptors for VEGF-A, while VEGF-B only interacts with VEGFR-1 [17]. Most functional VEGF-A signaling is mediated via VEGFR-2 and upon VEGF-A-induced stimulation of this receptor, there are major proangiogenic signals generated [18], while protective mechanisms in both the brain and the heart can involve signaling mediated through VEGFR-1 receptors [19, 20]. These different interactions determine downstream effects and allow for the comparison between VEGF-A and VEGF-B functions in various processes. Though VEGF-A is the most extensively studied of the VEGF family, multiple studies determined the protective role of VEGF-B in diseases such as ischemic heart disease and neurodegenerative diseases.

3. Why VEGF-B?

VEGF family members are key regulators of vascular biology, modulating angiogenesis, vasculogenesis, and maintaining vasculature during embryogenesis and in adults. VEGF-A has been considerably studied on the account of its ability to promote angiogenic effects via one of its receptors, VEGFR-2 [16]. VEGF-A can be induced when cells are subjected to hypoxic conditions and plays a central role in neovascularization, increasing energy substrates and oxygen. Hypoxia induces hypoxia inducible factor-1 expression, which binds to the enhancer sequence of the VEGF-A gene and mediates its physiological functions [21]. In contrast, VEGF-B does not contain a hypoxia response element in the promoter region and is not transcriptionally induced by hypoxia. However, VEGF-B is induced by ischemia in the brain but another unidentified mechanism must be involved in the stimulation of VEGF-B. VEGF-A is one of the strongest inducers of vascular permeability [22] and has also been shown to have neuroprotective effects in both *in vitro* and *in vivo* PD models [23]. For example, a study conducted by Yasuhara et al. suggested that VEGF-A effectively protects against 6-hydroxydopamine-induced cell death within cultures of embryonic rat mesencephalic dopaminergic neurons. Likewise, the continuous injection of VEGF-A, via encapsulated VEGF-A secreting cells (engineered baby hamster kidney cells), into the right striatum of adult rats resulted in a neuroprotective effect. There was a rescue of dopaminergic neurons demonstrated by an increase in tyrosine hydroxylase- (TH-) positive neurons in the striatum as well as a functional improvement demonstrated by a significant decrease in amphetamine-induced rotational behavior [23]. Another study supported the protective effect of VEGF-A, concluding that the intrastriatal delivery of VEGF-expressing adeno-associated virus demonstrated favorable effects on dopaminergic neurons in a rat Parkinson's disease model [24]. A direct neurotrophic effect on dopaminergic neurons by VEGF-A was suggested given that VEGF-A increased both tyrosine hydroxylase-immunoreactive cell survival and neurite outgrowth *in vitro* [25]. Similar protective effects were demonstrated in a study by Silverman et al. where VEGF-A promoted survival particularly of dopaminergic neurons in rat midbrain explant cultures [26].

While neuroprotective effects of VEGF-A have been identified, administering VEGF-A at high levels may lead to unwanted side effects such as an increase in vessel density [27] and cerebral edema [28], due to its angiogenic activity. VEGF-A has also been recently indicated in contributing to the development of L-DOPA-induced dyskinesia (LID), a dose limiting side effect of the gold standard treatment for PD, by increasing microvascular density [29]. Given these side effects, other studies investigated another VEGF isoform, VEGF-B, which may have a similar action in certain diseases but without these unwanted effects, due to the lack of angiogenic function. In contrast to VEGF-A, VEGF-B does not contain a hypoxia response element in the promoter region and is not transcriptionally induced by hypoxia. However, VEGF-B is induced by ischemia in the brain. VEGF-B upregulation in other pathological processes such as cortical cord injury in rats [30], motor neuron degeneration [31], and a cell-culture model of PD has also been shown [32]. In both ALS and peripheral neuron disease, VEGF-B mediated protective effects against neuronal degeneration [31, 33, 34]. VEGF-B evidently plays a role in various pathological processes, some of which will be discussed further in this review. The mechanisms of action, however, remain unclear and not well established. Nonetheless, VEGF-B protective function is an active area of research that merits investigation given its differences in safety profile.

4. Tissue Expression of VEGF-B and VEGFR-1

In order to elaborate on the action of VEGF-B and consider VEGFR-1 as part of its signaling pathway in certain diseases, it is important to determine expression of both VEGF-B and VEGR-1 in areas of interest, such as the heart and brain. *VEGF-B* expression in mouse tissues and human tissues was determined by Northern blot analysis. In mouse tissues, *VEGF-B* transcript expression was most abundant in heart, brain, lung, skeletal muscle, and kidney. In human tissues, *VEGF-B* transcript expression was most abundant in heart, skeletal muscle, pancreas, and prostate [35]. In a study by Muhl et al. the expression of both *VEGF-B* and *VEGFR-1* was explored in the murine heart, lung, and kidney. In all organs, there was a cell-specific pattern with VEGFR-1 expression restricted to endothelial cells and VEGF-B expression was found in cardiomyocytes, pulmonary myocardium of the lung, and renal epithelial cells of the kidney [36]. During ischemic stroke, VEGF-B expression was increased in neurons and inflammatory (macrophage/microglial) cells of the ischemic border zone after cerebral artery occlusion in a rat model [37]. In order for VEGF-B to affect motor neurons, VEGF-B must be expressed in the ventral horn of the spinal cord. Immunohistochemistry revealed VEGF-B expression in large neurons in the ventral horn, which were considered to be motor neurons given their size and location; expression was also shown in dorsal root ganglion neurons and in blood vessels [31]. VEGF-B was not detectable in quiescent astroglia in SOD1 mice, but its expression became prominent in activated astrocytes thought to maintain survival of motor neurons after injury [31]. Another example of VEGF-B expression in pathological states comes from a study by Boer et al. in which expression of VEGF-B and its receptor VEGFR-1 was demonstrated in resected human brain tissue from patients undergoing epilepsy surgery for focal cortical dysplasia type IIB [38]. Histologically normal cortex displayed only weak VEGF-B immunoreactivity, but an increased expression in the dysplastic cortex. Expression was shown in pyramidal neurons, in endothelial cells, and in CD68+ macrophages, while glial cells did not show VEGF-B staining. VEGF-B and VEGFR-1 are also expressed in neuromelanin-containing neurons in the SNpc of both healthy controls and PD patients; microglial and vascular immunoreactivity was also present in the SNpc [19, 39]. There were no overt differences between control subjects and PD patients in this small cohort.

5. Link between Cardiovascular System and Nervous System

Cells in both the heart and the brain are energy dependent cells, requiring tight control of mitochondria and subsequent cell functions. Perhaps if nonfunctional or damaged

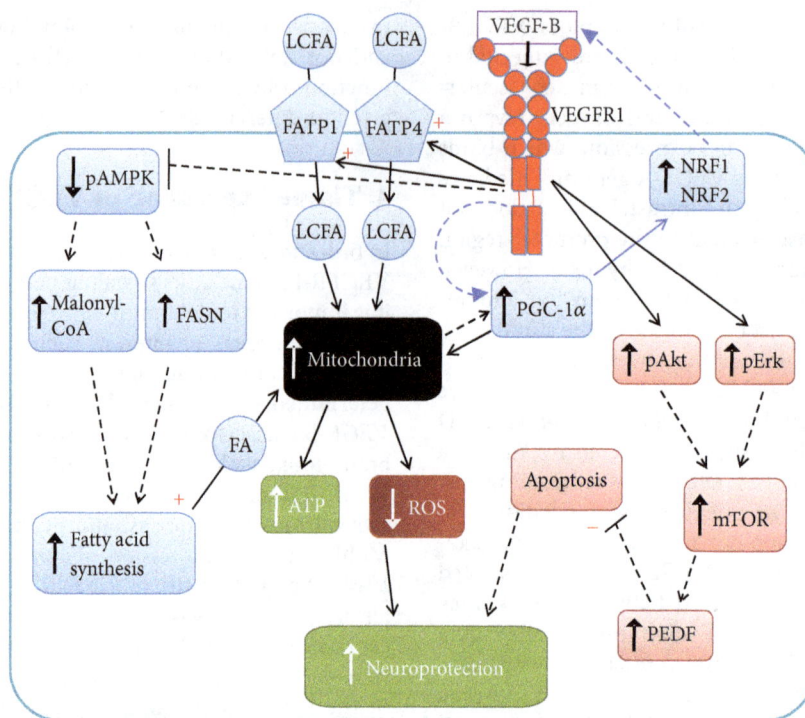

FIGURE 1: Proposed mechanisms of VEGF-B's protective effects in dopaminergic neurons. Black solid lines indicate pathways previously shown for DA cells. Black dashed lines indicate hypothesized pathways, based on other cell types. Blue lines indicate a possible feedback loop between VEGF-B and PGC-1α. Arrowheads and + signs: activation, − signs: inhibition. LCFA: long chain fatty acids; FA: fatty acids. In neuron survival, VEGF-B via VEGFR-1 upregulates pAkt and to a lesser extent pErk. Given data seen in cardiac tissue and sensory neurons, we propose that mTOR is increased downstream and generates antiapoptotic effects via upregulation of PEDF. Previous data also shows that VEGF-B mediated upregulation of fatty acid transporters FATP1 and FATP4 via VEGFR-1, leading to LCFA uptake and increasing mitochondrial function. This could generate more ATP and decreases ROS, promoting neuronal protection. Additionally, given VEGF-B action on pAMPK in cardiac cell protection, reduced AMPK phosphorylation may be involved in neuroprotection and serves as another way of improving mitochondrial function during neuron injury. The nuclear respiratory factors, NRF1 and NRF2, are downstream of PGC-1α in neuroprotection, and given findings in skeletal muscle, VEGF-B may be regulated by PGC-1α, via NRF1 and NRF2. Applying data from prior work in cardiac cells, we also suggest that VEGF-B may increase PGC-1α expression, providing an autocrine feedback loop in which either VEGF-B is directly upregulating PGC-1α followed by increased mitochondrial activity or VEGF-B could be increasing mitochondrial activity that is then feeding back to increase PGC-1α in order to maintain increased ATP production.

mitochondria begin to accumulate in neurons or cardiomyocytes, the energy required to maintain proper cell function is insufficient to promote cell survival in the presence of a pathological process. VEGF-B has been found to have protective capabilities for cells during injury in various contexts [33, 40, 41], and given its role in pathology involving both systems, future studies should continue elucidating the molecular links associated with cardiovascular and neurological diseases. Since mitochondrial dysfunction is central in PD, for example, VEGF-B mediated increases in fatty acid transport could help during disturbances in oxidative stress that cause mitochondrial dysfunction by providing an energy source for viable cells [42]. Generally, VEGFR-1, VEGF-B's receptor, activates downstream pathways used to aid with protective processes during cellular stress [16]. These pathways include regulation of the Akt pathway and Fatty Acid Transport Proteins (FATP), downstream factors that have been involved in VEGF-B protective function (Figure 1). This shared feature can potentially serve as a link between both systems that can provide a learning opportunity about

new areas of research and more insight into the development of new therapeutic agents that target specific pathways in certain disease processes.

6. Neuroprotective Role of VEGF-B in Parkinson's Disease

Growth factors have shown preclinical promise for treatment of PD, as reviewed in [43, 44], but have not yet been translated into the clinic. Combinations of more than one neurotrophic factor might be ultimately necessary for clinical efficacy [45]. To help with identifying additional protective factor candidates with distinct mechanisms of action, a study by Falk et al. used a rat midbrain culture model to identify genes that are changed after the addition of a neurotoxin, rotenone. Rotenone is a naturally occurring toxin and a commonly used pesticide that reproduces the neuropathological and behavioral features of PD in rats and is a well-characterized model for this disease [46]. In this study a gene chip array analysis demonstrated several genes were upregulated after treatment with rotenone and transcriptional activation of VEGF-B was evident. To verify these results, a semiquantitative western analysis was conducted, which demonstrated increased protein expression of VEGF-B, proving VEGF-B to be an inducible factor in a model of neurodegeneration [32]. To investigate the role of VEGF-B specifically, this same study utilized a rat midbrain *in vitro* PD model. In one series of experiments, there was a concentration dependent protective effect of VEGF-B on primary neurons in culture, with a mean effect of 30% increase in TH-positive cell number when compared to untreated cells. This reflected VEGF-B's protective effect against the natural loss of dopaminergic neurons in culture. Another series of experiments in the same study involved testing additional exogenous VEGF-B in the midbrain culture model using a severe rotenone challenge. This rotenone challenge resulted in a significant reduction of TH-positive neurons per culture dish compared to untreated cells (control). One hour prior to rotenone challenge, VEGF-B was administered and a neuroprotective effect of VEGF-B rescuing cell loss was demonstrated [32]. Based on the results using an *in vitro* PD model, VEGF-B's neuroprotective effect was investigated in an *in vivo* PD model. This study by Falk et al. involved utilizing a mildly progressive unilateral 6-hydroxydopamine (OHDA) rat PD model with an intrastriatal injection of VEGF-B prior to the neurotoxic 6-OHDA treatment. In VEGF-B treated animals, there was an improvement in PD behavior, indicating a protective effect of VEGF-B [19, 47]. Further analysis demonstrated that VEGF-B partially protected dopaminergic fibers in the striatum and partially rescued dopaminergic neurons in the SNpc [19, 47]. To identify genes that are coexpressed with *VEGF-B* and establish links to known signaling pathways or metabolic networks, Hagberg et al. clustered microarray data, which showed a significant coexpression of *VEGF-B* with nuclear encoded mitochondrial genes involved in fatty acid metabolism [42]. To identify potential mechanisms of VEGF-B's neuroprotective action on dopaminergic neurons, Yue et al. used the human neuroblastoma cell line SH-SY5Y, which exhibits hallmark characteristics of dopaminergic cells [48] and is a common cellular PD model. Certain pathways were chosen as potential targets of VEGFR-1 based on evidence from other tissue types. Among these targets are fatty acid transport protein 1 (FATP1), fatty acid transport protein 4 (FATP4), and Akt.

Transport of long chain fatty acids (LCFA) across the plasma membrane is facilitated by FATPs, providing an important source of energy for most organisms. FATPs have been shown to be expressed in a variety of tissues [49], and of particular importance is the expression of the murine FATP1 and FATP4 in the brain [49]. This expression of FATP1 and FATP4 in the brain is fundamental, as this was the primary area of interest. Taking also into consideration the regulation FATP transcription by VEGF-B [42], FATP1 and FATP4 were of specific interest.

In addition to exploring FATP1 and FATP4, investigating pathways involved in regulating transcription of antiapoptotic genes was another objective. In a study by Li et al. Akt pathways were shown to play a role in VEGF-B's inhibitory effect on apoptosis using different cell lines [50]. Given these

findings, the potential role of Akt and Erk 1/2 in VEGF-B's neuroprotective effect on dopaminergic cells was also investigated.

After investigating these pathways it was determined that the neuroprotective mechanisms of VEGF-B involve upregulation of FATP1 and FATP4 and activation of Akt and Erk1/2 signaling pathways. There was an evident upregulation of FATP1 and FATP4 with VEGF-B cotreatment after rotenone-induced stress [19], and the VEGF-B-induced increase of FATP1 and FATP4 mediated by VEGFR-1 may facilitate the translocation of long chain fatty acids across the plasma membrane, increasing mitochondrial function and allowing cells to recover from rotenone-induced mitochondrial damage by providing an additional energy source.

This is especially interesting since the mitochondria are thought to be at the center of both genetic and potential environmental causes for PD, and dopaminergic neurons in the SNpc are known to have a high mitochondrial oxidant stress, due to their high metabolic demands to maintain dopamine release [8, 51].

VEGF-B cotreatment significantly reversed rotenone-induced downregulation of total Akt and phospho-Akt protein levels, at both phosphorylation sites that are required together for maximal activation, and to a minimal degree, VEGF-B activated Erk 1/2. The increased Akt and Erk 1/2 signaling could be a parallel or additive process leading directly to activation of antiapoptotic cellular cascades, as has been shown in other tissues, including neuronal cells [50].

In summary, it was shown that the mechanisms of VEGF-B's neuroprotective action can involve VEGFR-1 mediated upregulation of FATP1 and FATP4 and activation of the Akt and Erk 1/2 signaling pathways [19] (Figure 1). By characterization of downstream targets of VEGF-B that are important in regulating cell processes in the brain, especially dopaminergic neurons, it may be possible to develop more effective clinical interventions to promote neuronal protection in PD and other neurodegenerative diseases involving mitochondrial dysfunction.

7. Neuroprotective Role of VEGF-B in Amyotrophic Lateral Sclerosis

Amyotrophic Lateral Sclerosis (ALS), a fatal and devastating adult-onset neurodegenerative disorder characterized by rapidly progressive degeneration of motor neurons in the spinal cord, brainstem, and primary motor cortex, is another disorder in which VEGF-A has been shown to play a major role. In one particular study, VEGF-A had promising results, with neuroprotection of motor neurons significantly improving neuronal survival in animal models [52]. However, as previously mentioned, the issues with VEGF-A's safety profile remain. The undesirable effects of VEGF-A on capillary permeability and the inflammatory response in the brain warrant studying another therapeutic pathway with a higher safety potential. In a study by Poesen et al. the role of VEGF-B and VEGFR-1 in motor degeneration in rodent models of ALS was investigated [31]. VEGF-B should be present in the ventral horn of the spinal cord, for it to affect motor neurons;

therefore, expression was determined in WT mice and real time PCR analysis revealed VEGF-B was present in WT mice embryos and adult mice. Mice lacking VEGF-B developed a more severe form of motor neuron degeneration when intercrossed with mutant superoxide dismutase 1 (SOD1) mice, a model for ALS. And intracerebroventricular VEGF-B recombinant protein injection prolonged survival of SOD1 mice, without causing blood vessel growth or blood-brain barrier leakiness. VEGF-B was not detectable in quiescent glial cells in presymptomatic SOD1 mice, but its expression was progressively upregulated in activated glial cells in symptomatic SOD1 mice, indicating a possible stress-induced paracrine effect. Given VEGFR-1 is the receptor for VEGF-B; this study also confirmed expression of VEGFR-1 in mouse spinal cord by RT-PCR analysis of VEGFR-1 transcript levels. After isolating primary motor neurons from embryonic mice embryos, VEGF-B was added to determine if it protected motor neurons from cell death, which came from deprivation of growth supplements. After comparing the percentage of surviving motor neurons to the initial number of motor neurons, VEGF-B was shown to significantly increase survival in a dose dependent manner. To investigate how VEGF-B mediated its neuroprotective effects, Poesen et al. used mice expressing a tyrosine kinase-dead VEGFR-1, which cannot conduct the biological effect of VEGF-B. As predicted, they found that VEGF-B failed to protect embryonic VEGF-1R-TK$^{-/-}$ motor neurons, indicating that VEGF-B exerts neuroprotective activity through VEGFR-1 mediated signaling [31]. The signaling cascade downstream of VEGFR-1, however, is not well understood.

The pathological mechanism in ALS is multifactorial and complex. Oxidative phosphorylation in mitochondria is the major source for reactive oxygen species and oxidative stress and mitochondrial damage are just one link that has been investigated in the pathogenesis of ALS [53]. Given the multiple functions of the mitochondria, damage to this organelle or alteration of its properties might confer susceptibility of motor neurons to stress and result in cell death. If mitochondria accumulate in the cell in a dysfunctional state, it is no longer able to supply ATP to the neuromuscular junction or to the cell body, eventually resulting in the degeneration of distal synapses and death of motor neurons [53]. Using information from VEGF-B action in PD, we could hypothesize the mechanism of neuroprotection in ALS as well. There is a possible role for VEGF-B in helping mitochondria with compromised function survive by mediating upregulation of fatty acid transport into cells to be utilized for energy production by intact mitochondria [19]. This may be a common avenue in the pathways involved with neuron protection in PD and ALS.

As previously mentioned, VEGF-A's role in ALS has been extensively studied, compared to VEGF-B, and the mechanism of motor neuron protection by VEGF-A primarily involves VEGFR-2 and Akt/PI3 K activation downstream of VEGFR-2 [54], or suppression of cell death pathways mediated by caspases [55]. With this knowledge, we can get some insight into other pathways involved with VEGFR-1 mediated neuroprotective effects on motor neurons in ALS. There

is potential for crosstalk between VEGFR-1 and VEGFR-2 and similar signaling pathways, such as Akt, could be involved. However, knowing that VEGF-A has a prominent effect on vascular permeability compared to VEGF-B and understanding the pathway through which that affect is elicited, then it may be possible to narrow the downstream signals involved in neuroprotection of motor neurons by VEGF-B.

8. VEGF-B Action in the Peripheral Nervous System

Studies reveal VEGF-B protection primarily in CNS-derived neurons and actions on the peripheral nervous system have been less characterized. Peripheral nerve injury is major neurological disorder that can cause multiple sensory and motor disturbances. There is a greater capacity of nerves in the peripheral nervous system to regenerate compared to nerves in the central nervous system and successful regeneration requires several factors for axonal regrowth [56]. The family of VEGFs has been associated as a potent mediator of adult nerve regeneration [57]. A study by Guaiquil et al. examined whether VEGF-B mediates peripheral nerve repair after injury from trauma or disease in a mouse model. They revealed restoration of the innervation of target tissues by VEGF-B mediated nerve growth and regeneration and that mice lacking VEGF-B had impaired peripheral nerve regeneration. Additionally, this study showed VEGF-B effects are specific for injured nerves and independent of any vascular effect [34]. Results revealed VEGF-B signaling led to neurite growth in a dose dependent manner and this effect was inhibited by VEGFR-1 antibodies, indicating VEGFR-1 mediated VEGF-B's effects. Additionally, addition of VEGF-B was found to protect against cell death. To further investigate the mechanism by which VEGF-B induces nerve growth, RNA sequencing analysis showed that important elements of the Notch, Wnt, and Plexin signaling pathways may play a role in VEGF-B mediated neurite growth in trigeminal neurons [34]. Previous studies demonstrated that VEGF-A signaling involved PI3 K/Akt [58, 59] so this pathway was also investigated in the context of VEGF-B's mechanism using a specific PI3 K inhibitor. Trigeminal ganglion neurons were pretreated with a PI3 K inhibitor and then incubated with VEGF-B. Neurite growth was followed and the number of neurons showing elongation patterns was analyzed. This analysis revealed that cells treated with the inhibitor formed nascent or short neurites compared to cells treated with VEGF-B alone and elongation of neurites was inhibited as well, proving signaling through PI3 K is required for VEGF-B-induced peripheral neuron growth [34]. Overall, this data demonstrated VEGF-B promotes proper nerve regeneration without affecting undamaged nerves or neovascularization and gave insight into the mechanisms involved, making it an important therapeutic target for treating injured peripheral nerves. In a recent study, VEGF-B improved corneal sensation and epithelial regeneration in both normal and diabetic mice, accompanied with the elevated corneal content of pigment epithelium-derived factor (PEDF). PEDF knockdown partially abolished trophic function of VEGF-B in diabetic corneal reinnervation [60]. PEDF is known to be a master regulator of apoptosis in many tissues and therefore could be driving the antiapoptotic effects of VEGF-B (Figure 1) [61]. This is of particular interest for dopaminergic neurons, as McKay et al. had shown in prior work that PEDF accounts for over 50% of the trophic potential of conditioned media from human retinal pigment epithelial (RPE) cells [62]. And in a follow-up study our group demonstrated that *in vitro* in rat midbrain cultures PEDF protected against both 6-OHDA and rotenone challenges, leading to increased survival and neurite length in dopaminergic neurons [63]. Remarkably, a study that investigated striatal levels of PEDF in PD patients suggests upregulation of PEDF in response to acute insult to the dopaminergic pathway and that such response might be disturbed in patients with advanced PD [64].

9. VEGF-B and Cerebral Ischemic Injury

Cerebral ischemia is very common in adults, especially the elderly, and some studies have addressed the potential of VEGF-B to protect against ischemic injury. In this setting, the limited ability of VEGF-B to induce vascular permeability could be advantageous in limiting stroke-related cerebral edema [65].

The effect of cerebral ischemia on other growth factors, such as VEGF-C and PlGF, has been reported. Ischemic injury upregulates VEGF-C in a rat stroke model [66] and PlGF expression was increased in response to oxygen and glucose deprivation in a rat model [67]. The effect on VEGF-B, however, is less clear. To address this, VEGF-B protein expression and protein distribution were measured up to 1-week after middle cerebral artery occlusion in rats. VEGF-B expression was increased in the border zone after injury and was associated with neurons. Therefore, VEGF-B may contribute to adaptive mechanisms that limit ischemic cerebral injury [37].

In a study by Sun et al. the middle cerebral artery was occluded in VEGF-B knockout, heterozygous (HZ), and wild type (WT) mice and the volume of resulting cerebral infarcts in addition to the associated neurological function impairment was measured. To investigate the protective effects of VEGF-B, middle cerebral artery occlusion was produced and infarct areas were measured 24 hours later. Infarct volume was increased approximately 40% in VEGF-B$^{-/-}$ mice compared to VEGF-B$^{+/+}$ mice and confirmed with hematoxylin staining. To assess neurological function, neurological scores were used, which reflect the severity of brain dysfunction after ischemia with higher values indicating more severe impairment. VEGF-B$^{-/-}$ mice received higher scores than did WT and HZ mice 24 hours after middle cerebral artery occlusion. This study concluded the size of cerebral infarcts as well as the severity of neurologic deficits increased in mice lacking the *Vegf-b* gene suggesting that VEGF-B limits the extent of cerebral ischemic injury [37].

The mechanism underlying this neuroprotection is unclear but previous studies as well as the study conducted by Sun et al. provide some insight. VEGFR-1 receptors are involved, as these are the receptors VEGF-B preferentially binds to [68] and it may have a direct action at this site. Comparing VEGF-A and VEGF-B mediated signaling pathways can also provide information on the downstream activity in this context. Protection of neurons from cerebral ischemia by VEGF-A likely involves VEGFR-2 and PI3 K/Akt signaling transduction pathways may be activated [69]. It is possible that VEGF-A and VEGF-B exhibit an additive effect on neurons and protection involves crosstalk between downstream signals of both VEGFR-1 and VEGFR-2.

From another perspective, mitochondrial damage during cerebral ischemia is a possibility due to the effects of increased arachidonic acid levels in the brain. Accumulation of arachidonic acid may inhibit mitochondrial ATP production during cerebral ischemia [70]. This process could be an area in which VEGF-B also plays a role and is a potential area of future investigation. Since VEGF-B expression is upregulated in neurons after ischemic injury [37], VEGF-B might coordinate mitochondrial function via long chain fatty acid uptake, providing an energy source for viable cells. This way, VEGF-B protects against further mitochondrial damage and increases survival of cells during ischemic injury.

10. VEGF-B and Cardiac Disease

VEGF-B is expressed in many tissues, including the heart, but the role of VEGF-B in vascular biology is somewhat elusive. It seems VEGF-B is required for normal cardiac function in adult animals. In VEGF-B$^{-/-}$ mice there were no observed gross abnormalities but when assessing cardiac function, ECG showed that VEGF-B$^{-/-}$ mice have an atrioventricular conduction defect, which was characterized by a prolonged QT interval [71]. Despite appearing overtly normal, VEGF-B deficient mice had mild cardiac phenotypes such as smaller heart size and displayed slight vascular dysfunction after coronary occlusion in one strain. Additionally, VEGF-B$^{-/-}$ mice showed clinical symptoms of compromised recovery from induced myocardial ischemia [72]. These results suggest an essential role of VEGF-B in establishing a fully functional cardiovascular system.

Several studies have indicated a role for VEGF-B in cardioprotection. Heart failure is a staggering clinical health problem and is associated with significant mortality and morbidity, particularly among those aged 65 and over, and its prevalence is rapidly increasing [73]. About half of patients with heart failure have diastolic dysfunction [74] but the mechanisms responsible for diastolic heart failure are not well defined. *Vegf-b* gene transfer in rats resulted in prevention of angiotensin II induced left ventricular diastolic dysfunction [75]. Rats were subjected to pressure overload by angiotensin II infusion for 2 weeks, which decreased *E/A* ratio and prolonged left ventricular isovolumic relaxation time. To evaluate the effect of VEGF-B on cardiac function, an echocardiogram was performed, which showed gene transfer ameliorated angiotensin II induced diastolic dysfunction and normalized *E/A* ratio. Additionally, an increased number of cells positive for phosphorylated Akt were induced by

VEGF-B gene transfer at 2 weeks [75]. This study demonstrated the association of VEGF-B with induction of the Akt pathway and the important role of VEGF-B in preventing the progression to heart failure. Though there are several drugs that have been reported to influence diastolic function, such as angiotensin-converting enzyme inhibitors and angiotensin receptor blockers, left ventricular hypertrophy occasionally persists and patients are at risk for developing heart failure; thus, VEGF-B serves as a potential therapeutic option.

Normal cardiac development and function as well as repair of damaged and diseased myocardium heavily rely on signaling between cardiomyocytes, endothelial cells, smooth muscle cells, and fibroblasts [76]. Recently, a link was found between VEGF-B and tissue metabolism regulation [77]. A better understanding of factors regulating myocardial angiogenesis and metabolism could lead to the development of new therapies for treatment of heart failure, which, as mentioned, is one of the most common causes of morbidity and mortality in developed countries. Elucidating on the role that VEGF-B plays in this process was the goal of a study conducted by Kivelä et al. in which VEGF-B was shown to increase functional coronary vasculature, reprogram cardiomyocyte metabolic pathways, and protect the rat heart from ischemic damage [40].

An experiment was conducted in which VEGF-B transgenic rats and WT rats were subjected to experimental myocardial infarction by ligating the left coronary artery. Positron emission topography showed a significantly smaller infarct region, 4 weeks after infarction. Furthermore, there was less oxygen consumption in noninfarct transgenic myocardium and transgenic hearts showed a better perfusion of noninfarcted septum as well as a better residual perfusion of the infarcted and border areas. Postmortem histological analysis confirmed the infarct areas and scar tissue areas were smaller in VEGF-B transgenic hearts.

Additional results revealed VEGF-B greatly expands the coronary vasculature and increases functional coronary reserve in VEGF-B transgenic hearts in which there was at least a doubling of number of arteries of all size classes. Lastly, the cardiac hypertrophy seen in VEGF-B transgenic rats is physiologic and the nature of this hypertrophy was determined by analyzing the expression of pathological remodeling genes. There were no differences in gene expression, confirming VEGF-B induced hypertrophy was physiological rather than pathological [40]. The study by Kivelä et al. provided evidence for VEGF-B as a protective and repair-enhancing protein in ischemic heart failure, as its overexpression increases coronary vasculature and reprogramming of myocardial metabolism to improve cardiac function [40].

Mechanisms involved in the protective role of VEGF-B are mediated through several signaling pathways. VEGF-B activated Erk 1/2, Akt, and mammalian target of rapamycin complex 1 (mTORC1) pathway components, indicating VEGF-B signaling engages major regulators of metabolism and cell growth [78] (Figure 1). Activation of mTOR regulates apoptotic pathways that can be dependent on activation of Akt and Erk 1/2. The protective pathways of mTOR can limit

cell death to promote cardiac repair and regeneration [40, 79] (Figure 1).

Oxidative stress plays a crucial role in onset of cardiovascular injury and can affect multiple systems that affect metabolic homeostasis. Oxidative stress can be caused by reactive oxygen species and promote cell injury [80]. The mTORC1 pathway has been related to the regulation of cardiac response to stress and myocyte survival [81]. On the other hand, prolonged activation of mTOR can lead to vascular dysfunction [82]; therefore, a balance is crucial to promote favorable effects.

Cardiac fatty acid uptake was also analyzed since it was reported that VEGF-B upregulates endothelial fatty acid transport via FATP3 and FATP4 [42]. Though results from Kivelä et al. confirm VEGF-B has metabolic effects in the heart, it does not occur at the substrate level. Rather, VEGF-B mediates metabolic signaling pathways via $5'$ AMP-activated protein kinase (AMPK) and mTORC1 and directs fatty acids to synthetic pathways rather than oxidation of fatty acids [40].

This information provided a better understanding of the signals involved in VEGF-B mediated protection of cardiomyocytes from cardiac injury and can be used to hypothesize the role of VEGF-B in pathways involving mTOR in neurodegenerative disease, specifically PD. In PD, mTOR activation can prevent injury of dopaminergic neurons during oxidative stress [83, 84]. Given that mTOR is a downstream target of the Akt and Erk 1/2 pathways as previously mentioned, and VEGF-B has been shown to upregulate these pathways in a PD model system [19], it is possible that VEGF-B's protective effects involve mTOR downstream of increased Akt and Erk, reducing apoptosis and protecting neurons from injury (Figure 1).

Overexpression of VEGF-B in the heart also leads to increased fatty acid synthesis via downregulation of phosphorylated $5'$ AMP-activated protein kinase (pAMPK) and an increase in Malonyl-CoA and fatty acid synthase (FASN) downstream. The increase in fatty acid synthesis provides fatty acids for mitochondrial use and energy production and serves as another mechanism of cardiomyocyte survival [85]. Again, this is another potential area of future research for VEGF-B's mechanism of action in neuroprotection (Figure 1) identified using information about VEGF-B's action in the cardiac system. A caveat for this mechanism contributing to ATP generation is that in neurons this could constitute a "futile" cycle in terms of energy production, as the concomitant increase of Malonyl-CoA will drain the mitochondria of citric acid, whereby more NADH but no additional ATP might be generated. On the other hand, AMPK could be involved in dopaminergic neurons in a separate way, as Kang et al. demonstrated that α-synuclein binds phosphoinositide-3 kinase enhancer L in a phosphorylation dependent manner and sequesters it in Lewy bodies, leading to dopaminergic cell death via AMPK hyperactivation [86]. Given the role of Lewy bodies and abnormal aggregation of α-synuclein in the pathogenesis of PD, reduction of pAMPK could be an alternative way in which VEGF-B could be protective for dopaminergic neurons.

11. VEGF-B and PGC-1α

These effects of VEGF-B as a homeostatic metabolic regulator are complex and much remains to be learned about the specific role of VEGF-B in metabolic regulation. To elucidate on this role, data from a study looking into peroxisome proliferator-activated receptor gamma coactivator 1-α (PGC-1α) in skeletal muscle was taken into consideration, where VEGF-B was shown to be a downstream target of the PGC-1α signaling pathway [87]. Additionally, in a study by Huusko et al., AAV9-VEGF-B gene transfer was able to postpone the development of heart failure, and to evaluate the degree of metabolic remodeling, the mRNA levels of PGC-1α were measured. Interestingly, after the AAV9-VEGF-B gene therapy, mRNA expression of PGC-1α was significantly increased [88]. This is suggestive of a positive feedback loop in which VEGF-B is directly upregulating PGC-1α followed by increased mitochondrial activity, or VEGF-B could be increasing mitochondrial activity that is then feeding back to increase PGC-1α in order to maintain increased production of ATP (Figure 1). Since PGC-1α can upregulate NRF1 and NRF2 (vide infra), it is possible that these transcription factors are involved in this direct positive feedback regulation in the center of VEGF-B-induced neuroprotection (Figure 1).

Given that PGC-1α is a central regulator within mitochondrial function that provides a protective effect in both cardiomyocytes and neurons, we propose that VEGF-B may tie into these pathways in several ways. In cardiac cells, transcription factors NRF1 and NRF2 are activated by PGC-1α, contributing to mitochondrial membrane biogenesis [89]. In neuroprotection, PGC-1α also increases activity of these transcription factors [90]. In postmortem brains of PD patients, in both the SNpc and blood cells, PGC-1α levels are decreased [91] and in PGC-1α knockout mice, dopaminergic cells are more sensitive to MPTP [92]. Another study demonstrated PGC-1α overexpression reduced α-synuclein levels, in addition to protecting cells from toxic effects of α-synuclein [93]. Overall, these studies reveal PGC-1α's neuroprotective role.

In both systems, it is possible that VEGF-B not only is a downstream target of PGC-1α, but also is linked with it in a feedback loop. In the context of neuroprotection of dopaminergic neurons, PGC-1α reduces ROS and provides positive effects on mitochondrial function. VEGF-B may play a role in this PGC-1α regulated event by increasing long chain fatty acid uptake via FATP1 and FATP4, improving mitochondrial function and reducing oxidative injury (Figure 1). This could be further enhanced if the increase of fatty acid syntheses, described for cardiac cells above, also happens in dopaminergic neurons. A recent small pilot study from our group does indicate that long-term viral overexpression of VEGF-B [94] might lead to increased striatal dopamine content in PINK1-knockout rats [95], a rodent model for a familial form of PD thought to involve mitochondrial defects. This could indicate long-term neuroprotective activity of VEGF-B for dopaminergic neurons with impaired mitochondrial function and needs further study.

12. VEGF-B and the Inverse Warburg Effect

There is an intriguing recent theoretical framework that could explain the protective action of VEGF-B on a systems level, involving the inverse Warburg effect [96]. A proposed model by Warburg postulates that cancer is a metabolic disease induced by abnormalities in mitochondria. The subsequent metabolic alteration in this model is the upregulation of glycolysis to compensate for diminished energy. This reprogramming is known as the Warburg effect and is derived from the observation that most cancer cells can switch to a less efficient form of metabolism and produce energy necessary for proliferation via glycolysis [97]. The concept of the inverse Warburg effect was introduced by Demetrius and colleagues to describe a complementary mode of metabolic reprogramming occurring in Alzheimer's disease [96, 98]. It has since been hypothesized to also be a contributing factor to the mitochondrial dysfunction seen in dopaminergic neurons that leads to PD, since a hypermetabolic state, as predicted by the inverse Warburg effect, has been detected in the brains of individuals during the presymptomatic phase of PD [99]. This effect initiates a neurodegenerative cascade, which involves a disproportionate upregulation of oxidative phosphorylation in mitochondria of certain neurons to compensate for energy production impairment. Cells not only are dependent on carbohydrate-derived pyruvate but also become critically dependent on lactate-derived pyruvate, with the lactate provided by astrocytes, ultimately leading to a competition for lactate among normal and impaired neurons. This resource constraint allows impaired neurons with upregulated oxidative phosphorylation activity to outcompete intact neurons with normal oxidative phosphorylation activity. Subsequently, there is a change in the overall neuronal population distribution, with an increase in the proportion of impaired neurons compared to healthy neurons [98]. While the inverse Warburg effect is still quite hypothetical in PD, particularly because there is no evidence for an upregulation of complexes of the respiratory chain in dopaminergic neurons in PD, it does provide an intriguing novel theoretic framework to help explain protective effects mediated via enhanced fatty acid metabolism. Providing alternative fuel sources, such as fatty acids, may reduce this resource constraint and alleviate the advantage of impaired neurons. The homeostatic regulator VEGF-B, in a feedback loop together with PGC-1α, could increase mitochondrial function via fatty acid uptake and usage, such that lactate is no longer a limiting resource for the neurons. This process could help prevent deleterious effects on initially healthy neurons and potentially serve to suppress the inverse Warburg effect, reducing the neurodegeneration of the starved neurons.

13. Conclusion

The aim of this review was to elucidate the mechanism of VEGF-B action in different systems and by taking data from both heart and skeletal muscle, we can infer possible functions and mechanisms of VEGF-B in neurons, particularly in the case of dopaminergic neurons in PD. Despite the complex etiology of neurodegenerative diseases, a common theme among them is mitochondrial dysfunction and apoptotic neuronal death. Numerous studies demonstrate VEGF-B is a potent protective factor with a unique safety profile. Ultimately, VEGF-B seems to possess a greater safety advantage, given the lack of angiogenic function, which is an important consideration for its potential therapeutic use in human diseases. There is evidence that VEGF-B promotes energy metabolism and a common observation between the pathogenesis of the diseases discussed in this review is the energy dependent nature of the cells involved. VEGF-B is a factor involved in the crosstalk between oxidative metabolism and mitochondrial biogenesis. There is strong evidence suggesting VEGF-B plays a crucial protective role, whether in context of heart failure or neurodegeneration. Though mechanistically there are differences in VEGF-B action in different tissues, there are also similarities in the downstream regulators involved in VEGF-B's effect. These similarities are a point of convergence, which strongly supports the importance of further illuminating the role of VEGF-B and its use as a therapeutic agent during neuronal injury. Therefore, it would be worth investigating VEGF-B's mechanisms of action further in dopaminergic neurons in the future to ultimately develop a VEGF-B targeted therapy that results in improving mitochondrial dysfunction in the context of cardiac disease and neurodegenerative disorders, including Parkinson's disease.

Disclosure

Parts of the review have been based on a Masters Dissertation Thesis by the 1st author [100].

Acknowledgments

The authors would like to acknowledge Dr. Paul St. John for his input and advice in the preparation of this review.

References

[1] L. S. Forno, "Neuropathology of Parkinson's disease," *Journal of Neuropathology and Experimental Neurology*, vol. 55, no. 3, pp. 259–272, 1996.

[2] A. G. Vidal-Gadea and J. T. Pierce-Shimomura, "Conserved role of dopamine in the modulation of behavior," *Communicative and Integrative Biology*, vol. 5, no. 5, pp. 440–447, 2012.

[3] A. Bose and M. F. Beal, "Mitochondrial dysfunction in Parkinson's disease," *Journal of Neurochemistry*, vol. 139, supplement 1, pp. 216–231, 2016.

[4] J. W. Langston, P. Ballard, J. W. Tetrud, and I. Irwin, "Chronic parkinsonism in humans due to a product of meperidine-analog synthesis," *Science*, vol. 219, no. 4587, pp. 979–980, 1983.

[5] R. S. Burns, P. A. LeWitt, M. H. Ebert, H. Pakkenberg, and I. J. Kopin, "The clinical syndrome of striatal dopamine deficiency. Parkinsonism induced by 1-methyl-4-phenyl-1,2,3,6-tetrahydropyridine (MPTP)," *The New England Journal of Medicine*, vol. 312, no. 22, pp. 1418–1421, 1985.

[6] R. K. Chaturvedi and M. F. Beal, "Mitochondrial approaches for neuroprotection," *Annals of the New York Academy of Sciences*, vol. 1147, pp. 395–412, 2008.

[7] D. Sulzer, "Multiple hit hypotheses for dopamine neuron loss in Parkinson's disease," *Trends in Neurosciences*, vol. 30, no. 5, pp. 244–250, 2007.

[8] D. J. Surmeier, J. N. Guzman, J. Sanchez-Padilla, and P. T. Schumacker, "The role of calcium and mitochondrial oxidant stress in the loss of substantia nigra pars compacta dopaminergic neurons in Parkinson's disease," *Neuroscience*, vol. 198, pp. 221–231, 2011.

[9] P. R. Angelova and A. Y. Abramov, "Alpha-synuclein and beta-amyloid—different targets, same players: calcium, free radicals and mitochondria in the mechanism of neurodegeneration," *Biochemical and Biophysical Research Communications*, vol. 483, no. 4, pp. 1110–1115, 2017.

[10] S. M. Jin and R. J. Youle, "PINK1-and Parkin-mediated mitophagy at a glance," *Journal of Cell Science*, vol. 125, no. 4, pp. 795–799, 2012.

[11] V. S. Van Laar and S. B. Berman, "The interplay of neuronal mitochondrial dynamics and bioenergetics: implications for Parkinson's disease," *Neurobiology of Disease*, vol. 51, pp. 43–55, 2013.

[12] C. Pacelli, N. Giguère, M.-J. Bourque, M. Lévesque, R. S. Slack, and L.-É. Trudeau, "Elevated mitochondrial bioenergetics and axonal arborization size are key contributors to the vulnerability of dopamine neurons," *Current Biology*, vol. 25, no. 18, pp. 2349–2360, 2015.

[13] E. Storkebaum, D. Lambrechts, and P. Carmeliet, "VEGF: once regarded as a specific angiogenic factor, now implicated in neuroprotection," *BioEssays*, vol. 26, no. 9, pp. 943–954, 2004.

[14] D. R. Senger, S. J. Galli, A. M. Dvorak, C. A. Perruzzi, V. Susan Harvey, and H. F. Dvorak, "Tumor cells secrete a vascular permeability factor that promotes accumulation of ascites fluid," *Science*, vol. 219, no. 4587, pp. 983–985, 1983.

[15] N. Ferrara, H.-P. Gerber, and J. LeCouter, "The biology of VEGF and its receptors," *Nature Medicine*, vol. 9, no. 6, pp. 669–676, 2003.

[16] A.-K. Olsson, A. Dimberg, J. Kreuger, and L. Claesson-Welsh, "VEGF receptor signalling—in control of vascular function," *Nature Reviews Molecular Cell Biology*, vol. 7, no. 5, pp. 359–371, 2006.

[17] T. Falk, R. T. Gonzalez, and S. J. Sherman, "The Yin and Yang of VEGF and PEDF: multifaceted neurotrophic factors and their potential in the treatment of Parkinson's disease," *International Journal of Molecular Sciences*, vol. 11, no. 8, pp. 2875–2900, 2010.

[18] M. Shibuya, "Vascular endothelial growth factor (VEGF) and its receptor (VEGFR) signaling in angiogenesis: a crucial target for anti- and pro-angiogenic therapies," *Genes and Cancer*, vol. 2, no. 12, pp. 1097–1105, 2011.

[19] X. Yue, D. J. Hariri, B. Caballero et al., "Comparative study of the neurotrophic effects elicited by VEGF-B and GDNF in preclinical in vivo models of Parkinson's disease," *Neuroscience*, vol. 258, pp. 385–400, 2014.

[20] X. Li, C. Lee, Z. Tang et al., "VEGF-B: a survival, or an angiogenic factor?" *Cell Adhesion and Migration*, vol. 3, no. 4, pp. 332–327, 2009.

[21] Y. Tsuzuki, D. Fukumura, B. Oosthuyse et al., "Vascular Endothelial Growth Factor (VEGF) modulation by targeting hypoxia-inducible factor-1α $\rightarrow$ hypoxia response element $\rightarrow$ VEGF cascade differentially regulates vascular response and growth rate in tumors," *Cancer Research*, vol. 60, pp. 6248–6252, 2000.

[22] S. Ylä-Herttuala, T. T. Rissanen, I. Vajanto, and J. Hartikainen, "Vascular endothelial growth factors: biology and current status of clinical applications in cardiovascular medicine," *Journal of the American College of Cardiology*, vol. 49, no. 10, pp. 1015–1026, 2007.

[23] T. Yasuhara, T. Shingo, K. Kobayashi et al., "Neuroprotective effects of vascular endothelial growth factor (VEGF) upon dopaminergic neurons in a rat model of Parkinson's disease," *The European Journal of Neuroscience*, vol. 19, no. 6, pp. 1494–1504, 2004.

[24] Y.-Y. Tian, C.-J. Tang, J.-N. Wang et al., "Favorable effects of VEGF gene transfer on a rat model of Parkinson disease using adeno-associated viral vectors," *Neuroscience Letters*, vol. 421, no. 3, pp. 239–244, 2007.

[25] M. R. Pitzer, C. E. Sortwell, B. F. Daley et al., "Angiogenic and neurotrophic effects of vascular endothelial growth factor (VEGF165): studies of grafted and cultured embryonic ventral mesencephalic cells," *Experimental Neurology*, vol. 182, no. 2, pp. 435–445, 2003.

[26] W. F. Silverman, J. M. Krum, N. Mani, and J. M. Rosenstein, "Vascular, glial and neuronal effects of vascular endothelial growth factor in mesencephalic explant cultures," *Neuroscience*, vol. 90, no. 4, pp. 1529–1541, 1999.

[27] M. R. Harrigan, S. R. Ennis, T. Masada, and R. F. Keep, "Intraventricular infusion of vascular endothelial growth factor promotes cerebral angiogenesis with minimal brain edema," *Neurosurgery*, vol. 50, no. 3, pp. 589–598, 2002.

[28] H. J. Schoch, S. Fischer, and H. H. Marti, "Hypoxia-induced vascular endothelial growth factor expression causes vascular leakage in the brain," *Brain*, vol. 125, no. 11, pp. 2549–2557, 2002.

[29] K. E. Ohlin, V. Francardo, H. S. Lindgren et al., "Vascular endothelial growth factor is upregulated by L-dopa in the parkinsonian brain: Implications for the development of dyskinesia," *Brain*, vol. 134, no. 8, pp. 2339–2357, 2011.

[30] S. Nag, M. R. Eskandarian, J. Davis, and J. H. Eubanks, "Differential expression of vascular endothelial growth factor-A (VEGF-A) and VEGF-B after brain injury," *Journal of Neuropathology and Experimental Neurology*, vol. 61, no. 9, pp. 778–788, 2002.

[31] K. Poesen, D. Lambrechts, P. Van Damme et al., "Novel role for vascular endothelial growth factor (VEGF) receptor-1 and its ligand VEGF-B in motor neuron degeneration," *Journal of Neuroscience*, vol. 28, no. 42, pp. 10451–10459, 2008.

[32] T. Falk, S. Zhang, and S. J. Sherman, "Vascular endothelial growth factor B (VEGF-B) is up-regulated and exogenous VEGF-B is neuroprotective in a culture model of Parkinson's disease," *Molecular Neurodegeneration*, vol. 4, article 49, 7 pages, 2009.

[33] J. Dhondt, E. Peeraer, A. Verheyen et al., "Neuronal FLT1 receptor and its selective ligand VEGF-B protect against retrograde degeneration of sensory neurons," *The FASEB Journal*, vol. 25, no. 5, pp. 1461–1473, 2011.

[34] V. H. Guaiquil, Z. Pan, N. Karagianni, S. Fukuoka, G. Alegre, and M. I. Rosenblatt, "VEGF-B selectively regenerates injured peripheral neurons and restores sensory and trophic functions,"

Proceedings of the National Academy of Sciences of the United States of America, vol. 111, no. 48, pp. 17272–17277, 2014.

[35] B. Olofsson, K. Pajusola, A. Kaipainen et al., "Vascular endothelial growth factor B, a novel growth factor for endothelial cells," *Proceedings of the National Academy of Sciences of the United States of America*, vol. 93, no. 6, pp. 2576–2581, 1996.

[36] L. Muhl, C. Moessinger, M. Z. Adzemovic et al., "Expression of vascular endothelial growth factor (VEGF)-B and its receptor (VEGFR1) in murine heart, lung and kidney," *Cell and Tissue Research*, vol. 365, no. 1, pp. 51–63, 2016.

[37] L. Xie, X. Mao, K. Jin, and D. A. Greenberg, "Vascular endothelial growth factor-B expression in postischemic rat brain," *Vascular Cell*, vol. 5, no. 1, article 8, 2013.

[38] K. Boer, D. Troost, W. G. M. Spliet, P. C. Van Rijen, J. A. Gorter, and E. Aronica, "Cellular distribution of vascular endothelial growth factor A (VEGFA) and B (VEGFB) and VEGF receptors 1 and 2 in focal cortical dysplasia type IIB," *Acta Neuropathologica*, vol. 115, no. 6, pp. 683–696, 2008.

[39] K. Wada, H. Arai, M. Takanashi et al., "Expression levels of vascular endothelial growth factor and its receptors in Parkinson's disease," *NeuroReport*, vol. 17, no. 7, pp. 705–709, 2006.

[40] R. Kivelä, M. Bry, M. R. Robciuc et al., "VEGF-B-induced vascular growth leads to metabolic reprogramming and ischemia resistance in the heart," *EMBO Molecular Medicine*, vol. 6, no. 3, pp. 307–321, 2014.

[41] M. H. Dijkstra, E. Pirinen, J. Huusko et al., "Lack of cardiac and high-fat diet induced metabolic phenotypes in two independent strains of vegf-b knockout mice," *Scientific Reports*, vol. 4, article 6238, 2014.

[42] C. E. Hagberg, A. Falkevall, X. Wang et al., "Vascular endothelial growth factor B controls endothelial fatty acid uptake," *Nature*, vol. 464, no. 7290, pp. 917–921, 2010.

[43] J. H. Kordower and A. Bjorklund, "Trophic factor gene therapy for Parkinson's disease," *Movement Disorders*, vol. 28, no. 1, pp. 96–109, 2013.

[44] R. T. Bartus and E. M. Johnson Jr., "Clinical tests of neurotrophic factors for human neurodegenerative diseases, part 1: where have we been and what have we learned?" *Neurobiology of Disease*, vol. 97, pp. 156–168, 2017.

[45] J. D. Jaumotte, S. L. Wyrostek, and M. J. Zigmond, "Protection of cultured dopamine neurons from MPP$^+$ requires a combination of neurotrophic factors," *European Journal of Neuroscience*, vol. 44, no. 1, pp. 1691–1699, 2016.

[46] M. Alam and W. J. Schmidt, "Rotenone destroys dopaminergic neurons and induces parkinsonian symptoms in rats," *Behavioural Brain Research*, vol. 136, no. 1, pp. 317–324, 2002.

[47] T. Falk, X. Yue, S. Zhang et al., "Vascular endothelial growth factor-B is neuroprotective in an in vivo rat model of Parkinson's disease," *Neuroscience Letters*, vol. 496, no. 1, pp. 43–47, 2011.

[48] X. Wang, Z.-H. Qin, Y. Leng et al., "Prostaglandin A1 inhibits rotenone-induced apoptosis in SH-SY5Y cells," *Journal of Neurochemistry*, vol. 83, no. 5, pp. 1094–1102, 2002.

[49] D. Hirsch, A. Stahl, and H. F. Lodish, "A family of fatty acid transporters conserved from mycobacterium to man," *Proceedings of the National Academy of Sciences of the United States of America*, vol. 95, no. 15, pp. 8625–8629, 1998.

[50] Y. Li, F. Zhang, N. Nagai et al., "VEGF-B inhibits apoptosis via VEGFR-1-mediated suppression of the expression of BH3-only protein genes in mice and rats," *Journal of Clinical Investigation*, vol. 118, no. 3, pp. 913–923, 2008.

[51] C. W. Olanow, M. B. Stern, and K. Sethi, "The scientific and clinical basis for the treatment of Parkinson disease," *Neurology*, vol. 72, no. 21, supplement 4, pp. S1–S136, 2009.

[52] A. C. Pronto-Laborinho, S. Pinto, and M. De Carvalho, "Roles of vascular endothelial growth factor in amyotrophic lateral sclerosis," *BioMed Research International*, vol. 2014, Article ID 947513, 14 pages, 2014.

[53] M. Cozzolino and M. T. Carrì, "Mitochondrial dysfunction in ALS," *Progress in Neurobiology*, vol. 97, no. 2, pp. 54–66, 2012.

[54] B. Li, W. Xu, C. Luo, D. Gozal, and R. Liu, "VEGF-induced activation of the PI3-K/Akt pathway reduces mutant SOD1-mediated motor neuron cell death," *Molecular Brain Research*, vol. 111, no. 1-2, pp. 155–164, 2003.

[55] M. Li, V. O. Ona, C. Guégan et al., "Functional role of caspase-1 and caspase-3 in an ALS transgenic mouse model," *Science*, vol. 288, no. 5464, pp. 335–339, 2000.

[56] F. Bosse, "Extrinsic cellular and molecular mediators of peripheral axonal regeneration," *Cell and Tissue Research*, vol. 349, no. 1, pp. 5–14, 2012.

[57] T. Licht and E. Keshet, "Delineating multiple functions of VEGF-A in the adult brain," *Cellular and Molecular Life Sciences*, vol. 70, no. 10, pp. 1727–1737, 2013.

[58] Ü. Kilic, E. Kilic, A. Järve et al., "Human vascular endothelial growth factor protects axotomized retinal ganglion cells in vivo by activating ERK-1/2 and Akt pathways," *Journal of Neuroscience*, vol. 26, no. 48, pp. 12439–12446, 2006.

[59] N. M. Fournier, B. Lee, M. Banasr, M. Elsayed, and R. S. Duman, "Vascular endothelial growth factor regulates adult hippocampal cell proliferation through MEK/ERK- and PI3K/Akt-dependent signaling," *Neuropharmacology*, vol. 63, no. 4, pp. 642–652, 2012.

[60] G. Di, X. Zhao, X. Qi et al., "VEGF-B promotes recovery of corneal innervations and trophic functions in diabetic mice," *Scientific Reports*, vol. 7, article 40582, 2017.

[61] J. Tombran-Tink and C. J. Barnstable, "PEDF: a multifaceted neurotrophic factor," *Nature Reviews Neuroscience*, vol. 4, no. 8, pp. 628–636, 2003.

[62] B. S. McKay, B. Goodman, T. Falk, and S. J. Sherman, "Retinal pigment epithelial cell transplantation could provide trophic support in Parkinson's disease: results from an in vitro model system," *Experimental Neurology*, vol. 201, no. 1, pp. 234–243, 2006.

[63] T. Falk, S. Zhang, and S. J. Sherman, "Pigment epithelium derived factor (PEDF) is neuroprotective in two in vitro models of Parkinson's disease," *Neuroscience Letters*, vol. 458, no. 2, pp. 49–52, 2009.

[64] T. Yasuda, M. Fukuda-Tani, T. Nihira et al., "Correlation between levels of pigment epithelium-derived factor and vascular endothelial growth factor in the striatum of patients with Parkinson's disease," *Experimental Neurology*, vol. 206, no. 2, pp. 308–317, 2007.

[65] D. A. Greenberg and K. Jin, "Vascular endothelial growth factors (VEGFs) and stroke," *Cellular and Molecular Life Sciences*, vol. 70, no. 10, pp. 1753–1761, 2013.

[66] W. Gu, T. Brännström, W. Jiang, A. Bergh, and P. Wester, "Vascular endothelial growth factor-A and -C protein up-regulation and early angiogenesis in a rat photothrombotic ring stroke model with spontaneous reperfusion," *Acta Neuropathologica*, vol. 102, no. 3, pp. 216–226, 2001.

[67] H. Du, P. Li, Y. Pan et al., "Vascular endothelial growth factor signaling implicated in neuroprotective effects of placental growth factor in an in vitro ischemic model," *Brain Research*, vol. 1357, pp. 1–8, 2010.

[68] B. Olofsson, E. Korpelainen, M. S. Pepper et al., "Vascular endothelial growth factor B (VEGF-B) binds to VEGF receptor-1 and regulates plasminogen activator activity in endothelial cells," *Proceedings of the National Academy of Sciences of the United States of America*, vol. 95, no. 20, pp. 11709–11714, 1998.

[69] K. L. Jin, X. O. Mao, T. Nagayama, P. C. Goldsmith, and D. A. Greenberg, "Induction of vascular endothelial growth factor receptors and phosphatidylinositol 3'-kinase/Akt signaling by global cerebral ischemia in the rat," *Neuroscience*, vol. 100, no. 4, pp. 713–717, 2000.

[70] Y. Takeuchi, H. Morii, M. Tamura, O. Hayaishi, and Y. Watanabe, "A possible mechanism of mitochondrial dysfunction during cerebral ischemia: inhibition of mitochondrial respiration activity by arachidonic acid," *Archives of Biochemistry and Biophysics*, vol. 289, no. 1, pp. 33–38, 1991.

[71] K. Aase, G. Von Euler, X. Li et al., "Vascular endothelial growth factor-B-deficient mice display an atrial conduction defect," *Circulation*, vol. 104, no. 3, pp. 358–364, 2001.

[72] D. Bellomo, J. P. Headrick, G. U. Silins et al., "Mice lacking the vascular endothelial growth factor-B gene (Vegfb) have smaller hearts, dysfunctional coronary vasculature, and impaired recovery from cardiac ischemia," *Circulation Research*, vol. 86, no. 2, pp. 29–35, 2000.

[73] V. L. Roger, "Epidemiology of heart failure," *Circulation Research*, vol. 113, no. 6, pp. 646–659, 2013.

[74] J. Wang and S. F. Nagueh, "Current perspectives on cardiac function in patients with diastolic heart failure," *Circulation*, vol. 119, no. 8, pp. 1146–1157, 2009.

[75] R. Serpi, A.-M. Tolonen, J. Huusko et al., "Vascular endothelial growth factor-B gene transfer prevents angiotensin II-induced diastolic dysfunction via proliferation and capillary dilatation in rats," *Cardiovascular Research*, vol. 89, no. 1, pp. 204–213, 2011.

[76] D. Tirziu, F. J. Giordano, and M. Simons, "Cell communications in the heart," *Circulation*, vol. 122, no. 9, pp. 928–937, 2010.

[77] Z. Arany, S.-Y. Foo, Y. Ma et al., "HIF-independent regulation of VEGF and angiogenesis by the transcriptional coactivator PGC-1α," *Nature*, vol. 451, no. 7181, pp. 1008–1012, 2008.

[78] B. Ren, Y. Deng, A. Mukhopadhyay et al., "ERK1/2-Akt1 crosstalk regulates arteriogenesis in mice and zebrafish," *Journal of Clinical Investigation*, vol. 120, no. 4, pp. 1217–1228, 2010.

[79] Z. Z. Chong, Y. C. Shang, and K. Maiese, "Cardiovascular disease and mTOR signaling," *Trends in Cardiovascular Medicine*, vol. 21, no. 5, pp. 151–155, 2011.

[80] K. Maiese, Z. Z. Chong, J. Hou, and Y. C. Shang, "Oxidative stress: biomarkers and novel therapeutic pathways," *Experimental Gerontology*, vol. 45, no. 3, pp. 217–234, 2010.

[81] D. Zhang, R. Contu, M. V. Latronico et al., "MTORC1 regulates cardiac function and myocyte survival through 4E-BP1 inhibition in mice," *Journal of Clinical Investigation*, vol. 120, no. 8, pp. 2805–2816, 2010.

[82] D. Mancini, S. Pinney, D. Burkhoff et al., "Use of rapamycin slows progression of cardiac transplantation vasculopathy," *Circulation*, vol. 108, no. 1, pp. 48–53, 2003.

[83] K.-C. Choi, S.-H. Kim, J.-Y. Ha, S.-T. Kim, and J. H. Son, "A novel mTOR activating protein protects dopamine neurons against oxidative stress by repressing autophagy related cell death," *Journal of Neurochemistry*, vol. 112, no. 2, pp. 366–376, 2010.

[84] K. Maiese, Z. Z. Chong, Y. C. Shang, and S. Wang, "MTOR: on target for novel therapeutic strategies in the nervous system," *Trends in Molecular Medicine*, vol. 19, no. 1, pp. 51–60, 2013.

[85] M. Bry, R. Kivelä, V.-M. Leppänen, and K. Alitalo, "Vascular endothelial growth factor-B in physiology and disease," *Physiological Reviews*, vol. 94, no. 3, pp. 779–794, 2014.

[86] S. S. Kang, Z. Zhang, X. Liu et al., "α-Synuclein binds and sequesters PIKE-L into Lewy bodies, triggering dopaminergic cell death via AMPK hyperactivation," *Proceedings of the National Academy of Sciences of the United States of America*, vol. 114, no. 5, pp. 1183–1188, 2017.

[87] A. Mehlem, I. Palombo, X. Wang, C. E. Hagberg, U. Eriksson, and A. Falkevall, "PGC-1α coordinates mitochondrial respiratory capacity and muscular fatty acid uptake via regulation of VEGF-B," *Diabetes*, vol. 65, no. 4, pp. 861–873, 2016.

[88] J. Huusko, L. Lottonen, M. Merentie et al., "AAV9-mediated VEGF-B gene transfer improves systolic function in progressive left ventricular hypertrophy," *Molecular Therapy*, vol. 20, no. 12, pp. 2212–2221, 2012.

[89] G. C. Rowe, A. Jiang, and Z. Arany, "PGC-1 coactivators in cardiac development and disease," *Circulation Research*, vol. 107, no. 7, pp. 825–838, 2010.

[90] J. C. Corona and M. R. Duchen, "PPARγ and PGC-1α as therapeutic targets in Parkinson's," *Neurochemical Research*, vol. 40, no. 2, pp. 308–316, 2015.

[91] B. Zheng, Z. Liao, J. J. Locascio et al., "PGC-1α, a potential therapeutic target for early intervention in Parkinson's disease," *Science Translational Medicine*, vol. 2, no. 52, Article ID 52ra73, 2010.

[92] J. St-Pierre, S. Drori, M. Uldry et al., "Suppression of reactive oxygen species and neurodegeneration by the PGC-1 transcriptional coactivators," *Cell*, vol. 127, no. 2, pp. 397–408, 2006.

[93] J. Eschbach, B. Schwalenstocker, S. M. Soyal et al., "PGC-1α is a male-specific disease modifier of human and experimental amyotrophic lateral sclerosis," *Human Molecular Genetics*, vol. 22, no. 17, pp. 3477–3484, 2013.

[94] M. J. Bartlett, B. D. Silashki, D. C. Muller et al., "AAV-mediated over-expression of VEGF-B in PINK1 gene knockout rats: a behavioral evaluation," *Society for Neuroscience Abstracts*, vol. 575, 13, 2016.

[95] K. D. Dave, S. De Silva, N. P. Sheth et al., "Phenotypic characterization of recessive gene knockout rat models of Parkinson's disease," *Neurobiology of Disease*, vol. 70, pp. 190–203, 2014.

[96] L. A. Demetrius and D. K. Simon, "An inverse-Warburg effect and the origin of Alzheimer's disease," *Biogerontology*, vol. 13, no. 6, pp. 583–594, 2012.

[97] O. Warburg, "On the origin of cancer cells," *Science*, vol. 123, no. 3191, pp. 309–314, 1956.

[98] L. A. Demetrius, P. J. Magistretti, and L. Pellerin, "Alzheimer's disease: the amyloid hypothesis and the Inverse Warburg effect," *Frontiers in Physiology*, vol. 5, article 522, pp. 2–28, 2015.

[99] C. C. Tang, K. L. Poston, V. Dhawan, and D. Eidelberg, "Abnormalities in metabolic network activity precede the onset of motor symptoms in Parkinson's disease," *The Journal of Neuroscience*, vol. 30, no. 3, pp. 1049–1056, 2010.

[100] B. Caballero, *Insights into the Mechanisms Involved in Protective Effects of VEGF-B in Neurons*, The University of Arizona, Tucson, Ariz, USA, 2016, http://hdl.handle.net/10150/621894.

8

Correlation of Visuospatial Ability and EEG Slowing in Patients with Parkinson's Disease

Dominique Eichelberger,[1] Pasquale Calabrese,[1] Antonia Meyer,[2] Menorca Chaturvedi,[2] Florian Hatz,[2] Peter Fuhr,[2] and Ute Gschwandtner[2]

[1]*Division of Molecular and Cognitive Neuroscience, Neuropsychology and Behavioural Neurology Unit, University of Basel, Basel, Switzerland*
[2]*Department of Neurology, Hospital of the University of Basel, Petersgraben 4, 4031 Basel, Switzerland*

Correspondence should be addressed to Pasquale Calabrese; pasquale.calabrese@unibas.ch

Academic Editor: Ivan Bodis-Wollner

Background. Visuospatial dysfunction is among the first cognitive symptoms in Parkinson's disease (PD) and is often predictive for PD-dementia. Furthermore, cognitive status in PD-patients correlates with quantitative EEG. This cross-sectional study aimed to investigate the correlation between EEG slowing and visuospatial ability in nondemented PD-patients. *Methods.* Fifty-seven nondemented PD-patients (17 females/40 males) were evaluated with a comprehensive neuropsychological test battery and a high-resolution 256-channel EEG was recorded. A median split was performed for each cognitive test dividing the patients sample into either a normal or lower performance group. The electrodes were split into five areas: frontal, central, temporal, parietal, and occipital. A linear mixed effects model (LME) was used for correlational analyses and to control for confounding factors. *Results.* Subsequently, for the lower performance, LME analysis showed a significant positive correlation between ROCF score and parietal alpha/theta ratio ($b = .59$, $p = .012$) and occipital alpha/theta ratio ($b = 0.50$, $p = .030$). No correlations were found in the group of patients with normal visuospatial abilities. *Conclusion.* We conclude that a reduction of the parietal alpha/theta ratio is related to visuospatial impairments in PD-patients. These findings indicate that visuospatial impairment in PD-patients could be influenced by parietal dysfunction.

1. Introduction

Cognitive decline is common in patients with Parkinson's disease (PD) and may range from mild impairment to overt dementia [1]. The cognitive symptoms are highly relevant as they go hand in hand with quality of life, disease prognosis, and caregiver burden [2]. The cognitive impairment generates far-reaching individual and health economic implications. Cognitive impairment in PD was mainly characterised by executive dysfunction, attentional, memory, and visuospatial deficits [3, 4]. Previous studies showed that visuospatial disturbances are among the first symptoms of cognitive decline to appear in PD [5, 6]. These deficits become more pronounced as the disease progresses [7] and they are independent of the severity of motor dysfunction and of the overall intellectual status. Interestingly, PD-patients with visuospatial deficits or memory impairment show a higher conversion rate

to Parkinson's disease dementia (PDD) than individuals with executive deficits [8, 9].

The cause of the visuospatial deficits remains unclear [10]. Pereira et al. [11] showed that patients with Parkinson's disease and mild cognitive impairment (PD-MCI) have a greater grey matter atrophy in both occipitotemporal and dorsoparietal cortices compared to healthy controls. Furthermore, previous research found that these patterns correlate with visuoperceptual and visuospatial abilities. These results are in line with the dual-stream hypothesis of visual processing which differentiates between two linked visual projection systems [12]. The first system expands from the area 17 (primary visual cortex) over the dorsal visual route towards the areas of the upper temporal lobe and the parietal lobe (occipitoparietal projection system). These areas participate in the analysis of visuospatial information such as movement, depth, position, orientation, and 3D characteristics of objects. The second projection system, the ventral visual stream, is responsible for pattern recognition (analysis of shapes, colours, objects, and faces). It connects area 17 to the lower temporal lobe.

Biomarker-based detection might lead to a better understanding of the cause of the visuospatial decline in PD-patients. Slowing of oscillatory brain activity (as measured by EEG and MEG) has been proposed as a surrogate marker of cognitive dysfunction [1, 13–15]. Soikkeli et al. [15] and also Olde Dubbelink et al. [16] demonstrated significantly different patterns in EEG frequencies between PD-patients and healthy controls. The authors found a decrease of beta and alpha activity and an analogous increase of theta and delta activity. In PDD-patients, the results are even more marked. A previous study showed that the alpha1/theta ratio is a reliable marker for PD-MCI [17]. Furthermore, Schmidt et al. [18] found that alpha/theta ratio discriminates Alzheimer's disease patients from healthy controls. The study of Kamei et al. [13] verified a positive correlation between deficient executive functions in PD and frontal EEG slowing. This relationship indicates that the deficits in executive tasks in PD could be due to a frontal dysfunction. Based on these findings, it would be interesting to investigate whether visuospatial abilities are related to parietal and occipital EEG activity in PD-patients.

More precisely, it is hypothesized that PD-patients with a visuospatial deficit manifest an EEG slowing which should be particularly pronounced in the parietal and the occipital lobe, compared to frontal, central, and temporal areas. To avoid confounding with overall cognitive performance the EEG slowing is matched with a test of memory span measures (short-term memory). This association in turn, is expected to be stronger in the frontal lobe compared to central, temporal, parietal, and occipital areas.

2. Materials and Methods

2.1. Subjects and Clinical Assessments. Participants were recruited between 2011 and 2015 from the outpatient clinic for movement disorders of the University Hospital Basel or through announcements in the Journal of the Swiss Parkinson's Disease Association. Altogether 72 patients with PD participated in the study. The data used in this study were baseline data collected from two studies. The first study was a computer-based, multidimensional and disease specific training of cognition in patients with PD that has already been published [20]. The second study is an ongoing group-based stress management training in patients with PD. Clinical assessment was performed with optimally medicated patients by means of the sum score of the motor section of the Unified Parkinson's Disease Rating Scale (UPDRS) subscale III [21]. Depression was assessed by Beck's Depression Inventory (BDI) [22]. The levodopa-equivalent (LED) was estimated according to Tomlinson et al. [23]. Inclusion criteria for the study were idiopathic PD according to UK Parkinson's disease Brain Bank Criteria [24] and signed informed consent was obtained from patients. Patients were excluded if they had other severe brain disorders and insufficient knowledge of the German language or if the EEG and the neuropsychology measurement were set apart more than 60 days.

For this study, the data of 57 patients with PD were included. Fifteen patients were excluded due to a Mini-Mental State Examination (MMSE) score of <24 ($n = 3$), because of undergoing a deep brain stimulation ($n = 6$) or due to insufficient EEG quality ($n = 6$, see below).

2.2. Neuropsychological Assessments. Patients were assessed with a comprehensive neuropsychological test battery. The following tests of this battery were used for this study; Clock Drawing Test, Rey-Osterrieth Complex Figure Test (ROCF) copy task [25], Block Design Test [26], and verbal Digit Span forward [27].

The *Clock Drawing Test* was scored according to Thalmann et al. [28]. It is a reliable measure of cognitive dysfunction [29, 30]. The Clock Drawing Test correlates with visuospatial tests like the ROCF and the Block Design [31, 32].

The *ROCF* is a common neuropsychological screening method for visuospatial abilities [33, 34]. Particularly, the copy variant of the task measures visuospatial construction while the delayed variant indicates visuospatial memory performance [34]. In the ROCF, the patients had to copy a complex figure. Afterwards, they had to reproduce it as complete as possible after a delay of 30 minutes. The ROCF was evaluated according to Aebi and Mistridis [35] based on Spreen and Strauss [36]. The sum score ranges from 0 to 36 points. The data were transformed into education and age controlled z-scores according to Aebi and Mistridis [35].

Block Design is a subtest of the revised Hamburg Wechsler Intelligence Scale for Adults [26]. The patients received at the beginning 4 and later 9 blocks, with different colour patterns on each side. With the blocks the patients had to build a predetermined pattern within a restricted period of time. The sum score ranges from 0 to 51 points; lower values are indicating more severe visuospatial disabilities.

Verbal Digit Span was applied to measure short-term memory. This test is a subtest of the Wechsler Memory Scale German adaption [27]. The examiner reads a series of digits aloud which have to be repeated by the subject afterwards. Each correctly repeated series granted a point, adding up to a sum score ranging from 0 to 12 points, where higher values indicate better short-term memory performance.

2.3. EEG Data. During 15 min an eyes-closed, resting-state, 256-channel EEG was recorded (Netstation 300; EGI Inc., Eugene, Oregon, USA). The reference electrode was Cz and rereferenced to the average. The sampling frequency was 1 kHz. Segments of >35 s without artifacts or signs of sleep were visually selected. EEGs were filtered (2,500 order least-square filter; band pass: 0.5–70 Hz, notch: 50 Hz) and bad electrodes were automatically detected (using TAPEEG software) [19] and visually checked for plausibility. Artifacts such as ECG and eye blinks were detected and removed by an application of an independent component analysis. Channels with bad activation were interpolated (spherical spline method). Frequency analysis was performed with the "Welch"-method [37]. Sliding windows of 4 s with 80% Hanning windows and the detection of bad windows were analysed with automated routines [19]. Semiautomatic processing of the data was applied in order to calculate the relative power in alpha (8–18 Hz) and theta (4–8 Hz) frequency bands across the 10 brain regions (see Figure 4). Relative alpha/theta ratios were calculated from the frequency results.

2.4. Statistical Procedure. The R software version 3.2.3 was used for statistical analysis [38]. The level of statistical significance was set at $p = .05$.

A linear mixed effects model (LME) with the alpha/theta ratio as the dependent variable was used to test the association between EEG slowing and visuospatial test scores. The test performance was used as fixed factor and the patients as random factor. Consequently, a b-value below zero indicates that the worse the alpha/theta ratio, the lower the test performance. The LME is a linear model that allows repeated measurement. This model was adopted due to the repeated measurements, resulting from EEG electrode subdivision into the five brain areas. An exhaustive search, according to Stöcklin [39], with age, gender, years of education, motor symptoms (UPDRS III), disease duration, depression scale (BDI), MMSE, and LED showed that gender and age were confounding factors for alpha/theta ratio. The assumptions for LME are homoscedasticity (homogeneous variance), linearity, no influential data points, and independence (collinearity). The plot of the standardized residuals showed a heterogeneous variance relating to the fitted values. A logarithmic transformation was performed in order to achieve a normal distribution as proposed by Crawley [40]. After the logarithmic transformation the residuals in the used LME models were normally distributed around zero and therefore the requested homogeneous variance was achieved [41]. Plots of the random effects showed an unsystematic arrangement around zero. This confirmed a normal distribution of the errors (linearity) [41]. Influential data points were not found. Furthermore, there was no correlation between the predictor variables.

In a first step, the LME calculations showed no correlation between alpha/theta ratio and the task performance. Because of this finding, a median split was used to separate potentially clinically conspicuous from inconspicuous patients in regard to the visuospatial ability. The median split was calculated separately for each neuropsychological test. Group A included patients from the lowest tasks performance up to the median and group B included patients from the median up to the best tasks performance. Clinical and demographic variables between the median split groups were analysed by means of X^2-test or Mann–Whitney U-test as appropriate. The difference in relative alpha/theta ratio between the left and the right cerebral hemisphere was calculated by a Wilcoxon's matched-pairs signed rank test. There were no significant differences in the relative alpha/theta ratio between the right- and left-sided electrode in the PD-patients ($p = .316$). Therefore, the analyses were based on combined data of the alpha/theta ratio for the right- and left-sided electrode locations. Furthermore, to compare the results, the LME were calculated with z-scaled Block Design and the Digit Span scores.

TABLE 1: Descriptive statistics and tasks performance of total group.

Parkinson patient $N = 57$	M	SD
Sex (M/F)	40/17	
Age (years)	67.21	(6.96)
Education (years)	14.67	(3.01)
UPDRS III	14.77	(11.13)
MMSE	28.70	(1.06)
Disease duration (years)	5.25	(0.50)
Dose of L-dopa (mg/day)	597.60	(372.06)
BDI	7.22	(4.47)
Clock Drawing Test (incorrectly/correctly drawn)	16/41	
ROCF	28.83	(4.19)
Block Design Test	24.79	(7.56)
Verbal Digit Span forward	7.49	(1.72)

Note. Means and standard deviations relate to raw values. UPDRS III = Unified Parkinson's Disease Rating Scale subscale III (range 0–108); MMES = Mini-Mental State Examination (range 0–30); BDI = Beck Depression Inventory (range 0–63); ROCF = Rey-Osterrieth Complex Figure Test.

3. Results

The visuospatial decrease which would be expected in PD-patients was weak in this population (see Table 1). The descriptive statistics of the clinical performance, split in the two median groups A and B, are shown in Table 2. Significant differences between group A and B had been obtained in the Clock Drawing Test with regard to the MMSE and the BDI and in the Digit Span with regard to the disease duration. Otherwise there were no significant differences between the groups. The exhaustive search had shown that gender and age were confounding factors for all used neuropsychological tests. The EEG alpha/theta ratio was different between males and females in all areas [parietal $U(57/57) = 211$, $p = .024$, frontal $U(57/57) = 200$, $p = .014$, central $U(57/57) = 205$, $p = .018$, temporal, $U(57/57) = 210$, $p = .023$, and occipital $U(57/57) = 194$, $p = .010$].

3.1. Clock Drawing. The LME results for the Clock Drawing Test are shown in Table 3. A significant lower alpha/theta ratio was recognised in PD-patients with an incorrectly drawn clock compared to PD-patients, who had produced a correctly drawn clock. The group difference was more distinct in parietal areas than in central, temporal, and occipital areas.

3.2. ROCF. As shown in Table 4, in group A of the ROCF, the results revealed that the deeper the parietal alpha/theta ratio the worse the ROCF performance. An increase of 1.0 z-score in the ROCF increased the parietal alpha/theta ratio by $b = 0.59$, $t(24) = 2.73$, and $p = .012$. There was also a significant positive association between occipital alpha/theta ratio and the ROCF performance in the ROCF group A. An increase of 1.0 z-score in the ROCF increased the occipital alpha/theta ratio [$b = 0.50$, $t(24) = 2.31$, $p = .030$]. No significant association was found in the other cortical areas

TABLE 2: Descriptive statistics of median split groups.

Allocation	Clock Drawing Test			ROCF			Block Design Test			Digit Span		
	Incorrectly drawn	Correctly drawn		A	B		A	B		A	B	
	$N = 16$	$N = 41$		$N = 26$	$N = 29$		$N = 29$	$N = 27$		$N = 29$	$N = 28$	
	Median	Median	p	Median	Median	p	Median	Median	p	Median	Median	p
Sex (M/F)	11/5	29/12	1.000	19/9	20/7	.833	20/9	19/8	1.000	20/9	20/8	1.000
Age	67.5	67	.930	66.5	69.0	.295	67.0	69.0	.384	67.0	67.5	.994
Education	15	15	.964	14	15	.572	14	15	.092	15	15	.413
UPDRS III	13.5	13.5	.765	17.0	10.0	.166	15.5	13.0	.511	14.0	13.5	.818
MMSE	28.5	29	.036*	29	29	.347	29	29	.209	29	29	.322
Disease duration	5.27	3.37	.160	4.30	3.24	.508	4.12	3.37	.558	2.94	4.74	.038*
Dose of L-dopa	666	510	.247	650	495	.206	590	550	.906	510	585	.296
BDI	4.5	8.0	.024*	6.5	7.18	.901	6.5	7.35	.655	7	7	.941

Note. Values are expressed by median; UPDRS III = Unified Parkinson's Disease Rating Scale subscale III (range 0–108); MMES = Mini-Mental State Examination (range 0–30); BDI = Beck Depression Inventory (range 0–63); ROCF = Rey-Osterrieth Complex Figure Test; A = group with lower tasks performance; B = group with higher tasks performance; * $p < .050$, · $p < .1$.

TABLE 3: Correlation between alpha/theta ratio and Clock Drawing Test.

Brain area	Δ incorrectly and correctly drawn		Comparison b parietal/other areas
	b	p	b
Parietal	0.54 (0.18)	**.003***	
Frontal	0.44 (0.18)	**.016***	0.134
Central	0.40 (0.18)	**.025***	**0.046***
Temporal	0.40 (0.18)	**.027***	**0.040***
Occipital	0.36 (0.18)	**.045***	**0.009***

Note. b = beta coefficient (standard errors); using a linear mixed effects model (LME); *$p < .05$.

(see Table 4). Furthermore, the associations in the parietal areas were different from the frontal [$b = -.19$, $t(104) = -2.28$, and $p = .025$], central [$b = -.24$, $t(104) = -2.88$, and $p = .005$], and temporal [$b = -.24$, $t(104) = -2.88$, and $p = .005$] areas. There was no significant difference between the association in parietal areas and the association in occipital areas [$b = -.09$, $t(104) = -1.06$, and $p = .290$]. In the ROCF group B there was neither an association between alpha/theta ratio and the ROCF z-score nor a significant difference between the association in parietal areas and the associations in the remaining areas.

3.3. Block Design Test. The LME results for the Block Design Test are shown in Table 5. No significant correlation was found between the alpha/theta ratio and the Block Design performance. In the Block Design group A there was simply a tendency towards a positive correlation between the parietal alpha/theta ratio and the Block Design performance. An increase of 1.0 z-score in the Block Design Test increased the alpha/theta ratio [$b = 0.48$, $t(25) = 1.96$, and $p = .062$]. No associations were found in the other cortical areas. The association in the parietal areas differed from the association in temporal areas [$b = -.24$, $t(108) = -2.54$, and $p = .013$]. Furthermore, there was a trend towards a difference between the association in parietal areas and the association in frontal [$b = -.16$, $t(108) = -1.71$, and $p = .090$] and central areas [$b = -.16$, $t(108) = -1.68$, and $p = .096$].

3.4. Verbal Digit Span forward. The results in both Digit Span groups, A and B, showed no correlation between the alpha/theta ratio and the Digit Span performance (see Table 6). However, in the Digit Span group A a slight tendency towards a negative correlation between the alpha/theta ratio and the Digit Span performance was observable in frontal [$b = -.35$, $t(25) = -2.05$, and $p = .051$], central, [$b = -.29$, $t(25) = -1.73$, and $p = .096$], and parietal areas, [$b = -.34$, $t(25) = -2.02$, and $p = .054$]. There were no associations in the other cortical areas. Furthermore, the association in the parietal areas was different from the occipital areas, [$b = .14$, $t(108) = 2.21$, and $p = .030$] in group A. In group B a difference between the association in parietal areas and the

association in central areas, [$b = -.16$, $t(104) = -2.07$, and $p = .041$] was observable (see Table 6).

4. Discussion

The aim of this study was to investigate possible relationships between parietal and occipital EEG slowing and visuospatial deficit in nondemented PD-patients. The EEG slowing was measured by determining the alpha/theta ratio in the frontal, central, temporal, parietal, and occipital lobe. The visuospatial ability was assessed by three different neuropsychological tests: Clock Drawing Test, ROCF, and Block Design Test. A LME was used to explore the association between visuospatial performances and alpha/theta ratio.

In contrast to previous findings, the PD-patients in our study showed only slight deficits in visuospatial ability [3, 4]. This might be explained by the high education level of the patients in our sample. Recent studies indicated that a high education is predictive for a slower cognitive decline [42–44]. In order to separate potentially clinically conspicuous from inconspicuous patients in regard to the visuospatial ability a median split was used.

The results of this study show that PD-patients with a parietal EEG slowing manifest a visuospatial deficit. This result is in line with findings from voxel-based morphometry MRI analysis, indicating correlations between visuospatial ability in PDD-patients and changes in the occipitotemporal and dorsoparietal cortices in comparison to healthy controls [11]. Nombela et al. [45] also reported a correlation between parietal activity and visuospatial performance. In line with our hypothesis, the association between the EEG slowing and the visuospatial task performance is particularly pronounced in parietal areas compared to frontal, central, and temporal areas (see Figure 3). In addition, no differences between the association in parietal and occipital areas were detected in our sample. This finding indicates that the association is not explained by the global EEG slowing, as has been shown in previous studies in patients with PD [46, 47]. Though other previous studies also indicated that the visuospatial ability is not correlated with global EEG slowing measured by median frequency [48], more research is needed to substantiate this point. Our present findings are also in line with the dual-stream hypothesis of the visual processing claiming the occipitoparietal projection system to be responsible for visuospatial performance [12].

In all groups with test scores above the median (i.e., unimpaired visuospatial abilities), no correlations were found between the alpha/theta ratio and the task performances, indicating that a relationship between the visuospatial ability and the EEG is only measurable if the visuospatial ability score decreases below the median.

In contrast to the results of the ROCF and the Block Design Test, the results of the Clock Drawing Test showed that PD-patients drawing an incorrect clock had lower alpha/theta ratio not only in parietal and occipital brain areas but also in all other brain areas. PD-patients with a flawless CDT-performance did not show this association (see Figure 2). The neuroanatomical correlates of Clock Drawing Test performance were investigated in several studies, but

TABLE 4: Correlation between alpha/theta ratio and Rey-Osterrieth Complex Figure Test.

brain areas	b	p	ROCF A Comparison b parietal/other areas p	b	p	ROCF B Comparison b parietal/other areas p
Parietal	0.59 (0.21)	.012*		−0.06 (0.17)	.738	
Frontal	0.39 (0.21)	.079˙	.025*	−0.08 (0.17)	.653	.724
Central	0.34 (0.21)	.123	.005*	−0.00 (0.17)	.984	.337
Temporal	0.34 (0.21)	.123	.005*	−0.01 (0.17)	.967	.372
Occipital	0.50 (0.21)	.030*	.290	−0.02 (0.17)	.900	.530

Note. b = beta coefficient (standard errors); using a linear mixed effects model (LME); $^*p < .05$, $˙p < .1$.

TABLE 5: Correlation between alpha/theta ratio and Block Design Test.

brain areas	b	p	Block Design A Comparison b parietal/other areas p	b	p	Block Design B Comparison b parietal/other areas p
Parietal	0.49 (0.25)	.062˙		0.02 (0.15)	.886	
Frontal	0.32 (0.25)	.202	.090˙	−0.01 (0.15)	.938	.588
Central	0.33 (0.25)	.198	.096˙	0.05 (0.15)	.711	.578
Temporal	0.25 (0.25)	.328	.013*	0.05 (0.15)	.735	.631
Occipital	0.40 (0.25)	.121	.353	−0.01 (0.15)	.962	.640

Note. b = beta coefficient (standard errors); using a linear mixed effects model (LME); $^*p < .05$, $˙p < .1$.

TABLE 6: Correlation between alpha/theta ratio and verbal Digit Span forward.

Brain areas	b	p	Digit Span A Comparison b parietal/other areas p	b	p	Digit Span B Comparison b parietal/other areas p
Parietal	−0.34 (0.17)	.054˙		0.25 (0.22)	.272	
Frontal	−0.35 (0.17)	.051˙	.944	0.13 (0.22)	.548	.156
Central	−0.29 (0.17)	.096˙	.469	0.08 (0.22)	.707	.041*
Temporal	−0.28 (0.17)	.107	.381	0.15 (0.22)	.505	.218
Occipital	−0.19 (0.17)	.265	.030*	0.13 (0.22)	.510	.210

Note. b = beta coefficient (standard errors); using a linear mixed effects model (LME); $^*p < .05$, $˙p < .1$.

the findings are inconsistent [49–52]. This discrepancy might probably stem from the fact that the Clock Drawing Test measures also executive function, numerical and verbal memory, and visuospatial ability [34, 53]. Furthermore, Matsuoka et al. [52] explored the relationship between regional cerebral blood flow and different scoring criteria of the Clock Drawing Test in patients with Alzheimer's disease, revealing that different criteria correlate with different brain regions. Consequently, it can be concluded that for a correlative analysis between different brain areas and CDT-performance an overall classification into errorless and incorrect CDT-performance might be too simple. Hence, future studies should adopt differential scoring CDT-scoring criteria to unravel this relationship.

In our study, the results of the ROCF and the Block Design Test are consistent. In line with our findings, for both tests, neuroanatomical correlations in parietal and occipital areas were also found in previous studies [54–57]. However, the results are more specific in ROCF than in the Block Design Test. This result could be partly explained by the somewhat different cognitive processes required by the different tasks. Hence, while the ROCF is mainly a visuo-constructive task, with a preponderance on visuoperceptive, visuospatial as well as graphomotor abilities without time limitation, the Block Design Test on the other hand requires mental rotation as well as geometric fragmentation analysis under time-restriction [26].

The Digit Span measures working memory. Studies on healthy subjects, using either transcranial magnetic stimulation [58] or functional neuroimaging [59], were able to show an involvement of the right dorsolateral prefrontal cortex in Digit Span processing. Furthermore, Gerton et al.

[59] reported that parietal and occipital areas are activated during the Digit Span forward task. In the present study no association was found between EEG slowing and the Digit Span performance. Nevertheless, a slight tendency towards a negative correlation between the alpha/theta ratio and the Digit Span performance was observed in frontal, central, and parietal areas (see Figure 3). The involvement of parietal areas could be explained by the use of the visual imagination strategies the subjects used during the Digit Span test [34]. An explanation for the negative tendency could be that the Digit Span performance is not relating to EEG slowing caused by a shifting in alpha/theta ratio but by a shifting in others frequency range (e.g., theta/delta ratio or beta/alpha).

The results from our present study do not reveal significant differences regarding confounding factors between the median split groups of the ROCF and Block Design Test. However, there were significant differences between the subgroups according to their Clock Drawing Test performance. Patients with an incorrectly drawn clock had a lower MMSE score than patients with a flawless CDT-performance. This finding is not surprising since both CDT and MMSE are also measures of global cognitive dysfunction [28–30, 60]. In addition, many studies found a correlation between these two tests [53, 61–63]. Furthermore, PD- Patients with an incorrectly drawn clock had a lower BDI score than PD-patients with a correctly drawn clock. These findings were unexpected as it is well-known that there is an association between depression and cognitive performance [64]. The results exploring the association between severity of depression and the performance in the Clock Drawing Test are inconsistent. Some authors have reported a significant negative relation [65, 66], whereas others have found minimal or no effect between the severity of depression and the Clock Drawing performance [61, 67–70]. In the present study, the BDI score has no significant influence on the used LME model. Nevertheless, the results cannot predict whether severity of depression has an influence on the cognitive performance. Another group difference is found between Digit Span performance and disease duration. Patients in the Digit Span group A have a shorter disease duration than patients in the Digit Span group B. This result contrasts with some recent findings which have shown a reduction of working memory capacity in PD-patients as the disease progresses [71, 72]. Hence, our result might be caused by the sampling process based on a right-skewed sample..

While in the present study gender (see Figure 1) and age are identified as confounding factors and were consequently controlled in the LME, other authors have found only a small influence for these variables on the EEG activity [46, 73]. Hence, further studies are needed to determine the influence of gender and age on EEG slowing in PD-patients.

One limitation of our study is that the calculation of z-scores for the ROCF was based on a norm population whereas the calculations of z-scores for the Block Design Test and the Digit Span were based on our study population, limiting a comparison of the tests. Moreover, since only 17 of 57 patients in our sample were female, the gender influence on EEG limits a generalization. Although the unequal distribution of gender is well-known in PD [74, 75] an equal gender

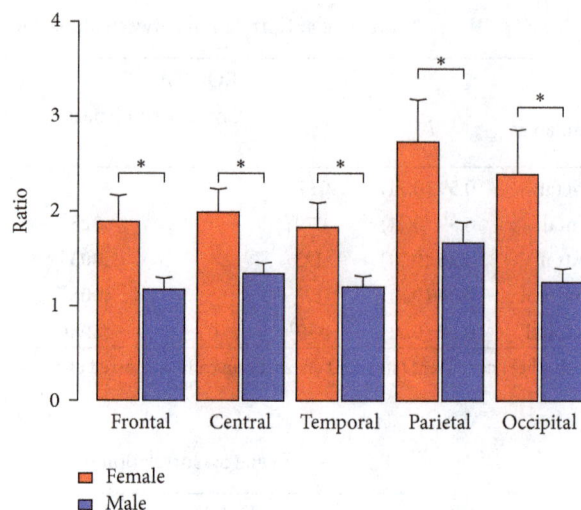

FIGURE 1: Difference alpha/theta ratio between gender in the different brain areas. $^*p < .050$.

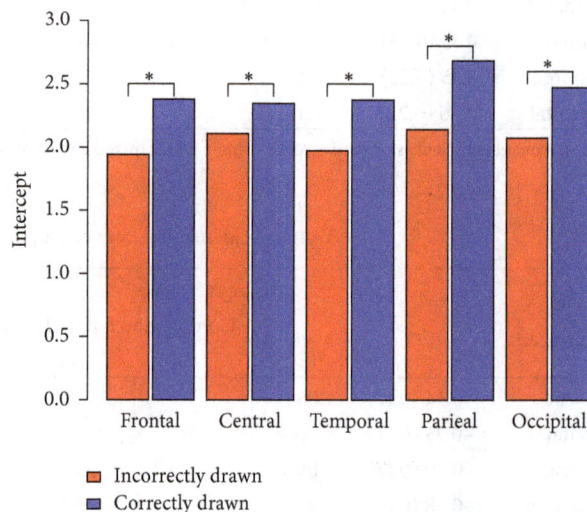

FIGURE 2: Comparison intercept between incorrectly and correctly drawn Clock Drawing Test groups related to the alpha/theta ratio in the different brain areas. $^*p < .050$.

distribution should be considered in future studies. Another limitation of this study is that there were no healthy controls included. Therefore, the conclusion that the findings are specific for patients with PD cannot be drawn. Moreover, since we adopted a priori hypothesis based models, we relinquished to account for multiple comparisons. Therefore the interpretation of the results should be treated with caution, bearing in mind that the probability of correlative findings increases with the number of tests performed. In conclusion, in PD-patients with only slight deficits in visuospatial abilities the visuospatial performance is related to parietal and occipital EEG slowing. The association between the EEG slowing and the visuospatial task performance is particularly pronounced in parietal areas compared to frontal, central, and temporal areas.

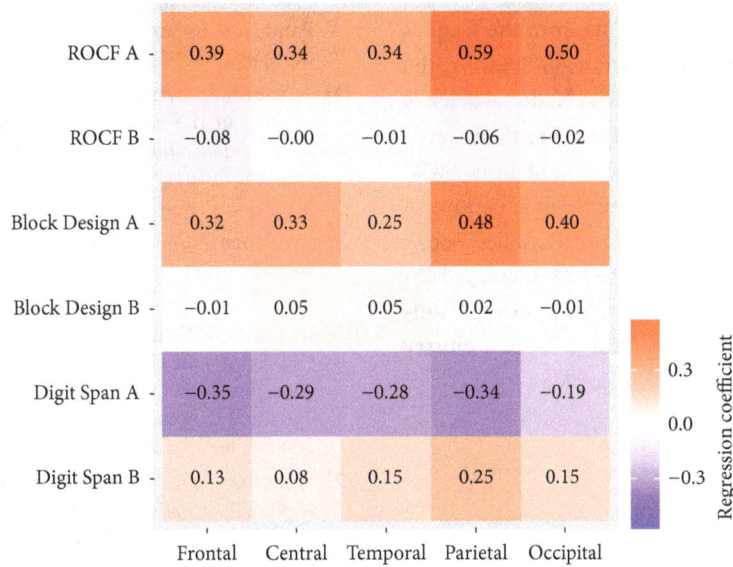

FIGURE 3: Correlation between alpha/theta ratio and tasks performance in different brain areas; ROCF is Rey-Osterrieth Complex Figure Test; A is group with lower tasks performance; B is group with higher tasks performance.

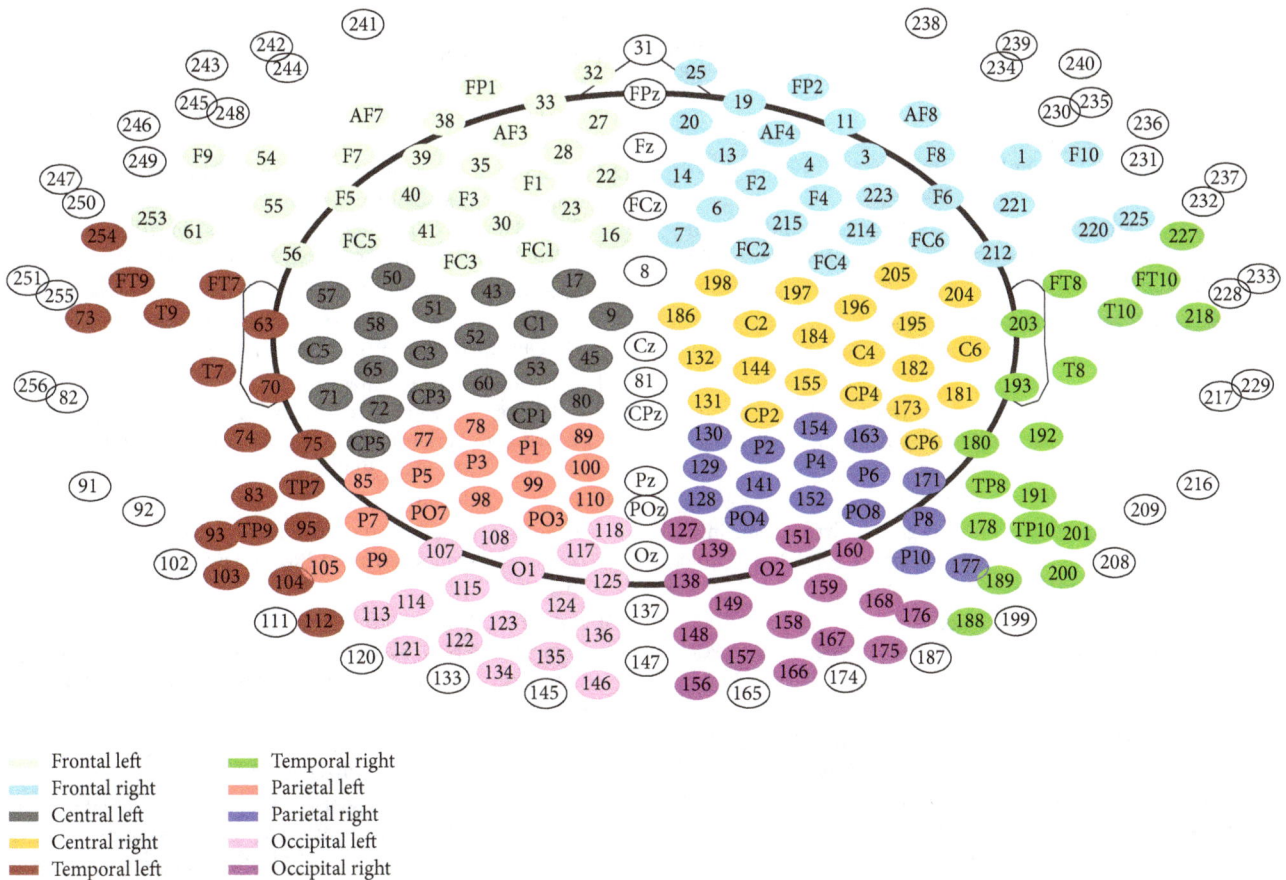

FIGURE 4: Electrodes allocation for frequency analyse [19].

Acknowledgments

The study was supported in part by grants from the Jacques and Gloria Gossweiler Foundation, Parkinson Schweiz, the Hedwig Widmer Foundation, and the Swiss National Science Foundation (SPUM 33CM30_140338). Peter Fuhr's research is supported by Swiss National Science Foundation, Swiss Multiple Sclerosis Society, Synapsis Foundation, Parkinson Schweiz, Novartis Research Foundation, Gossweiler Foundation, Freiwillige Akademische Gesellschaft Basel, Mach-Gaensslen-Stiftung, Botnar Foundation, Bangerter Foundation, and unconditional research grants from industry (Roche, AbbVie, Biogen, and General Electric).

References

[1] J. N. Caviness, J. G. Hentz, V. G. Evidente et al., "Both early and late cognitive dysfunction affects the electroencephalogram in Parkinson's disease," *Parkinsonism and Related Disorders*, vol. 13, no. 6, pp. 348–354, 2007.

[2] E. Kalbe and A. Petrelli, "Leichte kognitive Störungen und Demenz bei Patienten mit Morbus Parkinson," *Zeitschrift für Neuropsychologie*, vol. 25, no. 1, pp. 17–30, 2014.

[3] M. Emre, "Dementia associated with Parkinson's disease," *Lancet Neurology*, vol. 2, no. 4, pp. 229–237, 2003.

[4] J. Gratwicke, M. Jahanshahi, and T. Foltynie, "Parkinson's disease dementia: a neural networks perspective," *Brain*, vol. 138, no. 6, pp. 1454–1476, 2015.

[5] A. Antal, F. Bandini, S. Kéri, and I. Bodis-Wollner, "Visuo-cognitive dysfunctions in Parkinson's disease," *Clinical Neuroscience*, vol. 5, no. 2, pp. 147–152, 1998.

[6] F. Girotti, P. Soliveri, F. Carella et al., "Dementia and cognitive impairment in Parkinson's disease," *Journal of Neurology, Neurosurgery & Psychiatry*, vol. 51, no. 12, pp. 1498–1502, 1988.

[7] B. E. Levin, M. M. Llabre, S. Reisman et al., "Visuospatial impairment in Parkinson's disease," *Neurology*, vol. 41, no. 3, pp. 365–369, 1991.

[8] D. Muslimović, B. Post, J. D. Speelman, and B. Schmand, "Cognitive profile of patients with newly diagnosed Parkinson disease," *Neurology*, vol. 65, no. 8, pp. 1239–1245, 2005.

[9] C. H. Williams-Gray, T. Foltynie, C. E. G. Brayne, T. W. Robbins, and R. A. Barker, "Evolution of cognitive dysfunction in an incident Parkinson's disease cohort," *Brain*, vol. 130, no. 7, pp. 1787–1798, 2007.

[10] S. Laatu, A. Revonsuo, L. Pihko, R. Portin, and J. O. Rinne, "Visual object recognition deficits in early Parkinson's disease," *Parkinsonism & Related Disorders*, vol. 10, no. 4, pp. 227–233, 2004.

[11] J. B. Pereira, C. Junqué, M.-J. Martí, B. Ramirez-Ruiz, N. Bargalló, and E. Tolosa, "Neuroanatomical substrate of visuospatial and visuoperceptual impairment in Parkinson's disease," *Movement Disorders*, vol. 24, no. 8, pp. 1193–1199, 2009.

[12] L. G. Ungerleider and J. V. Haxby, "'What' and 'where' in the human brain," *Current Opinion in Neurobiology*, vol. 4, no. 2, pp. 157–165, 1994.

[13] S. Kamei, A. Morita, K. Serizawa, T. Mizutani, and K. Hirayanagi, "Quantitative EEG analysis of executive dysfunction in Parkinson disease," *Journal of Clinical Neurophysiology*, vol. 27, no. 3, pp. 193–197, 2010.

[14] A. Morita, S. Kamei, and T. Mizutani, "Relationship between slowing of the EEG and cognitive impairment in Parkinson disease," *Journal of Clinical Neurophysiology*, vol. 28, no. 4, pp. 384–387, 2011.

[15] R. Soikkeli, J. Partanen, H. Soininen, A. Pääkkönen, and P. Riekkinen Sr., "Slowing of EEG in Parkinson's disease," *Electroencephalography and Clinical Neurophysiology*, vol. 79, no. 3, pp. 159–165, 1991.

[16] K. T. E. Olde Dubbelink, D. Stoffers, J. B. Deijen, J. W. R. Twisk, C. J. Stam, and H. W. Berendse, "Cognitive decline in Parkinson's disease is associated with slowing of resting-state brain activity: a longitudinal study," *Neurobiology of Aging*, vol. 34, no. 2, pp. 408–418, 2013.

[17] H. Bousleiman, M. Chaturvedi, U. Gschwandtner et al., "P122. Alpha1/theta ratio from quantitative EEG (qEEG) as a reliable marker for mild cognitive impairment (MCI) in patients with Parkinson's disease (PD)," *Clinical Neurophysiology*, vol. 126, no. 8, pp. e150–e151, 2015.

[18] M. T. Schmidt, P. A. M. Kanda, L. F. H. Basile et al., "Index of alpha/theta ratio of the electroencephalogram: A new marker for Alzheimer's disease," *Frontiers in Aging Neuroscience*, vol. 5, 2013.

[19] F. Hatz, M. Hardmeier, H. Bousleiman, S. Rüegg, C. Schindler, and P. Fuhr, "Reliability of fully automated versus visually controlled pre- and post-processing of resting-state EEG," *Clinical Neurophysiology*, vol. 126, no. 2, pp. 268–274, 2015.

[20] R. Zimmermann, U. Gschwandtner, N. Benz et al., "Cognitive training in Parkinson disease: cognition-specific vs nonspecific computer training," *Neurology*, vol. 82, no. 14, pp. 1219–1226, 2014.

[21] S. Fahn and R. I. Elton, "Unified Parkinson's disease rating scale," in *Recent Developments in Parkinson's Disease*, S. Fahn, C. D. Marsden, D. B. Calne, and M. Goldstein, Eds., vol. 2, Macmillan Health Care Information, Florham Park, NJ, USA, 1987.

[22] A. Schrag, P. Barone, R. G. Brown et al., "Depression rating scales in Parkinson's disease: critique and recommendations," *Movement Disorders*, vol. 22, no. 8, pp. 1077–1092, 2007.

[23] C. L. Tomlinson, R. Stowe, S. Patel, C. Rick, R. Gray, and C. E. Clarke, "Systematic review of levodopa dose equivalency reporting in Parkinson's disease," *Movement Disorders*, vol. 25, no. 15, pp. 2649–2653, 2010.

[24] W. R. G. Gibb and A. J. Lees, "The relevance of the Lewy body to the pathogenesis of idiopathic Parkinson's disease," *Journal of Neurology, Neurosurgery and Psychiatry*, vol. 51, no. 6, pp. 745–752, 1988.

[25] J. F. Duley, J. W. Wilkins, S. L. Hamby, D. G. Hopkins, R. D. Burwell, and N. S. Barry, "Explicit scoring criteria for the Rey-Osterrieth and Taylor complex figures," *Clinical Neuropsychologist*, vol. 7, no. 1, pp. 29–38, 1993.

[26] D. Wechsler, *Hamburger Wechsler Intelligenztest für Erwachsene Revision*, Huber, Bern, Switzerland, 1991.

[27] C. Härting, H. J. Markowitsch, H. Neufeld, P. Calabrese, K. Deisinger, and J. Kessler, *Wechsler Gedächtnistest-Revidierte Fassung (WMS-R), Testmanual, Deutsche Adaptation der Revidierten Fassung der Wechsler Memory Scale von David Wechsler*, Hans Huber, Bern, Switzerland, 2000.

[28] B. Thalmann, R. Spiegel, H. B. Stahelin et al., "Dementia screening in general practice: optimised scoring for the clock drawing test," *Brain Aging*, vol. 2, no. 2, pp. 36–43, 2002.

[29] D. A. Cahn-Weiner, E. V. Sullivan, P. K. Shear et al., "Brain structural and cognitive correlates of clock drawing performance in Alzheimer's disease," *Journal of the International Neuropsychological Society*, vol. 5, no. 6, pp. 502–509, 1999.

[30] O. Riedel, J. Klotsche, H. Förstl, and H.-U. Wittchen, "Clock drawing test: is it useful for dementia screening in patients having parkinson disease with and without depression?" *Journal of Geriatric Psychiatry and Neurology*, vol. 26, no. 3, pp. 151–157, 2013.

[31] E. Pinto and R. Peters, "Literature review of the Clock Drawing Test as a tool for cognitive screening," *Dementia and Geriatric Cognitive Disorders*, vol. 27, no. 3, pp. 201–213, 2009.

[32] A. Hochrein, L. Jonitz, E. Plaum, and R. R. Engel, *Kompetenzbeurteilung und Kompetenzmessung bei Dementen—ein Vergleich zwischen Verfahren zur Quantifizierung demenzbedingter Beeinträchtigungen des Alltagsverhaltens*, Springer, Berlin, Germany, 1996.

[33] K. Karádi, T. Lucza, Z. Aschermann et al., "Visuospatial impairment in Parkinson's disease: the role of laterality," *Laterality*, vol. 20, no. 1, pp. 112–127, 2015.

[34] M. D. Lezak, D. B. Howieson, E. D. Bigler, and D. Tranel, *Neuropsychological Assessment*, Oxford University Press, New York, NY, USA, 2012.

[35] S. Aebi and P. Mistridis, "Die komplexe Figur von Rey-Osterrieth. Eine Normierungsstudie zur Bewertung der Reproduktionsgenauigkeit nach deutschen Kriterien," in *Unveröffentlichte Masterarbeit*, Universität Basel, Basel, Switzerland, 2009.

[36] O. Spreen and E. Strauss, *A Compendium of Neuropsychological Tests: Administration, Norms, and Commentary*, University Press, New York, NY, USA, 1991.

[37] P. D. Welch, "The use of fast fourier transform for the estimation of power spectra: a method based on time averaging over short, modified periodograms," *IEEE Transactions on Audio and Electroacoustics*, vol. 15, no. 2, pp. 70–73, 1967.

[38] R-Core-Team, *R: A Language and Environment for Statistical Computing*, R Foundation for Statistical Computing, Vienna, Austria, 2015, https://www.r-project.org/.

[39] M. Stöcklin, *Statistik 3 Eine Einführung mit R*, Fakultät für Psychologie-Universität Basel, Basel, Switzerland, 2014.

[40] M. J. Crawley, *Statistik mit R*, John Wiley & Sons, New York, NY, USA, 2012.

[41] R. Leonhart and S. Lichtenberg, *Lehrbuch Statistik*, H. Huber, 2009.

[42] H. H. Kornhuber, "Prävention von Demenz (einschließlich Alzheimer-Krankheit)," *Das Gesundheitswesen*, vol. 66, no. 5, pp. 346–351, 2004.

[43] Y. Stern, "Cognitive reserve," *Neuropsychologia*, vol. 47, no. 10, pp. 2015–2028, 2009.

[44] X. Meng and C. D'Arcy, "Education and dementia in the context of the cognitive reserve hypothesis: a systematic review with meta-analyses and qualitative analyses," *PLoS ONE*, vol. 7, no. 6, Article ID e38268, 2012.

[45] C. Nombela, J. B. Rowe, S. E. Winder-Rhodes et al., "Genetic impact on cognition and brain function in newly diagnosed Parkinson's disease: ICICLE-PD study," *Brain*, vol. 137, no. 10, pp. 2743–2758, 2014.

[46] B. T. Klassen, J. G. Hentz, H. A. Shill et al., "Quantitative EEG as a predictive biomarker for Parkinson disease dementia," *Neurology*, vol. 77, no. 2, pp. 118–124, 2011.

[47] K. T. E. O. Dubbelink, A. Hillebrand, J. W. R. Twisk et al., "Predicting dementia in Parkinson disease by combining neurophysiologic and cognitive markers," *Neurology*, vol. 82, no. 3, pp. 263–270, 2014.

[48] R. Zimmermann, U. Gschwandtner, F. Hatz et al., "Correlation of EEG slowing with cognitive domains in nondemented patients with Parkinson's disease," *Dementia and Geriatric Cognitive Disorders*, vol. 39, no. 3-4, pp. 207–214, 2014.

[49] T. Matsuoka, J. Narumoto, K. Shibata et al., "Neural correlates of performance on the different scoring systems of the clock drawing test," *Neuroscience Letters*, vol. 487, no. 3, pp. 421–425, 2011.

[50] D. Y. Lee, E. H. Seo, I. H. Choo et al., "Neural correlates of the clock drawing test performance in Alzheimer's disease: a FDG-PET study," *Dementia and Geriatric Cognitive Disorders*, vol. 26, no. 4, pp. 306–313, 2008.

[51] J. M. Shon, D. Y. Lee, E. H. Seo et al., "Functional neuroanatomical correlates of the executive clock drawing task (CLOX) performance in Alzheimer's disease: a FDG-PET study," *Neuroscience*, vol. 246, pp. 271–280, 2013.

[52] T. Matsuoka, J. Narumoto, A. Okamura et al., "Neural correlates of the components of the clock drawing test," *International Psychogeriatrics*, vol. 25, no. 8, pp. 1317–1323, 2013.

[53] K. I. Shulman, "Clock-drawing: is it the ideal cognitive screening test?" *International Journal of Geriatric Psychiatry*, vol. 15, no. 6, pp. 548–561, 2000.

[54] R. J. Melrose, D. Harwood, T. Khoo, M. Mandelkern, and D. L. Sultzer, "Association between cerebral metabolism and Rey-Osterrieth Complex Figure Test performance in Alzheimer's disease," *Journal of Clinical and Experimental Neuropsychology*, vol. 35, no. 3, pp. 246–258, 2013.

[55] T. N. Chase, P. Fedio, N. L. Foster, R. Brooks, G. Chiro, and L. Mansi, "Wechsler adult intelligence scale performance: cortical localization by fluorodeoxyglucose F18-positron emission tomography," *Archives of Neurology*, vol. 41, no. 12, pp. 1244–1247, 1984.

[56] E. K. Warrington, M. James, and C. Maciejewski, "The WAIS as a lateralizing and localizing diagnostic instrument: a study of 656 patients with unilateral cerebral lesions," *Neuropsychologia*, vol. 24, no. 2, pp. 223–239, 1986.

[57] M. C. Wilde, C. Boake, and M. Sherer, "Wechsler adult intelligence scale-revised block design broken configuration errors in nonpenetrating traumatic brain injury," *Applied Neuropsychology*, vol. 7, no. 4, pp. 208–214, 2000.

[58] A. Aleman and M. van't Wout, "Repetitive transcranial magnetic stimulation over the right dorsolateral prefrontal cortex disrupts digit span task performance," *Neuropsychobiology*, vol. 57, no. 1-2, pp. 44–48, 2008.

[59] B. K. Gerton, T. T. Brown, A. Meyer-Lindenberg et al., "Shared and distinct neurophysiological components of the digits forward and backward tasks as revealed by functional neuroimaging," *Neuropsychologia*, vol. 42, no. 13, pp. 1781–1787, 2004.

[60] C. Ploenes, S. Sharp, and M. Martin, "The Clock Test: drawing a clock for detection of cognitive disorders in geriatric patients," *Zeitschrift für Gerontologie und Geriatrie*, vol. 27, no. 4, pp. 246–252, 1994.

[61] L. K. Klein, *Vergleichende neuropsychologische Untersuchungen bei älteren Patienten mit früh und spät beginnenden depressiven Störungen unter besonderer Berücksichtigung von Uhrentests*, Universität Tübingen, Tübingen, Germany, 2015.

[62] H. Brodaty and C. M. Moore, "The clock drawing test for dementia of the Alzheimer's type: a comparison of three scoring

methods in a memory disorders clinic," *International Journal of Geriatric Psychiatry*, vol. 12, no. 6, pp. 619–627, 1997.

[63] J. Heinik, I. Solomesh, and P. Berkman, "Correlation between the CAMCOG, the MMSE, and three clock drawing tests in a specialized outpatient psychogeriatric service," *Archives of Gerontology and Geriatrics*, vol. 38, no. 1, pp. 77–84, 2004.

[64] D. C. Steffens and G. G. Potter, "Geriatric depression and cognitive impairment," *Psychological Medicine*, vol. 38, no. 2, pp. 163–175, 2008.

[65] P. O. Harvey, G. Le Bastard, J. B. Pochon et al., "Executive functions and updating of the contents of working memory in unipolar depression," *Journal of Psychiatric Research*, vol. 38, no. 6, pp. 567–576, 2004.

[66] C. Sarapas, S. A. Shankman, M. Harrow, and J. F. Goldberg, "Parsing trait and state effects of depression severity on neurocognition: evidence from a 26-year longitudinal study," *Journal of Abnormal Psychology*, vol. 121, no. 4, pp. 830–837, 2012.

[67] V. Elderkin-Thompson, K. B. Boone, S. Hwang, and A. Kumar, "Neurocognitive profiles in elderly patients with frontotemporal degeneration or major depressive disorder," *Journal of the International Neuropsychological Society*, vol. 10, no. 5, pp. 753–771, 2004.

[68] C. R. Quinn, A. Harris, K. Felmingham, P. Boyce, and A. Kemp, "The impact of depression heterogeneity on cognitive control in major depressive disorder," *Australian and New Zealand Journal of Psychiatry*, vol. 46, no. 11, pp. 1079–1088, 2012.

[69] M. Kirby, A. Denihan, I. Bruce, D. Coakley, and B. A. Lawlor, "The clock drawing test in primary care: sensitivity in dementia detection and specificity against normal and depressed elderly," *International Journal of Geriatric Psychiatry*, vol. 16, no. 10, pp. 935–940, 2001.

[70] N. Herrmann, D. Kidron, K. I. Shulman et al., "Clock tests in depression, Alzheimer's disease, and elderly controls," *International Journal of Psychiatry in Medicine*, vol. 28, no. 4, pp. 437–447, 1998.

[71] C. Warden, J. Hwang, A. Marshall, M. Fenesy, and K. L. Poston, "The effects of dopamine on digit span in Parkinson's disease," *Journal of Clinical Movement Disorders*, vol. 3, no. 1, article 5, 2016.

[72] D. K. Johnson, Z. Langford, M. Garnier-Villarreal, J. C. Morris, and J. E. Galvin, "Onset of mild cognitive impairment in parkinson disease," *Alzheimer Disease and Associated Disorders*, vol. 30, no. 2, pp. 127–133, 2016.

[73] M. L. Morgan, E. A. Witte, I. A. Cook, A. F. Leuchter, M. Abrams, and B. Siegman, "Influence of age, gender, health status, and depression on quantitative EEG," *Neuropsychobiology*, vol. 52, no. 2, pp. 71–76, 2005.

[74] M. Baldereschi, A. Di Carlo, W. A. Rocca et al., "Parkinson's disease and parkinsonism in a longitudinal study: two-fold higher incidence in men," *Neurology*, vol. 55, no. 9, pp. 1358–1363, 2000.

[75] S. K. Van Den Eeden, C. M. Tanner, A. L. Bernstein et al., "Incidence of Parkinson's disease: variation by age, gender, and race/ethnicity," *American Journal of Epidemiology*, vol. 157, no. 11, pp. 1015–1022, 2003.

Cognitive Function Characteristics of Parkinson's Disease with Sleep Disorders

Jing Huang,[1] Wenyan Zhuo,[1] Yuhu Zhang,[2] Hongchun Sun,[1] Huan Chen,[1] Peipei Zhu,[1] Xiaobo Pan,[1] Jianhao Yang,[1] and Lijuan Wang[2]

[1]*Department of Neurology, Zhuhai People's Hospital, Zhuhai 519000, China*
[2]*Department of Neurology, Guangdong Neuroscience Institute, Guangdong General Hospital and Guangdong Academy of Medical Sciences, Guangzhou 510080, China*

Correspondence should be addressed to Lijuan Wang; wljgd68@163.com

Academic Editor: Hélio Teive

Objective. The aim of this study was to investigate the cognitive function characteristics of Parkinson's disease (PD) with sleep disorders. *Methods.* Consecutive patients with PD ($n = 96$), patients with primary sleep disorders ($n = 76$), and healthy control subjects ($n = 66$) were assessed. The patients with PD were classified into sleep disorder (PD-SD) and non-sleep disorder (PD-NSD) groups. *Results.* Among 96 patients with PD, 69 were diagnosed with a sleep disorder. There were 38 sleep disorder cases, 31 RBD cases, and 27 NSD cases. On the Mini-Mental State Examination (MMSE), Montreal Cognitive Assessment (MoCA), and MoCA subtests, patients in the PD-SD, primary sleep disorder, and PD-NSD groups exhibited lower scores than those in the control group. Moreover, the PD-SD patients exhibited more significant cognitive impairment than was observed in the primary sleep disorder patients. In the PD-SD subgroup, the attention scores on the MoCA and on MoCA subtests were lower in the PD with RBD group than in the PD with insomnia group. *Conclusion.* PD with sleep disorders may exacerbate cognitive dysfunction in patients. PD associated with different types of sleep disorders differentially affects cognitive functions, and patients with PD with RBD exhibited poorer cognitive function than was seen in patients with PD with insomnia.

1. Introduction

Parkinson's disease (PD) is a typical movement disorder. In addition to motor symptoms, it is characterized by its nonmotor symptoms, including sleep disorders, cognitive dysfunction, autonomic dysfunction, and mental disorders, which seriously affect the quality of life of PD patients [1]. The most common nonmotor symptoms include sleep disorders and cognitive dysfunction. Sleep disorders affect up to 98% of PD patients [2]. At the time of PD diagnosis, 30–50% of patients may have mild cognitive impairment (MCI), but they usually do not show dementia unless the patient is diagnosed in the advanced stage of PD [3], and 60–80% of PD cases develop complete dementia within 10 years [4, 5]. Sleep quality is strongly correlated with health-related quality of life [6]. Sleep disorders include insomnia, sleep fragmentation, rapid eye movement sleep behavior disorder (RBD), sleep apnea syndrome, restless legs syndrome, and nocturnal enuresis [7]. In PD patients, insomnia and RBD, particularly the latter, are the most common and widely studied sleep disorders. RBD is not only a sleep disorder but also the preclinical manifestation of several neurodegenerative diseases (such as PD, multiple system atrophy, and Lewy body dementia) [8]. RBD includes a series of clinical symptoms (e.g., screaming, cursing and waving limbs, kicking, and falling out of bed). It accelerates the disease progression and affects the quality of sleep in PD patients, and it may lead to harm or death to patients or bedfellows [9].

The Braak pathological grade hypothesis drew attention to the fact that sleep disorders appear prior to cognitive impairment; moreover, there is a mutual influence between sleep disorders and cognitive impairment. It has been shown that chronic insomnia is an independent risk factor for cognitive impairment in nondepressed older men, whereas occasional insomnia does not increase the risk of cognitive impairment [10]. Similar to other neurodegenerative diseases (e.g., Alzheimer's disease), significant sleep problems occur in PD in combination with significant cognitive dysfunction [11]. Postuma et al. performed a 4-year follow-up study of nondementia PD patients. In their study, 27 cases of PD were associated with RBD, and the incidence of dementia in PD patients with RBD was 15% after 2 years, 29% after 3 years, and 48% after 4 years. In contrast, none of the 15 PD patients who did not present with RBD developed dementia [12]. Sleep disorders may represent an independent risk factor for cognitive impairment; however, most recent studies have only focused on sleep or cognitive conditions for PD patients. The relationship between cognitive function and PD with sleep disorders remains unclear, as do the effects of different types of sleep disorders on cognitive function.

Therefore, this study focused on PD with sleep disorders and comprehensively assessed the sleep quality and cognitive function in PD patients. We classified PD patients according to their sleep disorder types and analyzed the cognitive function characteristics of each subgroup to better characterize the relationship between PD with sleep disorders and cognitive function. Our study provides a novel theoretical basis and clinical application for the treatment, prevention, and early intervention of cognitive impairment in PD patients.

2. Materials and Methods

2.1. Study Population

2.1.1. General Information. PD patients admitted to the Neurology Department of Guangdong General Hospital and Zhuhai People's Hospital from April 2013 to May 2016 were enrolled in our study. We also assessed a primary sleep disorder group and a healthy control group with the same age, sex distribution, and education level as the PD patients. All subjects were examined by experienced neurologists; they met the United Kingdom PD Society Brain Bank criteria [13] and did not receive anti-PD medication before the evaluation of sleep and the cognition scale. Exclusion criteria were as follows: (1) excessive daytime sleepiness (EDS), sleep attacks, sleep apnea syndrome, restless legs syndrome, parasomnia, and other types of sleep disorders; (2) other serious or unstable physical conditions that affect sleep and cognitive function assessment; (3) pain disorders, drug or alcohol addicts with severe physical illness, or sleep problems being directly a result of physical or mental effects; (4) severe anxiety or depression history and other mental disorders; (5) active epilepsy; (6) history of acute cerebrovascular disease in the previous 3 months; (7) use of sedative or hypnotic drugs within 2 weeks prior to enrollment; (8) presence of aphasia, delirium, or consciousness disorders that affect sleep and cognitive function assessment.

2.1.2. Population Classification. According to the diagnostic criteria of sleep disorders, we classified the PD patients into 2 subgroups, the PD with sleep disorders (PD-SD) group and the PD with no sleep disorders (PD-NSD) group. The PD-SD group included the PD with insomnia group and

the PD with RBD group [14], whereas the primary sleep disorder group was divided into the primary insomnia group and the primary RBD group. All patients with primary insomnia met the American Psychiatric Association Mental Disorders Diagnostic and Statistical Manual IV diagnostic criteria for primary sleep disorders [15], whereas all primary RBD patients fulfilled the International Sleep Disorders Classification II diagnostic criteria for RBD [16].

2.2. Study Methods

2.2.1. Survey Demographics. We administered demographic surveys to all PD patients and to the control group, thereby obtaining general information regarding age, sex, height, weight, and education level and potential associations with other diseases (e.g., recent infection, high blood pressure, diabetes, cancer, and surgical history), age of onset, duration, drug treatment, family history, and concomitant symptoms.

2.2.2. Clinical Assessments

(a) Motor Function Assessment. The motor function was assessed using the Unified PD Rating Scale Part III (UPDRS-III), and the disease severity was assessed using the Hoehn-Yahr (H-Y) grade.

(b) Daily Capacity Assessment. Activities of Daily Living Scale (ADL) was used.

(c) Anxiety and Depression Assessment. The Hamilton Anxiety Scale (HAMA) and the Hamilton Depression Scale (HAMD) were used.

(d) Sleep Assessment. The PDSS-2, PSQI, and ESS scales were administered to assess the quality of sleep.

(e) Cognitive Function Assessment. The Mini-Mental State Examination [MMSE] and Montreal Cognitive Assessment [MoCA] were used.

2.3. Statistical Methods. SPSS 13.0 statistical software was used for the statistical analysis. Measurement data are presented as the mean ± standard deviation (±sd). The Kolmogorov-Smirnov test method was adopted for the normality test. For two samples that exhibited a normal distribution, the means were compared using the two independent samples' t-test. In contrast, the samples noncompliant with a normal distribution were tested using the Mann–Whitney U test. When multiple samples obeyed the normal distribution and multiple sample averages were compared, one-way ANOVA (analysis of variance) was implemented. Levene's test for equality of variance and Welch's t-test for unequal variance were also utilized. The homogeneity of variance was analyzed by the LSD multiple comparison method, and unequal variance was evaluated by Dunnett's T3 multiple comparisons. Comparisons of multiple samples that were not normally distributed were performed using the nonparametric Kruskal-Wallis H test with count data tested using a chi-square test. When $P < 0.05$, we considered the difference to be statistically significant.

TABLE 1: Comparison of subjective sleep in PD-SD and PD-NSD.

	PD-SD (69)	PD-NSD (27)	Z	P value
PDSS-2-T	20.69 ± 10.54	10.00 ± 5.90	−4.130	0.000
ESS-T	6.21 ± 4.39	4.39 ± 3.65	−1.496	0.135
PSQI-T	9.08 ± 4.22	6.44 ± 3.88	−2.329	0.020

TABLE 2: Comparison between PD-NSD and PD with sleep disorders.

	PD-SD (69)	PD-NSD (27)	$t/Z/\chi^2$	P value
Age, y	61.27 ± 11.38	56.28 ± 13.81	1.496	0.139
Gender, M/F (%)	32/37	11/16	0.091	0.763
Education, y	10.27 ± 3.92	12.39 ± 3.79	−1.805	0.071
Age of onset, y	57.25 ± 11.24	53.06 ± 12.87	1.298	0.199
PD duration, y	3.52 ± 2.96	3.31 ± 4.48	−1.042	0.297
UPDRS-III	28.23 ± 10.10	24.50 ± 10.84	−2.017	0.067
Hoehn-Yahr scale	2.68 ± 4.11	1.81 ± 0.94	−1.868	0.062
HAMA	9.33 ± 6.77	7.11 ± 3.61	−0.846	0.397
HAMD	9.69 ± 7.33	9.39 ± 6.09	−0.253	0.800
ADL	20.23 ± 9.87	19.83 ± 8.42	−0.610	0.701

TABLE 3: Cognitive function characteristic analysis comparing the PD-SD, PD-NSD, primary sleep disorder, and normal control groups.

	PD-SD (69)	PD-NSD (27)	Primary sleep disorders (76)	Normal controls (66)	χ^2	P value
MMSE	25.48 ± 3.82	28.44 ± 1.79	27.15 ± 3.65	28.92 ± 1.50	25.512	0.000
MoCA	19.00 ± 4.99	25.50 ± 3.20	22.54 ± 5.75	27.00 ± 2.49	47.963	0.000
Visuospatial and execution	2.50 ± 1.38	3.72 ± 1.02	3.15 ± 1.71	4.50 ± 0.83	34.282	0.000
Naming	2.35 ± 0.67	2.78 ± 0.55	2.87 ± 0.54	3.00 ± 0.00	37.522	0.000
Attention	4.50 ± 1.35	5.39 ± 0.92	5.48 ± 0.91	5.75 ± 0.44	27.669	0.000
Language	2.25 ± 0.91	2.78 ± 0.55	2.54 ± 0.59	2.75 ± 0.53	9.312	0.025
Abstract	0.96 ± 0.82	1.39 ± 0.70	1.15 ± 0.76	1.54 ± 0.66	10.108	0.018
Delayed recall	1.38 ± 1.10	3.61 ± 1.24	1.91 ± 1.76	3.58 ± 1.28	41.662	0.000
Orientation	5.08 ± 1.11	5.83 ± 0.38	5.70 ± 0.89	5.92 ± 0.28	26.226	0.000

3. Results

3.1. General Information. The 96 PD patients included 41 males and 55 females (mean age 58.91 ± 12.19 years); 76 patients were included in the primary sleep disorders group, including 43 males and 33 females (mean age 57.30 ± 13.36 years). The normal control group consisted of 66 subjects, including 36 males and 30 females (mean age 56.63 ± 9.84 years).

According to the diagnostic criteria for PD sleep disorders, the PD patients included a PD-SD group of 69 cases, which accounted for 72.7% of the total PD patients (38 cases in the PD with insomnia group, or 40.1% of the total PD patients; 31 cases in the PD with RBD group, or 31.8%). There were 27 cases in the PD-NSD group, accounting for 27.3% of the total PD patients. The PD-SD and PD-NSD groups showed significant differences in the PDSS-2-T and PSQI-T scores but no significant differences in the ESS scores (Table 1). There were no significant differences in the age,

age of onset, duration, years of education, UPDRS-III, H-Y classification, HAMA score, HAMD score, or ADL score ($P > 0.05$) (Table 2).

3.2. Cognitive Function Analysis in PD with Sleep Disorders. (1) There were significant differences in cognitive function among the PD-SD, PD-NSD, primary sleep disorder, and normal control groups. For the PD-SD and primary sleep disorder groups, the MMSE scores were only 25.48 ± 3.82 and 27.15 ± 3.65, and the MoCA scores were only 19.00 ± 4.99 and 22.54 ± 5.75, respectively, when using multiple independent samples. Similarly, for the overall cognitive function (MMSE and MoCA) and MoCA subtest assessments, the PD-SD and primary sleep disorder groups showed significantly lower scores (Table 3). Furthermore, using one-way ANOVA with the LSD test for cases in which Levene's test showed homogeneity of variance and with Dunnett's T3 method for cases of nonhomogeneous variance, we found that the PD-SD group showed more significant impairment of cognitive

TABLE 4: Cognitive function characteristic analysis comparing the PD-SD, PD-NSD, primary sleep disorders, and normal control groups.

	A versus B	A versus C	A versus D	B versus C	B versus D	C versus D
MMSE	0.004	0.038	0.000	0.590	0.922	0.043
MoCA	0.000	0.001	0.000	0.196	0.414	0.000
Visuospatial and execution	0.012	0.044	0.000	0.890	0.066	0.000
Naming	0.021	0.000	0.000	0.910	0.383	0.403
Attention	0.042	0.000	0.000	0.998	0.715	0.791
Language	0.052	0.816	0.062	0.345	1.000	0.440
Abstract	0.261	0.843	0.014	0.812	0.972	0.163
Delayed recall	0.000	0.427	0.000	0.000	1.000	0.000
Orientation	0.005	0.000	0.000	1.000	0.965	0.860

A: PD-SD; B: PD-NSD; C: primary sleep disorders; D: normal control.

TABLE 5: Cognitive function characteristic analysis comparing two subtypes of PD-SD.

	PD with insomnia (38)	PD with RBD (31)	Z	P value
MMSE	26.11 ± 3.86	24.67 ± 3.71	-1.914	0.056
MoCA	20.07 ± 5.36	17.62 ± 4.20	-2.187	0.029
Visuospatial and execution	2.74 ± 1.32	2.19 ± 1.44	-1.668	0.095
Naming	2.41 ± 0.69	2.29 ± 0.64	-0.746	0.456
Attention	4.93 ± 1.27	3.95 ± 1.28	-2.686	0.007
Language	2.26 ± 0.94	2.24 ± 0.89	0.161	0.872
Abstract	1.11 ± 0.80	0.76 ± 0.83	-1.466	0.143
Delayed recall	1.41 ± 1.25	1.33 ± 0.91	-0.011	0.991
Orientation	5.19 ± 1.18	4.95 ± 1.02	-1.247	0.212

function than did the primary sleep disorder group, based on measures such as the MMSE and MoCA scores and the Naming, Attention, and Orientation subitems in the MoCA (Table 4).

(2) Comparing the subtypes of PD-SD, the MoCA score was lower in the PD with RBD group than in the PD with insomnia group. Similarly, the attention score of the MoCA subtest was lower in the PD with RBD group than in the PD with insomnia group (Table 5).

4. Discussion

To date, the combination of PD with sleep disorders and cognitive function has been poorly investigated, particularly regarding the difference between the effects of different types of sleep disorders on cognitive function. Adequate sleep is an important requirement for good memory and efficient executive function. The cognitive changes that occur in early-to-moderate PD are primarily deficits in executive function and memory [17–19], which are the same domains as those affected in individuals with insomnia [20]. Studies have investigated the impact of PD with RBD on cognitive function, but how PD with insomnia affects cognitive function remains poorly understood. To address these gaps, our study compares cognitive functions between PD patients with RBD and PD patients with insomnia. Gagnon et al. determined that the MCI incidence rate was 73% in PD

patients with RBD but only 50% in primary RBD patients. Moreover, in the PD without RBD group, 11% of patients developed MCI, compared with an 8% incidence rate in the normal control group [21]. Furthermore, studies have indicated that there was no significant difference in motor function between PD with and without RBD. However, PD patients with RBD performed worse in memory, visuospatial, and executive functions [22]. Postuma et al. determined that PD patients with RBD were more likely to develop dementia than were PD patients without RBD [12]. Sleep quality in PD is significantly correlated with cognition, and it differentially impacts attention and executive function, thereby furthering our understanding of the link between sleep and cognition [23]. Our results were consistent with previous studies, and there were no significant differences in motor function or daily living ability between the PD with sleep disorder and PD with normal sleep groups. Interestingly, both PD with sleep disorder and primary sleep disorder patients showed significant impairments in the overall cognitive function and MoCA subtests compared with the PD with normal sleep and normal control groups. Moreover, the scores of the PD patients with sleep disorders were significantly lower than those of the primary sleep disorder patients. Thus, patients with PD with sleep disorders have a greater risk of cognitive dysfunction. Clinicians need to solve PD patients' sleep problems as early as possible in order to delay the associated cognitive decline.

In the analysis of the subtypes of PD with sleep disorders, the total MoCA score was lower in the PD with RBD group than in the PD with insomnia group. Furthermore, for the MoCA subtests, the PD patients with RBD had lower attention scores and more significant cognitive impairment compared with the PD patients with insomnia, particularly regarding attention. Therefore, poor sleepers exhibited worse performance on tests of global cognition. A sleep disorder is considered as an independent risk factor for PD-related cognitive impairment, whereas the impact of RBD on cognitive function is more obvious.

Cognitive function in patients with primary RBD has received increasing attention. RBD may be associated with preclinical presentation of a number of neurodegenerative diseases (multiple system atrophy, Lewy body dementia, and Parkinson's disease). The cognitive function of PD with RBD is also currently receiving substantial attention in the study of Parkinson's disease. Primary RBD patients often present with visuospatial impairment, attention dysfunction, executive dysfunction, or verbal memory loss [24]. Studies have indicated that 73% of PD patients with RBD present with MCI [25]. As previously discussed, RBD is considered an independent risk factor for PD-associated cognitive impairment. Consistent with other research results, our study demonstrated that PD patients with RBD have poorer cognitive function. To date, the pathophysiology underlying the effects of RBD on cognitive function remains unclear. First, the pathological mechanism of RBD may be related to the abnormalities of the tegmentum and the ascending reticular activating system [26]. Second, Braak et al. have suggested that the pathological evolution of PD that involves the medulla oblongata and pontine tegmentum occurs via a two-phase pathological process, and these are common regions of RBD occurrence [27]. The damaged regions of the cerebral cortex in PD or RBD patients are believed to regulate neural activity, and nervous system conduction disorders may affect cognitive function. It has been demonstrated that the brain metabolism perfusion patterns differ between PD and PD cognitive impairment patients. In PD cognitive impairment patients, there have been reports of reduced perfusion in the frontal and parietal regions and increased perfusion in the brain stem and cerebellum [28]. This abnormal metabolic perfusion has also been identified in studies of primary RBD [29]. The clinical manifestations of PD are significantly heterogeneous and may be related to the position and degree of neuronal injury. Furthermore, the mechanisms of neurodegeneration may differ between PD patients with and without RBD. However, there are no well-established imaging studies to elucidate the neuropathological mechanisms in PD with RBD; thus, additional studies are required to further illustrate its pathogenesis.

In summary, sleep disorders may exacerbate the occurrence and development of PD. Neurologists should focus on sleep disorders in PD patients and be fully aware of different types of sleep disorders to achieve early diagnosis, early intervention, and early treatment. This knowledge is essential for improving patient quality of life, reducing the risk of cognitive impairment, and slowing the progression of cognitive decline.

Authors' Contributions

Jing Huang and Wenyan Zhuo contributed equally to this work.

References

[1] K. R. Chaudhuri, C. Prieto-Jurcynska, Y. Naidu et al., "The non-declaration of nonmotor symptoms of Parkinson's disease to health care professionals: An international study using the nonmotor symptoms questionnaire," *Movement Disorders*, vol. 25, no. 6, pp. 704–709, 2010.

[2] C. H. Adler and M. J. Thorpy, "Sleep issues in Parkinson's disease," *Neurology*, vol. 64, no. 12, pp. S12–S20, 2005.

[3] D. Aarsland, J. T. Kvaløy, K. Andersen et al., "The effect of age of onset of PD on risk of dementia," *Journal of Neurology*, vol. 254, no. 1, pp. 38–45, 2007.

[4] D. Aarsland, K. Andersen, J. P. Larsen, A. Lolk, and P. Kragh-Sørensen, "Prevalence and characteristics of dementia in Parkinson disease: An 8-year prospective study," *Archives of Neurology*, vol. 60, no. 3, pp. 387–392, 2003.

[5] T. C. Buter, A. Van Den Hout, F. E. Matthews, J. P. Larsen, C. Brayne, and D. Aarsland, "Dementia and survival in Parkinson disease: A 12-year population study," *Neurology*, vol. 70, no. 13, pp. 1017–1022, 2008.

[6] T. Scaravilli, E. Gasparoli, F. Rinaldi, G. Polesello, and F. Bracco, "Health-related quality of life and sleep disorders in Parkinson's disease," *Neurological Sciences*, vol. 24, no. 3, pp. 209–210, 2003.

[7] E. Havlikova, J. P. V. Dijk, I. Nagyova et al., "The impact of sleep and mood disorders on quality of life in Parkinson's disease patients," *Journal of Neurology*, vol. 258, no. 12, pp. 2222–2229, 2011.

[8] A. Iranzo, A. Fernández-Arcos, E. Tolosa et al., "Neurodegenerative disorder risk in idiopathic REM sleep behavior disorder: Study in 174 patients," *PLoS ONE*, vol. 9, no. 2, Article ID e89741, 2014.

[9] C. H. Schenck, S. A. Lee, M. A. C. Bornemann, and M. W. Mahowald, "Potentially lethal behaviors associated with rapid eye movement sleep behavior disorder: Review of the literature and forensic implications," *Journal of Forensic Sciences*, vol. 54, no. 6, pp. 1475–1484, 2009.

[10] S. Beaulieu-Bonneau and C. Hudon, "Sleep disturbances in older adults with mild cognitive impairment," *International Psychogeriatrics*, vol. 21, no. 4, pp. 654–666, 2009.

[11] M. V. Vitiello and S. Borson, "Sleep disturbances in patients with alzheimer's disease: Epidemiology, pathophysiology and treatment," *CNS Drugs*, vol. 15, no. 10, pp. 777–796, 2001.

[12] R. B. Postuma, J.-A. Bertrand, J. Montplaisir et al., "Rapid eye movement sleep behavior disorder and risk of dementia in Parkinson's disease: A prospective study," *Movement Disorders*, vol. 27, no. 6, pp. 720–726, 2012.

[13] A. J. Hughes, S. E. Daniel, L. Kilford, and A. J. Lees, "Accuracy of clinical diagnosis of idiopathic Parkinsons disease: a clinico-pathological study of 100 cases," *Journal of Neurology, Neurosurgery & Psychiatry*, vol. 55, no. 3, pp. 181–184, 1992.

[14] M. Louter, W. C. C. A. Aarden, J. Lion, B. R. Bloem, and S. Overeem, "Recognition and diagnosis of sleep disorders in Parkinson's disease," *Journal of Neurology*, vol. 259, no. 10, pp. 2031–2040, 2012.

[15] American Psychiatric Association, *Diagnostic and Statistical Manual of Mental Disorders: DSM-IV*, American Psychiatric

Association, Washington, DC, USA, 4th edition, 1994.

[16] American Academy of Sleep Medicine, *International Classification of Sleep Disorders Diagnostic and Coding Manual*, American Academy of Sleep Medicine, Westchester, Ill, USA, 2nd edition, 2005.

[17] A. E. Taylor, J. A. Saint-Cyr, and A. E. Lang, "Memory and learning in early Parkinson's disease: Evidence for a "frontal lobe syndrome"," *Brain and Cognition*, vol. 13, no. 2, pp. 211–232, 1990.

[18] A. M. Owen, M. James, P. N. Leigh et al., "Fronto-striatal cognitive deficits at different stages of parkinson's disease," *Brain*, vol. 115, no. 6, pp. 1727–1751, 1992.

[19] D. Muslimović, B. Post, J. D. Speelman, and B. Schmand, "Cognitive profile of patients with newly diagnosed Parkinson disease," *Neurology*, vol. 65, no. 8, pp. 1239–1245, 2005.

[20] É. Fortier-Brochu, S. Beaulieu-Bonneau, H. Ivers, and C. M. Morin, "Insomnia and daytime cognitive performance: A meta-analysis," *Sleep Medicine Reviews*, vol. 16, no. 1, pp. 83–94, 2012.

[21] J.-F. Gagnon, M. Vendette, R. B. Postuma et al., "Mild cognitive impairment in rapid eye movement sleep behavior disorder and Parkinson's disease," *Annals of Neurology*, vol. 66, no. 1, pp. 39–47, 2009.

[22] J.-R. Zhang, J. Chen, Z.-J. Yang et al., "Rapid eye movement sleep behavior disorder symptoms correlate with domains of cognitive impairment in parkinson's disease," *Chinese Medical Journal*, vol. 129, no. 4, pp. 379–385, 2016.

[23] K. Stavitsky, S. Neargarder, Y. Bogdanova, P. McNamara, and A. Cronin-Golomb, "The impact of sleep quality on cognitive functioning in Parkinson's disease," *Journal of the International Neuropsychological Society*, vol. 18, no. 1, pp. 108–117, 2012.

[24] M. L. Fantini, E. Farini, P. Ortelli et al., "Longitudinal study of cognitive function in idiopathic REM sleep behavior disorder," *Sleep*, vol. 34, no. 5, pp. 619–625, 2011.

[25] I. Djonlagic, M. Guo, P. Matteis, A. Carusona, R. Stickgold, and A. Malhotra, "Untreated sleep-disordered breathing: Links to aging-related decline in sleep-dependent memory consolidation," *PLoS ONE*, vol. 9, no. 1, Article ID e85918, 2014.

[26] J.-F. Gagnon, R. B. Postuma, S. Mazza, J. Doyon, and J. Montplaisir, "Rapid-eye-movement sleep behaviour disorder and neurodegenerative diseases," *Lancet Neurology*, vol. 5, no. 5, pp. 424–432, 2006.

[27] H. Braak, K. Del Tredici, U. Rüb, R. A. I. De Vos, E. N. H. Jansen Steur, and E. Braak, "Staging of brain pathology related to sporadic Parkinson's disease," *Neurobiology of Aging*, vol. 24, no. 2, pp. 197–211, 2003.

[28] C. Huang, P. Mattis, K. Perrine, N. Brown, V. Dhawan, and D. Eidelberg, "Metabolic abnormalities associated with mild cognitive impairment in Parkinson disease," *Neurology*, vol. 70, no. 16, pp. 1470–1477, 2008.

[29] S. Mazza, J. P. Soucy, P. Gravel et al., "Assessing whole brain perfusion changes in patients with REM sleep behavior disorder," *Neurology*, vol. 67, no. 9, pp. 1618–1622, 2006.

Management of Psychosis in Parkinson's Disease: Emphasizing Clinical Subtypes and Pathophysiological Mechanisms of the Condition

Raquel N. Taddei, Seyda Cankaya, Sandeep Dhaliwal, and K. Ray Chaudhuri

Maurice Wohl Clinical Neuroscience Institute and NIHR Biomedical Research Centre, Institute of Psychiatry, Psychology and Neuroscience, King's College Hospital, London, UK

Correspondence should be addressed to Raquel N. Taddei; raqueltaddei@hotmail.com

Academic Editor: Giovanni Mirabella

Investigation into neuropsychiatric symptoms in Parkinson's disease (PD) is sparse and current drug development is mainly focused on the motor aspect of PD. The tight association of psychosis with an impaired quality of life in PD, together with an important underreporting of this comorbid condition, contributes to its actual insufficient assessment and management. Furthermore, the withdrawal from access to readily available treatment interventions is unacceptable and has an impact on PD prognosis. Despite its impact, to date no standardized guidelines to the adequate management of PD psychosis are available and they are therefore highly needed. Readily available knowledge on distinct clinical features as well as early biomarkers of psychosis in PD justifies the potential for its timely diagnosis and for early intervention strategies. Also, its specific characterisation opens up the possibility of further understanding the underlying pathophysiological mechanisms giving rise to more targeted therapeutic developments in the nearer future. A literature review on the most recent knowledge with special focus on specific clinical subtypes and pathophysiological mechanisms will not only contribute to an up to date practical approach of this condition for the health care providers, but furthermore open up new ideas for research in the near future.

1. Introduction

Nonmotor symptoms have an important impact on quality of life in PD patients and their caregivers and are largely recognized as such by a growing number of health care providers [1, 2]. Psychosis is recognized as one of the most frequent and disabling nonmotor symptoms in PD with prevalences of 20% up to 70% in advanced stages of the condition [3]. Its relevance is such that it has even been named as the main feature of one of the seven proposed nonmotor subtypes of PD described by Sauerbier et al. [4]. In this review we aim at providing an up to date practical approach to psychosis in PD, with especial emphasis on clinical subtypes and pathophysiological mechanisms underlying this condition with the aim of leading to better intervention strategies in the nearer future.

2. Defining PD Psychosis

2.1. History. The history of psychosis in PD goes back to the early 19th century, where the presence of mental disturbances among PD patients was described as being rare and was accounted for as either a consequence of a chronic disease evolution or regarded as coincidental [5]. After an outbreak of encephalitis lethargica between 1915 and 1926, a condition of unknown origin with acute onset and often chronic persistence of various neurological symptoms, including headache, lethargy, catatonia, parkinsonism, and tremor, a potential link between an altered mental state and parkinsonism was proposed and the first idea of complex psychotic symptoms in postencephalitic parkinsonism (PEP) cases was described [6, 7]. In more recent years however, the etiologic relationship between the encephalitis outbreak and the

(G1) An acute onset of delusions, hallucinations, incomprehensible or incoherent speech, or any combination of these. The time interval between the first appearance of any psychotic symptoms and the presentation of the fully developed disorder should not exceed two weeks.

(G2) If transient states of perplexity, misidentification, or impairment of attention and concentration are present, they do not fulfill the criteria for organically caused clouding of consciousness.

(G3) The disorder does not meet the symptomatic criteria for manic episode (F30), depressive episode (F32), or recurrent depressive disorder.

(G4) No evidence of recent psychoactive substance use sufficient to fulfil the criteria of intoxication, harmful use, dependence, or withdrawal states. The continued moderate and largely unchanged use of alcohol or drugs in amounts or frequencies to which the subject is accustomed does not necessarily rule out the use of F23; this must be decided by clinical judgement and the requirements of the research project in question.

(G5) Most commonly used exclusion criteria: absence of organic brain disease or serious metabolic disturbances affecting the central nervous system (this does not include childbirth).

Box 1: The ICD-10 classification of mental and behavioural disorders: definition criteria for acute and transient psychosis. F23, F30, F32: diagnosis codes of psychotic (F23) and mood disorders (F30 and F32) taken from ICD-10 guidelines; reference: taken from WHO International classifications, ICD-10 guidelines [15].

alleged PEP has been discussed as controversial due to a lack of consistency in clinical features and in the onset of symptoms and the possibility of other causes of parkinsonism has been postulated [7, 8]. Moreover, in subsequent years, confusional states were reported under treatment with L-Dopa and later under dopamine agonist therapy in PD patients, giving rise to this new core feature in PD. In 1995 the first review on drug-induced psychosis in PD was published by Factor et al., leading to the first international awareness of this PD complication [9].

Currently, under various searching terms on psychotic symptoms in PD, including the terms hallucinations, psychotic symptoms, illusions, delusions, and misperceptions among others, over 4000 articles and reviews can be found, dated back as far as 1945 in the current literature (PubMed), being the first description found in a book published in 1921.

2.2. General Psychosis and PD Psychosis. With regard to the clinical definition of the main features of psychosis, which include hallucinations, illusions, and delusions, current ICD-10 guidelines define hallucinations as a disorder characterised by a false sensory perception in the absence of an external stimulus, whereas an illusion is regarded as a misperception of an externally present stimulus. In contrast to classical hallucinations and illusions, delusions are a false interpretation of the experienced misperceptions, often involving topics of persecution, imposters, or grandiosity. Some specific forms of delusions such as the Cotard syndrome (implying nihilistic delusions, hypochondriacal delusions, and delusions of immortality) [10–12], Capgras syndrome (including having the conviction that a family member or friend has been replaced by another), and Othello syndrome (being described as a delusional jealousy) have further been named [13, 14], the latter showing an association with dopamine agonist therapy and an improvement after its reduction. The current diagnostic criteria from ICD-10 based guidelines for acute and transient psychosis are shown in Box 1; other definitions of psychosis falling under the term of schizoaffective disorders will not be further developed in this review.

With regard to psychosis arising in PD patients, it is defined as the occurrence of hallucinations, delusions, or both, most of the psychotic symptoms being of visual character, with the potential of other sensory modalities to be involved as well [16]. They can be subdivided into minor and nonminor hallucinations [17] and minor symptoms can be subdivided into three forms, known as illusions (meaning that real objects are seen transformed into other shapes/figures), passage hallucinations (implying, e.g., hallucinated objects or dots of light passing in the peripheral visual field), or presence hallucinations (including the sense of a nearby person or animal) [18, 19].

As to the clinical presentation of the psychotic features in PD, they are mostly of visual character, including complex perceptions containing animals, persons, or objects, and are normally not frightening to the patients, who clearly recognize them as being abnormal [17, 20]. Most occur in poor light conditions and reduced stimulus environment, more often at night, and last for seconds to minutes [17]. The visual hallucination might be in black and white or in colour and is perceived by most of the patients as "bothersome." A common form of visual hallucination is the perception of bugs on the walls or on the floor. Later occurring auditory hallucinations are mostly described as indistinct sounds (e.g., a radio playing in the room, a band performing on the street, or a conversation taking place outside the room) and are therefore distinct to the symptoms of psychosis in schizophrenia patients, where a threatening or denigrating character is typical.

In early PD stages, hallucinations typically occur with preserved insight, whereas in later disease stages this characteristic is lost and patients might not recognize the misperceptions as unreal anymore, giving rise to the above-mentioned term of (secondary) delusions [17]. When other sensory modalities are involved, auditory but also more rarely olfactory or tactile hallucinations may occur [21]. Proposed diagnostic criteria for psychosis in PD arose from a consensus conference in 2007 by the NONDS/NIMH work group [22] and are shown in Box 2.

(A) Characteristic symptoms
Presence of at least one of the following symptoms (specify which of the symptoms fulfill the criteria)
    (i) Illusions
    (ii) False sense of presence
    (iii) Hallucinations
    (iv) Delusions
(B) Primary diagnosis
        UK brain bank criteria for PD
(C) Chronology of the onset of symptoms of psychosis
        The symptoms in Criterion (A) occur after the onset of PD
(D) Duration
        The symptom(s) in Criterion (A) are recurrent or continuous for 1 month
(E) Exclusion of other causes
        The symptoms in Criterion (A) are not better accounted for by another cause of Parkinsonism
such as dementia with Lewy bodies, psychiatric disorders such as schizophrenia, schizoaffective
disorder, delusional disorder, or mood disorder with psychotic features, or a general medical condition
including delirium
(F) Associated features (specify if associated)
    (i) With/without insight
    (ii) With/without dementia
    (iii) With/without treatment for PD (specify drug, surgical, other)

Box 2: Proposed criteria for psychosis in Parkinson's disease. PD, Parkinson's disease; UK, United Kingdom; references: Ravina et al., 2007, and Fenelon et al., 2008 [22, 23].

The prevalence of PD psychosis varies widely; among untreated PD patients it is reported to occur "rarely" [24], whereas in treated patients prevalence widely differs in the literature, with reported illusions or hallucinations occurring in 15–40% of treated PD patients [25] and an estimated development of psychosis in up to 60% of PD patients after a 12-year disease duration [26] or even 70% in "advanced" PD stages [3]. The occurrence of minor phenomena is reported to range between 17% and 72% in the current literature [27–30]. A recently published study on 423 drug-naïve PD patients followed up for 3-4 years showed an overall prevalence of psychotic symptoms in 27% of the PD patients after a median time of 19 months [19]. Table 1 shows the different prevalence rates of PD psychosis reported among various studies.

Various risk factors have been linked with the development of PD psychosis, such as the use of dopaminergic drugs as one of the first described ones. A recent study by the Parkinson's Progression Markers Initiative (PPMS) found that there were no significant differences with regard to occurrence of PD psychosis after starting L-Dopa or dopamine agonists, but a higher proportion of PD psychosis was observed over time after a period of 24 months in PD patients treated with dopamine agonists compared to the ones treated with L-Dopa [19].

Nowadays, emphasis on various other related factors has been attributed to leading to psychosis in PD patients, including higher age, later disease onset, higher PD severity (H&Y state), longer PD duration [27, 32], hyposmia [33], cognitive impairment, depression [34], diurnal somnolence, REM sleep behaviour disorder [28], visual disorders, severe axial impairment, autonomic dysfunction, and high medical comorbidity and polypharmacy, especially including the use of psychoactive drugs [3, 23, 35].

To assess the risk of developing psychosis, several scales are accessible either to address the presence of psychosis or to establish its severity. These include the PD nonmotor symptom scale developed by Chaudhuri et al. [36] and subscores of the MDS-UPDRS scale [37], as well as more specific scales directed towards assessing specifically psychiatric comorbidity in PD, including the Parkinson Psychosis Questionnaire [38], the Scale for Assessment of Positive Symptoms [39], and the Scale for Evaluation of Neuropsychiatric Disorders in PD [40]. These available scales are summarised in Table 2.

2.3. Other Psychotic Syndromes. In the following section, we will revise three specific subtypes of psychosis that may cooccur or contribute to the "classical" PD psychosis described above, in order to provide a complete revision on this topic.

2.3.1. Charles-Bonnet Syndrome. This syndrome with an estimated prevalence of 0.4% up to 30% in the overall population [41–45] dates back to a Swiss scientist named Charles-Bonnet, who described the occurrence of detailed visual hallucinations including figures, persons, and animals in his visually impaired grandfather, after losing his sight due to a bilateral cataract surgery. But it was not until 1967 that another Swiss scientist called G. de Morsier described this syndrome with the currently used term Charles-Bonnet syndrome. Diagnostic criteria for this syndrome are yet a topic of controversy, the current definition being the presence of visual hallucinations occurring as a result of ocular or visual pathway disease. The visual hallucinations can be of simple or complex nature, including hallucinations of faces or people-like figures [46], and normally last for seconds to a few hours. Most patients do not describe a negative or fearful experience during their visual hallucinations [41] and partial or full insight of

TABLE 1: Studies on the prevalence of psychotic symptoms in PD.

Study	N	Setting/design	Assessment instruments	Main findings
Celesia et al., 1970	45	Outpatient/prospective longitudinal	Columbia disability scale	17.7% developed psychosis (delusions, hallucinations, behavioral disorder)
Sweet et al., 1976	100	Outpatient/retrospective	Cornell, weighted scale, WAIS	60% agitated confusion
Moskovitz et al., 1978	88	Outpatient/retrospective	No	48% experienced vivid dreams (30.7%), hallucinations (29.5%), illusions (5.7%), and nonconfusional (9.1%), confusional psychoses (3.4%)
de Smet et al., 1982	75	Inpatient/retrospective	No	31% confusional states
Tanner et al., 1983	775	Outpatient/retrospective	HY	33% hallucinations
Fischer et al., 1990	25	Inpatient/retrospective	HY, MMSE	80% at least one episode of "pharmacotoxic psychosis"
Sanchez-Ramos et al., 1996	214	Outpatient/prospective cross-sectional	HY, MMSE	25.7% visual hallucinations
Inzelberg et al., 1998	121	Outpatient/prospective cross-sectional	HY, SMT	29% visual, 8% visual and auditory hallucinations
Aarsland et al., 1999	245	Community/prospective cross-sectional	UPDRS, MMSE, DSM-III-R, MADRAS	25.5% vivid dreaming, 9.8% hallucinations with insight retained, and 6% severe hallucinations or delusions
Fenelon et al., 2000	216	Outpatient/prospective cross-sectional	UPDRS, HY, MMP, CES-D, DSM-IV	39.8% hallucinations. Minor hallucinations 25.5%, formed visual hallucinations 22.2%, and auditory hallucinations 9.7%
Giladi et al., 2000	172	Outpatient/prospective cross-sectional	HY, MMSE, DSM-IV, ADAS-cog	27% had psychosis
Goetz et al., 2001	60	Outpatient/prospective longitudinal	UPDRS, HY, RHI	Hallucinations increased from 33% at baseline to 44% at 18 months and 63% at 48 months
Holroyd et al., 2001	102	Outpatient/prospective cross-sectional	DSM-IV, TICS, GDS	29.4% had hallucinations or delusions
Doe De Maindreville, 2004		Outpatient/prospective longitudinal	UPDRS, HY, MMP, CES-D, DSM-IV	Hallucinations increased from 41.7% to 49.6% over 12 months

HY: Hoehn and Yahr staging; SMT: Short Mental Test; MMSE: Mini Mental State Examination; UPDRS: Unified PD Rating Scale; MMP: Mini Mental Parkinson; DSM-III-R: Diagnostic and Statistical Manual for Psychiatric Disorders, revised third edition; DSM-IV: Diagnostic and Statistical Manual of Mental Disorders, 4th edition; MADRAS: Montgomery and Asberg Depression Rating Scale; RHI: Rush Hallucination Inventory; ADAS-cog: Alzheimer's Disease Assessment Scale (ADAS) Cognitive Section; TICS: Telephone Interview for Cognitive Status; GDS: Geriatric Depression Scale; WAIS: Wechsler Adult Intelligence Scale; CES-D: Center for Epidemiologic Studies-Depression self-rating scale; reference: Papapetropoulos and Mash, 2005 [31].

TABLE 2: Recommended scales for the assessment of psychosis in Parkinson's disease.

Scale	Objective	References
PD nonmotor symptom scale	Risk of developing psychosis	Chaudhuri et al., 2007
MDS-UPDRS I, item 1.2	Presence and severity of psychosis	Goetz et al., 2007
Parkinson Psychosis Questionnaire (PPQ)	Presence and severity of psychosis	Sawada and Oeda, 2013
Scale for Evaluation of Neuropsychiatric Disorders in Parkinson's disease (SEND-PD)	Presence, severity of psychosis, and other neuropsychiatric symptoms	Rodriguez-Violante et al., 2014
Scale for Assessment of Positive Symptoms (SAPS)	Presence, severity, and impact of psychosis	Voss et al., 2013

PD, Parkinson's disease; MDS-UPDRS 1: Movement Disorder Society Unified Parkinson's Disease Rating Scale 1; SEND-PD: Scale for Evaluation of Neuropsychiatric Disorders in Parkinson's disease; SAPS: Scale for Assessment of Positive Symptoms; reference: Levin et al., 2016 [3].

their unreal character, absence of coexisting psychological disorders, and preserved intellectual capacity is typically observed [47]. This condition has been described at different ages with no specific age dependent prevalence.

In PD patients, the loss of dopaminergic neurons in the brainstem leading to a deficiency of dopamine has been linked with an impairment in visual pathways, involving mainly the retina, as well as central pathways [48]. Whether the presence of visual hallucinations in PD patients could be at least partially explained by a visual impairment due to dopaminergic loss in form of a Charles-Bonnet syndrome needs to be further elucidated. Currently, impaired vision has been associated with the occurrence of visual hallucinations in PD patients as described above [49].

2.3.2. "Malignant": DLB/PD Dementia with Psychosis.
Dementia with Lewy bodies (DLB) and PD associated dementia (PDD) are two separate entities, yet both involving a similar pathological pathway of deposition of Alpha-synuclein within the brain in form of Lewy bodies. Presence of hallucinations is a common hallmark in both entities, being described in as many as 25–30% of DLB and PDD patients [22] and being most commonly of visual character, although also acoustic and haptic (tactile) hallucinations can occur [46]. In the progress of more severe presence of cognitive decline, visual hallucinations tend to shift from a blurred character among PD and PDD patients to fully formed complex visual hallucinations among DLB patients [46]. The distinction between both types of dementia is nonetheless a challenge and often complicated by an overlap of the clinical presentations and an unclear time window. DLB is commonly diagnosed, when cognitive impairment occurs within a year of development of parkinsonian symptoms, whereas PDD is defined as dementia occurring at least 1 year after motor symptom onset [50]. A recent study by Fritz et al. could additionally find some clinical features that differ between DLB and PD which included a slower speed, shorter stride length, and increased stance phases of gait as well as a higher frequency of falls among DLB when compared to PD patients [51]. The differentiation and correct recognition thus pose a challenge to the clinician.

With regard to the presence of hallucinations, in DLB these tend to occur early in the disease course and are not associated with dopaminergic medication, whereas in PDD they tend to develop in later stages and to be related to intake of dopaminergic therapy, mostly of dopamine agonists

[52]. Autopsy series in DLB with hallucinations showed a deposition of Lewy bodies in the inferior temporal cortex, with similar anatomical correlates found in autopsies of PD patients with hallucinations, so that hallucinations were correlated with the presence of Lewy body pathology in the temporal lobes [53]. Nonetheless, a more recent study assessing structural changes in dementia by means of MRI scans could correlate the presence of hallucinations with a cortical atrophy in visual pathways, rather than an anatomical correlate in temporal regions [54]. As a potential further biomarker of hallucinations in PDD, a study on the effect of fluctuating cognition in DLB and PDD showed a significantly higher prevalence of hallucinations among DLB and PDD patients when fluctuating cognition features were present [55].

2.3.3. Acute Psychosis in PD Patients.
Psychosis normally develops in the course of PD, gradually increasing in severity over time. If isolated visual hallucinations manifest independently or before the onset of "classical" PD psychosis, which is defined as lasting for over 1 month, it has been described as mostly resulting from medication [56]. An acute setting with sudden onset of psychotic symptoms must be regarded as an emergency situation [57]. Apart from recent changes in PD medication and acute intoxications associated with dehydration or other metabolic disorders, less frequent differential diagnosis such as cerebral infarction, intracranial haemorrhage, or CNS infections needs to be addressed. It is well known that some specific medical comorbidities can acutely trigger a psychotic episode or influence the severity of its symptoms [3], including infections, dehydration, sleep deprivation, irregular nutrition, psychosocial stress, deprivation or overload of sensory inputs, operations, metabolic alterations, dopaminergic drugs, and some other not antiparkinsonian drugs such as beta-blockers or corticosteroids. Under benzodiazepines a paradoxical reaction with restlessness, excitation, and euphoria may occur.

Another associated acute neuropsychiatric disturbance in PD is delirium, which implies a fluctuating alteration of attention accompanied by an additional disturbance in cognition, as defined by the DSM-V criteria [58] and has been considered as an acute decompensation occurring in ageing and/or dementia, particularly among vulnerable brains such as PD affected individuals. The estimated prevalence is of 8 to 24% [59–61] and a 5 times higher risk of developing delirium among PD patients when compared to healthy controls has been described in a recent study by Lubomski et al. [59]. A

TABLE 3: Features of delirium versus psychosis in PD.

Features	Delirium	Psychosis
Onset	Acute	Insidious
Course	Fluctuating, usually resolving over days to weeks	Progressive
Conscious level	Often impaired; can fluctuate rapidly; can be drowsy or hyperaroused	Clear
Cognitive defects	Poor short-term memory, poor attention span	Subtle
Hallucinations	Common, especially visual	Common especially complex visual or auditory
Key symptoms	Inattention, thought disorganisation, day-night reversal	Hallucinations, delusions, thought insertion, withdrawal or broadcast, passivity phenomena, phantom boarder
Medical status	Abnormal	Normal

Reference: Vardy et al., 2015 [58].

differentiation of delirium and psychosis, although challenging and not thoroughly studied in the current literature, can be considered with the features in Table 3.

A further acutely occurring alteration of mental status is the acute confusional state, which overlaps with delirium and has to date no condensed distinctive features from it. In fact the terms acute confusional state and encephalopathy are commonly used synonymously with the term delirium. While the symptom confusion itself refers more specifically to an inability to think coherently and an overall depressed sensorium, it poses an essential feature of the above defined term delirium [62, 63].

Another acutely occurring complication in PD is acute akinesia or akinetic crisis, which primarily involves worsening of motor performance lasting for ≥48 hours despite treatment [64] but is frequently associated with psychotic and cognitive symptoms as well [65]. It poses a life-threatening but rare complication in PD, having an estimated prevalence of 0.3% and mainly arising secondary to infections, surgical interventions, or changes in treatment [66]. The main clinical features imply a severe rigidity and akinesia associated with hyperthermia, dysautonomia, dysphagia, and/or increased serum muscle enzymes levels. Although frequently severe and associated with a high mortality rate of around 15%, also less severe forms known as "forme frusta" have been described [67, 68]. The clinical similarities to the malignant neuroleptic syndrome led this condition to also be named as neuroleptic malignant-like syndrome, malignant syndrome, or parkinsonism-hyperpyrexia [67], although some of these terms might be misleading, since an independent occurrence from neuroleptic drug use has been reported [64]. A study specifically addressing the adverse events arising from antipsychotic use in PD patients found an overall highest incidence of adverse reactions under quetiapine therapy, followed by clozapine and olanzapine but when addressing the occurrence of the adverse event "neuroleptic malignant syndrome," quetiapine was the most frequently concomitantly given medication [69], which goes along other published case reports on the association of quetiapine and the occurrence of neuroleptic malignant syndrome in PD [70].

3. Pathophysiology and Potential Biomarkers of Psychosis in PD

3.1. Introduction. Psychosis in PD patients is mostly arising in patients with a clear sensorium in a chronic setting after a long disease duration and is triggered or enhanced by pharmacological factors. Nonetheless, other recent risk factors have been studied, giving rise to a potential multifactorial underlying aetiology and thus physiopathology. The differentiation between early and late onset psychosis in general, and also specifically in PD, is not currently validated, having some studies randomly set cut-off values at 2–4 years of PD onset to determine early versus late onset psychosis [71]. More interestingly, the assessment of psychosis as a potential prodromal feature could give rise to finding biomarkers in PD, in order to predict its occurrence and treat it at early stages. In this section we will review the pathophysiology of psychosis, focusing on prodromal/premotor psychosis and on psychosis arising in the course of PD (with no differentiation between early and late onset), and then address potential biomarkers of PD psychosis.

3.2. Premotor versus Late Occurring PD Psychosis. To our knowledge only one study has been performed and recently published to analyze the presence of psychotic symptoms as a feature of the premotor state of PD; Pagonabarraga et al. studied a cohort of 50 drug-naïve PD patients and compared them with 100 healthy controls to assess the presence of hallucinations [72]. They found an overall prevalence of minor hallucinations in the untreated PD group of 42%, the onset of these being 7 months to 8 years prior to motor symptom onset. The prevalence of hallucinations in the control group was 5%. When comparing the cohort of PD patients and healthy controls, the groups did not differ in baseline characteristics, apart from a significant impairment in global cognitive function in the PD group compared with the control group. Nonetheless, dementia criteria were not met in any of the subjects included in the study. When then comparing the PD patients with and without hallucinations, older age and the presence of rapid-eye-movement behaviour disorder

TABLE 4: Clinical and demographic features of PD patients with and PD patients without hallucinations after following up prospectively.

	PD-mH ($n = 21$)	PD-NH ($n = 29$)	P
Age, y	71.1 ± 7	65.8 ± 12	0.06 (t-test)
Education, y	8.4 ± 4	9.4 ± 5	0.45 (t-test)
Sex, ♂	57.10%	55.60%	0.91 (χ^2)
Disease duration, months from onset of motor symptoms	22.8 ± 10	28.8 ± 14	0.12 (t-test)
UPDRS-III, at baseline	18.3 ± 9	20.1 ± 8	0.47 (t-test)
Hoehn & Yahr, at baseline	1.9 ± 0.2	2.1 ± 0.5	0.19 (t-test)
Predominance of motor symptoms, right%	52.3	65.5	0.23 (χ^2)
Depression, %	52.3	41.40%	0.39 (χ^2)
Anxiety, %	47.6	48.2	0.91 (χ^2)
Apathy, %	42.8	55.1	0.47 (χ^2)
Insomnia, %	38.1	41.3	0.68 (χ^2)
Daytime sleepiness, %	38.1	27.5	0.45 (χ^2)
RBD, %	38.1	10.3	0.03 (χ^2)
Hyposmia, %	33.3	27.5	0.80 (χ^2)

PD-mH: Parkinson's disease with minor hallucinations; PD-NH: PD without hallucinations; UPDRS-III: Unified PD Rating Scale, motor section; RBD: REM sleep behaviour disorder; reference: Pagonabarraga et al., 2016 [72].

(RBD) were statistically significantly correlated ($P < 0.05$) as seen in Table 4. This preliminary study sheds light on a potential prodromal occurrence of PD psychosis and proposes risk factors that could help recognize at-risk PD patients. Further studies with wider sample sizes are nonetheless needed.

As mentioned previously, the prevalence of psychosis in the course of PD varies widely in the literature. Psychosis itself represents a relevant burden in PD, involving their caregivers and health professionals, since it has been associated with a higher morbidity and mortality [73]. Additionally, together with depression and dementia, it poses one of the most prevalent nonmotor features in PD [74], accounting for up to one-fifth of the complications arising over time [75].

As to potential biomarkers, a strong correlation of psychosis with depression and REM behaviour disorders has been described by Lee and Weintraub in a study on 191 nondemented PD patients [74], where the risk of developing psychosis with comorbid depression and sleep related disorders was 5 times higher. In this study they identified an overall prevalence for psychotic symptoms in 21% of PD patients. The variables associated with the occurrence of psychosis were similar to previous studies, Hoehn and Yahr (H&Y) stage, disease duration, Unified PD Rating Scale (UPDRS) motor score, depression, anxiety, RBD symptoms, daytime sleepiness, and apathy. A nonstatistically significant trend towards psychosis under higher L-Dopa dosages was found, but no correlation with dopamine agonist therapy could be established, in contrast to previous studies. A lower Mini Mental State Examination (MMSE) score also indicated a trend towards psychosis.

The risk factors of psychosis thus seem to be related to multiple pathways involving different neurotransmitter systems, complicating the understanding of the underlying processes taking place.

3.3. Pathophysiology of PD Psychosis. The pathophysiological processes underlying PD psychosis can be subdivided into intrinsic (neurotransmitter-dysfunction related and thus not externally induced) and extrinsic (drug-related and thus a direct result of the use of pharmacological agents). While intrinsic PD psychosis is thought to be caused by alterations in dopamine, serotonin, and acetylcholine systems involving subcortical projections as well as synaptic and neuronal changes in limbic and cortical structures [76], extrinsic PD mainly involves dopaminergic or anticholinergic therapies, especially dopamine agonists [35, 72].

To better understand the neurotransmitter dysfunctions underlying the development of hallucinations, the effect of hallucinogenic agents with known mechanisms of actions is of advantage. Classically, hallucinogenic agents were subdivided into those affecting the cholinergic system and those involving the aminergic system, herein dopaminergic and serotoninergic agents being included [77]. The described clinical characteristics and associated hallucinations caused by these two distinct systems also differ: while the effects caused by anticholinergic agents are associated with peripheral autonomic features, confusion, disorientation, and visual hallucinations, mostly poorly formed and of a threatening nature, the symptoms caused by aminergic agents are characterised by a heightened awareness of objects, forms, and colours with a clear sensorium, sometimes involving the presence of hypnagogic phenomena of a dream-like quality [77].

A novel model to clarify the underlying mechanism of psychosis in PD proposed by Wolters [78] suggests that the DA stimulated orbitofrontal output activates dorsal raphe neurons, which release serotonin and activate 5HT2a receptors. These receptors stimulate GABAergic neurons which influence dopamine neurons in the ventral tegmental area [79] through the neurotransmitter glutamate. Finally excitation of the limbic system and inhibition of the prefrontal cortex take place, giving rise to an impaired selection and weighing of external environmental stimuli, thus leading to a mis/overinterpretation of external inputs.

Other hypotheses come from a combination of neurotransmitters from Birkmayer and Riederer [80], shedding light on a dopamine/serotonin imbalance as an underlying mechanism of psychosis. This goes along postmortem studies, which found a loss of serotonin among PD patients [81] and the evidence on the positive effect of pharmacological agents which act by activating the 5-HT2 receptors, such as pimavanserin.

Since cholinergic deficiency is present not only in Alzheimer's disease, but also in PDD and DLB [82], and there is a close link between cognitive impairment and psychosis, a potential implication of this neurotransmitter could be considered. This led to a further hypothesis on the pathophysiology of psychosis by Perry et al., who proposes a cholinergic/serotoninergic imbalance [83, 84]. Cholinergic depletion is already regarded as a potential underlying cause of psychosis in DLB alongside visuospatial processing deficits, which could therefore be thought of having a similar mechanism in PD psychosis.

Papapetropoulos and Mash propose, based on the above-mentioned findings, a neurochemical pathway for PD psychosis pathogenesis [31], with a disruption in mesolimbic dopaminergic pathways that lead to a supersensitivity of the implicated DA neurons in the striatum along with facilitating systems involving the serotoninergic/dopaminergic and serotoninergic/cholinergic balance as seen in Figure 1. Other factors, such as genetic variances or environmental factors, were also postulated in this study; studies on potential DA receptor genes variants implicated in hallucinations in PD have nonetheless shown controversial results, 2 studies suggesting an influence on psychosis by some genes [85, 86], but one other study not being conclusive on this relationship [87].

It is well known that treatment with antiparkinsonian drugs may induce psychotic features in PD patients, posing a limitation in their application and even leading to their discontinuation if severe symptoms arise. Dopamine replacement therapy is the current mainstay treatment of PD but its pulsatile administration leads to an increase in both tonic and phasic dopamine signalling [88, 89]. While the externally administered replacement of dopamine in areas of dopaminergic cell loss is of beneficial effect, the stimulation of relatively unaffected areas such as the ventral tegmental area and the ventral striatum can impair the functioning of these areas.

In a study conducted on PD patients with marked hallucinations under antiparkinsonian treatment, a clear sensorium even after long-term anticholinergic treatment and a precipitation of psychosis after increases of dopaminergic or anticholinergic drugs with a typically similar appearance of hallucinations within each patient could be found, whereas decreases in the dosage of dopaminergic or anticholinergic treatment showed to improve hallucinations [90]. These findings support a pathophysiological mechanism directly related to changes in both dopamine and acetylcholine levels within the brain related to externally administered medication.

Animal models on the effect of long-term L-Dopa therapy have also shown changes at dopamine receptor sites along behavioural changes. Particularly mesolimbic areas, with a known high density of dopaminergic and cholinergic nerve terminals, have been implicated in the pathophysiology of these underlying neuronal changes [90]. Furthermore, animal studies on MPTP-treated monkeys showed upregulations of D1 and D2 receptors in the denervated striatum [91], which could be replicated in humans in further studies, showing a potential compensatory upregulation of DA receptors presumably due to nigrostriatal DA denervation (so-called denervation supersensitivity) [92, 93].

Interestingly, abnormal dopaminergic transmission has also been observed in schizophrenia and schizotypal trails and has been considered a main characteristic of its underlying pathophysiology [94]. In PD patients receiving dopaminergic therapy, some positive schizotypal trails could be found, postulating a potentially, at least partially common pathway of psychosis development [95, 96]. Externally administered dopamine therapy is thought to stimulate supersensitive striatal and mesolimbic dopamine receptors thus leading to the generation of visual hallucinations, the connections to frontal regions being specifically implicated and thus an anatomically/topologically comprehensive pathway for the induction of PD psychosis [77]. Nonetheless, a small study on intravenous L-Dopa infusions in 5 nondemented PD patients with daily hallucinations did not trigger visual hallucinations, postulating that high levels of L-Dopa and thus DA receptor activation alone do not cause visual hallucinations solely, so that more complex systems might be involved [97].

The link between cognitive impairment and PD psychosis has been thoroughly described in the literature [74, 98] with a recent review stating a correlation of PD psychosis in patients with impairment in mainly cognitive executive, attentional, and visuospatial domains [98]. Further, PD psychosis has also been described as a risk factor for the development of PD dementia [32, 74], giving rise to a potential link between both complications. Accordingly, a recent study by Factor et al. [99] confirmed an association between hallucinations in PD and global cognitive decline but also described for the first time a lack of correlation between delusions and cognition in PD patients. Structural neuroimaging studies have shown evidence of pronounced atrophies in frontal and limbic areas, as well as in the visual pathways and cortex in PD patients with hallucinations and cognitive impairment [100], although some controversy within the results has also been reported [101]. With regard to neurotransmitter systems implied in the pathophysiology of both conditions, cholinergic and dopaminergic pathways are thought to be involved [102]. Evidence in favour of an underlying cholinergic degeneration in PD psychosis among cognitively impaired patients has been supported by the fact that choline acetyl transferase reduction has been found in the neocortex of hallucinating PD as well as Lewy body dementia patients [103, 104] and the fact that cholinesterase inhibitors improve psychotic symptoms in some cases of Lewy body dementia patients [105, 106]. With regard to the dopaminergic system, the finding of a missing relation between delusions and cognitive decline [107, 108], the reported cases were found to be described

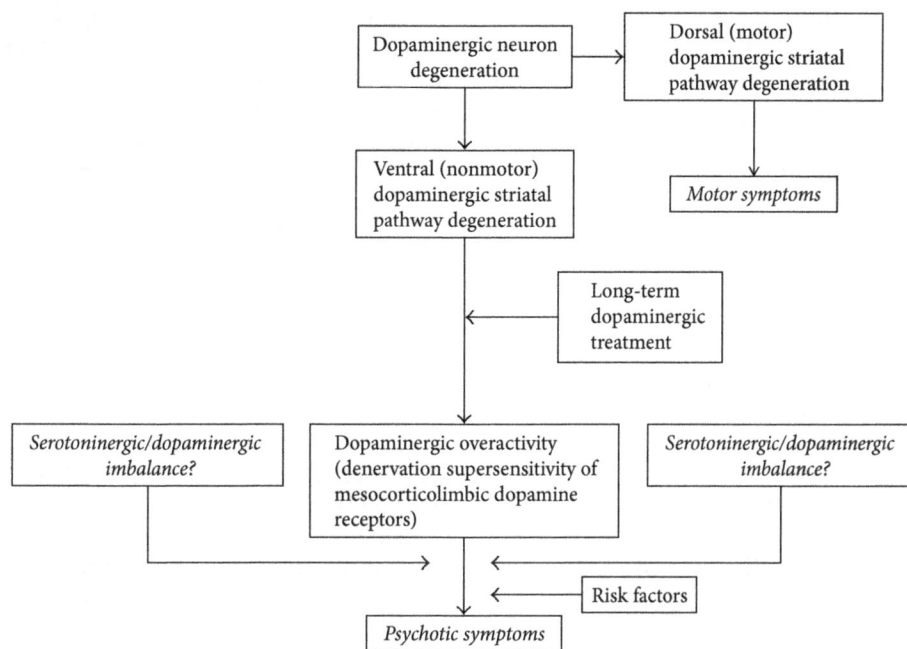

FIGURE 1: Proposed neurochemical pathways in the pathogenesis of psychosis in PD. DA, dopamine. Reference: Papapetropoulos et al., 2005 [31].

in PD patients on dopamine agonists and the symptoms as reversible after dopaminergic drug discontinuation, shedding light on a direct and strong involvement of the dopaminergic pathways in the development of psychotic features defined as delusions. The complexity and controversy among clinical presentations, imaging findings, and neurotransmitter imbalance thought to be involved [18] have been recently addressed in a thorough review and have shed light on the need of future research into this field.

3.4. Potential Biomarkers of PD Psychosis.
A biomarker is defined as a characteristic that can be objectively measured and that can indicate a normal biological process, a pathogenic process, or a pharmacologic response to a specific therapy [109]. Biomarkers can range from clinical, neuroimaging, and biochemical to genetic or proteomic characteristics and their purpose can be to confirm a diagnosis, serve for epidemiological screening, predict an outcome, monitor disease progression, or assess and predict response to a treatment. In the thorough search for a therapy for PD in the past 30 years, next to the complexity of the disease itself, the lack of reliable tools available to monitor progression and to observe the effects of the interventions has been a major drawback. Screening for biomarkers in PD is therefore highly relevant, but no reliable ones are readily available [110]. To this purpose, the PPMI (Parkinson Progression Marker Initiative) is currently undergoing an observational, multicentre, international study designed to evaluate potential biomarkers of PD progression comprising 400 recently diagnosed PD patients and 200 healthy subjects among a total of 21 centres [111].

Apart from the above-mentioned associated risk factors in PD, specific biomarkers for PD psychosis have to our

knowledge not been studied so far; nonetheless biomarkers for cognitive decline, which is a risk factor for the development of psychosis in PD, have been recently published. In a study by Skogseth et al. [112], cerebrospinal fluid (CSF) parameters and cognition in PD were assessed, finding a significant correlation between reduced Alpha-synuclein and reduced composite cognition and executive-attention domain scores. Associations between T-Tau and A-beta42 were not significantly associated with PD-MCI. Alongside this finding, another recent study by Stav et al. showed a significant correlation between A-beta38, A-beta40, and also Alpha-synuclein in PD patients with MCI [113]. In the current literature on biomarkers in cognitive decline in PD, the most consistent finding is an association of reduced A-Beta 42 in CSF, while the findings on T-/P-Tau are inconsistent [114]. With regard to biomarkers for psychosis (in non-PD subjects), a recent study on leukocytic miRNA comparing healthy subjects with persons who were at high risk of psychosis without progressing to psychosis and individuals who did develop psychosis over a course of 2 years showed a specific pattern of expression of small regulatory miRNAs in people who developed psychosis compared to those who did not [115]. They could not find individual miRNAs with statistically significant power; nonetheless a sum of 5 miRNAs was proposed to indicate a progression towards psychosis. This goes along another study by Gardiner et al., in which miRNAs were found to be downregulated in 112 schizophrenia patients when compared to 76 healthy controls [116]. Whether these findings could be extrapolated to PD psychosis remains open and needs further studies.

Along this biochemical biomarkers, imaging studies in schizoid and schizotypal personality disorders have found greater volume loss in the superior part of the corona radiata [117] as well as smaller neocortical grey matter volumes with larger sulcal CSF relative volumes [118], as a potential further biomarker of psychotic trails in schizotypal individuals compared to healthy controls. As in the case of the mentioned biochemical biomarkers, further studies are needed with regard to imaging biomarkers as well.

4. Management of PD Psychosis

4.1. Nonpharmacological Treatment. The importance of a multidisciplinary approach for the treatment of PD psychosis has been revised by several authors in the literature and implies the involvement of psychiatrists and other mental health professionals, neurologists, and functional neurosurgeons [119]. With regard to noninterventional treatments, psychoeducation and cognitive behavioural therapy (CBT) have shown efficacy in schizophrenia [120] but have not specifically been assessed in PD psychosis. Active music therapy in PD patients showed benefits in behavioural, as well as in motor and affective functions [121]; however more systematic studies with a higher number of patients are required to study its potential effect as well as its long-term outcome.

4.2. Pharmacological Treatment. It is important to differentiate the treatment strategy of an acute and potentially life-threatening PD psychosis from a chronic setting.

The treatment strategy of acute psychotic episodes in PD is primarily to address and treat the underlying cause, including general measures, treatment of specific triggers, adaptation of medication, and/or addition of cholinesterase inhibitors in cognitively impaired PD patients (rivastigmine, donepezil, or galantamine) and antipsychotic agents such as clozapine or quetiapine when not manageable with the previous steps as shown in Table 5. If there is no response to neuroleptic agents, further investigations such as the measurement of amphetamines, methamphetamines, digoxin, T3, T4, TSH, and protoporphyrin should be considered. A transition from an acute to a chronic state can follow. In the chronic setting of a PD psychosis on the other hand, the first pharmacological approach is the optimization of the administered antiparkinsonian therapy, aiming at the lowest effective dose. The order in which the medication should be reduced is as follows: anticholinergic agents, selegiline, amantadine, dopamine receptor agonists, COMT-inhibitors, and lastly L-Dopa [124]. If reduction of medication however does not improve psychosis, the use of cholinesterase inhibitors or antipsychotic medication similarly as in the treatment strategy of the acute onset PD psychosis needs to be evaluated.

The main antipsychotic drugs used in PD psychosis are clozapine and quetiapine. Clozapine is slightly stronger than quetiapine but has a greater risk to induce agranulocytosis, with an estimated overall prevalence of 1-2% [125].

4.2.1. Clozapine. Clozapine is an atypical antipsychotic whose mechanism of action is only partially understood, being thought to mainly act as an antagonist of dopamine D2 receptors and serotonin 2A receptors. It was first produced in 1958 and sold commercially after 1972. A double-blind,

placebo-controlled study on clozapine for the treatment of drug-induced psychosis in PD (PSYCLOPS trial) showed an effectiveness of low-dose clozapine without worsening of motor function and response maintenance over at least 4 months in PD patients with psychosis [126]. A further double-blind, placebo-controlled study by Pollak et al. could find a statistically significant improvement in psychosis scores when compared to placebo, without significant motor function worsening, when using a low dose of clozapine of 50 mg/day. They also found wearing-off of the effect after discontinuation of the therapy [127]. These studies support the effectiveness of low-dose clozapine for the management of psychosis in PD.

4.2.2. Other Antipsychotics. The use of newer antipsychotics was to follow the discovery of clozapine. The beneficial use of atypical antipsychotics in PD has been associated with a statistically significant increased risk of mortality, quetiapine being the weakest one associated with this fatal outcome, as studied in a recent trial by Weintraub et al. [128], so that studies to assess its efficacy in PD psychosis have been sought after.

Quetiapine is a dibenzothiazepine derivative structurally related to clozapine and was approved by the FDA in 1997 [129]. A study by Morgante et al. analyzed in a randomized, rater-blinded trial the effect of clozapine versus quetiapine in 45 PD patients with drug-induced psychosis over 12 weeks and concluded an equally efficacious potential of both drugs with unchanged motor scores among both groups [130]. A further study comparing the two medications by Merims et al. in 27 PD patients with recent-onset psychosis showed similar results but showed an overall trend of clozapine over quetiapine to control hallucinations ($P = 0.097$) and an advantage in reducing delusions ($P = 0.011$). Nonetheless the relatively high incidence of agranulocytosis under clozapine therapy poses a limitation in its use and the alternative of using quetiapine remains of importance [131]. Nonetheless, other studies comparing quetiapine to placebo in a total of 31 subjects [132], 58 subjects [133], and 24 subjects [134] failed to show efficacy on hallucinations when comparing quetiapine with placebo.

Studies on olanzapine, another atypical antipsychotic agent with dopamine D2 receptor and serotonin 2A receptor antagonism, could show no significant improvements in drug-induced PD psychosis and significant worsening in motor function in PD patients when compared to placebo in two placebo-controlled trials [135, 136].

Summarising the above-mentioned antipsychotic drugs as shown in Table 6, clozapine is efficacious for the treatment of psychosis in PD with an acceptable risk of side effects, if blood cell count is monitored. For quetiapine there is currently insufficient evidence to conclude on its efficacy for PD psychosis, but its safety profile shows benefit with no need of monitoring. For olanzapine, there is no evidence of efficacy in PD psychosis and an unacceptable motor function deterioration consequently making this compound not recommended for use in PD psychosis.

Less commonly used compounds such as risperidone have shown to be effective in the treatment of PD psychosis, nonetheless worsening motor function [138], so that it is currently not recommended as a treatment for PD psychosis.

TABLE 5: Proposed treatment strategies of acute, secondary psychosis in Parkinson's disease.

Step	Action	
I	General measures	Reestablishment of circadian rhythms
		Reestablishment of normal-level sensory inputs
		Hearing and vision aids
		Reestablishment of familial environment
II	Treatment of specific triggers	Treatment of infection, dehydration
		Balancing electrolytes, glucose, vitamins, hormones
		Treatment of heart insufficiency
III	Elimination of nonessential medication	Particularly anticholinergic, antiglutamatergic, sedating drugs
IV	Reduction of anti-Parkinson medication	Anticholinergics > amantadine > MAO-B-inhibitors > dopamine agonists > COMT-inhibitors > L-dopa retard > L-dopa nonretarded
V	Cholinesterase inhibitors in cognitively impaired patients	For example, rivastigmine 6–12 mg/d 2-3/d, or donepezil 5–10 mg/d 1/d (off-label), or galantamine 4–32 mg/d 2-3/d (off-label)
VI	Antipsychotic medication	Clozapine 12.5–62.5 mg/d (first-line), or quetiapine 12.5–75 mg/d (off-label)

COMT, catechol-O-methyltransferase; MAO-B, monoamine oxidase B; reference: Levin et al., 2016 [3], taken from Seppi et al., 2011 [122] and Connolly and Lang, 2014 [123].

TABLE 6: Summary of commonly used antipsychotic drugs to treat PD psychosis.

Drug	Efficacy	Safety	Practice Implications
Clozapine	Efficacious	Acceptable risk with specialized monitoring	Clinically useful
Olanzapine	Unlikely efficacious	Unacceptable risk	Not useful
Quetiapine	Insufficient evidence	Acceptable risk without specialized monitoring	Investigational

Reference: Seppi et al., 2011 [122].

Ziprasidone has shown to improve PD psychosis symptoms in one small randomized single-blind parallel comparison study between ziprasidone and clozapine in 14 patients by Pintor et al., with no worsening of motor scores or cognitive function when comparing both intervention arms [139]. But to draw clinically relevant conclusions further studies with higher sample sizes are needed. Finally, melperone, another atypical antipsychotic of the butyrophenone chemical class, showed no benefit in the treatment of PD psychosis when compared to placebo in an unpublished double-blind, placebo-controlled trial by Friedman [140].

4.2.3. Pimavanserin. Pimavanserin, a selective 5-HT2A inverse agonist without dopaminergic, adrenergic, histaminergic, or muscarinic effect [141], has been approved by the FDA [142] in September 2014 and has shown to be effective and safe in the treatment of PD psychosis, reducing hallucinations and delusions without affecting motor function [143, 144], which is a commonly observed drawback of most antipsychotic drugs due to dopamine antagonism. Recent studies have shown the potential of this drug to improve psychotic symptoms among PD patients [144, 145]. Results showed a significant improvement in measures of psychosis

in PD patients without impairing motor function in one study by Meltzer et al. [145] and a statistically significant decrease in SAPS-PD scores in a bigger cohort of 199 PD patients in a randomized, double-blind, placebo-controlled phase 3 trial by Cummings et al. [144]. But pimavanserin and commonly used antipsychotics have up to now not been systematically compared.

4.2.4. Cholinesterase Inhibitors. Clinical trials to assess the potential benefit of the widely used cholinesterase inhibitors for the treatment of dementia have been studied in PD psychosis due to its close relationship but have shown no beneficial effect on PD psychosis to date [73]. A randomized, placebo-controlled trial of donepezil in cognitive impaired PD patients showed a beneficial effect in memory, with no differences in psychiatric status or motor function [146] and an overall reduced tolerability with the recommendation of careful monitoring when used in PD patients. Another placebo-controlled study of rivastigmine in cognitive impaired PD patients showed moderate improvements in cognitive function but also higher rates of side effects, such as nausea, vomiting, and tremor [106]. Nonetheless, treatment of hallucinations in DLB has been reported to be

TABLE 7: Clinical evaluation with scales before and after the sessions of electroconvulsive therapy (ECT).

Scales	Before ECT (mean ± SD)	After ECT (mean ± SD)	P
UPDRS III ($n = 23$)	45.2 ± 14.1	27.6 ± 11.9	<0.001
UPDRS IV ($n = 23$)	7 ± 3.1	2.7 ± 1.1	<0.001
HY ($n = 21$)	3.2 ± 0.6	2.1 ± 0.5	<0.001
MMSE ($n = 27$)	26.5 ± 3.9	26.3 ± 4.2	0.79
CGI ($n = 27$)	4.7 ± 0.8	2.9 ± 1	<0.001
BPRS ($n = 27$)	18.4 ± 8.6	9.6 ± 5.7	<0.001
HDRS ($n = 27$)	21.1 ± 2.2	10.5 ± 3	<0.001

ECT: electroconvulsive therapy; SD: standard deviation; UPDRS: Unified Parkinson's Disease Rating Scale; HY: Hoehn and Yahr; MMSE: Mini Mental Status Examination; CGI: clinical global impression; BPRS: Brief Psychiatric Rating Scale; HDRS: Hamilton Depression Rating Scale; reference: Calderón-Fajardo et al., 2015 [137].

efficacious with cholinesterase inhibitors such as donepezil [147, 148] and a clinical trial on the effect of donepezil in PD psychosis is currently under way [149]. Recommendation to use cholinesterase inhibitors in PD psychosis in cognitively impaired patients is currently supported by some authors [122, 123].

4.3. Electroconvulsive Therapy (ECT) and Deep Brain Stimulation (DBS). Electroconvulsive therapy has shown beneficial effects in the treatment of neuropsychiatric symptoms in PD in some studies in the literature. The most recently published study on the effect of ECT in 29 drug-refractory PD patients with psychiatric symptoms, 12 of them having psychosis and depression and one having isolated psychosis, showed an improvement in measures of motor as well as nonmotor function assessed by means of different scales as seen in Table 7 [137].

This goes along other previous studies on ECT performed on PD patients with psychiatric comorbidities as summarised in Table 8, where most of the studies showed improvements in clinical impression and in the used scales. The mechanism of action of ECT is currently not known; potential postsynaptic dopamine receptor upregulation in the striatum, an increase in postsynaptic dopamine responsiveness, and an increase in levels of L-Dopa in the central nervous system by disrupting the blood-brain-barrier are thought to be underlying [150, 151]. As to its antipsychotic and antidepressant effect, enhancement of serotoninergic neurotransmission and mesocorticolimbic pathway activation has been postulated [152]; a PET study in PD patients with psychosis and depression showed that ECT led to an increase in metabolism in the anterior cingulate cortex and hippocampus, the latter of both showing correlation with a reduction of positive symptoms assessed by the Hamilton Depression Rating Scale (HDRS) [153]. Safety and tolerability issues have not been reported under ECT so far; nonetheless the performed studies to date are only small sample sized, have not been blinded, and have not assessed long-term efficacy. A large, sham-controlled study on the effect of ECT for the treatment of neuropsychiatric symptoms in PD is therefore highly needed. Studies on the effect of ECT in patients with deep brain stimulators have so far not been assessed; an undergoing collection of data to that purpose is under way [154].

Deep brain stimulation (DBS) has been reported as causing psychosis as a potential severe adverse event in PD patients [155], but the direct link to this complication is often overlapped by comorbid conditions and therefore contradictory in the actual literature [155, 156]. Its potential to treat psychiatric disorders in non-PD patients has furthermore shown some promising results in psychiatric conditions such as obsessive compulsive disorders [157]. Nonetheless, current evidence of DBS effect on PD psychosis is scarce and knowledge on its effect, whether improving or worsening the symptoms, cannot be stated at this point of time [19]. A clinical trial for the assessment of DBS for the treatment of resistant schizophrenia is currently under way; whether, if positive, the results could be potentially extrapolated to PD in the future remains open.

5. Conclusion

Although psychosis was thoroughly studied in recent years after being identified as one of the most relevant nonmotor features in PD, standardized guidelines for the management of PD psychosis are not available. Interestingly, psychosis, being one of the hallmarks of psychiatric illnesses such as schizophrenia with patients typically presenting with auditory features [21], presents rather differently in PD patients, where visual hallucinations clearly predominate, implicating a potentially different entity and thus underlying pathophysiological mechanism, further challenging the actual use of the same treatment options for both. In addition, current hypotheses on the underlying pathophysiological mechanisms including neurotransmitter dysregulation, structural/functional brain imaging abnormalities, and blood and CSF based biochemical measurements are sparse and inconsistent, supporting the lack of knowledge and the need of further investigation in order to potentially develop target oriented drugs in the nearer future. Currently undergoing studies on novel drugs for PD psychosis are expected to produce results in due time; ideas of further intervention strategies such as deep brain stimulation or stem cell therapy are being addressed for other causes of psychosis and could, if efficient, pose further options in the future. For now it remains clear that much more effort needs to be put into understanding this condition.

TABLE 8: Summary of published reports of electroconvulsive therapy for the management of neuropsychiatric symptoms in subjects with Parkinson's disease.

Study	Sample	Neuropsychiatric disorder	Measurements	Findings
Nishioka et al., 2014	4	Psychosis	NPI HAM-D	Improvement of 89.8% in the NPI / Improvement of 81.1% in the HAM-D
Sadananda et al., 2013	1	Psychosis	PANNS	Improvement of 77.3% in the PANNS
Muhammad et al., 2012	1	Obsessive-compulsive disorder	Clinical impression	Improvement
Usui et al., 2011	8	Psychosis	SAPS	Improvement of 65.8% in the mean SAPS total
Ducharme et al., 2011	1	Depression	Clinical impression	Improvement
Ueda et al. 2010	5	Psychosis	BPRS HAM-D	Improvement of 89.2% in the BPRS / Improvement of 83.8% in the HAM-D
Bailine et al. 2008	1	Psychotic depression	Clinical impression	Improvement
Lance et al., 1998	1	Depression	Clinical impression	Improvement
Mollentine et al., 1998	25	Depression and/or psychosis, dementia	BPRS HAM-D	
Nymeyer et al., 1997	1	Depression	Clinical impression	Improvement
Factor et al., 1995	2	Depression and/or psychosis	Clinical impression	Improvement
Sandky et al., 1993	1	Psychotic depression	Clinical impression	Modest improvement
Oh et al., 1992	11	Depression and/or psychosis	Clinical impression	82% of the patients improved
Zwil et al., 1992	8	Depression and/or psychosis		
Friedman et al., 1992	5	Depression and/or psychosis	Clinical impression	Improvement
Stern, 1991	1	Depression	Clinical impression	Improvement
Liberzon et al., 1990	1	Psychotic depression	Clinical impression	Improvement

NPI: neuropsychiatric inventory; HAM-D: Hamilton Depression Rating Scale; PANNS: Positive and Negative Syndrome Scale; SAPS: Scale for the Assessment of Positive Symptoms; BPRS: Brief Psychiatric Rating Scale; reference: Calderón-Fajardo et al., 2015 [137].

References

[1] J. G. Goldman and S. Holden, "Treatment of psychosis and dementia in Parkinson's disease," *Current Treatment Options in Neurology*, vol. 16, no. 3, article 281, 2014.

[2] W.-M. Liu, R.-J. Lin, R.-L. Yu, C.-H. Tai, C.-H. Lin, and R.-M. Wu, "The impact of nonmotor symptoms on quality of life in patients with parkinson's disease in Taiwan," *Neuropsychiatric Disease and Treatment*, vol. 11, pp. 2865–2873, 2015.

[3] J. Levin, A. Hasan, and G. U. Höglinger, "Psychosis in Parkinson's disease: identification, prevention and treatment," *Journal of Neural Transmission*, vol. 123, no. 1, pp. 45–50, 2016.

[4] A. Sauerbier, P. Jenner, A. Todorova, and K. R. Chaudhuri, "Non motor subtypes and Parkinson's disease," *Parkinsonism and Related Disorders*, vol. 22, pp. S41–S46, 2016.

[5] A. Souqes, *Rapport sur les syndromes parkinsoniens. Revue neurologique*, Masson, Paris, France, 1921.

[6] J. De Ajuriaguerra, *Ajuriaguerra, Etude psychopathologique des parkinsoniens in Monoamines, noyaux gris centraux et syndromes parkinsoniens*, Masson, Paris, France, 1971.

[7] M. Onofrj, D. Carrozzino, A. D'Amico et al., "Psychosis in parkinsonism: an unorthodox approach," *Neuropsychiatric Disease and Treatment*, vol. Volume 13, pp. 1313–1330, 2017.

[8] J. A. Vilensky, S. Gilman, and S. McCall, "Does the historical literature on encephalitis lethargica support a simple (direct) relationship with postencephalitic Parkinsonism?" *Movement Disorders*, vol. 25, no. 9, pp. 1124–1130, 2010.

[9] S. A. Factor, E. S. Molho, G. D. Podskalny, and D. Brown, "Parkinson's disease: drug-induced psychiatric states," *Advances in Neurology*, vol. 65, pp. 115–138, 1995.

[10] K. A. Josephs, "Capgras syndrome and its relationship to neurodegenerative disease," *Archives of Neurology*, vol. 64, no. 12, pp. 1762–1766, 2007.

[11] S. A. Factor and E. S. Molho, "Threatening auditory hallucinations and cotard syndrome in Parkinson disease," *Clinical Neuropharmacology*, vol. 27, no. 5, pp. 205–207, 2004.

[12] N. Moschopoulos, S. Kaprinis, and J. Nimatoudis, "Cotard's syndrome: case report and a brief review of literature," *Psychiatriki*, vol. 27, no. 4, pp. 296–302, 2016.

[13] M. Poletti, G. Perugi, C. Logi et al., "Dopamine agonists and delusional jealousy in Parkinson's disease: A cross-sectional prevalence study," *Movement Disorders*, vol. 27, no. 13, pp. 1679–1682, 2012.

[14] D. Georgiev, A. Danieli, L. Ocepek et al., "Othello syndrome in patients with parkinson's disease," *Psychiatria Danubina*, vol. 22, no. 1, pp. 94–98, 2010.

[15] World Health Organization, "The ICD-10 Classification of Mental and Behavioural Disorders," http://www.who.int/classifications/icd/en/GRNBOOK.pdf, 1993.

[16] J. MacK, P. Rabins, K. Anderson et al., "Prevalence of psychotic symptoms in a community-based parkinson disease sample," *American Journal of Geriatric Psychiatry*, vol. 20, no. 2, pp. 123–132, 2012.

[17] J. H. Friedman, "Parkinson disease psychosis: update," *Behavioural Neurology*, vol. 27, no. 4, pp. 469–477, 2013.

[18] D. H. Ffytche, B. Creese, M. Politis et al., "The psychosis spectrum in Parkinson disease," *Nature Reviews Neurology*, vol. 13, no. 2, pp. 81–95, 2017.

[19] D. H. Ffytche, J. B. Pereira, C. Ballard, K. R. Chaudhuri, D. Weintraub, and D. Aarsland, "Risk factors for early psychosis in PD: Insights from the Parkinson's Progression markers initiative," *Journal of Neurology, Neurosurgery and Psychiatry*, vol. 88, no. 4, pp. 325–331, 2017.

[20] B. R. Thanvi, T. C. N. Lo, and D. P. Harsh, "Psychosis in Parkinson's disease," *Postgraduate Medical Journal*, vol. 81, no. 960, pp. 644–646, 2005.

[21] S. Chaudhury, "Hallucinations: clinical aspects and management," *Industrial Psychiatry Journal*, vol. 19, no. 1, p. 5, 2010.

[22] B. Ravina, K. Marder, H. H. Fernandez et al., "Diagnostic criteria for psychosis in Parkinson's disease: report of an NINDS, NIMH Work Group," *Movement Disorders*, vol. 22, no. 8, pp. 1061–1068, 2007.

[23] G. Fenelon, "Psychosis in parkinson's disease: phenomenology, frequency, risk factors, and current understanding of pathophysiologic mechanisms," *CNS Spectrums*, vol. 13, no. 3, pp. 18–25, 2008.

[24] J. L. Cummings, "Behavioral complications of drug treatment of Parkinson's disease," *Journal of the American Geriatrics Society*, vol. 39, no. 7, pp. 708–716, 1991.

[25] D. Weintraub and H. I. Hurtig, "Presentation and management of psychosis in Parkinson's disease and dementia with lewy bodies," *American Journal of Psychiatry*, vol. 164, no. 10, pp. 1491–1498, 2007.

[26] E. B. Forsaa, J. P. Larsen, T. Wentzel-Larsen et al., "A 12-year population-based study of psychosis in Parkinson disease," *Archives of Neurology*, vol. 67, no. 8, pp. 996–1001, 2010.

[27] G. Fenelon, F. Mahieux, R. Huon, and M. Ziegler, "Hallucinations in Parkinson's disease. prevalence, phenomenology and risk factors," *Brain, American Journal of Ophthalmology*, vol. 130, no. 2, pp. 261-262, 2000.

[28] C. Pacchetti, R. Manni, R. Zangaglia et al., "Relationship between hallucinations, delusions, and rapid eye movement sleep behavior disorder in Parkinson's disease," *Movement Disorders*, vol. 20, no. 11, pp. 1439–1448, 2005.

[29] D. R. Williams, J. D. Warren, and A. J. Lees, "Using the presence of visual hallucinations to differentiate Parkinson's disease from atypical parkinsonism," *Journal of Neurology, Neurosurgery and Psychiatry*, vol. 79, no. 6, pp. 652–655, 2008.

[30] G. Fenelon, T. Soulas, F. Zenasni, and L. C. de Langavant, "The changing face of Parkinson's disease-associated psychosis: a cross-sectional study based on the new NINDS-NIMH criteria," *Movement Disorders : Official Journal of The Movement Disorder Society*, vol. 25, no. 6, pp. 755–759, 2010.

[31] S. Papapetropoulos and D. C. Mash, "Psychotic symptoms in Parkinson's disease. From description to etiology," *Journal of Neurology*, vol. 252, no. 7, pp. 753–764, 2005.

[32] S. A. Factor, P. J. Feustel, and J. H. Friedman, "Longitudinal outcome of Parkinson's disease patients with psychosis," *Neurology*, vol. 60, no. 11, pp. 1756–1761, 2003.

[33] A. Lenka, S. Hegde, K. R. Jhunjhunwala, and P. K. Pal, "Interactions of visual hallucinations, rapid eye movement sleep behavior disorder and cognitive impairment in Parkinson's disease: A review," *Parkinsonism and Related Disorders*, vol. 22, pp. 1–8, 2016.

[34] D. H. Hepp, C. C. da Hora, T. Koene et al., "Cognitive correlates of visual hallucinations in non-demented Parkinson's disease patients," *Parkinsonism and Related Disorders*, vol. 19, no. 9, pp. 795–799, 2013.

[35] G. Fenelon, "Psychotic symptoms in Parkinson's disease," in *Psychologie & Neuropsychiatrie Du Vieillissement*, pp. S17–S24, 2006.

[36] K. R. Chaudhuri, P. Martinez-Martin, R. G. Brown et al., "The metric properties of a novel non-motor symptoms scale for Parkinson's disease: results from an international pilot study," *Movement Disorders*, vol. 22, no. 13, pp. 1901–1911, 2007.

[37] C. G. Goetz, S. Fahn, P. Martinez-Martin et al., "Movement disorder society-sponsored revision of the unified Parkinson's disease rating scale (MDS-UPDRS): process, format, and clinimetric testing plan," *Movement Disorders*, vol. 22, no. 1, pp. 41–47, 2007.

[38] H. Sawada, T. Oeda, K. Yamamoto et al., "Trigger medications and patient-related risk factors for Parkinson disease psychosis requiring anti-psychotic drugs: A retrospective cohort study," *BMC Neurology*, vol. 13, article no. 145, 2013.

[39] T. Voss, D. Bahr, J. Cummings, R. Mills, B. Ravina, and H. Williams, "Performance of a shortened scale for assessment of positive symptoms for parkinson's disease psychosis," *Parkinsonism and Related Disorders*, vol. 19, no. 3, pp. 295–299, 2013.

[40] M. Rodriguez-Violante, A. Cervantes-Arriaga, S. Velázquez-Osuna et al., "Independent validation of the SEND-PD and correlation with the MDS-UPDRS part IA," *Parkinson's Disease*, vol. 2014, Article ID 260485, 5 pages, 2014.

[41] E. M. Kester, "Charles bonnet syndrome: case presentation and literature review," *Optometry*, vol. 80, no. 7, pp. 360–366, 2009.

[42] B. W. Rovner, "The charles bonnet syndrome: a review of recent research," *Current Opinion in Ophthalmology*, vol. 17, no. 3, pp. 275–277, 2006.

[43] J. C. Khan, H. Shahid, D. A. Thurlby, J. R. W. Yates, and A. T. Moore, "Charles Bonnet syndrome in age-related macular degeneration: The nature and frequency of images in subjects with end-stage disease," *Ophthalmic Epidemiology*, vol. 15, no. 3, pp. 202–208, 2008.

[44] G. Schultz and R. Melzack, "The Charles Bonnet syndrome: 'phantom visual images'.," *Perception*, vol. 20, no. 6, pp. 809–825, 1991.

[45] R. J. Teunisse, F. G. Zitman, and D. C. M. Raes, "Clinical evaluation of 14 patients with the Charles Bonnet syndrome (isolated visual hallucinations)," *Comprehensive Psychiatry*, vol. 35, no. 1, pp. 70–75, 1994.

[46] M. Onofrj, J. P. Taylor, D. Monaco et al., "Visual Hallucinations in PD and Lewy body dementias: old and new hypotheses," *Behavioural Neurology*, vol. 27, no. 4, pp. 479–493, 2013.

[47] L. Pang, "Hallucinations experienced by visually impaired: Charles bonnet syndrome," *Optometry and Vision Science*, vol. 93, no. 12, pp. 1466–1478, 2016.

[48] M. Manford and F. Andermann, "Complex visual hallucinations. Clinical and neurobiological insights," *Brain*, vol. 121, no. 10, pp. 1819–1840, 1998.

[49] V. Biousse, B. C. Skibell, R. L. Watts, D. N. Loupe, C. Drews-Botsch, and N. J. Newman, "Ophthalmologic features of Parkinson's disease," *Neurology*, vol. 62, no. 2, pp. 177–180, 2004.

[50] D. Aarsland, B. Creese, M. Politis et al., "Cognitive decline in Parkinson disease," *Nature Reviews Neurology*, 2017.

[51] N. E. Fritz, D. A. Kegelmeyer, A. D. Kloos et al., "Motor performance differentiates individuals with Lewy body dementia, Parkinson's and Alzheimer's disease," *Gait and Posture*, vol. 50, pp. 1–7, 2016.

[52] A. J. Harding, G. A. Broe, and G. M. Halliday, "Visual hallucinations in Lewy body disease relate to Lewy bodies in the temporal lobe," *Brain*, vol. 125, no. 2, pp. 391–403, 2002.

[53] D. A. Gallagher, L. Parkkinen, S. S. O'Sullivan et al., "Testing an aetiological model of visual hallucinations in Parkinson's disease," *Brain*, vol. 134, no. 11, pp. 3299–3309, 2011.

[54] J. G. Goldman, G. T. Stebbins, V. Dinh et al., "Visuoperceptive region atrophy independent of cognitive status in patients with Parkinson's disease with hallucinations," *Brain*, vol. 137, no. 3, pp. 849–859, 2014.

[55] S. Varanese, B. Perfetti, D. Monaco et al., "Fluctuating cognition and different cognitive and behavioural profiles in Parkinson's disease with dementia: Comparison of dementia with Lewy bodies and Alzheimer's disease," *Journal of Neurology*, vol. 257, no. 6, pp. 1004–1011, 2010.

[56] A. Moser, J. Hagenah, and D. Kömpf, "Hallucinations in Parkinson's disease," *Nervenarzt*, vol. 74, no. 4, pp. 376–386, 2003.

[57] T. Müller, H. Baas, J. Kassubek et al., "Laboratory assessments in the course of Parkinson's disease: a clinician's perspective," *Journal of Neural Transmission*, vol. 123, no. 1, pp. 65–71, 2016.

[58] E. R. L. C. Vardy, A. Teodorczuk, and A. J. Yarnall, "Review of delirium in patients with Parkinson's disease," *Journal of Neurology*, vol. 262, no. 11, pp. 2401–2410, 2015.

[59] M. Lubomski, R. L. Rushworth, and S. Tisch, "Hospitalisation and comorbidities in Parkinson's disease: a large Australian retrospective study," *Journal of Neurology, Neurosurgery and Psychiatry*, vol. 86, no. 3, pp. 324–329, 2015.

[60] OH. Gerlach, MP. Broen, and WE. Weber, "Motor outcomes during hospitalization in Parkinson's disease patients: a prospective study," *Parkinsonism & related disorders*, vol. 19, pp. 737–741, 2013.

[61] M. Boorsma, K. J. Joling, D. H. M. Frijters, M. E. Ribbe, G. Nijpels, and H. P. J. Van Hout, "The prevalence, incidence and risk factors for delirium in Dutch nursing homes and residential care homes," *International Journal of Geriatric Psychiatry*, vol. 27, no. 7, pp. 709–715, 2012.

[62] J. Francis, "Diagnosis of delirium and confusional states," 2017.

[63] L. Patti and S. Dulebohn, *Change, Mental Status*, StatPearls Publishing, FL, USA, 2017.

[64] M. Onofrj and A. Thomas, "Acute akinesia in Parkinson disease," *Neurology*, vol. 64, no. 7, pp. 1162–1169, 2005.

[65] A. Thomas, D. Iacono, A. L. Luciano, K. Armellino, and M. Onofrj, "Acute akinesia or akinetic crisis in Parkinson's disease," *Neurological Sciences*, vol. 24, no. 3, pp. 219–220, 2003.

[66] M. Simonetto, L. Ferigo, L. Zanet et al., "Acute akinesia, an unusual complication in Parkinson's Disease: A case report," *Neurological Sciences*, vol. 29, no. 3, pp. 181–183, 2008.

[67] V. Kaasinen, J. Joutsa, T. Noponen, and M. Päivärinta, "Akinetic crisis in parkinson's disease is associated with a severe loss of striatal dopamine transporter function: A report of two cases," *Case Reports in Neurology*, vol. 6, no. 3, pp. 275–280, 2014.

[68] M. Onofrj, L. Bonanni, G. Cossu, D. Manca, F. Stocchi, and A. Thomas, "Emergencies in parkinsonism: akinetic crisis, life-threatening dyskinesias, and polyneuropathy during L-Dopa gel treatment," *Parkinsonism and Related Disorders*, vol. 15, no. 3, pp. S233–S236, 2009.

[69] U. Lertxundi, A. I. Ruiz, M. Á. S. Aspiazu et al., "Adverse reactions to antipsychotics in parkinson disease: An analysis of the Spanish Pharmacovigilance database," *Clinical Neuropharmacology*, vol. 38, no. 3, pp. 69–84, 2015.

[70] A. Schattner, E. Kitroser, and J. D. Cohen, "Fatal Neuroleptic Malignant Syndrome Associated with Quetiapine," *American Journal of Therapeutics*, vol. 23, no. 5, pp. e1209–e1210, 2016.

[71] Y. T. Kwak, Y. Yang, and M. Koo, "Late-Onset Psychosis; Is It Real?" *Dementia and Neurocognitive Disorders*, vol. 14, no. 1, p. 1, 2015.

[72] J. Pagonabarraga, S. Martinez-Horta, R. Fernández de Bobadilla et al., "Minor hallucinations occur in drug-naive Parkinson's disease patients, even from the premotor phase," *Movement Disorders*, vol. 31, no. 1, pp. 45–52, 2016.

[73] N. Samudra, N. Patel, K. B. Womack, P. Khemani, and S. Chitnis, "Psychosis in parkinson disease: a review of etiology, phenomenology, and management," *Drugs and Aging*, vol. 33, no. 12, pp. 855–863, 2016.

[74] A. H. Lee and D. Weintraub, "Psychosis in Parkinson's disease without dementia: Common and comorbid with other non-motor symptoms," *Movement Disorders*, vol. 27, no. 7, pp. 858–863, 2012.

[75] D. A. Gallagher and A. Schrag, "Psychosis, apathy, depression and anxiety in Parkinson's disease," *Neurobiology of Disease*, vol. 46, no. 3, pp. 581–589, 2012.

[76] E. Oikonomou and T. Paparrigopoulos, "Neuropsychiatric manifestations in Parkinson's disease," *Psychiatrike = Psychiatriki*, vol. 26, no. 2, pp. 116–130, 2015.

[77] C. G. Goetz, C. M. Tanner, and H. L. Klawans, "Pharmacology of hallucinations induced by long-term drug therapy," *American Journal of Psychiatry*, vol. 139, no. 4, pp. 494–497, 1982.

[78] E. C. Wolters, "Intrinsic and extrinsic psychosis in Parkinson's disease," *Journal of Neurology*, vol. 248, no. S3, pp. 22–27, 2001.

[79] T. H. Svensson, J. M. Mathé, J. L. Andersson, B. G. Nomikos, B. E. Hildebrand, and M. Marcus, "Mode of action of atypical neuroleptics in relation to the phencyclidine model of schizophrenia: role of 5-HT2 receptor and α1-adrenoreceptor antagonism," *Journal of Clinical Psychopharmacology*, vol. 15, pp. 11S–18S, 1995.

[80] W. Birkmayer and P. Riederer, "Responsibility of extrastriatal areas for the appearance of psychotic symptoms (Clinical and biochemical human post-mortem findings)," *Journal of Neural Transmission*, vol. 37, no. 2, pp. 175–182, 1975.

[81] K. Jellinger, "Neuropathological substrates of Alzheimer's disease and Parkinson's disease.," *Journal of Neural Transmission, Supplement*, vol. 24, pp. 109–129, 1987.

[82] P. J. Whitehouse, J. C. Hedreen, C. L. White, and D. L. Price, "Basal forebrain neurons in the dementia of Parkinson disease," *Annals of Neurology*, vol. 13, no. 3, pp. 243–248, 1983.

[83] E. K. Perry, E. Marshall, J. Kerwin et al., "Evidence of a Mono-aminergic-Cholinergic Imbalance Related to Visual Hallucinations in Lewy Body Dementia," *Journal of Neurochemistry*, vol. 55, no. 4, pp. 1454–1456, 1990.

[84] E. K. Perry, I. McKeith, P. Thompson et al., "Topography, extent, and clinical relevance of neurochemical deficits in dementia of Lewy body type, Parkinson's disease, and Alzheimer's disease," *Annals of the New York Academy of Sciences*, vol. 640, pp. 197–202, 1991.

[85] C. G. Goetz, P. F. Burke, S. Leurgans et al., "Genetic variation analysis in Parkinson disease patients with and without hallucinations: Case-control study," *Archives of Neurology*, vol. 58, no. 2, pp. 209–213, 2001.

[86] A. J. Makoff, J. M. Graham, M. J. Arranz et al., "Association study of dopamine receptor gene polymorphisms with drug-induced hallucinations in patients with idiopathic Parkinson's disease," *Pharmacogenetics*, vol. 10, no. 1, pp. 43–48, 2000.

[87] J. Wang, C. Zhao, B. Chen, and Z.-L. Liu, "Polymorphisms of dopamine receptor and transporter genes and hallucinations in Parkinson's disease," *Neuroscience Letters*, vol. 355, no. 3, pp. 193–196, 2004.

[88] M. J. Frank, L. C. Seeberger, and R. C. O'Reilly, "By carrot or by stick: cognitive reinforcement learning in Parkinsonism," *Science*, vol. 306, no. 5703, pp. 1940–1943, 2004.

[89] D. G. Harden and A. A. Grace, "Activation of dopamine cell firing by repeated L-DOPA administration to dopamine-depleted rats: Its potential role in mediating the therapeutic response to L-DOPA treatment," *Journal of Neuroscience*, vol. 15, no. 9, pp. 6157–6166, 1995.

[90] H. L. Klawans Jr., "The pharmacology of extrapyramidal movement disorders," *Monographs in Neural Sciences*, vol. 2, pp. 1–136, 1973.

[91] R. Betarbet and J. T. Greenamyre, "Regulation of dopamine receptor and neuropeptide expression in the basal ganglia of monkeys treated with MPTP," *Experimental Neurology*, vol. 189, no. 2, pp. 393–403, 2004.

[92] J. O. Rinne, A. Laihinen, A. Ruottinen et al., "Increased density of dopamine D2 receptors in the putamen, but not in the caudate nucleus in early Parkinson's disease: a PET study with [11C]raclopride," *Journal of the Neurological Sciences*, vol. 132, no. 2, pp. 156–161, 1995.

[93] L. Rioux, P. A. Frohna, J. N. Joyce, and J. S. Schneider, "The effects of chronic levodopa treatment on pre- and postsynaptic markers of dopaminergic function in striatum of Parkinsonian monkeys," *Movement Disorders*, vol. 12, no. 2, pp. 148–158, 1997.

[94] O. D. Howes and S. Kapur, "The dopamine hypothesis of schizophrenia: version III—the final common pathway," *Schizophrenia Bulletin*, vol. 35, no. 3, pp. 549–562, 2009.

[95] C. R. Housden, S. S. O'Sullivan, E. M. Joyce, A. J. Lees, and J. P. Roiser, "Intact reward learning but elevated delay discounting in Parkinson's disease patients with impulsive-compulsive spectrum behaviors," *Neuropsychopharmacology*, vol. 35, no. 11, pp. 2155–2164, 2010.

[96] H. Nagy, E. Levy-Gigi, Z. Somlai, A. Takáts, D. Bereczki, and S. Kéri, "The effect of dopamine agonists on adaptive and aberrant salience in Parkinson's disease," *Neuropsychopharmacology*, vol. 37, no. 4, pp. 950–958, 2012.

[97] C. G. Goetz, E. J. Pappert, L. M. Blasucci et al., "Intravenous levodopa in hallucinating Parkinson's disease patients: high-dose challenge does not precipitate hallucinations," *Neurology*, vol. 50, no. 2, pp. 515–517, 1998.

[98] A. Lenka, S. Hegde, S. S. Arumugham, and P. K. Pal, "Pattern of cognitive impairment in patients with Parkinson's disease and psychosis: a critical review," *Parkinsonism and Related Disorders*, vol. 37, pp. 11–18, 2017.

[99] S. A. Factor, W. M. McDonald, and F. C. Goldstein, "The role of neurotransmitters in the development of Parkinson's disease-related psychosis," *European Journal of Neurology*.

[100] A. Lenka, K. R. Jhunjhunwala, J. Saini, and P. K. Pal, "Structural and functional neuroimaging in patients with Parkinson's disease and visual hallucinations: A critical review," *Parkinsonism and Related Disorders*, vol. 21, no. 7, pp. 683–691, 2015.

[101] A. M. Meppelink, B. M. de Jong, L. K. Teune, and T. van Laar, "Regional cortical grey matter loss in Parkinson's disease without dementia is independent from visual hallucinations," *Movement Disorders*, vol. 26, no. 1, pp. 142–147, 2011.

[102] A. A. Kehagia, R. A. Barker, and T. W. Robbins, "Neuropsychological and clinical heterogeneity of cognitive impairment and dementia in patients with Parkinson's disease," *The Lancet Neurology*, vol. 9, no. 12, pp. 1200–1213, 2010.

[103] E. K. Perry and R. H. Perry, "Acetylcholine and Hallucinations - Disease-Related Compared to Drug-Induced Alterations in Human Consciousness," *Brain and Cognition*, vol. 28, no. 3, pp. 240–258, 1995.

[104] E. K. Perry, D. Irving, J. M. Kerwin et al., "Cholinergic transmitter and neurotrophic activities in lewy body dementia: similarity to parkinson's and distinction from alzheimer disease," *Alzheimer Disease and Associated Disorders*, vol. 7, no. 2, pp. 69–79, 1993.

[105] I. McKeith, T. del Ser, P. Spano et al., "Efficacy of rivastigmine in dementia with Lewy bodies: a randomised, double-blind, placebo-controlled international study," *The Lancet*, vol. 356, no. 9247, pp. 2031–2036, 2000.

[106] M. Emre, D. Aarsland, A. Albanese et al., "Rivastigmine for dementia associated with Parkinson's disease," *The New England Journal of Medicine*, vol. 351, no. 24, pp. 2509–2518, 2004.

[107] N. Stefanis, M. Bozi, C. Christodoulou et al., "Isolated delusional syndrome in Parkinson's Disease," *Parkinsonism and Related Disorders*, vol. 16, no. 8, pp. 550–552, 2010.

[108] S. A. Factor, M. K. Scullin, A. B. Sollinger et al., "Cognitive correlates of hallucinations and delusions in Parkinson's disease," *Journal of the Neurological Sciences*, vol. 347, no. 1-2, pp. 316–321, 2014.

[109] A. J. Atkinson Jr., W. A. Colburn, V. G. DeGruttola et al., "Biomarkers and surrogate endpoints: preferred definitions and conceptual framework," *Clinical Pharmacology and Therapeutics*, vol. 69, no. 3, pp. 89–95, 2001.

[110] M. Gerlach, W. Maetzler, K. Broich et al., "Biomarker candidates of neurodegeneration in Parkinson's disease for the evaluation of disease-modifying therapeutics," *Journal of Neural Transmission*, vol. 119, no. 1, pp. 39–52, 2012.

[111] K. Marek, D. Jennings, S. Lasch et al., "The parkinson progression marker initiative (PPMI)," *Progress in Neurobiology*, vol. 25, no. 4, pp. 629–635, 2011.

[112] R. E. Skogseth, K. Bronnick, J. B. Pereira et al., "Associations between cerebrospinal fluid biomarkers and cognition in early Untreated Parkinson's Disease," *Journal of Parkinson's Disease*, vol. 5, no. 4, pp. 783–792, 2015.

[113] A. L. Stav, D. Aarsland, K. K. Johansen, E. Hessen, E. Auning, and T. Fladby, "Amyloid-β and α-synuclein cerebrospinal fluid biomarkers and cognition in early Parkinson's disease," *Parkinsonism and Related Disorders*, vol. 21, no. 7, pp. 758–764, 2015.

[114] C.-H. Lin and R.-M. Wu, "Biomarkers of cognitive decline in Parkinson's disease," *Parkinsonism & Related Disorders*, vol. 21, no. 5, pp. 431–443, 2015.

[115] C. D. Jeffries, D. O. Perkins, S. D. Chandler et al., "Insights into psychosis risk from leukocyte microRNA expression," *Translational Psychiatry*, vol. 6, no. 12, p. e981, 2016.

[116] C.-Y. Lai, S.-L. Yu, and M. H. Hsieh, "MicroRNA expression aberration as potential peripheral blood biomarkers for Schizophrenia," *PLoS ONE*, vol. 6, no. 6, Article ID e21635, 2011.

[117] E. Via, C. Orfila, C. Pedreño et al., "Structural alterations of the pyramidal pathway in schizoid and schizotypal cluster A personality disorders," *International Journal of Psychophysiology*, vol. 110, pp. 163–170, 2016.

[118] M.-S. Koo, C. C. Dickey, H.-J. Park et al., "Smaller neocortical gray matter and larger sulcal cerebrospinal fluid volumes in neuroleptic-naive women with schizotypal personality disorder," *Archives of General Psychiatry*, vol. 63, no. 10, pp. 1090–1100, 2006.

[119] J. Taylor, W. S. Anderson, J. Brandt, Z. Mari, and G. M. Pontone, "Neuropsychiatric complications of parkinson disease treatments: importance of multidisciplinary care," *American Journal of Geriatric Psychiatry*, vol. 24, no. 12, pp. 1171–1180, 2016.

[120] P. D. McGorry, "Psychoeducation in first-episode psychosis: a therapeutic process," *Psychiatry (New York)*, vol. 58, no. 4, pp. 313–328, 1995.

[121] C. Pacchetti, F. Mancini, R. Aglieri, C. Fundaró, E. Martignoni, and G. Nappi, "Active music therapy in Parkinson's disease: an integrative method for motor and emotional rehabilitation," *Psychosomatic Medicine*, vol. 62, no. 3, pp. 386–393, 2000.

[122] K. Seppi, D. Weintraub, M. Coelho et al., "The movement disorder society evidence-based medicine review update: treatments for the non-motor symptoms of Parkinson's disease," *Movement Disorders*, vol. 26, no. 3, pp. S42–S80, 2011.

[123] B. S. Connolly and A. E. Lang, "Pharmacological treatment of Parkinson disease: a review," *Journal of the American Medical Association*, vol. 311, no. 16, pp. 1670–1683, 2014.

[124] S. Grover, M. Somaiya, S. Kumar, and A. Avasthi, "Psychiatric aspects of Parkinson's disease," *Journal of Neurosciences in Rural Practice*, vol. 6, no. 1, pp. 65–76, 2015.

[125] S. Chen, P. Chan, S. Sun et al., "The recommendations of Chinese Parkinson's disease and movement disorder society consensus on therapeutic management of Parkinson's disease," *Translational Neurodegeneration*, vol. 5, no. 1, p. 12, 2016.

[126] S. A. Factor, J. H. Friedman, M. C. Lannon, D. Oakes, and K. Bourgeois, "Clozapine for the treatment of drug-induced psychosis in Parkinson's disease: results of the 12 week open label extension in the PSYCLOPS trial," *Movement Disorders*, vol. 16, no. 1, pp. 135–139, 2001.

[127] P. Pollak, F. Tison, O. Rascol et al., "Clozapine in drug induced psychosis in Parkinson's disease: a randomised, placebo controlled study with open follow up," *Journal of Neurology, Neurosurgery and Psychiatry*, vol. 75, no. 5, pp. 689–695, 2004.

[128] D. Weintraub, C. Chiang, H. M. Kim et al., "Association of antipsychotic use with mortality risk in patients with Parkinson disease," *JAMA Neurology*, vol. 73, no. 5, pp. 535–541, 2016.

[129] J. L. Goren and G. M. Levin, "Quetiapine, an atypical antipsychotic," *Pharmacotherapy*, vol. 18, no. 6 I, pp. 1183–1194, 1998.

[130] L. Morgante, A. Epifanio, E. Spina et al., "Quetiapine and clozapine in parkinsonian patients with dopaminergic psychosis," *Clinical Neuropharmacology*, vol. 27, no. 4, pp. 153–156, 2004.

[131] D. Merims, M. Balas, C. Peretz, H. Shabtai, and N. Giladi, "Rater-blinded, prospective comparison: quetiapine versus clozapine for parkinson's disease psychosis," *Clinical Neuropharmacology*, vol. 29, no. 6, pp. 331–337, 2006.

[132] W. G. Ondo, R. Tintner, K. D. Voung, D. Lai, and G. Ringholz, "Double-blind, placebo-controlled, unforced titration parallel trial of quetiapine for dopaminergic-induced hallucinations in Parkinson's disease," *Movement Disorders*, vol. 20, no. 8, pp. 958–963, 2005.

[133] J. M. Rabey, T. Prokhorov, A. Miniovitz, E. Dobronevsky, and C. Klein, "Effect of quetiapine in psychotic Parkinson's disease patients: a double-blind labeled study of 3 months' duration," *Movement Disorders*, vol. 22, no. 3, pp. 313–318, 2007.

[134] P. Shotbolt, M. Samuel, C. Fox, and A. S. David, "A randomized controlled trial of quetiapine for psychosis in Parkinson's disease," *Neuropsychiatric Disease and Treatment*, vol. 5, no. 1, pp. 327–332, 2009.

[135] A. Breier, V. K. Sutton, P. D. Feldman et al., "Olanzapine in the treatment of dopamimetic-induced psychosis in patients with

Parkinson's disease," *Biological Psychiatry*, vol. 52, no. 5, pp. 438–445, 2002.

[136] W. G. Ondo, J. K. Levy, K. D. Vuong, C. Hunter, and J. Jankovic, "Olanzapine treatment for dopaminergic-induced hallucinations," *Movement Disorders*, vol. 17, no. 5, pp. 1031–1035, 2002.

[137] H. Calderón-Fajardo, A. Cervantes-Arriaga, R. Llorens-Arenas, J. Ramírez-Bermudez, Á. Ruiz-Chow, and M. Rodríguez-Violante, "Electroconvulsive therapy in Parkinson's disease," *Arquivos de Neuro-Psiquiatria*, vol. 73, no. 10, pp. 856–860, 2015.

[138] G. Meco, A. Alessandri, P. Giustini, and V. Bonifati, "Risperidone in levodopa-induced psychosis in advanced Parkinson's disease: an open-label, long-term study," *Movement Disorders*, vol. 12, no. 4, pp. 610–612, 1997.

[139] L. Pintor, F. Valldeoriola, E. Baillés, M. J. Martí, A. Muñiz, and E. Tolosa, "Ziprasidone versus clozapine in the treatment of psychotic symptoms in Parkinson disease: a randomized open clinical trial," *Clinical Neuropharmacology*, vol. 35, no. 2, pp. 61–66, 2012.

[140] J. H. Friedman, "Melperone is ineffective in treating Parkinson's disease psychosis," *Movement Disorders*, vol. 27, no. 6, pp. 803-804, 2012.

[141] K. E. Vanover, D. M. Weiner, M. Makhay et al., "Pharmacological and behavioral profile of N-(4-fluorophenylmethyl)-N-(1-methylpiperidin-4-yl)-N/-(4-(2- methylpropyloxy)phenylmethyl) carbamide (2R,3R)-dihydroxybutanedioate (2:1) (ACP-103), a novel 5-hydroxytryptamine2A receptor inverse agonist," *Journal of Pharmacology and Experimental Therapeutics*, vol. 317, no. 2, pp. 910–918, 2006.

[142] N. S. Hunter, K. C. Anderson, and A. Cox, "Pimavanserin," *Drugs of Today*, vol. 51, no. 11, pp. 646–652, 2015.

[143] A. Abbas and B. L. Roth, "Pimavanserin tartrate: A 5-HT2A inverse agonist with potential for treating various neuropsychiatric disorders," *Expert Opinion on Pharmacotherapy*, vol. 9, no. 18, pp. 3251–3259, 2008.

[144] J. Cummings, S. Isaacson, R. Mills et al., "Pimavanserin for patients with Parkinson's disease psychosis: a randomised, placebo-controlled phase 3 trial," *The Lancet*, vol. 383, no. 9916, pp. 533–540, 2014.

[145] H. Y. Meltzer, R. Mills, S. Revell et al., "Pimavanserin, a serotonin 2A receptor inverse agonist, for the treatment of Parkinson's disease psychosis," *Neuropsychopharmacology*, vol. 35, no. 4, pp. 881–892, 2010.

[146] I. Leroi, J. Brandt, S. G. Reich et al., "Randomized placebo-controlled trial of donepezil in cognitive impairment in Parkinson's disease," *International Journal of Geriatric Psychiatry*, vol. 19, no. 1, pp. 1–8, 2004.

[147] K. Szigeti and M. U. Hafeez, "Exploring the role of donepezil in Dementia with Lewy Bodies," *Drugs of Today*, vol. 51, no. 10, pp. 579–590, 2015.

[148] J. Cummings, T.-J. Lai, S. Hemrungrojn et al., "Role of Donepezil in the Management of Neuropsychiatric Symptoms in Alzheimer's Disease and Dementia with Lewy Bodies," *CNS Neuroscience and Therapeutics*, vol. 22, no. 3, pp. 159–166, 2016.

[149] H. Sawada and T. Oeda, "Protocol for a randomised controlled trial: Efficacy of donepezil against psychosis in Parkinson's disease (EDAP)," *BMJ Open*, vol. 3, no. 9, Article ID e003533, 2013.

[150] D. Popeo and C. H. Kellner, "ECT for Parkinson's disease," *Medical Hypotheses*, vol. 73, no. 4, pp. 468-469, 2009.

[151] R. Kennedy, D. Mittal, and J. O'Jile, "Electroconvulsive Therapy in Movement Disorders: An Update," *Journal of Neuropsychiatry and Clinical Neurosciences*, vol. 15, no. 4, pp. 407–421, 2003.

[152] P. Baldinger, A. Lotan, R. Frey, S. Kasper, B. Lerer, and R. Lanzenberger, "Neurotransmitters and electroconvulsive therapy," *Journal of ECT*, vol. 30, no. 2, pp. 116–121, 2014.

[153] L. M. McCormick, L. L. Boles Ponto, R. K. Pierson, H. J. Johnson, V. Magnotta, and M. C. Brumm, "Metabolic correlates of antidepressant and antipsychotic response in patients with psychotic depression undergoing electroconvulsive therapy," *Journal of ECT*, vol. 23, no. 4, pp. 265–273, 2007.

[154] F. Vila-Rodriguez, A. McGirr, J. Tham, G. Hadjipavlou, and C. R. Honey, "Electroconvulsive therapy in patients with deep brain stimulators," *Journal of ECT*, vol. 30, no. 3, pp. e16–e18, 2014.

[155] S. Piccoli, G. Perini, S. Pizzighello et al., "A long term effects of a new onset psychosis after DBS treated with Quetiapine in a patient with Parkinson's disease," *Psychiatry Investigation*, vol. 12, no. 1, pp. 146–149, 2015.

[156] A. A. Qureshi, J. J. Cheng, A. N. Sunshine et al., "Postoperative symptoms of psychosis after deep brain stimulation in patients with Parkinson's disease," *Neurosurgical Focus*, vol. 38, no. 6, article no. E5, 2015.

[157] P. Alonso, D. Cuadras, L. Gabriëls et al., "Deep brain stimulation for obsessive-compulsive disorder: a meta-analysis of treatment outcome and predictors of response," *PLoS ONE*, vol. 10, no. 7, Article ID e0133591, 2015.

11

Event-Related Potentials in Parkinson's Disease Patients with Visual Hallucination

Yang-Pei Chang,[1] Yuan-Han Yang,[1,2] Chiou-Lian Lai,[2,3] and Li-Min Liou[2,3]

[1]*Department of Neurology, Kaohsiung Municipal Ta-Tung Hospital, Kaohsiung Medical University, Kaohsiung, Taiwan*
[2]*Department of Neurology, Faculty of Medicine, College of Medicine, Kaohsiung Medical University, Kaohsiung, Taiwan*
[3]*Department of Neurology, Kaohsiung Medical University Hospital, Kaohsiung, Taiwan*

Correspondence should be addressed to Chiou-Lian Lai; cllai@kmu.edu.tw

Academic Editor: Jan Aasly

Using neuropsychological investigation and visual event-related potentials (ERPs), we aimed to compare the ERPs and cognitive function of nondemented Parkinson's disease (PD) patients with and without visual hallucinations (VHs) and of control subjects. We recruited 12 PD patients with VHs (PD-H), 23 PD patients without VHs (PD-NH), and 18 age-matched controls. All subjects underwent comprehensive neuropsychological assessment and visual ERPs measurement. A visual odd-ball paradigm with two different fixed interstimulus intervals (ISI) (1600 ms and 5000 ms) elicited visual ERPs. The frontal test battery was used to assess attention, visual-spatial function, verbal fluency, memory, higher executive function, and motor programming. The PD-H patients had significant cognitive dysfunction in several domains, compared to the PD-NH patients and controls. The mean P3 latency with ISI of 1600 ms in PD-H patients was significantly longer than that in controls. Logistic regression disclosed UPDRS-on score and P3 latency as significant predictors of VH. Our findings suggest that nondemented PD-H patients have worse cognitive function and P3 measurements. The development of VHs in nondemented PD patients might be implicated in executive dysfunction with altered visual information processing.

1. Introduction

Visual hallucinations (VHs) and cognitive impairment, which are nonmotor symptoms of Parkinson's disease (PD), have been an intriguing issue in recent years [1]. It is crucial to screen mild cognitive impairment and dementia in PD patients because dementia may cause nursing home placement, increased burden for health care and caregiver, and higher mortality [2]. In the mid-stage of PD, VHs act as a clinical predictor of dementia [3, 4] and correlate with disease progression and decline in Mini-Mental State Examination (MMSE) scores [5, 6]. Recent hypotheses suggest that the development of VHs in PD may result from an imbalance of external and internal inputs and impaired reality monitoring, while cognitive impairment may play a role in reality monitoring [7, 8]. Cognitive correlation of VHs in PD patients is evident [9–12]. A one-year neuropsychological follow-up study reported that nondemented PD patients with VHs have faster decline of complex visual function and multiple cognitive domains than patients without VHs [13]. Previous studies have also reported worse attention and visuospatial function in PD patients with VHs [14, 15]. However, another 4-year longitudinal observatory study showed that VHs may be more associated with longer disease duration, increased functional impairment, and premorbid psychiatry illness rather than cognitive impairment [16]. Accumulating evidence has demonstrated that cognitive dysfunction may contribute to the occurrence of VH symptoms of PD patients in nondemented PD patients with VHs regardless of the side effect of dopaminergic medication [17, 18]. Indeed, recent study using functional MRI technique suggests desynchronization between aberrant frontal circuit and posterior cortical areas during active visual hallucinations [19].

Event-related potential (ERP) is a developed sensitive and noninvasive tool to detect cognitive dysfunction in patients with mild cognitive impairment and dementia [20–22]. Early components of ERP (N1 and P2) are considered exogenous sensory components that have been associated with attention and sensory processing. The N2 component reflects an early detection of cognitive ability, such as target discrimination. P3 is a positive shift when a subject detects an informative task-relevant stimulus [23, 24]. While some studies have supported the correlation between ERP abnormality and cognitive impairment in PD patients with dementia, the role of ERP in nondemented PD patients is not confirmed [25–31]. One study found visual cognitive impairment and prolonged visual P3 latency especially in patients with PD dementia with hallucinations [32].

Since ERP may be a sensitive tool in the detection of cognitive impairment in PD in the absence of clinical dementia and VH is a potentially premonitory symptom of dementia in PD patients, it may be interesting to explore the ERP abnormality in nondemented PD patient with VHs. In the literature, few studies focused on the topic. We aim to assess the visual ERP and neuropsychological assessments in nondemented PD patients with (PD-H) and without VH (PD-NH) and healthy controls and find the linkage.

2. Materials and Methods

2.1. Participants. This study was conducted at the Kaohsiung Medical University Hospital (KMUH), a tertiary referral center in Southern Taiwan. The KMUH institution review board approved all procedures and written informed consent was obtained from study participants. The control subjects were recruited from volunteer in nearby community college. All PD participants had a presumptive clinical diagnosis of PD according to UKPD Brain Bank criteria. Individuals were inquired carefully and were assigned to groups according to whether they had experienced VHs in the past one year. No patient in the population sampled had a clinical diagnosis of either Alzheimer's disease or Lewy body dementia. Patients were excluded if Mini-Mental State Examination (MMSE) is less than 25. Patients with eye disease or migraine or other conditions like concurrent stroke, delirium, delusions, multiple sclerosis, and psychiatric illness or those under neuroleptics treatment were all excluded. Duration of illness and medication were recorded and stage of illness was scored according to the Hoehn and Yahr scale and United Parkinson's Disease Rating Scale (UPDRS) during "on" state. PD patients take neuropsychological assessment and event-related potential during "on" state after regular oral medications.

2.2. Neuropsychological Assessment. The neuropsychological assessment focusing on frontal lobe function [21] includes Mini-Mental State Examination (MMSE), Digit Span (Wechsler Adult Intelligence Scale-Revision (WAIS-R)), Digit Symbol (WAIS-R), Stroop Test, and Trail Making Tests (parts A and B) to assess attention and concentration; Block Design (WAIS-R) and Rey-Osterrieth Complex Figure Test-Copy to evaluate visuoconstructional ability; word list generation (Controlled Oral Word Association; Category Fluency Test) to assess semantic verbal fluency; word list learning-recall and Rey-Osterrieth Complex Figure Test-Recall to evaluate memory; Wisconsin Card Sorting Test-Modified (WCST),

Design Fluency (Five-Point Test), and Similarity (WAIS-R) to assess higher executive function; Luria's Hand Sequence to evaluate motor programming function.

2.3. Event-Related Potentials Measurements. A visual "oddball" stimulus paradigm (NeuroStim, NeuroScan, Inc.) was used to elicit visual event-related potentials, and an electroencephalograph (EEG) was recorded using Ag/AgCl electrodes placed at 5 scalp locations (FPz, Fz, Cz, Pz, and Oz), based on the 10–20 system. All were referenced to linked earlobes. The electrode impedance was kept below 5 kΩ. The EEG was amplified (band pass, 0.01–40 Hz) by a SynAmps amplifier (NeuroScan, Inc.), and continuous EEG records were kept for further offline analysis at a sampling rate of 256 Hz. The averaging epoch was 1024 ms, including 200 ms of prestimulus baseline [21, 22].

The subjects sat in a comfortable chair in a sound-attenuated room with dim lighting 100 cm in front of a 19-inch LCD computer screen. Stimuli were presented in the central of the screen. The stimuli consisted of two neutral pictures from the NeuroScan template on a dark ground. The participants were asked to centrally fixate throughout the recording. We adopted a visual odd-ball task, with a target stimulus and a nontarget stimulus. Mistrials including eyeball movement artifacts were excluded from the offline analysis.

Stimuli were presented randomly with the probability of 20% target stimulus and 80% nontarget stimuli. In each block a total of 250 stimuli (50 targets, 200 nontargets) were presented for 100 ms and interstimulus interval (ISI) of 1600 ms and 5000 ms. The experiment consisted of 4 blocks (2 blocks with ISI of 1600 ms and 2 blocks with ISI of 5000 ms). Participants performed a brief training session to ensure they were able to detect the target accurately. During the examination, participants were asked to press the button as quickly as possible when they saw the target. Reaction time was measured relative to target onset for correct trials, while accuracy was measured as the percentage of correct responses out of all responses to the target stimulus. Individual trials with eye blink artifacts (more than 250 μV of peak-to-peak amplitude), target trials for which the reaction time (RT) was more than 1.4 s, and nontarget trials with a response were all excluded from the averaging. Separate ERP averages were made for each trial type. For amplitudes analysis, the mean potential during the 200 ms period preceding the stimulus onset served as baseline. The N1, P2, N2, and P3 components at Pz recording were assessed for highest amplitude distribution. The latencies windows were N1 component as the maximum negativity between 75 and 160 ms, P2 component as the maximum positivity between 170 and 260 ms, N2 component as the maximum negativity between 190 and 360 ms, and P3 component as the maximum positivity between 250 and 500 ms.

2.4. Statistics. We performed statistical analysis with SPSS 12.0 package, and $p < 0.05$ was set to be statistically significant. We used two-tailed t-test for analyzing continuous data of disease characteristic of PD patients. We used analysis of

TABLE 1: Characteristics in PD-H, PD-NH, and controls.

	PD-H $n = 12$	PD-NH $n = 23$	Controls $n = 18$	p
Age[1], years	67.79 ± 7.93	66.36 ± 9.68	68.29 ± 6.83	0.753
Women[1], n (%)	5 (36)	7 (28)	10 (59)	0.107
Education[1], y	9.27 ± 6.65	10.88 ± 4.16	12.16 ± 3.32	0.245
Disease duration[2], y	**11.73 ± 6.41**	6.20 ± 4.86	n/a	**0.007**
Duration of levodopa[2], y	**8.44 ± 5.78**	3.04 ± 3.57	n/a	**0.004**
H&Y[2]	**2.65 ± 0.89**	1.52 ± 0.65	n/a	**<0.001**
MMSE[1] (score)	27.73 ± 2.20	27.58 ± 1.36	28.41 ± 1.37	0.472
HDI[1] (score)	**5.00 ± 4.67**	**4.125 ± 4.11**[*]	0.25 ± 0.79	**<0.001**
UPDRS-III motor[2] (score)	**27.92 ± 13.00**	14.20 ± 8.42	n/a	**<0.001**
Levodopa-equivalent dose	863.8 ± 390.6	311.2 ± 160.5	n/a	0.08

PD-H: PD patients with visual hallucinations; PD-NH: PD patients without visual hallucinations; H&Y: Hoehn and Yahr stage; HDI: Hamilton depression index; UPDRS: Unified Parkinson's Disease Rating Scale; n/a: not available.
p: p value, $p < 0.05$; by [1]ANOVA [2]t-test.

covariate (ANCOVA) to determine the differences of neuropsychological test between groups after adjusting disease duration, duration of levodopa use, Hoehn and Yahr stage, Hamilton depression index, and the scores of UPDRS-III. For P3 latency and amplitude, we used ANCOVA to determine the significant difference after adjusting age, gender, disease duration, duration of levodopa use, and Hoehn and Yahr stage with Tukey method used for post hoc analysis. One-way repeated measures analysis of variance (ANOVA) was used to explore the effect of ISI on P3 latency and amplitude. Pearson correlation coefficient was calculated to explore the relationship between neuropsychological function and N1, P2, N2, and P3 latency and amplitude at Pz recording. ERP components at Fz and Cz recordings were not analyzed because of artifacts. For our intent in analyzing the predictive risk factors of VH, logistic regression with the existence or absence of VHs as dependent variable was performed in four different models with different confounding factors. To clarify the role of UPDRS-on score in the development of VH, we adjusted age and gender in model 1, while we adjusted age, gender, and three cognitive domains in model 3. To further observe the role of P3 latency in the development of VH, age and gender and UPDRS-on score were adjusted in model 2, while age and gender, UPDRS-on score, and three cognitive domains were adjusted in model 4. The chosen cognitive domains (Trail Making Tests, R-O copy, or Luria Hand Sequence) were significantly different between PD-H and PD-NH patients. According to WAIS-III Chinese version, the cut-off values of three cognitive domains were chosen and were transformed to dichotomy dummy variable for logistic regression.

3. Results

3.1. Demographic Data. Twelve PD-H patients, twenty-three PD-NH patients, and eighteen healthy control subjects were recruited in this study (Table 1). The mean age, education level, and MMSE did not differ significantly between these three groups, while there were significant differences between

the PD patients with and without visual hallucinations with regard to disease duration, duration of levodopa use, Hoehn and Yahr stage, and the scores of UPDRS-III. We also found significant difference in Hamilton depression index in PD-H or PD-NH patients when comparing with normal controls.

3.2. Neuropsychological Assessment. The data of neuropsychological investigations in all participants are shown in Table 2. There were multiple domains of frontal dysfunction in PD patients, especially in PD-H patients. The PD-H patients performed significantly worse than normal controls at Trail Making Test, R-O copy, Wisconsin Card Sorting Test, and Luria Hand Sequence. Moreover, when comparing PD-H patients to PD-NH patients, significantly lower scores were found in the former group at Trail Making Test, R-O copy, Wisconsin Card Sorting Test, and Luria's Hand Sequence. When comparing to normal controls, PD-NH patients performed significantly worse in Wisconsin Card Sorting Test.

3.3. Visual ERP Data. For the highest amplitude distribution, the N1, P2, N2, and P3 components with two different ISI at Pz are outlined in Table 3. There was no significant difference between PD-H patients, PD-NH patients, and controls, regardless of different ISI (1600 ms and 5000 ms). However, the mean latency of P3 with ISI of 1600 ms in PD-H patients revealed significant prolongation when comparing with that in controls. The mean reaction time and error rate of PD-H patients, PD-NH patients, and controls revealed no significant difference.

We also assessed the effect of ISI on P3 latencies, P3 amplitude, and reaction time at Pz (Table 3) using one-way repeated measure ANOVA in PD-H patients, PD-NH patients, and controls. P3 latency was significantly prolonged at 5000 ms ISI compared to 1600 ms ISI in PD-NH patients and control (control, $F = 19.289$, $p = 0.003$; PD-NH, $F = 5.391$, $p = 0.04$), while PD-H patients did not show significant difference ($F = 0.025$, $p = 0.879$). P3 amplitude showed unremarkable difference in three groups

TABLE 2: Comparison of frontal test battery in PD patients and controls.

Demographic data mean ± SD	PD-H $n = 12$	PD-NH $n = 23$	Controls $n = 18$	p
Attention				
Stroop Test (errors)	7.92 ± 9.09	7.33 ± 8.45	3.41 ± 5.19	0.151
TMT-A (s)	**122.21 ± 87.47**[ab]	70.84 ± 41.47	52.76 ± 30.27	**0.018**
TMT-B (s)	241.21 ± 121.73	134.00 ± 106.8	124.76 ± 84.81	0.264
Digit Span	15.64 ± 4.24	15.88 ± 2.76	17.27 ± 4.54	0.198
Visual-constructional ability				
Block Design (score)	7.21 ± 4.16	12.08 ± 4.05	11.50 ± 3.78	0.255
R–O-copy (score)	**25.93 ± 10.17**[ab]	32.08 ± 6.55	33.47 ± 1.91	**<0.001**
Verbal fluency				
Word list generation	41.00 ± 14.81	44.21 ± 11.29	46.47 ± 8.68	0.122
Memory				
Wordlist learning recall (number)	17.21 ± 3.66	19.19 ± 3.76	22.29 ± 1.45	0.301
R–O-recall (score)	7.71 ± 6.76	11.96 ± 9.19	13.00 ± 8.32	0.549
Higher executive function				
Similarities (score)	9.29 ± 6.08	10.12 ± 7.11	13.53 ± 4.58	0.760
Five-Point Test (correct number)	2.79 ± 2.46	4.57 ± 2.92	5.35 ± 2.52	0.485
WCST-category (number)	5.21 ± 2.12	6.00 ± 1.71	6.24 ± 2.31	0.697
WCST-PN/total errors (%)	**63.00 ± 32.91**[b]	**72.80 ± 31.40**[c]	25.29 ± 20.95	**0.027**
Motor programming				
Luria's Hand Sequence (score)	**1.29 ± 1.07**[ab]	2.23 ± 1.14	2.12 ± 0.68	**0.019**

PD-H: PD patients with visual hallucinations; PD-NH: PD patients without visual hallucinations; TMT: Trail Making Test; R–O Complex Figure Test: Rey-Osterrieth Complex Figure Test; WCST: Wisconsin Card Sorting Test.
p: p value, by one-way analysis of covariance (ANCOVA) with age, gender, and education as covariates.
Post hoc analysis with Tukey method ([a]PD-H versus PD-NH, [b]PD-H versus controls, and [c]PD-NH versus controls).

when comparing 1600 ms ISI to 5000 ms ISI (PD-H, $F = 0.324$, $p = 0.585$; PD-NH, $F = 2.987$, $p = 0.112$; control, $F = 1.031$, $p = 0.344$). Reaction time was significantly prolonged at 5000 ms ISI compared to 1600 ms ISI in PD-NH and PD-H patients (PD-NH, $F = 0.359$, $p < 0.001$; PD-H, $F = 13.059$, $p = 0.005$), while there was no significant difference in controls ($F = 2.831$, $p = 0.111$).

3.4. The Correlations of Frontal Function and ERPs in PD-H Patients. The domains of frontal function in PD-H patients were analyzed for their correlation with measures of N1, P2, N2, and P3 at Pz lead. Pearson's r values of correlation between P3 latency, P3 amplitude, and neuropsychological scores are shown in supplementary Table 1 (in Supplementary Material available online at http://dx.doi.org/10.1155/2016/1863508). For higher executive function (Similarities, Wisconsin Card Sorting Test), attention (Trail Making Test-type B, Digit Span), visuo-constructional ability (Digit Span, Rey-Osterrieth Complex Figure copy test), verbal fluency (word list generation), and memory (Rey-Osterrieth Complex Figure recall test), there were significant correlations for P3. However, other earlier components of N1, P2, and N2 correlations with cognitive measures were not significantly evident (data not shown).

Supplementary Table 2 summarizes the odds ratio of binary logistic regression for UPDRS-on score and P3 latency

in different models. Overall, the results showed that increase of UPDRS-on scores in PD patients was associated with significantly increased risk of VH in four different models. After adjusting age, gender, and UPDRS-on scores, model 2 disclosed that one millisecond increase of P3 latency in PD patients was in line with 6% ($p = 0.046$) higher risk of having VH. By contrast, model 3 showed that there was nonsignificant trend where poor performance of Trail Making Tests, R-O copy, or Luria Hand Sequence was more likely to have VH.

4. Discussion

Our study showed that nondemented PD patients with VHs had worse cognitive function than those without VHs and age-matched controls. In addition to UPDRS scores, the latency of visual P3 was associated with VH after statistically adjusting the possible confounding factors and also correlated with cognitive impairment in PD patients. In accordance with previous studies using neuropsychological assessment or functional MRI [15–18, 33, 34], our finding suggests that frontal dysfunction may play a role in the development of VH in nondemented PD patients.

The term of P300 is composed of mainly two distinct subcomponents, P3a and P3b. Although the precise functional origin of P300 induced by visual stimuli is controversial,

TABLE 3: Comparisons of latencies and amplitude at Pz in visual ERPs of PD-H, PD-NH, and controls.

	PD-H n = 12	PD-NH n = 23	Controls n = 18	p
Amplitude, uV				
ISI = 1600 ms				
N1	−0.59 ± 3.19	−2.48 ± 4.75	−2.57 ± 5.18	0.479
P2	7.05 ± 3.81	10.87 ± 6.75	7.18 ± 5.73	0.164
N2	−0.07 ± 5.42	0.95 ± 7.77	−1.33 ± 6.04	0.388
P3	12.19 ± 4.74	14.14 ± 9.76	11.62 ± 7.86	0.934
ISI = 5000 ms				
N1	−1.44 ± 3.42	−2.02 ± 1.81	−2.26 ± 4.25	0.351
P2	6.40 ± 3.40	5.83 ± 3.81	6.18 ± 4.89	0.831
N2	−1.57 ± 5.08	−1.24 ± 4.39	−1.48 ± 4.32	0.836
P3	11.18 ± 5.21	12.38 ± 8.33	13.34 ± 6.50	0.831
Latency, ms				
ISI = 1600 ms				
N1	140.29 ± 13.03	139.43 ± 21.83	133.73 ± 15.34	0.585
P2	183.67 ± 15.40	185.57 ± 22.67	176.60 ± 8.09	0.643
N2	277.11 ± 33.45	262.85 ± 18.26	263.92 ± 18.67	0.288
P3	**396.44 ± 28.19**[a]	366.57 ± 21.58	359.89 ± 27.89	**0.005**
ISI = 5000 ms				
N1	152.86 ± 22.68	131.17 ± 20.25	135.63 ± 13.19	0.594
P2	215.14 ± 26.02	191.13 ± 29.20	197.11 ± 18.28	0.391
N2	282.75 ± 34.45	278.00 ± 22.94	265.17 ± 22.41	0.498
P3	397.38 ± 18.78	**395.89 ± 28.29**[b]	**404.44 ± 39.88**[b]	0.827
RT, ms				
ISI = 1600 ms	434.39 ± 71.49	395.65 ± 77.05	382.70 ± 52.97	0.145
ISI = 5000 ms	**480.81 ± 88.60**[b]	**450.64 ± 94.03**[b]	**421.29 ± 121.03**[b]	0.321
Error rate				
ISI = 1600 ms	0.03 ± 0.02	0.04 ± 0.05	0.19 ± 0.02	0.178
ISI = 5000 ms	0.03 ± 0.04	0.02 ± 0.02	0.02 ± 0.02	0.552

PD-H: PD patients with visual hallucinations; PD-NH: PD patients without visual hallucinations; RT: reaction time. Values are expressed as mean ± SD.
p: p value, by one-way analysis of covariance (ANCOVA) with age, gender as covariate for between-group comparison and by one-way repeated measures analysis of variance (ANOVA) for within-group comparison.
[a] $p < 0.05$, PD-H versus control, Tukey method for post hoc analysis,
[b] $p < 0.05$, ISI = 5000 ms versus 1600 ms, by paired t-test.

visual P3b represents parietal cortical distribution reflecting the top-down allocation of attention resources to relevant stimuli [35–37]. As we measured our visual P3 latency as P3b, our P3 latency may reflect the top-down attribution of visual processing.

In the present study, P3 latency with ISI of 1600 ms in PD-H patients was significantly longer than control and associated with VH after adjustment of confounding factors. As P3 latency of ERPs increases in line with cognitive decline in Lewy body dementia patients and demented PD patients with VHs [29, 32, 38], our finding implies that visual cognitive functions are particularly impaired in nondemented PD patients with visual hallucinations. It is accepted that VHs in PD could be related to central cholinergic dysfunction in pedunculopontine nucleus [33, 39]. On the basis of indirect pharmacological evidence, P3 ERPs in Alzheimer's disease could reflect central cholinergic function [40, 41]. Hence, a

possible explanation for our findings might be that nondemented PD patients with VHs might have more dysfunction over the frontobasal cholinergic pathways. In addition, visual ERP of fixed ISI with 1600 ms might be an auxiliary tool to detect cognitive dysfunction in nondemented PD.

There are several theoretical models implicated in the development of VHs in PD, and integrative approach may be needed to explore sensory, attention, and cognitive deficits [42]. Functional MRI during active VHs showed desynchronization between frontal and posterior cortical areas involved in visual processing [19], while Shine et al. suggest that decreased attentional network activity and increased primary visual system connectivity with default mode network may contribute to the development of VHs [43]. Our PD-H patient also showed significant deficits in tests about attention, visuoconstructional ability, executive function, and motor programming when comparing to PD-NH patients and control. However, latencies and amplitude of N1 ERP or P2 ERP, which may be more correlated with attentional network in brain, did not show significant differences between groups.

There were several limitations in our study. First, we collect PD patients from university-based hospital and the collection bias cannot be completely excluded. Secondly, visual ERP may be affected by excessive eyelid blinking related to blepharospasm, which is common in PD [44]. We did not exclude PD patients with blepharospasm in this study but the eyeball movement artifacts are excluded from the analysis. Thirdly, neuropsychological assessment may be affected by poor attention or decreased motor function in PD patients. We arranged the assessment in the morning and patients receive regular medications before the exam, but poor attention or motor fluctuation may still happen during the time-consuming tests.

5. Conclusion

We found that P3 ERPs measurements may be associated with visual hallucination and cognitive impairment in nondemented PD patients. Further longitudinal follow-up may be needed to confirm whether P3 ERP measurements and visual hallucinations might predict the development of dementia in PD patients

Acknowledgments

This study was supported by grants from Kaohsiung Medical University Hospital (KMUH97-7G30 and KMUH-IRB-980169). The authors are grateful for contributions from Professor Pang-Ying Shih. Professor Pang-Ying Shih passed away on September 1, 2013.

References

[1] D. R. Williams and A. J. Lees, "Visual hallucinations in the diagnosis of idiopathic Parkinson's disease: a retrospective autopsy study," *Lancet Neurology*, vol. 4, no. 10, pp. 605–610, 2005.

[2] G. Levy, M.-X. Tang, E. D. Louis et al., "The association of incident dementia with mortality in PD," *Neurology*, vol. 59, no. 11, pp. 1708–1713, 2002.

[3] N. Ibarretxe-Bilbao, B. Ramirez-Ruiz, C. Junque et al., "Differential progression of brain atrophy in Parkinson's disease with and without visual hallucinations," *Journal of Neurology, Neurosurgery & Psychiatry*, vol. 81, no. 6, pp. 650–657, 2010.

[4] G. Fénelon, C. G. Goetz, and A. Karenberg, "Hallucinations in Parkinson disease in the prelevodopa era," *Neurology*, vol. 66, no. 1, pp. 93–98, 2006.

[5] D. Aarsland, K. Andersen, J. P. Larsen, A. Lolk, and P. Kragh-Sørensen, "Prevalence and characteristics of dementia in Parkinson disease: an 8-year prospective study," *Archives of Neurology*, vol. 60, no. 3, pp. 387–392, 2003.

[6] D. Aarsland, K. Andersen, J. P. Larsen et al., "The rate of cognitive decline in Parkinson disease," *Archives of Neurology*, vol. 61, no. 12, pp. 1906–1911, 2004.

[7] N. J. Diederich, C. G. Goetz, and G. T. Stebbins, "Repeated visual hallucinations in Parkinson's disease as disturbed external/internal perceptions: Focused review and a new integrative model," *Movement Disorders*, vol. 20, no. 2, pp. 130–140, 2005.

[8] J. Barnes, L. Boubert, J. Harris, A. Lee, and A. S. David, "Reality monitoring and visual hallucinations in Parkinson's disease," *Neuropsychologia*, vol. 41, no. 5, pp. 565–574, 2003.

[9] K. Smulders, M. van Nimwegen, M. Munneke, B. R. Bloem, R. P. C. Kessels, and R. A. J. Esselink, "Involvement of specific executive functions in mobility in Parkinson's disease," *Parkinsonism & Related Disorders*, vol. 19, no. 1, pp. 126–128, 2013.

[10] J. Pagonabarraga and J. Kulisevsky, "Cognitive impairment and dementia in Parkinson's disease," *Neurobiology of Disease*, vol. 46, no. 3, pp. 590–596, 2012.

[11] Q. Wu, L. Chen, Y. Zheng et al., "Cognitive impairment is common in Parkinson's disease without dementia in the early and middle stages in a Han Chinese cohort," *Parkinsonism & Related Disorders*, vol. 18, no. 2, pp. 161–165, 2012.

[12] E. Y. Uc, M. P. McDermott, K. S. Marder et al., "Incidence of and risk factors for cognitive impairment in an early parkinson disease clinical trial cohort," *Neurology*, vol. 73, no. 18, pp. 1469–1477, 2009.

[13] B. Ramirez-Ruiz, C. Junque, M.-J. Marti, F. Valldeoriola, and E. Tolosa, "Cognitive changes in Parkinson's disease patients with visual hallucinations," *Dementia and Geriatric Cognitive Disorders*, vol. 23, no. 5, pp. 281–288, 2007.

[14] W. Reginold, M. J. Armstrong, S. Duff-Canning et al., "The pill questionnaire in a nondemented Parkinson's disease population," *Movement Disorders*, vol. 27, no. 10, pp. 1308–1311, 2012.

[15] B. Ramírez-Ruiz, C. Junqué, M.-J. Marti, F. Valldeoriola, and E. Toloso, "Neuropsychological deficits in Parkinson's disease patients with visual hallucinations," *Movement Disorders*, vol. 21, no. 9, pp. 1483–1487, 2006.

[16] G. Gibson, P. G. Mottram, D. J. Burn et al., "Frequency, prevalence, incidence and risk factors associated with visual hallucinations in a sample of patients with Parkinson's disease: a longitudinal 4-year study," *International Journal of Geriatric Psychiatry*, vol. 28, no. 6, pp. 626–631, 2013.

[17] D. Grossi, L. Trojano, M. T. Pellecchia, M. Amboni, N. A. Fragassi, and P. Barone, "Frontal dysfunction contributes to the genesis of hallucination in non-demented Parkinsonian patients," *International Journal of Geriatric Psychiatry*, vol. 20, no. 7, pp. 668–673, 2005.

[18] G. Llebaria, J. Pagonabarraga, M. Martínez-Corral et al., "Neuropsychological correlates of mild to severe hallucinations in Parkinson's disease," *Movement Disorders*, vol. 25, no. 16, pp. 2785–2791, 2010.

[19] C. G. Goetz, C. L. Vaughan, J. G. Goldman, and G. T. Stebbins, "I finally see what you see: Parkinson's disease visual hallucinations captured with functional neuroimaging," *Movement Disorders*, vol. 29, no. 1, pp. 115–117, 2014.

[20] T. Yamasaki, S. Horie, H. Muranaka, Y. Kaseda, Y. Mimori, and S. Tobimatsu, "Relevance of in vivo neurophysiological biomarkers for mild cognitive impairment and Alzheimer's disease," *Journal of Alzheimer's Disease*, vol. 31, supplement 3, pp. S137–S154, 2012.

[21] C.-L. Lai, R.-T. Lin, L.-M. Liou, Y.-H. Yang, and C.-K. Liu, "The role of cognitive event-related potentials in executive dysfunction," *Kaohsiung Journal of Medical Sciences*, vol. 29, no. 12, pp. 680–686, 2013.

[22] C.-L. Lai, R.-T. Lin, L.-M. Liou, and C.-K. Liu, "The role of event-related potentials in cognitive decline in Alzheimer's disease," *Clinical Neurophysiology*, vol. 121, no. 2, pp. 194–199, 2010.

[23] J. Polich, J. E. Alexander, L. O. Bauer et al., "P300 topography of Amplitude/Latency correlations," *Brain Topography*, vol. 9, no. 4, pp. 275–282, 1997.

[24] J. Polich and T. Bondurant, "P300 sequence effects, probability, and interstimulus interval," *Physiology & Behavior*, vol. 61, no. 6, pp. 843–849, 1997.

[25] H. Wang, Y. Wang, D. Wang, L. Cui, S. Tian, and Y. Zhang, "Cognitive impairment in Parkinson's disease revealed by event-related potential N270," *Journal of the Neurological Sciences*, vol. 194, no. 1, pp. 49–53, 2002.

[26] S. Prabhakar, P. Syal, and T. Srivastava, "P300 in newly diagnosed non-dementing Parkinson's disease: effect of dopaminergic drugs," *Neurology India*, vol. 48, no. 3, pp. 239–242, 2000.

[27] H. Tanaka, T. Koenig, R. D. Pascual-Marqui, K. Hirata, K. Kochi, and D. Lehmann, "Event-related potential and EEG measures in Parkinson's disease without and with dementia," *Dementia and Geriatric Cognitive Disorders*, vol. 11, no. 1, pp. 39–45, 2000.

[28] A. Aotsuka, S. J. Weate, M. E. Drake Jr., and G. W. Paulson, "Event-related potentials in Parkinson's disease," *Electromyography and Clinical Neurophysiology*, vol. 36, no. 4, pp. 215–220, 1996.

[29] K. Toda, H. Tachibana, M. Sugita, and K. Konishi, "P300 and reaction time in Parkinson's disease," *Journal of Geriatric Psychiatry and Neurology*, vol. 6, no. 3, pp. 131–136, 1993.

[30] D. O'Mahony, M. Rowan, J. Feely, D. O'Neill, J. B. Walsh, and D. Coakley, "Parkinson's dementia and Alzheimer's dementia: an evoked potential comparison," *Gerontology*, vol. 39, no. 4, pp. 228–240, 1993.

[31] S. Pang, J. C. Borod, A. Hernandez et al., "The auditory P300 correlates with specific cognitive deficits in Parkinson's disease," *Journal of Neural Transmission-Parkinson's Disease and Dementia Section*, vol. 2, no. 4, pp. 249–264, 1990.

[32] A. Kurita, M. Murakami, S. Takagi, M. Matsushima, and M. Suzuki, "Visual hallucinations and altered visual information processing in Parkinson disease and dementia with lewy bodies," *Movement Disorders*, vol. 25, no. 2, pp. 167–171, 2010.

[33] F. Manganelli, C. Vitale, G. Santangelo et al., "Functional involvement of central cholinergic circuits and visual hallucinations in Parkinson's disease," *Brain*, vol. 132, no. 9, pp. 2350–2355, 2009.

[34] C. Sanchez-Castaneda, R. Rene, B. Ramirez-Ruiz et al., "Frontal and associative visual areas related to visual hallucinations in dementia with lewy bodies and Parkinson's disease with dementia," *Movement Disorders*, vol. 25, no. 5, pp. 615–622, 2010.

[35] H. H. Fernandez and K. L. Lapane, "Predictors of mortality among nursing home residents with a diagnosis of Parkinson's disease," *Medical Science Monitor*, vol. 8, no. 4, pp. CR241–CR246, 2002.

[36] H. H. Fernandez, K. L. Lapane, B. R. Ott, and J. H. Friedman, "Gender differences in the frequency and treatment of behavior problems in Parkinson's disease. SAGE Study Group. Systematic Assessment and Geriatric drug use via Epidemiology," *Movement Disorders*, vol. 15, no. 3, pp. 490–496, 2000.

[37] V. T. Nasman and P. J. Dorio, "Reduced P3b category response in prefrontal patients," *International Journal of Psychophysiology*, vol. 14, no. 1, pp. 61–74, 1993.

[38] I. Kimura, A. Ohnuma, H. Seki, S.-I. Saso, and K. Kogure, "Cognitive impairment in Parkinson's disease assessed by visuomotor performance system and P300 potential," *The Tohoku Journal of Experimental Medicine*, vol. 161, pp. 155–165, 1990.

[39] J. Janzen, D. Van'T Ent, A. W. Lemstra, H. W. Berendse, F. Barkhof, and E. M. J. Foncke, "The pedunculopontine nucleus is related to visual hallucinations in Parkinson's disease: preliminary results of a voxel-based morphometry study," *Journal of Neurology*, vol. 259, no. 1, pp. 147–154, 2012.

[40] A. Thomas, D. Iacono, L. Bonanni, G. D'Andreamatteo, and M. Onofrj, "Donepezil, rivastigmine, and vitamin E in Alzheimer disease: a combined P300 event-related potentials/neuropsychologic evaluation over 6 months," *Clinical Neuropharmacology*, vol. 24, no. 1, pp. 31–42, 2001.

[41] M. Onofrj, A. Thomas, A. L. Luciano et al., "Donepezil versus vitamin E in Alzheimer's Disease part 2: mild versus moderate-severe Alzheimer's Disease," *Clinical Neuropharmacology*, vol. 25, no. 4, pp. 207–215, 2002.

[42] A. J. Muller, J. M. Shine, G. M. Halliday, and S. J. G. Lewis, "Visual hallucinations in Parkinson's disease: theoretical models," *Movement Disorders*, vol. 29, no. 13, pp. 1591–1598, 2014.

[43] J. M. Shine, C. O'Callaghan, G. M. Halliday, and S. J. G. Lewis, "Tricks of the mind: visual hallucinations as disorders of attention," *Progress in Neurobiology*, vol. 116, pp. 58–65, 2014.

[44] A.-Q. Rana, A. Kabir, O. Dogu, A. Patel, and S. Khondker, "Prevalence of blepharospasm and apraxia of eyelid opening in patients with parkinsonism, cervical dystonia and essential tremor," *European Neurology*, vol. 68, no. 5, pp. 318–321, 2012.

12

Genetic Variants in SNCA and the Risk of Sporadic Parkinson's Disease and Clinical Outcomes

Clarissa Loureiro das Chagas Campêlo[1] and Regina Helena Silva[2]

[1]Memory Studies Laboratory, Department of Physiology, Universidade Federal do Rio Grande do Norte, Natal, RN, Brazil
[2]Behavioral Neuroscience Laboratory, Department of Pharmacology, Universidade Federal de São Paulo, São Paulo, SP, Brazil

Correspondence should be addressed to Regina Helena Silva; reginahsilva@gmail.com

Academic Editor: Hao Deng

There is increasing evidence of the contribution of genetic susceptibility to the etiology of Parkinson's disease (PD). Genetic variations in the SNCA gene are well established by linkage and genome-wide association studies. Positive associations of single nucleotide polymorphisms (SNPs) in SNCA and increased risk for PD were found. However, the role of SNCA variants in individual traits or phenotypes of PD is unknown. Here, we reviewed the current literature and identified 57 studies, performed in fourteen different countries, that investigated SNCA variants and susceptibility to PD. We discussed the findings based on environmental factors, history of PD, clinical outcomes, and ethnicity. In conclusion, SNPs within the SNCA gene can modify the susceptibility to PD, leading to increased or decreased risk. The risk associations of some SNPs varied among samples. Of notice, no studies in South American or African populations were found. There is little information about the effects of these variants on particular clinical aspects of PD, such as motor and nonmotor symptoms. Similarly, evidence of possible interactions between SNCA SNPs and environmental factors or disease progression is scarce. There is a need to expand the clinical applicability of these data as well as to investigate the role of SNCA SNPs in populations with different ethnic backgrounds.

1. Introduction

Parkinson's disease (PD) is a neurodegenerative disorder that is characterized by motor dysfunction but also causes nonmotor deficits [1]. Although the etiology of PD remains unclear, the interaction between genetic and environmental factors has been implicated in the emergence of the disease [2, 3]. Genome-wide association studies (GWAS) have identified variants of many candidate genes that contribute to PD susceptibility, such as variations of the SNCA gene [4–6]. Moreover, certain polymorphisms of SNCA are among the major risk factors for sporadic PD [5].

The SNCA gene is located on human chromosome 4 and encodes the protein alpha-synuclein. The physiological function of alpha-synuclein is not completely understood. Studies have shown a key role for alpha-synuclein in the regulation of neurotransmitter release, synaptic function, and plasticity of dopaminergic neurons [7–9]. The involvement in dopaminergic transmission and the predominant presence of alpha-synuclein in Lewy bodies [10–12] denote the relationship of this protein with the etiology of PD. In addition, genetic data support the role of alpha-synuclein in the pathogenic process of the disease. For example, missense mutations in SNCA locus were identified in familial forms of PD (A53T, A30P, E46K, and H50Q) [13–17], as well as in sporadic PD patients (A18T and A29S) [18]. Further, duplications and triplications of the SNCA locus cause familial parkinsonism and correlate with disease severity [19, 20].

Single nucleotide polymorphism (SNP) analyses in case-control studies performed in different populations have shown an association between several SNCA polymorphisms and the risk of PD. For example, the dinucleotide repeat REP1 located in the SNCA promoter (SNCA-REP1) and the 3' untranslated region (UTR) variants are frequently investigated [21]. Variations in these regions may increase susceptibility to PD by interfering with transcription factor binding sites [22, 23] and creating or destroying microRNAs target sites, which in turn modifies gene expression [24–26].

In spite of the fact that this type of study is frequent, investigations of the association between SNPs and the risk of PD in different populations show conflicting results. Furthermore, the consequences of genetic variability on clinical phenotypes, as well the interaction between genetic and environmental substrates, are poorly elucidated. Ideally, data from SNP studies would improve knowledge of pathophysiological pathways and help to target the best therapeutic program. This review aims to identify and compare the main SNP association studies conducted in different populations. The role of SNCA polymorphisms as a risk factor for PD and their association with clinical outcomes are discussed.

2. Literature Search

We conducted a survey in the relevant databases PubMed/Medline and Scopus for studies up to July 2016 using combinations of the keywords "polymorphism", "alpha synuclein", "SNCA gene", and "Parkinson's disease". We selected articles that met the following inclusion criteria: (a) articles that are written in English; (b) articles that described investigations of SNPs in the SNCA gene; (c) articles that had available data of allele and genotype distributions; (d) studies that were conducted in humans; (e) studies including participants who were diagnosed with Parkinson's disease. 57 studies were selected to conduct the review. In addition, despite not necessarily meeting the selection criteria, other relevant publications were included throughout the article in order to foment discussion.

The following information was extracted from each study: authors, year of publication, country of the studied population, number of patients and control subjects, risk association with PD, and investigation of environmental factors and clinical outcomes. The association of SNCA polymorphisms and PD susceptibility was often assessed by comparing the frequency of risk allele and risk genotypes in patients and controls. Values of odds ratio (OR) and confidence interval (95% CI) indicated the characteristic and significance of the association (OR values higher than 1 indicated increased risk and values lower than 1 suggested reduced risk).

Table 1 summarizes the main data from the 57 selected studies. The majority of the studies were performed in Caucasian and Asian populations. The studies were carried out in fourteen different countries (Mexico, China, Russia, Germany, Taiwan, USA, Japan, Spain, Italy, Ireland, Netherlands, Norway, Australia, and Greece) assembling patients from twenty countries (Mexico, China, Russia, Germany, Taiwan, USA, Japan, Spain, Italy, Norway, Netherlands, Serbia, Ireland, Australia, France, Greece, Poland, Sweden, Iran, and Australia). Sample sizes varied from 91 to 5302 patients in PD groups. The mean age at onset of PD varied from 45.2 to 68.2 years old.

3. SNPs and the Risk for Parkinson's Disease

GWAS have identified 28 distinct loci that modify the individual risk to PD [85] and suggest that genetic factors contribute to at least one-fourth of the total variation in liability to PD [86]. The two most consistent genes for susceptibility to sporadic PD are the alpha-synuclein (SNCA) and microtubule-associated protein tau (MAPT) genes, which can exert independent or joint effects on the risk of PD [56, 59, 61, 62, 87]. In addition, variants in other genes previously linked with autosomal forms (LRRK2, PARK16–18, and GBA) have also shown association with PD risk [64, 88–90]. Based on odds ratio and confidence intervals values in the selected studies, thirty-nine different SNPs in the SNCA gene showed a statistically significant effect on PD susceptibility: nine variants in the 5' end, nine variants near the 3' end, and 25 intron variants (Table 2). The locations of the six more frequently investigated SNPs within the SNCA gene are illustrated in Figure 1.

Two major linkage disequilibrium blocks in the SNCA gene have been proposed: (1) a 5' block that extends from the promoter-enhancer region to exon 4 and (2) a 3' block that includes intron 4, 3' UTR, and the 3' end region of the gene [73, 80]. SNPs in the 3' block presented a more expressive association with PD. The largest number of significant markers in the 3' block across different populations suggests a major causal effect for variants located in the 3' end compared with the 5' end. The 3' block contains elements with higher conservation across species, which emphasize its biological relevance [25].

The polymorphic microsatellite REP1 (D4S3481) in the promoter region of SNCA is one of the most frequently investigated polymorphisms and was pointed out as a risk factor in thirteen of the articles [47, 50, 60, 64, 65, 68, 71–73, 75, 77, 79, 81]. REP1 region plays a crucial role in the regulation of alpha-synuclein protein expression. Variants in REP1 are the only putative functional polymorphism identified within the SNCA locus. The REP1 SNP is a triallelic polymorphism with the longest (263 bp) and intermediate length (261 bp) alleles usually associated with an increased risk for PD, as seen in studies with North American [47, 50, 60, 64, 65, 68, 71, 72, 75, 81], German [73], Greek [79], and Dutch [77] samples. In 2006, a meta-analysis including over 5000 subjects provided strong evidence that the 263 bp allele was more frequent in cases and that the 259 bp allele was more frequent in controls (indicating decreased risk of PD) [91]. The other four SNPs in the 5' region (rs2619362, rs2619363, rs2619364, and rs2583988) contributed to the increase in the risk of PD in North American [49, 65] and European [56, 61, 77] populations.

Twenty-five intronic variants were associated with PD susceptibility, although the precise function of those variants of human SNCA is still unknown. The SNP rs2736990 in intron 4 was the most frequent, with the exception of one study [40]; this SNP was a consistent risk factor for PD [27, 28, 41, 49, 52, 55]. Similarly, the SNPs rs2572324, rs7684318, and rs894278 also increased susceptibility to sporadic PD [49, 60, 64, 65]. In contrast, a significant reduction of PD risk was found for the SNP rs356186 in Italian [56], North American [60], and Irish [61] samples.

Recently, the SNPs located near the 3' end have also been identified as risk factors for PD. Within the 3' region, the majority of the studies focused on rs356219, rs11931074, and rs356165. Among them, the SNP rs356219 was the most

TABLE 1: Characterization of the reviewed studies.

Studies	Study ID	Country of participants	Sample size		Onset age (mean ± SD)
			PD	Ctr	
Davila-Ortiz de Montellano et al., 2016	[27]	Mexico	171	171	—
Davis et al., 2016	[28]	USA	418	150	60.4 ± 11.1
García et al., 2016	[29]	Mexico	106	135	56.2 ± 14.4
Shahmohammadibeni et al., 2016	[30]	Iran	489	489	—
Wang et al., 2016	[31]	China	296	—	—
Cheng et al., 2016	[32]	China	1053	1152	52.0 ± 10.4
Guella et al., 2016	[33]	Multicentric*	1492	971	60.3 ± 10.2
Chen et al., 2015	[34]	China	218	110	60.6 ± 07.4
Huang et al., 2015	[35]	China, Australia	402	—	—
Han et al., 2015	[36]	China	91	92	—
Chen et al., 2015	[37]	China	1276	846	56.3 ± 11.5
Gao et al., 2015	[38]	USA	507	1330	68.3 ± 5.8
Cardo et al., 2014	[39]	China	752	489	—
Guo et al., 2014	[40]	China	1011	721	56.6 ± 11.8
Pan et al., 2013	[41]	China	515	450	45.2 ± 04.6
Mata et al., 2014	[42]	USA	1191	—	59.46 ± 10.6
Markopoulou et al., 2014	[43]	USA	1098	—	62.2
Emelyanov et al., 2013	[44]	Russia	244	308	—
Wu-Chou et al., 2013	[45]	Taiwan	626	473	63.2 ± 07.8
Brockmann et al., 2013	[46]	Germany	1396	—	56.9 ± 01.9
Chung et al., 2013	[47]	USA	1098	1098	60.4
Pihlstrøm et al., 2013	[48]	Norway and Sweden	1380	1295	59.0
Heckman et al., 2012	[49]	USA	426	769	62.0 ± 12.0
Ritz et al., 2012	[50]	USA	232	—	—
Schmitt et al., 2012	[51]	Germany	980	1005	59.4 ± 12.2
Miyake et al., 2012	[52]	Japan	229	357	65.7 ± 08.8
Pan et al., 2012	[53]	China	403	315	57.8 ± 08.6
Cardo et al., 2012	[54]	Spain	727	480	—
Gao et al., 2012	[55]	USA	584	1571	68.2 ± 05.7
Trotta et al., 2012	[56]	Italy	904	891	56.1 ± 11.0
Hu et al., 2012	[57]	China	110	136	56.7 ± 10.8
Botta-Orfilla et al., 2012	[58]	Spain	84	—	—
Mata et al., 2011	[59]	Spain	1445	1161	60.0 ± 12.2
Chung et al., 2011	[60]	USA	1103	1103	62.2
Elbaz et al., 2011	[61]	Multicentric**	5302	4161	—
Wider er al., 2011	[62]	USA, Ireland, Norway	1020	1095	58.0 ± 12.0
Botta-Orfilla et al., 2011	[63]	Spain	757	708	—
Biernacka et al., 2011	[64]	USA	1098	1098	62.2
Mata et al., 2010	[65]	USA	1956	2112	58.7 ± 11.9
Yu et al., 2010	[66]	China	332	300	54.3 ± 11.1
Hu et al., 2010	[67]	China	330	300	52.6 ± 11.8
Gatto et al., 2010	[68]	USA	333	336	—
Rajput et al., 2009	[69]	Canada	452	245	—
Sutherland et al., 2009	[70]	Australia	331	296	60.1 ± 10.6
Brighina et al., 2009	[71]	USA	893	893	62.1
Kay et al., 2008	[72]	USA	1802	2192	—
Myhre et al., 2008	[73]	Netherlands	236	236	—
Verbaan et al., 2008	[74]	Netherlands	295	150	—
Brighina et al., 2008	[75]	USA	833	833	61.9
Ross et al., 2007	[76]	Ireland	186	186	50.0 ± 11.0
Winkler et al., 2007	[77]	Germany, Serbia	397	270	—

TABLE 1: Continued.

| Studies | Study ID | Country of participants | Sample size | | Onset age |
			PD	Ctr	(mean ± SD)
Goris et al., 2007	[78]	UK	659	2176	63.0
Hadjigeorgiou et al., 2006	[79]	Greece	178	186	63.3 ± 9.6
Mueller et al., 2005	[80]	Germany	669	1002	55.4 ± 19.1
Mamah et al., 2005	[81]	USA	557	557	63.0
Spadafora et al., 2003	[82]	Italy	186	182	—
Izumi et al., 2001	[83]	Japan	200	250	61.0 ± 09.1

ID: identification; PD: Parkinson's disease group; Ctr: control group; SD: standard deviation. *The countries of origin of participants were New Zeeland, Canada, UK, and USA. **The countries of origin of participants were Australia, France, Germany, Greece, Ireland, Italy, Norway, Poland, Sweden, and USA.

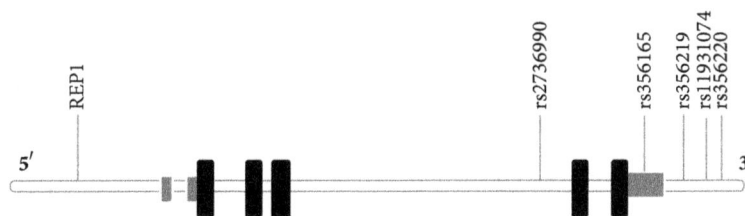

FIGURE 1: Diagram illustrating the locations of the main SNPs in human SNCA gene reviewed in the present study: SNCA-REP1 (promoter region), rs2736990 (intron 4), rs356165 (3' UTR), and rs356219, rs356220, and rs11931074 (3' end). Black boxes indicate translated exons, grey boxes indicate untranslated regions, and the white line indicates introns.

investigated, and it stands out as a consistent risk factor for PD in twelve of the studies. Variants in the 3' region possibly increase SNCA expression because of the misregulation of the posttranscriptional control. In the 3' untranslated region (UTR), there are target binding sites for two microRNAs (mir-7 and mir-153), and alterations in these regions might affect mRNA stability and translation [92]. Further, mir-7 and mir-153 were associated with SNCA mRNA expression in human studies [23, 24]. The SNP rs356219 showed a robust association as a common susceptibility marker in twelve studies with patients from Russia [44], Germany [46, 80], Spain [58, 59], Japan [52], China [53], USA [28, 65], United Kingdom [78], and Netherlands [73]. Similarly, the SNP rs11931074 showed a significant association with increased PD risk in seven studies, four of which were performed in Chinese samples [32, 34, 39, 40].

The variants rs356221, rs356165, and rs356182 in 3' UTR also contribute significantly to the increase in the PD risk in Germany [51, 77, 80], USA [28, 50], China [34], Taiwan [45], and Netherlands [73]. These findings reinforce the role of a posttranscriptional mechanism in PD etiology. The variant rs356165 was the most expressive [28, 50, 51, 54, 61, 73, 77, 80].

4. SNCA SNPs and Environmental Factors Interactions

Despite the relevance of environmental data to the understanding of the etiology of PD, the majority of studies contain little or no information on possible associations between SNCA SNPs and environmental factors (Table 3).

Sporadic PD is considered a result of complex interactions between genetic and environmental risk factors.

Professional pesticide exposure, rural living, and well-water drinking were reported to increase the risk of PD [93–95]. In contrast, cigarette smoking [96, 97] and caffeine intake [98] have been pointed out as protective factors. Furthermore, though less consistently, reduced PD risk was associated with alcohol drinking [99]. Potential interactions between SNCA SNPs and pesticide exposure, smoking habits, head injury, or coffee and alcohol drinking were investigated in a few of the studies [47, 50, 52, 55, 56]. Overall, data demonstrated some pairwise interactions, but without reaching significant levels after Bonferroni correction. For example, although Miyake et al. [52], Chung et al. [47], and Gao et al. [55] found a significant protective effect of smoking habits against PD, corroborating epidemiological data, only the first study found significant interactions between SNPs rs356219 and rs356220 and smoking.

Meta-analyses [96, 97] have reinforced the inverse association between cigarette smoking and PD risk more consistently than other environmental factors (rural living, well-water consumption, farming, and the use of pesticides). One of the mechanisms suggested to underlie this neuroprotection is the reduction of brain levels of the enzyme monoamine oxidase B (MAO B), an isoform that selectively metabolizes dopamine. This reduction would enhance the levels of dopamine and decrease the production of hydrogen peroxide and oxidative stress rates [100]. An alternative explanation is that smoke induces cytochrome P-450 enzyme activity. This enzyme is responsible for the metabolism of antipsychotic drugs and the detoxification of certain environmental toxins such as MPTP [101]. In this respect, a case-control study carried out in European countries investigated polymorphisms with relevance to brain expression and metabolism

TABLE 2: Single nucleotide polymorphisms (SNPs) in SNCA associated with Parkinson's disease.

Variant	Region	Alleles	Studies* with significant association with PD risk
REP1	Promoter	259 bp/261 bp/263 bp	[47, 50, 60, 64, 65, 68, 71–73, 75, 77, 79, 81] (↑) [43, 56, 76] (↓)
rs1372519	Promoter	A/G	[49] (↓)
rs2301134	Promoter	C/T	[45, 76] (↑)
rs2301135	Promoter	C/G	[45] (↓)
rs2619361	Promoter	A/C	[49] (↑)
rs2619362	5′ region	C/T	[49] (↑)
rs2619363	5′ region	G/T	[49, 77] (↑)
rs2619364	5′ region	A/G	[66, 77] (↑)
rs2583988	5′ region	C/T	[49, 56, 61, 77] (↑)
rs2119787	Intron	A/G	[65] (↓)
rs2197120	Intron	A/G	[56] (↓)
rs2572324	Intron	C/T	[49, 60, 64, 65] (↑)
rs2583959	Intron	C/G	[49, 64] (↑)
rs2736990	Intron	T/C	[27, 28, 41, 47, 49, 52, 55, 60] (↑) [40] (↓)
rs2737020	Intron	C/T	[76] (↓)
rs2737029	Intron	C/T	[56, 65, 80] (↑)
rs2737033	Intron	A/G	[46] (↑)
rs356164	Intron	C/G	[76] (↓)
rs356168	Intron	A/G	[64, 80] (↑)
rs356186	Intron	A/G	[56, 60, 76] (↓)
rs356203	Intron	A/G	[27, 80] (↑)
rs356204	Intron	A/G	[80] (↑)
rs3822086	Intron	C/T	[37] (↓)
rs3857057	Intron	A/G	[33] (↑)
rs3857059	Intron	A/G	[29, 80] (↑)
rs6848726	Intron	C/T	[80] (↓)
rs7684318	Intron	C/T	[27, 66] (↑)
rs7689942	Intron	C/T	[33] (↑)
rs894278	Intron	G/T	[35, 36] (↑)
rs1372520	Intron	C/T	[47, 49] (↑) [60] (↓)
rs10018362	Intron	C/T	[33] (↑)
rs2737012	Intron	C/T	[49] (↑)
rs3756063	Intron	C/G	[36] (↑)
rs3775423	Intron	C/T	[48, 60, 64] (↑)
rs356221	3′ region	A/T	[45, 48, 77] (↑)
rs356165	3′ region	A/G	[28, 50, 51, 54, 69, 73, 76, 77, 80] (↑)
rs356182	3′ region	A/G	[32] (↑)
rs356218	3′ region	A/G	[47, 49, 60] (↑)
rs356219	3′ region	A/G	[28, 42, 44, 46, 52, 53, 59, 61–63, 65, 73, 78, 80] (↑)
rs356220	3′ region	C/T	[27, 28, 30, 33, 52, 55, 80] (↑) [40] (↓)
rs356225	3′ region	C/T	[33] (↑)
rs181489	3′ region	C/T	[61, 76, 77] (↑)
rs11931074	3′ region	G/T	[30, 31, 34, 39, 55, 57, 61] (↑) [37, 45] (↓)

SNP: single nucleotide polymorphism. *See Table 1. Arrows indicate whether the SNP increased (↑) or reduced (↓) PD susceptibility in each study, based on values of odds ratio and confidence intervals.

TABLE 3: Association of environmental factors of PD with SNPs in SNCA.

Environmental factors	Studies*	Results
Smoking	[34, 38, 47, 50, 52, 55, 56, 68, 70]	Individuals with GG-rs356219 and TT-rs356220 genotypes [52] and carriers of allele REP1-263 bp [47] who never had smoked had a significantly increased risk of PD.
Coffee intake	[38, 47, 55, 56]	No SNPs were significantly associated with this factor.
Pesticide exposure	[47, 68, 70, 71]	Chung et al. [47] found a suggestive association between C-rs3775423 and pesticide exposure.
Alcohol drinking	[47, 75]	Brighina et al. [75] found independent effects to alcohol consumption and REP1-SNCA. Alcohol use was associated with a decreased PD risk.
Head injury	[38]	Head injury increases PD risk, especially when it happens before the age of 30; no significant association with SNCA SNPs.

*See Table 1.

TABLE 4: Association of clinical aspects of PD and SNPs within SNCA.

Variables	Studies*	Results
Age at onset	[28, 32, 35, 37, 40, 41, 46, 53, 54, 58, 66, 69, 70, 72, 79]	SNPs were associated with earlier PD onset: REP1-263 bp [35, 69, 79]; C-rs2736990 [41]; G-rs894278 [35]; G-rs356219 [46, 53, 58]; G-rs356215 [54]
Motor outcomes[a]	[28, 31, 32, 34, 43, 50, 51, 74]	Wang et al. [31] found a protective association between T-rs11931074 allele carriers and motor severity. Ritz et al. [50] found that REP1-263 bp and G-rs356165 alleles increased the risk of faster decline of motor function, whereas Markopoulou et al. [43] demonstrated that REP1-263 bp allele reduced the risk of developing motor impairments
Cognition outcomes[b]	[31–34, 37, 40, 42, 43, 74, 78]	Markopoulou et al. [43] showed an increased risk of cognitive impairment in carriers of REP1-259 bp allele. Guella et al. [33] found a significant association of C-rs10018362, T-rs7689942, and G-rs1348224 alleles with PD with dementia
Anxiety and depression[c]	[32, 34, 37, 40, 74]	No SNPs were significantly associated with symptoms
Autonomic and sleep disorders[d]	[34, 74]	No SNPs were significantly associated with symptoms
Hyposmia	[34, 74]	In Chen et al.'s study [34], TT-rs11931074 genotype increased the risk of hyposmia in PD

*See Table 1. [a]Questionnaires used: Unified Parkinson Disease Rating Scale-III and Hoehn and Yahr. [b]Questionnaires used: Mini-Mental State Examination, Frontal Assessment Battery, Montreal Cognitive Assessment, Scales for Outcomes in Parkinson's Disease Cognition, Hopkins Verbal Learning Test-Revised, Letter-Number Sequencing Test and Trail Making Test, Semantic and Phonemic Verbal Fluency Tests, and Benton Judgment of Line Orientation test. [c]Questionnaires used: Hamilton Rating Scale for Depression and Anxiety and Beck Depression Inventory. [d]Questionnaires used: REM Sleep Behavior Disorder Questionnaire, and Scales for Outcomes in Parkinson's Disease Autonomic, Nighttime Sleep, Daytime Sleepiness and Psychiatric Complications.

of substances contained in tobacco smoke and confirmed significant interactions of SNPs in cytochrome P-450 enzyme family genes (GSTM1, GSTP1, and NAT2). However, there is no information about the mechanisms that explain the biological interaction between SNCA genotypes and cigarette smoking.

5. SNCA SNPs and PD Clinical Outcomes Interactions

The influence of polymorphisms on PD phenotypic variability remains unclear. Indeed, few studies specifically investigated their associations with particular aspects of the disease, such as disease history and clinical outcomes (Table 4).

The age at onset is the most frequently investigated and well established aspect of disease history. Polymorphisms located in the promoter (REP1), introns (rs2736990, rs894278), and 3′ region (rs356219 and rs356165) are suggested to be predictors of earlier PD onset in Australian and Chinese [35], Spanish [54], German [46], and UK [61] samples. The identification of genetic features associated with the onset of PD has a relevant potential for therapeutic targeting. In view of the fact that neurodegeneration precedes the appearance of motor symptoms [102], it is critical to predict the risk of developing PD prior to clinical manifestations.

Even though it is expected that SNCA variants would influence individual traits or phenotypes of sporadic PD, this association was poorly explored in the studies. In a

TABLE 5: Interactions between alpha-synuclein levels and SNCA SNPs.

Study	SNP	Risk allele	Results
Hu et al. [57]	rs11931074	T	The allele was associated with reduced levels of alpha-synuclein in serum
	REP1		Different alleles and genotypes did not influence levels of alpha-synuclein in serum
Mata et al. [65]	rs356219	C	CC genotype was correlated with increased levels of alpha-synuclein in plasma
Fuchs et al. [84][a]	rs2583988	T	No correlation with alpha-synuclein mRNA or protein levels
	REP1	261 pb	256 pb/256 bp genotype was associated with lower alpha-synuclein levels assessed in blood samples; no effect in brain samples
	rs356219	C	CT genotype correlated with higher SNCA mRNA levels in the substantia nigra and TT genotype showed higher SNCA mRNA levels in the cerebellum; no effect in blood samples
McCarthy et al. [24][a]	rs2736990	G	In the 3 SNPs, the GG genotype correlated with an increased expression ratio of SNCA112 mRNA in the frontal cortex
	rs356165	G	
	rs356219	G	
McCarthy et al. [24][a]	rs3857059	G	No correlation between genotypes and the ratio expression levels of SNCA112 mRNA
	rs17016074	A	
Cardo et al. [39][a]	rs356165	G	No significant differences for the SNCA isoform levels between the different genotypes assessed in brain tissues
	rs11931074	T	

[a]Postmortem studies.

longitudinal study with a North American sample, Ritz et al. [50] showed that the REP1-263 bp promoter variant and the G-rs356165 allele are risk factors to faster motor progression in Caucasian and non-Caucasian PD patients (OR 1.66; 95% CI: 0.96–2.88). Wang et al. [31] found a protective association between T-rs11931074 allele and motor severity. However, in a larger sample of Caucasian patients, Markopoulou et al. [43] showed that REP1-263 pb allele reduced the risk of developing motor impairments. This divergence can be a result of differences in the methods of motor evaluation. According to Markopoulou et al. [43], the discrepancies may also suggest a dual and time-dependent role of SNCA.

Impairments in the olfactory function are a common early-stage nonmotor feature of PD, and the TT-rs11931074 genotype may increase the risk of hyposmia in PD cases [34].

Few other studies pointed out weak or absent associations with clinical outcomes such as anxiety or depression [32, 34, 37, 40, 74], sleep and autonomic disorders [34, 74], and cognitive impairments [31, 32, 34, 37, 40, 74]. Regarding cognitive features, Markopoulou et al. [43] demonstrated that the REP1-259 pb allele increased the risk of cognitive outcomes. Trotta et al. [56] found significant associations of C-rs10018362, T-rs7689942, and G-rs1348224 alleles with PD with dementia and also identified a specific haplotype in intron 4 of SNCA (C-rs62306323 and T-rs7689942) associated with increased risk of PD with dementia. It is important to mention that limited data of SNP associations with PD phenotype in cross-sectional studies might be related to a single event of clinical assessment, which could mask possible effects. Studies of such associations could provide important clinical applicability of the significant findings of genotyping studies. More studies evaluating specific clinical aspects, especially with longitudinal designs, are necessary to enhance the understanding of how genetic factors contribute to PD.

6. Biological Effects of SNCA SNPs

There is increasing evidence supporting the biological effects of genetic variants in SNCA, possibly by modifying alpha-synuclein expression. Among the studies listed in Table 5, the associations of SNCA-REP1 and 3′ variants (rs356219 and 11931074) and peripheral alpha-synuclein levels were investigated in Chinese [57] and North American [65] populations. Mata et al. [65] found an association of CC-356219 genotype with increased plasma levels of alpha-synuclein. A variation in the REP1 region might affect transcriptional activity by increasing the expression of alpha-synuclein and consequent protein accumulation [22, 23]. SNCA duplication and triplication in familial PD have been linked to increased mRNA expression levels [103] and to disease severity [19, 20].

In postmortem brain tissue studies, the 3′ region SNPs rs356219 [84], rs356165 [24], and rs11931074 [39] have been associated with increased gene expression. For rs356219, the heterozygote CT genotype correlated with higher levels of SNCA-mRNA in the substantia nigra of PD patients. However, the TT protective genotype was accompanied by higher expression in the cerebellum, a structure that is more preserved in the course of PD [84]. Similarly, G-rs356219 allele carriers presented higher levels of the SNCA112-mRNA isoform in the frontal cortex [24]. Further, PD patients presented higher levels of the SNCA-112 and SNCA-98 transcripts in the cerebellum and occipital cortex when compared to controls [39].

Linnertz et al. [104] investigated the effects of SNCA SNPs in 5′ and 3′ regions on SNCA expression in postmortem brains from neurologically normal subjects. For REP1, the 256 bp/256 bp genotype correlated with lower SNCA-mRNA levels, corroborating the hypotheses that decreased SNCA levels protect against the disease. Unexpectedly, the protective genotypes AA-rs356219 and AA-rs365165 in the $3'$ region correlated with higher levels of SNCA-mRNA in the temporal cortex and substantia nigra, which highlights an expanded regulatory effect of this region on total SNCA-mRNA levels.

Regarding in vivo studies, patients with SNP rs2583988 genotypes did not present alterations in alpha-synuclein levels in peripheral blood mononuclear cells, while the protein levels were reduced in the absence of the REP1 risk allele [84]. For SNPs in the $3'$ region, while carriers of T-rs11931074 allele presented reduced levels of protein in serum [57], a higher level of alpha-synuclein in plasma was observed in carriers of the C-rs356219 allele [65].

7. Genetical Background, Ethnicity, and the Effect of SNCA SNPs

Methodological aspects such as variations in the sample size, control of population stratification, and statistical analyses can explain the discrepancies in the effects of SNPs among the different studies. In addition, it is common to exclude the influence of confounder variables as sex, age, and ethnic background, which can modify the results substantially.

The majority of the studies were carried out in countries of Europe, North America, and Asia, that is, populations with mainly Caucasian and Asian genetic backgrounds. Despite the fact that ethnic differences can preclude the generalization of the results in genetic studies, many of the SNPs showed similar effects in groups with different genetic backgrounds. For example, the SNP rs356219 remained an important risk factor for PD in studies performed within North American [65], Spanish [63], Russian [44], and Chinese [41] populations. Nevertheless, given the significance of results and perspectives of clinical advancement, it seems necessary to extend these investigations to other continents, in order to confirm whether these genetic effects are consistent across different populations and to verify the implications of between-population heterogeneity.

Finally, apart from variants in the SNCA gene, it is necessary to consider the role of interactions between multiple genetic variants in disease risk and clinical profile. For example, investigations of phenotypic diversity in PD have identified an association between SNCA and MAPT. This association contributed to increased cognitive and motor severity in a Chinese sample [31] and influenced the development of cognitive impairment and dementia in a British sample [78]. In addition, polymorphisms in GAB [28] and LRRK2 [58] have been associated with earlier age at the onset in a European-American population and in a Spanish sample, respectively. Also, in North Americans, APOE variants predicted lower cognitive performance in PD patients [42].

8. Conclusions

This review collected the contributions of polymorphisms in the SNCA gene to PD susceptibility and clinical phenotypes. In most of the studies, the influence of polymorphisms in

multiple regions of SNCA gene was pointed out, such as the promoter region (REP1-SNCA), $3'$ end (e.g., rs11931074 and rs356219), $3'$ untranslated regions (e.g., rs356165), and introns (e.g., rs7684318, rs894278, and rs276990). In addition, we highlight that it is necessary to expand the clinical applicability of these data, as well as investigate the role of SNCA variations in populations with different ethnic backgrounds.

Acknowledgments

The authors would like to thank the funding agencies Conselho Nacional de Desenvolvimento Científico e Tecnológico (CNPq) (Grant no. 402054/2010-5), Coordenação de Aperfeiçoamento de Pessoal de Nível Superior (CAPES), Fundação de Apoio à Pesquisa do Estado do Rio Grande do Norte (FAPERN/PRONEX), and Fundação de Amparo à Pesquisa do Estado de São Paulo (FAPESP) (Grant no. 2015/12308-5).

References

[1] S. Fahn, "Description of Parkinson's disease as a clinical syndrome," *Annals of the New York Academy of Sciences*, vol. 991, pp. 1–14, 2003.

[2] K. Wirdefeldt, H. Adami, P. Cole, D. Trichopoulos, and J. Mandel, "Epidemiology and etiology of Parkinson's disease: a review of the evidence," *European Journal of Epidemiology*, vol. 26, no. 1, supplement, pp. S1–S58, 2011.

[3] L. M. de Lau and M. M. Breteler, "Epidemiology of Parkinson's disease," *The Lancet Neurology*, vol. 5, no. 6, pp. 525–535, 2006.

[4] W. Satake, Y. Nakabayashi, I. Mizuta et al., "Genome-wide association study identifies common variants at four loci as genetic risk factors for Parkinson's disease," *Nature Genetics*, vol. 41, no. 12, pp. 1303–1307, 2009.

[5] J. Simón-Sánchez, C. Schulte, J. M. Bras, M. Sharma, D. Gibbs Berg Jr. et al., "Genome-wide association study reveals genetic risk underlying Parkinsons disease," *Nature Genetics*, vol. 41, pp. 1308–1312, 2009.

[6] M. Sharma, J. P. A. Ioannidis, J. O. Aasly et al., "Large-scale replication and heterogeneity in Parkinson disease genetic loci," *Neurology*, vol. 79, no. 7, pp. 659–667, 2012.

[7] H. A. Lashuel, C. R. Overk, A. Oueslati, and E. Masliah, "The many faces of α-synuclein: from structure and toxicity to therapeutic target," *Nature Reviews Neuroscience*, vol. 14, no. 1, pp. 38–48, 2013.

[8] J. Bendor, T. Logan, and R. Edwards, "The function of α-synuclein," *Neuron*, vol. 79, no. 6, pp. 1044–1066, 2013.

[9] S. E. Eisbach and T. F. Outeiro, "Alpha-Synuclein and intracellular trafficking: Impact on the spreading of Parkinson's disease pathology," *Journal of Molecular Medicine*, vol. 91, no. 6, pp. 693–703, 2013.

[10] J. Q. Trojanowski and V. M.-Y. Lee, "Aggregation of neurofilament and α-synuclein proteins in Lewy bodies: implications for the pathogenesis of Parkinson disease and Lewy body dementia," *Archives of Neurology*, vol. 55, no. 2, pp. 151–152, 1998.

[11] M. G. Spillantini, M. L. Schmidt, V. M. Lee, J. Q. Trojanowski, R. Jakes, and M. Goedert, "α-synuclein in Lewy bodies," *Nature*, vol. 388, no. 6645, pp. 839-840, 1997.

[12] M. G. Spillantini, R. A. Crowther, R. Jakes, M. Hasegawa, and M. Goedert, "α-Synuclein in filamentous inclusions of Lewy bodies from Parkinson's disease and dementia with Lewy bodies," *Proceedings of the National Academy of Sciences of the United States of America*, vol. 95, no. 11, pp. 6469-6473, 1998.

[13] O. Khalaf, B. Fauvet, A. Oueslati et al., "The H50Q mutation enhances αα-synuclein aggregation, secretion, and toxicity," *Journal of Biological Chemistry*, vol. 289, no. 32, pp. 21856-21876, 2014.

[14] M. Bozi, D. Papadimitriou, R. Antonellou et al., "Genetic assessment of familial and early-onset Parkinson's disease in a Greek population," *European Journal of Neurology*, vol. 21, no. 7, pp. 963-968, 2014.

[15] R. Krüger, W. Kuhn, T. Müller et al., "Ala30Pro mutation in the gene encoding α-synuclein in Parkinson's disease," *Nature Genetics*, vol. 18, no. 2, pp. 106-108, 1998.

[16] M. H. Polymeropoulos, C. Lavedan, E. Leroy et al., "Mutation in the α-synuclein gene identified in families with Parkinson's disease," *Science*, vol. 276, no. 5321, pp. 2045-2047, 1997.

[17] J. J. Zarranz, J. Alegre, J. C. Gómez-Esteban et al., "The new mutation, E46K, of α-synuclein causes Parkinson and Lewy body dementia," *Annals of Neurology*, vol. 55, no. 2, pp. 164-173, 2004.

[18] D. Hoffman-Zacharska, D. Koziorowski, O. A. Ross et al., "Novel A18T and pA29S substitutions in α-synuclein may be associated with sporadic Parkinson's disease," *Parkinsonism and Related Disorders*, vol. 19, no. 11, pp. 1057-1060, 2013.

[19] P. Ibáñez, A.-M. Bonnet, B. Débarges et al., "Causal relation between α-synuclein gene duplication and familial Parkinson's disease," *The Lancet*, vol. 364, no. 9440, pp. 1169-1171, 2004.

[20] M. Chartier-Harlin, J. Kachergus, C. Roumier et al., "α-synuclein locus duplication as a cause of familial Parkinson's disease," *The Lancet*, vol. 364, no. 9440, pp. 1167-1169, 2004.

[21] P. Pals, S. Lincoln, J. Manning et al., "α-Synuclein promoter confers susceptibility to Parkinson's disease," *Annals of Neurology*, vol. 56, no. 4, pp. 591-595, 2004.

[22] O. Chiba-Falek and R. L. Nussbaum, "Effect of allelic variation at the NACP-Rep1 repeat upstream of the α-synuclein gene (SNCA) on transcription in a cell culture luciferase reporter system," *Human Molecular Genetics*, vol. 10, no. 26, pp. 3101-3109, 2001.

[23] O. Chib-Falek, J. W. Touchman, and R. L. Nussbaum, "Functional analysis of intra-allelic variation at NACP-Rep1 in the α-synuclein gene," *Human Genetics*, vol. 113, no. 5, pp. 426-431, 2003.

[24] J. J. McCarthy, C. Linnertz, L. Saucier et al., "The effect of SNCA 3′ region on the levels of SNCA-112 splicing variant," *Neurogenetics*, vol. 12, no. 1, pp. 59-64, 2011.

[25] S. Sotiriou, G. Gibney, A. D. Baxevanis, and R. L. Nussbaum, "A single nucleotide polymorphism in the 3′UTR of the SNCA gene encoding alpha-synuclein is a new potential susceptibility locus for Parkinson disease," *Neuroscience Letters*, vol. 461, no. 2, pp. 196-201, 2009.

[26] G. Wang, J. M. van der Walt, G. Mayhew et al., "Variation in the miRNA-433 binding site of FGF20 confers risk for Parkinson disease by overexpression of α-synuclein," *The American Journal of Human Genetics*, vol. 82, no. 2, pp. 283-289, 2008.

[27] D. J. Davila-Ortiz de Montellano, M. Rodriguez-Violante, A. Fresan, N. Monroy-Jaramillo, and P. Yescas-Gomez, "Frequency of single nucleotide polymorphisms and alpha-synuclein haplotypes associated with sporadic Parkinsons disease in the Mexican population," *Revue Neurologique*, vol. 63, pp. 345-350, 2016.

[28] A. A. Davis, K. M. Andruska, B. A. Benitez, B. A. Racette, J. S. Perlmutter, and C. Cruchaga, "Variants in GBA, SNCA, and MAPT influence Parkinson disease risk, age at onset, and progression," *Neurobiology of Aging*, vol. 37, pp. 209.e1-209.e7, 2016.

[29] S. García, G. Chavira-Hernández, M. Gallegos-Arreola et al., "The rs3857059 variant of the SNCA gene is associated with Parkinson's disease in Mexican Mestizos," *Arquivos de Neuro-Psiquiatria*, vol. 74, no. 6, pp. 445-449, 2016.

[30] N. Shahmohammadibeni, S. Rahimi-Aliabadi, J. Jamshidi et al., "The analysis of association between SNCA, HUSEYO and CSMD1 gene variants and Parkinson's disease in Iranian population," *Neurological Sciences*, vol. 37, no. 5, pp. 731-736, 2016.

[31] G. Wang, Y. Huang, Wei Chen et al., "Variants in the SNCA gene associate with motor progression while variants in the MAPT gene associate with the severity of Parkinson's disease," *Parkinsonism and Related Disorders*, vol. 24, pp. 89-94, 2016.

[32] L. Cheng, L. Wang, N.-N. Li et al., "SNCA rs356182 variant increases risk of sporadic Parkinson's disease in ethnic Chinese," *Journal of the Neurological Sciences*, vol. 368, pp. 231-234, 2016.

[33] I. Guella, D. M. Evans, C. Szu-Tu et al., "α-synuclein genetic variability: a biomarker for dementia in Parkinson disease," *Annals of Neurology*, vol. 79, no. 6, pp. 991-999, 2016.

[34] W. Chen, W.-Y. Kang, S. Chen et al., "Hyposmia correlates with SNCA variant and non-motor symptoms in Chinese patients with Parkinson's disease," *Parkinsonism and Related Disorders*, vol. 21, no. 6, pp. 610-614, 2015.

[35] Y. Huang, G. Wang, D. Rowe et al., "SNCA gene, but not MAPT, influences onset age of Parkinson's disease in Chinese and Australians," *BioMed Research International*, vol. 2015, Article ID 135674, 2015.

[36] W. Han, Y. Liu, Y. Mi, J. Zhao, D. Liu, and Q. Tian, "Alpha-synuclein (SNCA) polymorphisms and susceptibility to Parkinson's disease: a meta-analysis," *American Journal of Medical Genetics, Part B: Neuropsychiatric Genetics*, vol. 168, no. 2, pp. 123-134, 2015.

[37] Y. P. Chen, Q.-Q. Wei, R. W. Ou et al., "Genetic variants of snca are associated with susceptibility to Parkinson's disease but not amyotrophic lateral sclerosis or multiple system atrophy in a Chinese population," *PLoS ONE*, vol. 10, no. 7, Article ID e0133776, 2015.

[38] J. Gao, R. Liu, E. Zhao et al., "Head injury, potential interaction with genes, and risk for Parkinson's disease," *Parkinsonism and Related Disorders*, vol. 21, no. 3, pp. 292-296, 2015.

[39] L. F. Cardo, E. Coto, L. de Mena et al., "Alpha-synuclein transcript isoforms in three different brain regions from Parkinson's disease and healthy subjects in relation to the SNCA rs356165/rs11931074 polymorphisms," *Neuroscience Letters*, vol. 562, pp. 45-49, 2014.

[40] X. Y. Guo, Y. P. Chen, W. Song et al., "SNCA variants rs2736990 and rs356220 as risk factors for Parkinson's disease but not for amyotrophic lateral sclerosis and multiple system atrophy in a Chinese population," *Neurobiology of Aging*, vol. 35, no. 12, pp. 2882.e1-2882.e6, 2014.

[41] F. Pan, H. Ding, H. Dong et al., "Association of polymorphism in rs2736990 of the -synuclein gene with Parkinson's disease in a Chinese population," *Neurology India*, vol. 61, no. 4, pp. 360–364, 2013.

[42] I. F. Mata, J. B. Leverenz, D. Weintraub et al., "APOE, MAPT, and SNCA genes and cognitive performance in Parkinson disease," *JAMA Neurology*, vol. 71, no. 11, pp. 1405–1412, 2014.

[43] K. Markopoulou, J. M. Biernacka, S. M. Armasu et al., "Does α-synuclein have a dual and opposing effect in preclinical vs. clinical Parkinson's disease?" *Parkinsonism and Related Disorders*, vol. 20, no. 6, pp. 584–589, 2014.

[44] A. Emelyanov, P. Andoskin, A. Yakimovskii et al., "SNCA, LRRK2, MAPT polymorphisms and Parkinson's disease in Russia," *Parkinsonism and Related Disorders*, vol. 19, no. 11, pp. 1064-1065, 2013.

[45] Y.-H. Wu-Chou, Y.-T. Chen, T.-H. Yeh et al., "Genetic variants of SNCA and LRRK2 genes are associated with sporadic PD susceptibility: a replication study in a Taiwanese cohort," *Parkinsonism and Related Disorders*, vol. 19, no. 2, pp. 251–255, 2013.

[46] K. Brockmann, C. Schulte, A.-K. Hauser et al., "SNCA: major genetic modifier of age at onset of Parkinson's disease," *Movement Disorders*, vol. 28, no. 9, pp. 1217–1221, 2013.

[47] S. J. Chung, S. M. Armasu, K. J. Anderson et al., "Genetic susceptibility loci, environmental exposures, and Parkinson's disease: a case-control study of gene-environment interactions," *Parkinsonism and Related Disorders*, vol. 19, no. 6, pp. 595–599, 2013.

[48] L. Pihlstrøm, G. Axelsson, K. A. Bjørnarå et al., "Supportive evidence for 11 loci from genome-wide association studies in Parkinson's disease," *Neurobiology of Aging*, vol. 34, no. 6, pp. 1708.e7–1708.e13, 2013.

[49] M. G. Heckman, A. I. Soto-Ortolaza, N. N. Diehl et al., "Evaluation of the role of SNCA variants in survival without neurological disease," *PLoS ONE*, vol. 7, no. 8, Article ID e42877, 2012.

[50] B. Ritz, S. L. Rhodes, Y. Bordelon, and J. Bronstein, "α-Synuclein genetic variants predict faster motor symptom progression in idiopathic Parkinson disease," *PLoS ONE*, vol. 7, no. 5, Article ID e36199, 2012.

[51] I. Schmitt, U. Wüllner, J. P. Van Rooyen et al., "Variants in the 3′UTR of SNCA do not affect miRNA-433 binding and alpha-synuclein expression," *European Journal of Human Genetics*, vol. 20, no. 12, pp. 1265–1269, 2012.

[52] Y. Miyake, K. Tanaka, W. Fukushima et al., "SNCA polymorphisms, smoking, and sporadic Parkinson's disease in Japanese," *Parkinsonism and Related Disorders*, vol. 18, no. 5, pp. 557–561, 2012.

[53] F. Pan, H. Dong, H. Ding et al., "SNP rs356219 of the α-synuclein (SNCA) gene is associated with Parkinson's disease in a Chinese Han population," *Parkinsonism and Related Disorders*, vol. 18, no. 5, pp. 632–634, 2012.

[54] L. F. Cardo, E. Coto, L. de Mena et al., "A search for SNCA 3′ UTR variants identified SNP rs356165 as a determinant of disease risk and onset age in Parkinson's disease," *Journal of Molecular Neuroscience*, vol. 47, no. 3, pp. 425–430, 2012.

[55] J. Gao, M. A. Nalls, M. Shi et al., "An exploratory analysis on gene-environment interactions for Parkinson disease," *Neurobiology of Aging*, vol. 33, no. 10, pp. 2528.e1–2528.e6, 2012.

[56] L. Trotta, I. Guella, G. Soldà et al., "SNCA and MAPT genes: independent and joint effects in Parkinson disease in the Italian population," *Parkinsonism and Related Disorders*, vol. 18, no. 3, pp. 257–262, 2012.

[57] Y. Hu, B. Tang, J. Guo et al., "Variant in the 30 region of SNCA associated with Parkinson's disease and serum α-synuclein levels," *Journal of Neurology*, vol. 259, no. 3, pp. 497–504, 2012.

[58] T. Botta-Orfila, M. Ezquerra, P. Pastor et al., "Age at onset in LRRK2-associated PD is modified by SNCA variants," *Journal of Molecular Neuroscience*, vol. 48, no. 1, pp. 245–247, 2012.

[59] I. F. Mata, D. Yearout, V. Alvarez et al., "Replication of MAPT and SNCA, but not PARK16-18, as susceptibility genes for Parkinson's disease," *Movement Disorders*, vol. 26, no. 5, pp. 819–823, 2011.

[60] S. J. Chung, S. M. Armasu, J. M. Biernacka et al., "Common variants in PARK loci and related genes and Parkinson's disease," *Movement Disorders*, vol. 26, no. 2, pp. 280–288, 2011.

[61] A. Elbaz, O. A. Ross, J. P. A. Ioannidis et al., "Independent and joint effects of the MAPT and SNCA genes in Parkinson disease," *Annals of Neurology*, vol. 69, no. 5, pp. 778–792, 2011.

[62] C. Wider, C. Vilariño-Güell, M. G. Heckman et al., "SNCA, MAPT, and GSK3B in Parkinson disease: A gene-gene interaction study," *European Journal of Neurology*, vol. 18, no. 6, pp. 876–881, 2011.

[63] T. Botta-Orfila, M. Ezquerra, J. Ríos et al., "Lack of interaction of SNCA and MAPT genotypes in Parkinson's disease," *European Journal of Neurology*, vol. 18, no. 3, p. e32, 2011.

[64] J. M. Biernacka, S. M. Armasu, J. M. Cunningham, J. Eric Ahlskog, S. J. Chung, and D. M. Maraganore, "Do interactions between SNCA, MAPT, and LRRK2 genes contribute to Parkinson's disease susceptibility?" *Parkinsonism and Related Disorders*, vol. 17, no. 10, pp. 730–736, 2011.

[65] I. F. Mata, M. Shi, P. Agarwal et al., "SNCA variant associated with Parkinson disease and plasma α-synuclein level," *Archives of Neurology*, vol. 67, no. 11, pp. 1350–1356, 2010.

[66] L. Yu, P. Xu, X. He et al., "SNP rs7684318 of the α-synuclein gene is associated with Parkinson's disease in the Han Chinese population," *Brain Research*, vol. 1346, pp. 262–265, 2010.

[67] F.-Y. Hu, W.-B. Hu, L. Liu et al., "Lack of replication of a previously reported association between polymorphism in the 3′UTR of the alpha-synuclein gene and Parkinson's disease in Chinese subjects," *Neuroscience Letters*, vol. 479, no. 1, pp. 31–33, 2010.

[68] N. M. Gatto, S. L. Rhodes, A. D. Manthripragada et al., "Alpha-synuclein gene may interact with environmental factors in increasing risk of Parkinson's disease," *Neuroepidemiology*, vol. 35, no. 3, pp. 191–195, 2010.

[69] A. Rajput, C. Vilariño-Güell, M. L. Rajput et al., "Alpha-synuclein polymorphisms are associated with Parkinson's disease in a Saskatchewan population," *Movement Disorders*, vol. 24, no. 16, pp. 2411–2414, 2009.

[70] G. T. Sutherland, G. M. Halliday, P. A. Silburn et al., "Do polymorphisms in the familial parkinsonism genes contribute to risk for sporadic Parkinson's disease?" *Movement Disorders*, vol. 24, no. 6, pp. 833–838, 2009.

[71] L. Brighina, N. K. Schneider, T. G. Lesnick et al., "α-Synuclein, alcohol use disorders, and Parkinson disease: a case-control study," *Parkinsonism and Related Disorders*, vol. 15, no. 6, pp. 430–434, 2009.

[72] D. M. Kay, S. A. Factor, A. Samii et al., "Genetic association between α-synuclein and idiopathic Parkinson's disease," *American Journal of Medical Genetics, Part B: Neuropsychiatric Genetics*, vol. 147, no. 7, pp. 1222–1230, 2008.

[73] R. Myhre, M. Toft, J. Kachergus et al., "Multiple alpha-synuclein gene polymorphisms are associated with Parkinson's disease in a Norwegian population," *Acta Neurologica Scandinavica*, vol. 118, no. 5, pp. 320–327, 2008.

[74] D. Verbaan, S. Boesveldt, S. M. van Rooden et al., "Is olfactory impairment in Parkinson disease related to phenotypic or genotypic characteristics?" *Neurology*, vol. 71, no. 23, pp. 1877–1882, 2008.

[75] L. Brighina, R. Frigerio, N. K. Schneider et al., "α-Synuclein, pesticides, and Parkinson disease: a case-control study," *Neurology*, vol. 70, no. 16, pp. 1461–1469, 2008.

[76] O. A. Ross, D. Gosal, J. T. Stone et al., "Familial genes in sporadic disease: common variants of α-synuclein gene associate with Parkinson's disease," *Mechanisms of Ageing and Development*, vol. 128, no. 5-6, pp. 378–382, 2007.

[77] S. Winkler, J. Hagenah, S. Lincoln et al., "α-Synuclein and Parkinson disease susceptibility," *Neurology*, vol. 69, no. 18, pp. 1745–1750, 2007.

[78] A. Goris, C. H. Williams-Gray, G. R. Clark et al., "Tau and α-synuclein in susceptibility to, and dementia in, Parkinson's disease," *Annals of Neurology*, vol. 62, no. 2, pp. 145–153, 2007.

[79] G. M. Hadjigeorgiou, G. Xiromerisiou, V. Gourbali et al., "Association of α-synuclein Rep1 polymorphism and Parkinson's disease: Influence of Rep1 on age at onset," *Movement Disorders*, vol. 21, no. 4, pp. 534–539, 2006.

[80] J. C. Mueller, J. Fuchs, A. Hofer et al., "Multiple regions of α-synuclein are associated with Parkinson's disease," *Annals of Neurology*, vol. 57, no. 4, pp. 535–541, 2005.

[81] C. E. Mamah, T. G. Lesnick, S. J. Lincoln et al., "Interaction of α-synuclein and tau genotypes in Parkinson's disease," *Annals of Neurology*, vol. 57, no. 3, pp. 439–443, 2005.

[82] P. Spadafora, G. Annesi, A. A. Pasqua et al., "NACP-REP1 polymorphism is not involved in Parkinson's disease: a case-control study in a population sample from southern Italy," *Neuroscience Letters*, vol. 351, no. 2, pp. 75–78, 2003.

[83] Y. Izumi, H. Morino, M. Oda et al., "Genetic studies in Parkinson's disease with an α-synuclein/NACP gene polymorphism in Japan," *Neuroscience Letters*, vol. 300, no. 2, pp. 125–127, 2001.

[84] J. Fuchs, A. Tichopad, Y. Golub et al., "Genetic variability in the SNCA gene influences α-synuclein levels in the blood and brain," *FASEB Journal*, vol. 22, no. 5, pp. 1327–1334, 2008.

[85] M. A. Nalls, N. Pankratz, C. M. Lill et al., "Large-scale meta-analysis of genome-wide association data identifies six new risk loci for Parkinson's disease," *Nature Genetics*, vol. 46, no. 9, pp. 989–993, 2014.

[86] C. B. Do, J. Y. Tung, E. Dorfman et al., "Web-based genome-wide association study identifies two novel loci and a substantial genetic component for parkinson's disease," *PLoS Genetics*, vol. 7, no. 6, Article ID e1002141, 2011.

[87] Z. Wang, H. Lei, M. Zheng, Y. Li, Y. Cui, and F. Hao, "Meta-analysis of the association between alzheimer disease and variants in GAB2, PICALM, and SORL1," *Molecular Neurobiology*, vol. 53, no. 9, pp. 6501–6510, 2016.

[88] E. K. Tan, H. K. Kwok, L. C. Tan, W. T. Zhao, K. M. Prakash, W. L. Au et al., "Analysis of GWAS-linked loci in Parkinson disease reaffirms PARK16 as a susceptibility locus," *Neurology*, vol. 75, pp. 508–512, 2010.

[89] S. Lesage and A. Brice, "Parkinson's disease: from monogenic forms to genetic susceptibility factors," *Human Molecular Genetics*, vol. 18, no. R1, pp. R48–R59, 2009.

[90] J. N. Foo, S. J. Chung, L. C. Tan et al., "Linking a genome-wide association study signal to a LRRK2 coding variant in Parkinson's disease," *Movement Disorders*, vol. 31, no. 4, pp. 484–487, 2016.

[91] D. M. Maraganore, M. de Andrade, A. Elbaz et al., "Collaborative analysis of α-synuclein gene promoter variability and Parkinson disease," *The Journal of the American Medical Association*, vol. 296, no. 6, pp. 661–670, 2006.

[92] L. L. Venda, S. J. Cragg, V. L. Buchman, and R. Wade-Martins, "α-Synuclein and dopamine at the crossroads of Parkinson's disease," *Trends in Neurosciences*, vol. 33, no. 12, pp. 559–568, 2010.

[93] J. A. Firestone, T. Smith-Weller, G. Franklin, P. Swanson, W. T. Longstreth Jr., and H. Checkoway, "Pesticides and risk of parkinson disease: a population-based case-control study," *Archives of Neurology*, vol. 62, no. 1, pp. 91–95, 2005.

[94] K. M. Semchuk, E. J. Love, and R. G. Lee, "Parkinson's disease and exposure to rural environmental factors: a population based case-control study," *Journal Canadien des Sciences Neurologiques*, vol. 18, no. 3, pp. 279–286, 1991.

[95] M. F. Allam, A. S. Del Castillo, and R. Fernández-Crehuet Navajas, "Parkinson's disease risk factors: genetic, environmental, or both?" *Neurological Research*, vol. 27, no. 2, pp. 206–208, 2005.

[96] M. F. Allam, M. J. Campbell, A. Hofman, A. S. Del Castillo, and R. F.-C. Navajas, "Smoking and Parkinson's disease: systematic review of prospective studies," *Movement Disorders*, vol. 19, no. 6, pp. 614–621, 2004.

[97] X. Li, W. Li, G. Liu, X. Shen, and Y. Tang, "Association between cigarette smoking and Parkinson's disease: a meta-analysis," *Archives of Gerontology and Geriatrics*, vol. 61, no. 3, pp. 510–516, 2015.

[98] J. Costa, N. Lunet, C. Santos, J. Santos, and A. Vaz-Carneiro, "Caffeine exposure and the risk of Parkinson's disease: a systematic review and meta-analysis of observational studiess," *Journal of Alzheimer's Disease*, vol. 20, supplement 1, pp. S221–S238, 2010.

[99] S. S. Bettiol, T. C. Rose, C. J. Hughes, and L. A. Smith, "Alcohol consumption and Parkinson's disease risk: a review of recent findings," *Journal of Parkinson's Disease*, vol. 5, no. 3, pp. 425–442, 2015.

[100] P. Riederer, C. Konradi, G. Hebenstreit, and M. Youdim, "Neurochemical perspectives to the function of monoamine oxidase," *Acta Neurologica Scandinavica*, vol. 80, pp. 41–45, 1989.

[101] G. S. Shahi and S. M. Moochhala, "Smoking and Parkinson's disease—a new perspective," *Reviews on Environmental Health*, vol. 9, no. 3, pp. 123–136, 1991.

[102] R. Savica, W. A. Rocca, and J. E. Ahlskog, "When does Parkinson disease start?" *Archives of Neurology*, vol. 67, no. 7, pp. 798–801, 2010.

[103] M. Farrer, J. Kachergus, L. Forno et al., "Comparison of kindreds with Parkinsonism and α-synuclein genomic multiplications," *Annals of Neurology*, vol. 55, no. 2, pp. 174–179, 2004.

[104] C. Linnertz, L. Saucier, D. Ge et al., "Genetic regulation of α-synuclein mRNA expression in various human brain tissues," *PLoS ONE*, vol. 4, no. 10, Article ID e7480, 2009.

Patterns and Predictors of Depression Treatment among Older Adults with Parkinson's Disease and Depression in Ambulatory Care Settings in the United States

Sandipan Bhattacharjee ⓘ,[1] Nina Vadiei,[1] Lisa Goldstone,[2] Ziyad Alrabiah,[1,3] and Scott J. Sherman[4]

[1]Department of Pharmacy Practice and Science, College of Pharmacy, The University of Arizona, Tucson, AZ, USA
[2]University of Southern California School of Pharmacy, Los Angeles, CA, USA
[3]College of Pharmacy, King Saud University, Riyadh, Saudi Arabia
[4]Department of Neurology, College of Medicine, The University of Arizona, Tucson, USA

Correspondence should be addressed to Sandipan Bhattacharjee; bhattacharjee@pharmacy.arizona.edu

Academic Editor: Jan Aasly

Little is known regarding depression treatment patterns and predictors among older adults with comorbid Parkinson's disease and depression (dPD) in the United States (US). The objective of this study was to assess the patterns and predictors of depression treatment among older adults with dPD in the US. We adopted a cross-sectional study design by pooling multiple-year data (2005–2011) from the National Ambulatory Medical Care Survey (NAMCS) and the outpatient department of the National Hospital Ambulatory Medical Care Survey (NHAMCS). The final study sample consisted of visits by older adults with dPD. Depression treatment was defined as antidepressant use with or without psychotherapy. To identify predictors of depression treatment, multivariate logistic regression analysis was conducted adjusting for predisposing, enabling, and need factors. Individuals with dPD and polypharmacy were 74% more likely to receive depression treatment (odds ratio = 1.743, 95% CI 1.376–2.209), while dPD subjects with comorbid chronic conditions were 44% less likely (odds ratio = 0.559, 95% CI 0.396–0.790) to receive depression treatment. Approximately six out of ten older adults with PD and depression received depression treatment. Treatment options for dPD are underutilized in routine clinical practice, and further research should explore how overall medical complexity presents a barrier to depression treatment.

1. Introduction

Among neurodegenerative diseases, Parkinson's disease (PD) ranks second in frequency and importance [1]. Parkinson's disease is characterized by the well-studied motor symptoms: bradykinesia, tremor, rigidity, and postural imbalance [2]. Although less studied, the nonmotor symptoms are increasingly recognized as important targets of research due to their high prevalence and significant negative impact on the quality life of individuals with PD. Depression is one of the most common nonmotor symptoms of PD, with clinically significant depressive symptoms present in over one-third of individuals with PD [3]. It is

thought that this is not only due to the psychosocial stress and disability experienced by individuals with PD, but also due to underlying neuroanatomical degeneration [4]. This includes neurodegenerative processes of the brainstem monoamine and indolamine afferents, along with various subcortical nuclei (ventral tegmental area, hypothalamus, dorsal raphe, and locus coeruleus) that have been implicated in depression [5]. Additionally research has shown that depression precedes the onset of motor symptom development and that dPD patients have been shown to be more depressed than those with other disabling medical illnesses [6, 7]. A relationship between severity of PD and depression has also been observed [8], and treatment of motor symptoms of PD has not been shown to consistently correlate with changes in mood [9, 10]. Therefore, depressive symptoms experienced in dPD may be attributed to the illness neurobiology, increasing the likelihood that depression treatment will eventually be needed during the course of illness. Depression in PD (dPD) not only significantly decreases quality of life [11] but is also associated with sleep disturbances, reduced functional status, and limitations of activities of daily living [12].

Antidepressant medication [13] and psychotherapeutic approaches, such as cognitive behavior therapy (CBT) [14], have shown to decrease depression scores and improve the quality of life among individuals with dPD. Unfortunately, the majority of individuals with dPD are untreated [15–17], and even in the case of treatment, up to 50% may still remain depressed, suggesting inadequate or ineffective treatment [18]. To the best of our knowledge, no study is available to date that examines the depression treatment pattern and predictors at the United States (US) national-level among older adults with dPD. Hence, we undertook this cross-sectional study to assess the patterns and predictors of depression treatment among older adults with dPD seeking care in ambulatory settings in the US.

2. Materials and Methods

2.1. Study Design. We adopted a cross-sectional study design by using multiple years (2005–2011) of data from the National Ambulatory Medical Care Survey (NAMCS) and the outpatient department (OPD) of the National Hospital Ambulatory Medical Care Survey (NHAMCS). Human subjects review was not required for this study according to The University of Arizona Institutional Review Board.

2.2. Data Source. Nationally representative information related to ambulatory medical care services use and provisions in nonfederally employed physician offices and outpatient departments of noninstitutional general and short-stay hospitals are captured by NAMCS and NHAMCS, respectively. NAMCS and NHAMCS are ongoing yearly surveys administered by the National Center for Health Statistics (NCHS) of the Centers for Disease Control and Prevention (CDC) [19]. National-level estimates are obtained by using the weight assigned to each visit.

A visit, which serves as the basic sampling unit for NAMCS and NHAMCS, is defined as a direct, personal encounter between a physician or a staff member working under a physician's direction for the purpose of obtaining care and providing health services. A multistage probability design is used by NAMCS for data collection, where the initial stage involves drawing probability sample from primary sampling units (PSUs) such as counties, groups of counties, county equivalents, or towns and townships. Subsequent to this stage, a probability sample of practicing physicians from each of the PSUs is obtained. In the final stage, which involves a two-step process, patient visits from the yearly practices of sampled physicians are selected. In the first step, the whole physician sample is split into 52 random subsamples of approximately identical size, and each subsample is randomly assigned to one of the 52 weeks during the survey year. In the second step, during the assigned week a systematic random sample of visits are selected by the physicians. Using the Patient Record Form (PRF), which is the data collection form for NAMCS and NHAMCS, a wide array of information with respect to patient characteristics, physician characteristics, diagnoses, medications prescribed, and the delivery of therapeutic services are collected by NAMCS. NAMCS and NHAMCS can record up to three diagnoses codes and eight prescription medications for each visit.

Data collection is conducted using a multistage probability sample survey involving selection of probability samples of PSUs, hospitals from each PSU, some or all outpatient and emergency departments from hospitals, and patient visits within these departments. The final stage of sampling in the NHAMCS is similar to that of the NAMCS. Due to the similarity of the medical care provided in OPD and office-based settings, only the OPD portion of the NHAMCS was used for this study. Data collection of NHAMCS was conducted using a similar PRF as the NAMCS.

2.3. Study Population. The final study sample consisted of visits by older adults (age ≥ 65 years) with PD and depression. PD was identified by using International Classification of Diseases, Ninth Revision, Clinical Modification (ICD-9-CM) of 332.xx [20]. Depression diagnosis was identified if answer to the question "Regardless of the diagnoses written ... does the patient now have: depression?" was "yes" [21]. To supplement chronic conditions, this item was added since 2005, and the robustness of this item has been described elsewhere.

2.4. Dependent Variable. Depression treatment, which was the dependent variable for this study, was defined as antidepressant use with or without psychotherapy. Antidepressant use was determined using generic drug codes and Multum Lexicon Codes. Due to small sample size, antidepressants were classified into the selective serotonin reuptake inhibitors (SSRIs) and other antidepressants. Psychotherapy was ascertained from the variable (PSYCHOTH) available in NAMCS and NHAMCS.

2.5. Independent Variables. The Anderson Behavioral Model (ABM) was used as the conceptual framework for this study, and the independent variables were classified as (i) predisposing, (ii) enabling, and (iii) need factors [22]. Predisposing factors comprised of age (65–74 years and ≥75 years), gender (male/female), race/ethnicity (white only non-Hispanic and others), geographical region (south and others), and metropolitan status (metropolitan and nonmetropolitan). Enabling factors consisted of health insurance status (government-Medicaid/Medicare and others), new patient visit (yes/no), and physician/clinic specialty (general and family practice and others). Need factors constituted of receipt of new prescription during the visit (yes/no), total number of chronic conditions, and total number of medications used.

2.6. Statistical Analysis. Ambulatory visits at national-level were reported in terms of weighted frequencies (in millions) and weighted percentages. To identify the predictors of depression treatment, multivariate logistic regression analysis was conducted adjusting for predisposing, enabling, and need factors. Survey procedures (SURVEYFREQ, SURVEYMEANS, and SURVEYLOGISTIC) were used to adjust for the complex survey design of NAMCS-NHAMCS to obtain national-level estimates in SAS version 9.4 (SAS Institute Inc., Cary, NC, USA).

3. Results

According to NAMCS-NHAMCS 2005–2011, approximately 9.3 million ambulatory visits (national estimation) recorded PD diagnosis, among which approximately 1.7 million visits (18.18%, 95% confidence interval (CI): 13.03%–23.33%) recorded a concurrent depression diagnosis forming the final study sample.

Individual-level characteristics of the study sample in terms of predisposing, enabling, and need factors are provided in Table 1 as weighted frequencies of visits in millions (national level) and their corresponding weighted percentages. Majority of the visits by the study sample consisted of individuals aged 75 years and older (55.29%), men (54.45%), and whites (non-Hispanic) (87.03%), who resided in metropolitan areas (79.07%), had some form of government insurance (85.04%) and were from Southern US (48.59%). An overwhelming majority (86.59%) of the study sample visits were recorded in physician/clinic specialties other than general and family practice and involved patients already established with the physician/clinic (87.16%). Mean total number of medications used and total chronic conditions recoded was 4.79 (S.E. 0.36) and 3.20 (S.E. 0.28), respectively (data not presented in tabular form), in the study sample.

Depression treatment (antidepressant with or without psychotherapy) was recorded in 57.63% (95% CI: 44.30%–70.97%) of the study sample visits. Among antidepressants, SSRIs were the most prescribed class, accounting for approximately 70% of antidepressant use (69.57%, 95% CI: 49.36%–89.78%). We were not able to estimate the national-level percentage of older adults with dPD receiving psychotherapy due to small sample size ($N = 5$).

Table 2 summarizes findings from the multivariate logistic regression analyses to ascertain the predictors of depression treatment. Men were 64% less likely (adjusted odds ratio (AOR): 0.36, 95% CI: 0.14–0.93) than women to receive depression treatment. Individuals with dPD and polypharmacy were 74% more likely to receive depression treatment (odds ratio = 1.743, 95% CI 1.376–2.209), while dPD subjects with comorbid chronic conditions were 44% less likely (odds ratio = 0.559, 95% CI 0.396–0.790) to receive depression treatment.

4. Discussion

To the best of our knowledge, this is the first study to assess the depression treatment patterns and predictors among older adults with dPD at the national level in the US ambulatory care settings. Presence of depression has been associated with death or suicidal ideation [23], and hence, understanding depression treatment patterns in this vulnerable population is critical. Our study findings suggest that approximately six out of ten older adults with dPD received some form of depression treatment during their ambulatory visits. This estimate is higher compared to previous studies examining depression treatment patterns among individuals with dPD [18, 24]. A study by Weintraub et al. [18] using a convenience sample of patients at a PD center observed that among individuals with PD who met depressive disorder criteria, only one-third of them received antidepressant treatment. The study by Bega et al. [24] used the National Parkinson Foundation-Quality Improvement Initiative (NPF-QII) data and found that among individuals with PD meeting the depression diagnosis cut-off, only 33% used antidepressants, 6% used health services, and 14% used combination of antidepressants and health services. The convenience sample used by Weintraub et al. [18] or the NPF-QII data [24] are not nationally representative sample of US and as such lacks generalizability. Moreover, the data from Weintraub et al. [18] is more than a decade old. It is possible that the depression treatment patterns have changed since this published study. Although it is difficult to make direct comparisons between our study sample and these published studies, our findings show higher proportions of depression treatment.

Findings from our study indicate that SSRIs were the most prescribed antidepressant class (representing 70% of the overall antidepressant use) among older adults with dPD. This estimate is similar to the Weintraub et al. [18] study, which observed 69.6% of antidepressant use to be accounted by SSRIs. Despite the high use of SSRIs to treat depression among individuals with PD, a recent network meta-analysis [25] demonstrated that evidence to support efficacy and acceptability of SSRIs to treat depression in PD is insufficient and concluded that SSRIs may actually be the last treatment choice in these patients. Hence, findings from our study have implications for current practice. Tricyclic antidepressants can alternatively be considered given they have demonstrated ability to delay the need for dopaminergic therapy in early PD [26]. However, while anticholinergic medications such as tricyclic antidepressants can improve movement problems in PD, they carry the risk of adverse mental effects such as confusion, memory problems, hallucinations, and restlessness [27, 28]. In an existing literature review [29], it was summarized that while case reports have suggested SSRIs may worsen motor symptoms, these disturbances are reversible and generally not severe. A prior prospective study found no difference in serious extrapyramidal symptoms with the use of antidepressants versus dopaminergic drugs in dPD [30], and it is reported the potential benefit of SSRIs in dPD outweigh the risk [31]. Further studies are still needed to clarify whether SSRIs represent the best therapeutic index among available classes of agents.

Our study observed that males were less likely to receive depression treatment compared to females. Although studies

TABLE 1: Demographic and clinical characteristics and depression treatment of older adults with Parkinson disease and depression.

Characteristics	Wt. Freq. (millions)	Wt. %
Predisposing factors		
Age		
65–74	0.756	44.70
≥75	0.935	55.30
Gender		
Male	0.921	54.45
Female	0.770	45.55
Race/ethnicity		
White only, NH	1.472	87.03
Others	0.219	12.97
Geo region		
West	0.288	17.05
Northeast	0.384	22.72
Midwest	0.197	11.64
South	0.822	48.59
Metro status		
Metro	1.337	79.07
Nonmetro	0.354	20.93
Enabling factors		
Insurance		
Govt. insurance	1.438	85.04
Others	0.253	14.96
Physician/clinic specialty		
General and family practice	0.227	13.41
Others	1.464	86.59
Need factors		
New prescription during visit		
≥1	0.723	42.74
No	0.968	57.26
New patient		
Yes	0.217	12.84
No	1.474	87.16
Anti-Parkinson medication		
Yes	0.750	44.36
No	0.941	55.64
Chronic diseases		
Arthritis	0.411	24.31
Asthma	0.130	7.71
Cancer	0.084	4.97
CHF	0.556	3.29
COPD	0.194	11.49
Diabetes	0.624	36.91
HYPLIPID	0.649	38.36
HTN	0.832	49.17
IHD	0.338	19.96
CEBVD	0.199	11.78
Osteoporosis	0.088	5.19

TABLE 1: Continued.

Characteristics	Wt. Freq. (millions)	Wt. %
Overall depression treatment		
Depression treatment	0.975	57.63

Note. Based on unweighted N = 133 (nationally representative weighted N = 1.7 million) ambulatory visits of older adults (age ≥ 65 years) with Parkinson's disease and depression using NAMCS and NHAMCS 2005–2011 data; NAMCS: National Ambulatory Medical Care Survey; NHAMCS: National Hospital Ambulatory Medical Care Survey; Wt: weighted; Freq.: frequency; NH: non-Hispanic; Govt.: government; CHF: congestive heart failure; COPD: chronic obstructive pulmonary disease; HYPLIPID: hyperlipidemia; HTN: hypertension; IHD: ischemic heart disease; CEBVD: cerebrovascular disease.

specific to ambulatory settings are lacking, this finding is consistent with a study by Fernandez et al. [32] among nursing home PD residents, which observed that irrespective of behavioral symptoms, females with PD were more likely to receive antidepressants compared to males. This can partly be attributed to the fact that women with PD exhibit higher depression rates compared to men [33]. Our finding is also consistent with that of the general population that shows women to be two-and-half times more likely to receive antidepressants compared to men [34]. Piecing together findings from our study and existing studies, we can speculate presence of gender differences in terms of depression and antidepressant use among individuals with PD, and future research is warranted to elucidate and address this difference.

Our study findings indicate that the chances of receiving antidepressants were positively correlated with total number of medications recorded at the sampled visit. This may reflect a higher likelihood of prescribing antidepressants to PD patients with more advanced disease progression. It should be noted that this does not necessarily signify dPD patients having a delay in treatment, since psychotherapy is sometimes used in place of medication to avoid polypharmacy. Polypharmacy may lead to higher risk of adverse events such as fall frequency, fall severity, hyponatremia, bleeding, and drug-drug interactions [35]. Hence, healthcare providers should be aware of the overall medication burden and specific drug interactions when prescribing SSRIs for dPD. Finally, we observed that there was a lower likelihood of receiving depression treatment with increase in number of chronic diseases. This finding can be partially explained by competing demands arising from presence of other chronic conditions [36], having to rule out depression due to underlying untreated/unresolved medical conditions, as well as presence of drug-drug interactions [37].

The following limitations should be kept in mind while interpreting these findings. There is a possibility of statistical under power as the final unweighted study sample (N = 133) was small. Chances of underestimation of disease conditions are possible as NAMCS and NHAMCS provide up to only three diagnoses per visit. Our study did not adjust for sedation, pain, sleep, and appetite stimulation for which antidepressants are also prescribed. Existing literature suggests that the ICD-9-CM code of 332.0 is often used to identify

TABLE 2: Predictors of depression treatment among older adults with Parkinson disease and depression.

Characteristics	Odds ratio	95% CI	Significance
Predisposing factors			
Age			
65–74	Ref.		
≥75	1.008	0.24, 4.26	0.9909
Gender*			
Female	Ref.		
Male	0.359	0.14, 0.93	0.0361
Race/ethnicity			
White only, NH	1.044	0.18, 6.1	0.9611
Other	Ref.		
Geographic region			
South	0.519	0.23, 1.15	0.1025
Other	Ref.		
Metro			
Metro	Ref.		
Nonmetro	0.584	0.11, 3.22	0.5276
Enabling factors			
Physician/clinical specialty			
General and family practice	Ref.		
Others	2.943	0.57, 15.16	0.1903
Insurance			
Govt. insurance	Ref.		
Others	0.776	0.23, 2.63	0.6755
Need factors			
New prescription			
No	Ref.		
≥1	3.019	0.99, 9.12	0.0501
Patient established			
New	Ref.		
Yes	5.43	0.66, 44.97	0.1134
Number of medications*	1.743	1.38, 2.21	<0.0001
Number of chronic conditions*	0.559	0.39, 0.79	0.0016

Note. Based on unweighted $N = 133$ (nationally representative weighted $N = 1.7$ million) ambulatory visits of older adults (age ≥ 65 years) with Parkinson's disease and depression using NAMCS and NHAMCS 2005–2011 data; NAMCS: National Ambulatory Medical Care Survey; NHAMCS: National Hospital Ambulatory Medical Care Survey; Ref.: reference group; AOR: adjusted odds ratio; CI: confidence interval; NH: non-Hispanic; NUMMED: total number of medications; TOTCHRON: total number of chronic conditions; *statistically significant at $p < 0.05$.

other conditions such as atypical parkinsonism, drug-induced parkinsonism, and idiopathic PD, and this code is unable to differentiate between parkinsonism and PD [38]. Hence, another limitation of this study is that the use of the 332.xx code may not be able to distinguish between PD and other forms of parkinsonism. We did not have information related to duration and severity of PD and depression, antidepressant dose, activities of daily living, instrumental activities of daily living, and functional status. Patient and

physician preferences were also not available in the dataset. Furthermore, to achieve appropriate relative standard error, several variable categories (such as antidepressant classes) had to be combined to achieve reliable estimates, and we were not able to estimate the national-level estimate for psychotherapy use. Some other limitations include the possibility for reporting errors and coding errors, and interviewer effects should also be considered. Causal inferences cannot be reached due to the cross-sectional study design. Finally, we were able to use up to 2011 data, as the latest publically available OPD NHAMCS data is up to 2011.

5. Conclusion

Approximately six out of ten older adults in the US with PD and depression received depression treatment. SSRIs were most frequently prescribed, and gender, number of medications prescribed during visit, and number of chronic conditions were significantly associated with depression treatment among older adults with dPD. Psychotherapy is underutilized in this study sample. Future real-world long-term studies should investigate health outcomes associated with depression treatment in this vulnerable population.

Disclosure

A part of this work was presented as poster at the 2017 Annual International Meeting of the International Society for Pharmacoeconomics and Outcomes Research on May 20–24, Boston, MA, USA.

References

[1] C. M. Tanner and S. M. Goldman, "Epidemiology of Parkinson's disease," *Neurologic Clinics*, vol. 14, no. 2, pp. 317–335, 1996.

[2] J. Jankovic, "Parkinson's disease: clinical features and diagnosis," *Journal of Neurology, Neurosurgery & Psychiatry*, vol. 79, no. 4, pp. 368–376, 2008.

[3] J. S. Reijnders, U. Ehrt, W. E. Weber, D. Aarsland, and A. F. Leentjens, "A systematic review of prevalence studies of depression in Parkinson's disease," *Movement Disorders*, vol. 23, no. 2, pp. 183–189, 2008.

[4] W. M. McDonald, I. H. Richard, and M. R. DeLong, "Prevalence, etiology, and treatment of depression in Parkinson's disease," *Biological Psychiatry*, vol. 54, no. 3, pp. 363–375, 2003.

[5] F. Blandini, G. Nappi, C. Tassorelli, and E. Martignoni, "Functional changes of the basal ganglia circuitry in Parkinson's disease," *Progress in Neurobiology*, vol. 62, no. 1, pp. 63–88, 2000.

[6] M. A. Menza and M. H. Mark, "Parkinson's disease and depression: the relationship to disability and personality," *Journal of Neuropsychiatry and Clinical Neurosciences*, vol. 6, no. 2, pp. 165–169, 1994.

[7] T. S. Ehmann, R. J. Beninger, M. J. Gawel, and R. J. Riopelle, "Depressive symptoms in Parkinson's disease: a comparison

with disabled control subjects," *Journal of Geriatric Psychiatry and Neurology*, vol. 3, no. 1, pp. 3–9, 1990.

[8] S. Papapetropoulos, J. Ellul, A. A. Argyriou, E. Chroni, and N. P. Lekka, "The effect of depression on motor function and disease severity of Parkinson's disease," *Clinical Neurology and Neurosurgery*, vol. 108, no. 5, pp. 465–469, 2006.

[9] I. H. Richard, A. W. Justus, and R. Kurlan, "Relationship between mood and motor fluctuations in Parkinson's disease," *Journal of Neuropsychiatry and Clinical Neurosciences*, vol. 13, no. 1, pp. 35–41, 2001.

[10] R. A. Maricle, J. G. Nutt, and J. H. Carter, "Mood and anxiety fluctuation in Parkinson's disease associated with levodopa infusion: preliminary findings," *Movement Disorders*, vol. 10, no. 3, pp. 329–332, 1995.

[11] A. Schrag, "Quality of life and depression in Parkinson's disease," *Journal of the Neurological Sciences*, vol. 248, no. 1-2, pp. 151–157, 2006.

[12] L. C. Tan, "Mood disorders in Parkinson's disease," *Parkinsonism & Related Disorders*, vol. 18, no. 1, pp. S74–S76, 2012.

[13] M. Menza, R. D. Dobkin, H. Marin et al., "The impact of treatment of depression on quality of life, disability and relapse in patients with Parkinson's disease," *Movement Disorders*, vol. 24, no. 9, pp. 1325–1332, 2009.

[14] R. D. Dobkin, M. Menza, L. A. Allen et al., "Cognitive-behavioral therapy for depression in Parkinson's disease: a randomized, controlled trial," *American Journal of Psychiatry*, vol. 168, no. 10, pp. 1066–1074, 2011.

[15] T. C. van der Hoek, B. A. Bus, P. Matui, M. A. van der Marck, R. A. Esselink, and I. Tendolkar, "Prevalence of depression in Parkinson's disease: effects of disease stage, motor subtype and gender," *Journal of the Neurological Sciences*, vol. 310, no. 1-2, pp. 220–224, 2011.

[16] A. Althaus, O. A. Becker, A. Spottke et al., "Frequency and treatment of depressive symptoms in a Parkinson's disease registry," *Parkinsonism & Related Disorders*, vol. 14, no. 8, pp. 626–632, 2008.

[17] D. K. Worku, Y. M. Yifru, D. G. Postels, and F. E. Gashe, "Prevalence of depression in Parkinson's disease patients in Ethiopia," *Journal of Clinical Movement Disorders*, vol. 1, no. 1, p. 10, 2014.

[18] D. Weintraub, P. J. Moberg, J. E. Duda, I. R. Katz, and M. B. Stern, "Recognition and treatment of depression in Parkinson's disease," *Journal of Geriatric Psychiatry and Neurology*, vol. 16, no. 3, pp. 178–183, 2003.

[19] Centers for Disease Control and Prevention: National Center for Health Statistics, "Ambulatory health care data," August 2017, http://www.cdc.gov/nchs/ahcd/index.htm.

[20] J. R. Avasarala, C. A. O'Donovan, S. E. Roach, F. Camacho, and S. R. Feldman, "Analysis of NAMCS data for multiple sclerosis, 1998–2004," *BMC Medicine*, vol. 5, no. 1, p. 6, 2007.

[21] I. S. Zenlea, C. E. Milliren, L. Mednick, and E. T. Rhodes, "Depression screening in adolescents in the United States: a national study of ambulatory office-based practice," *Academic Pediatrics*, vol. 14, no. 2, pp. 186–191, 2014.

[22] J. G. Anderson and D. E. Bartkus, "Choice of medical care: a behavioral model of health and illness behavior," *Journal of Health and Social Behavior*, vol. 14, no. 4, pp. 348–362, 1973.

[23] S. Nazem, A. D. Siderowf, J. E. Duda et al., "Suicidal and death ideation in Parkinson's disease," *Movement Disorders*, vol. 23, no. 11, pp. 1573–1579, 2008.

[24] D. Bega, S. S. Wu, Q. Pei, P. N. Schmidt, and T. Simuni, "Recognition and treatment of depressive symptoms in Parkinson's disease: the NPF dataset," *Journal of Parkinson's Disease*, vol. 4, pp. 639–643, 2014.

[25] J. Liu, J. Dong, L. Wang, Y. Su, P. Yan, and S. Sun, "Comparative efficacy and acceptability of antidepressants in Parkinson's disease: a network meta-analysis," *PLoS One*, vol. 8, no. 10, article e76651, 2013.

[26] K. L. Paumier, A. D. Siderowf, P. Auinger et al., "Tricyclic antidepressants delay the need for dopaminergic therapy in early Parkinson's disease," *Movement Disorders*, vol. 27, no. 7, pp. 880–887, 2012.

[27] U. Ehrt, K. Broich, J. P. Larsen, C. Ballard, and D. Aarsland, "Use of drugs with anticholinergic effect and impact on cognition in Parkinson's disease: a cohort study," *Journal of Neurology, Neurosurgery & Psychiatry*, vol. 81, no. 2, pp. 160–165, 2010.

[28] R. Katzenschlager, C. Sampaio, J. Costa, and A. Lees, "Anticholinergics for symptomatic management of Parkinson's disease," *Cochrane Database of Systematic Reviews*, no. 3, article no. CD003735, 2002.

[29] T. A. Zesiewicz, M. Gold, G. Chari, and R. A. Hauser, "Current issues in depression in Parkinson's disease," *American Journal of Geriatric Psychiatry*, vol. 7, no. 2, pp. 110–118, 1999.

[30] M. Gony, M. Lapeyre-Mestre, J. L. Montastruc, and French Network of Regional Pharmacovigilance C, "Risk of serious extrapyramidal symptoms in patients with Parkinson's disease receiving antidepressant drugs: a pharmacoepidemiologic study comparing serotonin reuptake inhibitors and other antidepressant drugs," *Clinical Neuropharmacology*, vol. 26, no. 3, pp. 142–145, 2003.

[31] M. Menza, R. D. Dobkin, and H. Marin, "Treatment of depression in Parkinson's disease," *Current Psychiatry Reports*, vol. 8, no. 3, pp. 234–240, 2006.

[32] H. H. Fernandez, K. L. Lapane, B. R. Ott, J. H. Friedman, and SAGE Study Group, "Gender differences in the frequency and treatment of behavior problems in Parkinson's disease," *Movement Disorders*, vol. 15, no. 3, pp. 490–496, 2000.

[33] I. N. Miller and A. Cronin-Golomb, "Gender differences in Parkinson's disease: clinical characteristics and cognition," *Movement Disorders*, vol. 25, no. 16, pp. 2695–2703, 2010.

[34] L. A. Pratt, D. J. Brody, and Q. Gu, "Antidepressant use in persons aged 12 and over: United States, 2005–2008," August 2017, http://www.cdc.gov/nchs/data/databriefs/db76.pdf.

[35] K. Richardson, K. Bennett, and R. A. Kenny, "Polypharmacy including falls risk-increasing medications and subsequent falls in community-dwelling middle-aged and older adults," *Age and Ageing*, vol. 44, no. 1, pp. 90–96, 2015.

[36] K. Rost, P. Nutting, J. Smith, J. C. Coyne, L. Cooper-Patrick, and L. Rubenstein, "The role of competing demands in the treatment provided primary care patients with major depression," *Archives of Family Medicine*, vol. 9, no. 2, pp. 150–154, 2000.

[37] E. Spina, V. Santoro, and C. D'Arrigo, "Clinically relevant pharmacokinetic drug interactions with second-generation antidepressants: an update," *Clinical Therapeutics*, vol. 30, no. 7, pp. 1206–1227, 2008.

[38] K. Swarztrauber, J. Anau, and D. Peters, "Identifying and distinguishing cases of parkinsonism and Parkinson's disease using ICD-9 CM codes and pharmacy data," *Movement Disorders*, vol. 20, no. 8, pp. 964–970, 2005.

14

Programming for Stimulation-Induced Transient Nonmotor Psychiatric Symptoms after Bilateral Subthalamic Nucleus Deep Brain Stimulation for Parkinson's Disease

Xi Wu,[1] Yiqing Qiu,[1] Keith Simfukwe,[2] Jiali Wang,[1] Jianchun Chen,[1] and Xiaowu Hu[1]

[1]Department of Neurosurgery, Second Military Medical University, Changhai Hospital, No. 168 Changhai Road, Yangpu District, Shanghai, China
[2]Department of Neurosurgery, Changhai Hospital, Second Military Medical University, International College of Exchange, No. 800 Xiangyin Road, Shanghai 200433, China

Correspondence should be addressed to Xiaowu Hu; huxiaowu_smmu@sina.com

Academic Editor: Hélio Teive

Background. Stimulation-induced transient nonmotor psychiatric symptoms (STPSs) are side effects following bilateral subthalamic nucleus deep brain stimulation (STN-DBS) in Parkinson's disease (PD) patients. We designed algorithms which (1) determine the electrode contacts that induce STPSs and (2) provide a programming protocol to eliminate STPS and maintain the optimal motor functions. Our objective is to test the effectiveness of these algorithms. *Materials and Methods.* 454 PD patients who underwent programming sessions after STN-DBS implantations were retrospectively analyzed. Only STPS patients were enrolled. In these patients, the contacts inducing STPS were found and the programming protocol algorithms used. *Results.* Eleven patients were diagnosed with STPS. Of these patients, two had four episodes of crying, and two had four episodes of mirthful laughter. In one patient, two episodes of abnormal sense of spatial orientation were observed. Hallucination episodes were observed twice in one patient, while five patients recorded eight episodes of hypomania. There were no statistical differences between the UPDRS-III under the final stimulation parameter (without STPS) and previous optimum UPDRS-III under the STPSs ($p = 1.000$). *Conclusion.* The flow diagram used for determining electrode contacts that induce STPS and the programming protocol employed in the treatment of these symptoms are effective.

1. Introductions

Subthalamic nucleus deep brain stimulation (STN-DBS) is an effective therapy which ameliorates motor manifestations suffered by patients with idiopathic Parkinson's disease (PD). The hallmark symptoms in PD patients include tremor, rigidity, and bradykinesia. STN-DBS has been documented to be well tolerated by PD patients with marked improvement of motor functions even after over ten-year follow-up [1–3]. The limbic system innervates the limbic part of STN and other anatomic surrounding structures that lay in proximity [4]. As a result, the likelihood of accidental tempering of these nearby anatomical structures during STN-DBS may result in psychiatric symptoms called stimulation-induced transient nonmotor psychiatric symptoms (STPS), which are

clinically manifested as depression [5], anxiety [6], apathy [7], explosive-aggressive behavior [8], manic episode [9], mirthful laughter [10], impulse control disorders [11], and so forth. Like other nonmotor functions, in some instances, STPS may have a drastic impact on a patient's life quality of life. [12]. It has been noted that the stimulation parameters which induce STPS are usually higher than normal. Decreasing stimulation intensity on the Implantable Pulsar Generator (IPG) may eliminate STPS. However, patients' motor functions may also be exacerbated. Changhai Hospital Neurosurgery Department conducts more than 160 DBS implantation surgeries every year. Since December 2014, the therapeutic center for Parkinson's disease in Changhai Hospital, Shanghai, China, has designed and implemented (1) an algorithm that identifies specific electrode contacts

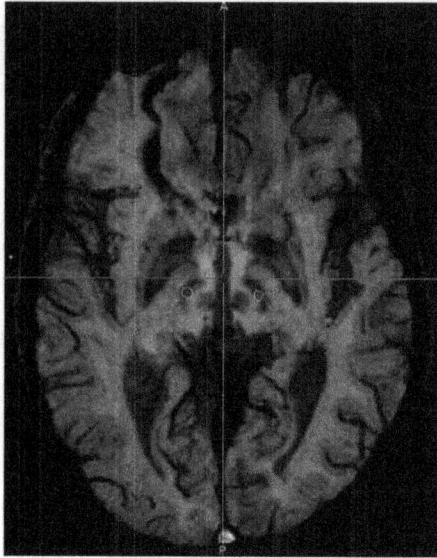

Figure 1: Merging SWI sequence with postoperation CT to determine the electrode position.

that induce STPS (2) a programming protocol to eliminate STPS. This study aim is to assess the effectiveness of these algorithms.

2. Materials and Methods

2.1. Patients. After acquiring approval from the Ethics Committee of Changhai Hospital, we retrospectively analyzed all patients with idiopathic Parkinson's disease who received clinical programming of implanted bilateral STN-DBS in the DBS programming clinic of Changhai Hospital, Shanghai, China, from January 1, 2015, to December 31, 2015. Patients who are being initiated on DBS, as well as those receiving follow-up programming sessions due to various reasons after achieving optimal stimulation parameters, were included in the present study. The UK PD Brain Bank diagnostic criteria were adopted for the diagnosis of idiopathic Parkinson's disease.

2.2. Mapping the Active Contact. If the active contact is not within the STN, the programming protocol may be less effective. Therefore we reviewed intraoperative MRI of all the patients with Leksell G frame and indicator to confirm the electrode location. The Medtronic S7 Neuro Navigation System (Medtronic Navigation, Louisville, USA) was used to merge preoperative 3.0T-MRI images with postoperative CT images. The CT scan images were calibrated at 1 mm thickness and without pneumocranium (Figure 1). It was essential that the active contact center is placed within the boundaries of the STN. Patients with the active contact center outside STN boundary were excluded from this study.

2.3. Motor Assessment. Patient's motor function was graded using the Unified Parkinson's Disease Rating Scale Part III (UPDRS-III, 1998 edition). All patients included in this study were assessed preoperatively, postoperatively and then, finally, before and after the occurrence of STPS. All clinicians who administered the Unified Parkinson's Disease Rating Scale in this study are board-certified with the International Parkinson and Movement Disorder Society.

2.4. Cognitive and Psychiatric Assessment. All patients with STPS were enrolled in this study. Patients that had any mild psychiatric episodes that occurred more than twice as a result of programming (increasing) the electrode power parameters at home by oneself or caregivers were enrolled in this study. Episodes of acute psychiatric symptoms during or after the clinic programming procedures were also enlisted. Patients with psychiatric symptoms similar to the preoperative ones or had changed medication dose in less than one month were excluded. This was because it would be difficult to confirm whether the symptoms were induced by electric stimulation or not. So, only new postoperative psychiatric symptoms were regarded as suspicious STPS. The litmus test for STPS identification was defined by (1) psychiatric symptoms of patients which improved after decreasing stimulation intensity in 30 minutes; however, this could also confirm that the STPS was induced by stimulation because it occurred at the time when stimulation intensity was increased to improve the patient's motor functions, (2) patients who must have no similar history of psychiatric symptoms and upon clinical programming have shown marked improvement within three months without any change in the medication, and (3) identification of causative STPS active contact.

Cognitive and depressive symptoms were evaluated preoperatively and graded using Unified Parkinson's Disease Rating Scale Parts I and II (UPDRS-I and UPDRS-II), the Mini-Mental State Examination (MMSE), and the 17-item Hamilton Depression Scale (HAM-D-17). Mania type STPS was graded using the Young Mania Rating Scale (YMRS) [13]. The YMRS was calculated using patient collateral history from caregivers and direct observation by the physicians. Patients with STPS while being initiated on IPG were recorded using preoperative evaluation results only.

2.5. Assessment of STPS and Recording of Stimulation Parameters. Patient's collateral history regarding unusual psychiatric symptoms recorded in programming sessions was reviewed. Stimulus parameters (active, stimulating contacts, stimulating pattern, voltage/current, pulse width, and frequency) were recorded following the occurrence of STPS. Changes and the final status of stimulation parameters in programming sessions were also recorded. Electrode contacts inducing STPS and programming protocols were determined according to previously established flow diagrams (Figures 2 and 3). The disappearance of STPS was determined by no relapse of similar psychiatric symptoms for three months after programming.

2.6. Statistical Analysis. Paired-sample t-test was used to examine for changes of variables in UPDRS-III during clinical evaluation. $p < 0.05$ was considered statistically significant.

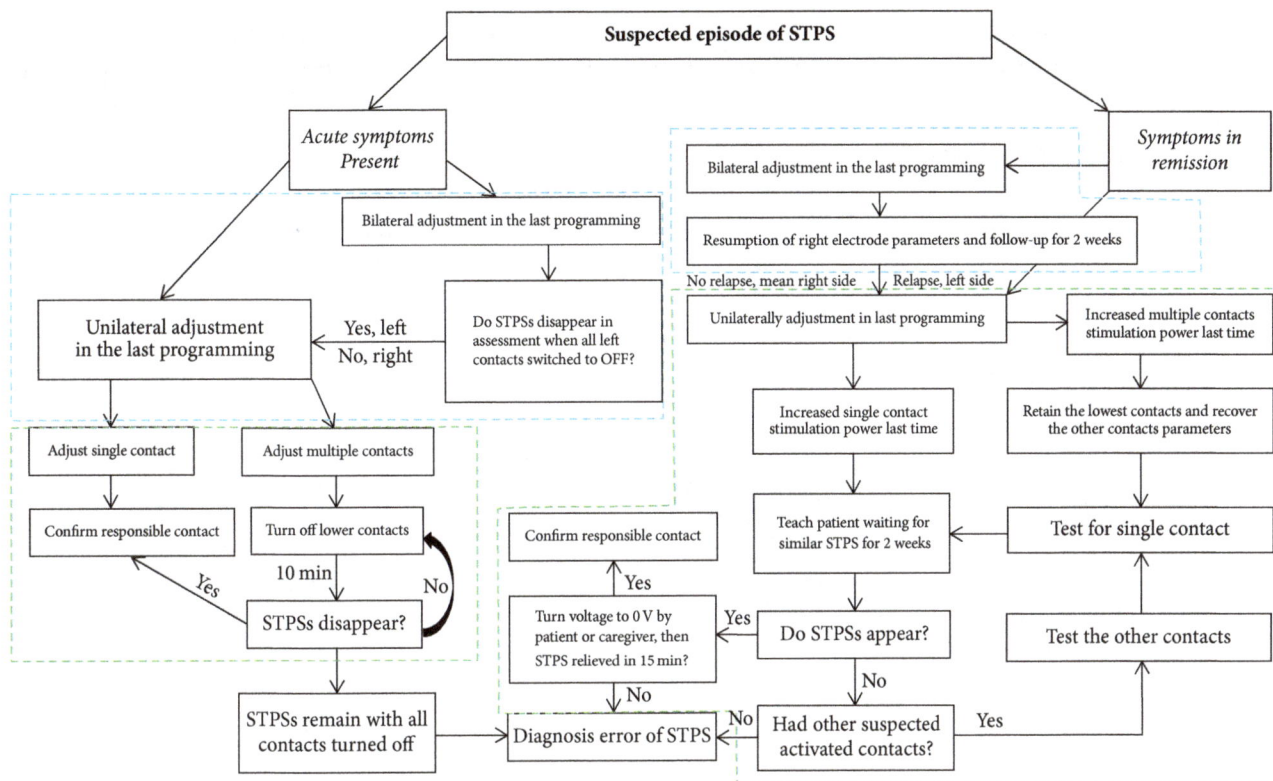

FIGURE 2: Flow diagram to determine electrode contacts inducing STPS.

3. Results

3.1. Baseline Data. There were three groups of patients enrolled in this study: (1) the first group is comprised of 145 patients undergoing DBS initiation 1 month postoperatively for optimal programming parameter; (2) the second group had 231 patients who underwent DBS less than one year postoperatively; (3) finally, the third group had 166 patients who underwent DBS more than one year postoperatively. There were a total number of 1142 episodes of clinical programming for the purpose of adjusting the stimulation parameters in the second and third groups. There were 20 episodes of STPS that occurred in 11 patients (6 females and 5 males). The mean age at the time of DBS surgery was 63.45 ± 8.27 years. The mean duration between identification of Parkinsonian symptoms and DBS surgery was 11.91 ± 3.33 years. Cognitive functional impairment was excluded in all patients. Only six patients received antidepressant drugs before and after surgery, while the rest of the patients had no obvious depression symptoms. Preoperatively, patients were given an average Levodopa Equivalent Daily Dose (LEDD) of 942.5 ± 232.7 mg. Postoperatively, before the STPS occurred, the LEDD was reduced to 404.5 ± 353.3 mg. By the time programming eliminated STPS at 3 months after programming,

the LEDD had further reduced to 284.5 ± 187.8 mg. The UPDRS-III improvement rate between postoperative (med-off time) status and preoperative (med-off time) status was 35.14~72.34% at 3 months after programming. When we compared the baseline data of STPS + patients versus STPS − patients to characterize patients inherent risk factors for STPS, no significant statistical difference was found between groups (see Table 1).

3.2. STPS Occurrence. During the programming, 20 episodes of STPS occurred in 11 patients. These psychiatric symptoms consisted of four (04) episodes of crying in two (02) patients, four (04) episodes of inexplicable euphoria or mirthful laughter in two (02) patients, two (02) episodes of spatial disorientation in one patient, two (02) episodes of hallucination in one patient, and eight (08) episodes of hypomania in five (05) patients. In five (05) patients, STPS occurred during titration adjustment for optimal programming parameter in the first year after devices were implanted, while two (02) patients showed psychiatric symptoms two days after being started on IPG and discharged from the hospital. For patients who had implanted devices for more than one year, three (03) developed STPS during programming sessions. Manifestations of patients during STPS episodes

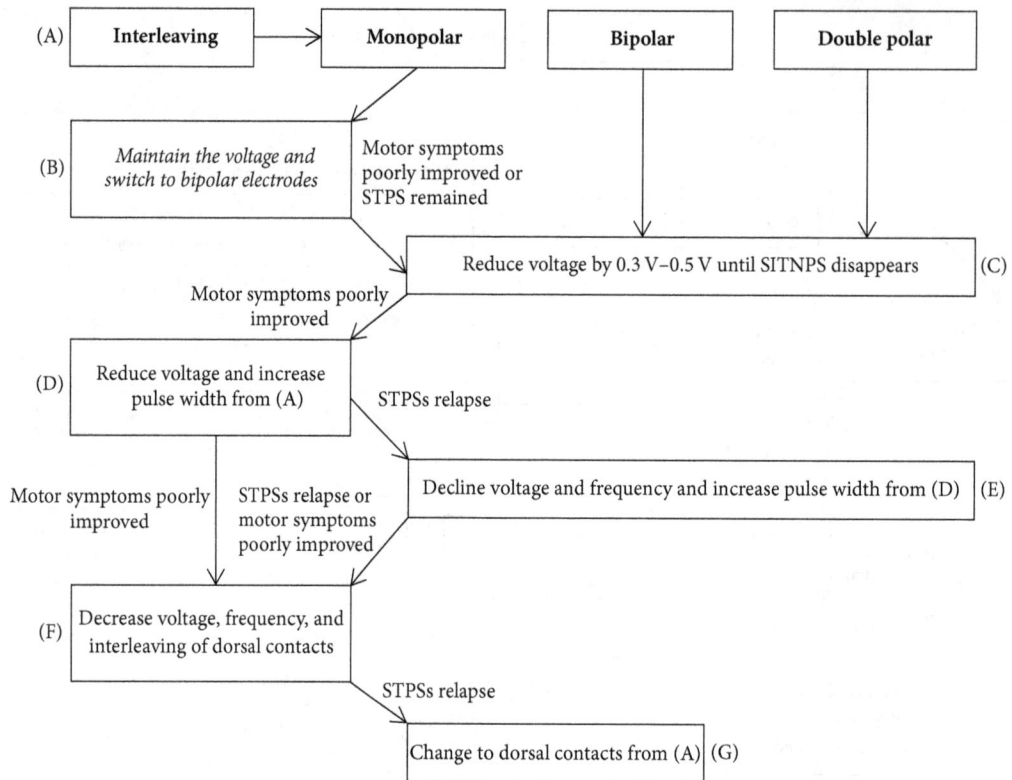

FIGURE 3: Programming protocol flow diagram (After determining STPS causative active contacts with Figure 2, (A) record the initial parameters and programming according to the stimulation mode; (D) recover the initial parameters and reduce voltage 0.3 V–0.5 V and increase pulse width by 10–20 μs; (E) if STPS relapsed, then reduce voltage 0.1–0.3 V and reduce frequency 10–30 Hz, increase pulse width 10–20 μs, and keep the total electrical energy delivered (TEED) equal to the counterpart of (D), TEED = voltage^2 × frequency × pulse width/impedance; (F) decrease frequency to 125 Hz and decrease voltage 0.3–0.5 V, and keep the TEED equal or slightly higher to the counterpart of (D) or (E); activate the other dorsal contact with interleaving mode.).

were described in Table 2. The stimulation parameters before the onset of STPS were listed in Table 3.

3.3. Programming of STPS and Motor Functions.

Following the adjustment of stimulation parameters (Table 3), ten patients maintained the improvement of motor functions with psychiatric symptoms eliminated. The adjustments were based on the algorithms as follows: (1) the stimulation voltage decreased while the pulse width increased in 2 patients (numbers 1 and 11); (2) the voltage was maintained while switching to bipolar stimulation in 2 patients (numbers 2 and 7); (3) voltage and frequency were decreased with pulse width increased in 1 patient (number 9); (4) voltage and frequency were decreased while switching to interleaving stimulation in 3 patients (numbers 3, 4, and 10); (5) the activation contacts were replaced with dorsal ones in 2 patients (numbers 5 and 8). One patient (number 6), after multiple programming sessions, developed concurrent motor and nonmotor functions, and UPDRS-III score increased by 2 points under the final stimulation parameters by her choice (see details of the programming duration in Table 4). There were no statistical differences between the UPDRS-III under the final stimulation parameter (without STPSs) and optimum UPDRS-III under the STPSs (26.45 ± 10.59 versus 26.45 ± 10.17, $p = 1.000$).

4. Discussion

4.1. The Clinical Value of Programming Algorithms for STPS.

Since the application of STN-DBS in the treatment of PD patients, there have been sporadic reports [10] noting STPSs, as one of the side effects. The development of these programming algorithms is aiming to reduce the ambiguity in the management of STPS. The ambiguity was on the predisposition of the following. (1) In earlier studies, STPS was implicated with stimulation of the medial and inferior part (limbic part) of STN. However, recent studies show their active contacts located in the dorsolateral (sensorimotor) area of STN [14] which also induces STPS. Because of this reason, the limbic and sensorimotor regions of the STN overlap were greater than what has been previously reported [15]. In this study, we also found that the active contacts which induced STPS were located at a medial and inferior part of the STN in seven (07) patients. In the other four (04) patients, the active contacts were located in the lateral part of STN which also induced STPS. This is similar to what was reported by Abulseoud and colleagues [14]. For this reason, we concluded that the side effects of STPS are difficult to avoid by just implanting contacts into dorsolateral STN. (2) Secondly, under the routine stimulation parameter, the spherical radius of active volume (without contacts volume)

TABLE 1

(a) Baseline clinical data of patients who developed STPS.

	Age	Gender	Duration (year)	MMSE	HAMD (α)	LEDD pre-op (mg)	LEED STPS Emerged	LEDD 3 m post-STPS (mg)	UPDRS I	UPDRS II	UPDRS-III Pre-op med-off	UPDRS-III Pre-op med-on	UPDRS IV
PD1	61	M	17	29	19 (14)	1200	1200	550	8	17	47	13	3
PD2	52	M	14	29	10	900	125	125	4	18	41	15	6
PD3	59	F	8	30	21 (16)	768	325	300	7	24	53	26	9
PD4	74	M	7	26	10	563	175	175	6	31	37	24	11
PD5	61	M	8	29	17 (10)	825	825	280	5	11	43	15	10
PD6	58	M	11	26	30 (17)	1100	325	325	10	18	75	42	4
PD7	52	F	15	27	11	963	75	75	2	13	70	34	3
PD8	75	F	13	27	16	1287	300	200	4	20	81	37	8
PD9	72	F	10	28	8	787	250	250	4	13	27	16	4
PD10	64	F	13	26	24 (13)	750	150	150	5	16	51	28	7
PD11	70	F	15	27	30 (16)	1225	700	700	9	22	63	31	10

α: post-antidepression treatment; LEDD: Levodopa Equivalent Daily Dose.

(b) Compare the baseline data of STPS positive Versus STPS negative patients.

	STPS+	STPS−	p value
Patient	11	443$^\beta$	
Age	63.45 ± 8.28	62.05 ± 7.78	0.555
Disease duration to DBS	11.91 ± 3.33	9.95 ± 4.03	0.112
LEDD pre-op (mg)	942.55 ± 232.67	836.32 ± 393.79	0.374
UPDRS-III med-off pre-op	53.45 ± 16.94	52.46 ± 14.24	0.819
UPDRS-III med-on pre-op	25.55 ± 9.91	25.80 ± 11.14	0.940
MMSE	27.64 ± 1.43	27.07 ± 2.57	0.463
HAMD before receiving antidepressant drug	17.82 ± 7.85	20.71 ± 6.21	0.130

β: 443 patients included three groups: 145 patients initiated the IPG and 99 of them achieved the optimal programming parameters before the study was finished; the 99 patients and other 132 patient who achieved the optimal programming parameters received STN-DBS for less than one year. 166 patients had received STN-DBS for more than one year: 145 + 132 + 166 = 443.

TABLE 2: Clinical manifestations of STPS.

| Number | Times | Description of episode | | Interval between episode and operation | Time of occurrence | Relationship with medication | Duration |
		Chief complaints and symptoms	YMRS				
(1)	1	Inexplicable euphoria (sense of floating)	22	Postoperative 1 month (newly activated)	Day 1 after hospital discharge	Med-on 1.5 h	2 h
	2	Inexplicable euphoria (sense of floating)			Day 2 after hospital discharge	Med-on 1 h	2.5 h
(2)	1	Wail	none	Postoperative 18 months	During programming	MED+ ON	20 min
(3)	1	Hallucination (cloud-like light and shadow)	none	Postoperative 2 months	First night after hospital discharge	Med-on	About 20 min
	2	Hallucination (cloud-like light and shadow)			Second morning after programming	Med-on	30 min
(4)	1	Hypomania (hard to restrain anger)	30	Postoperative 17 months	During programming	Med-off	10 min until adjustment of parameter
	2	Hypomania (sense of anger)	28		During programming	Med-off	10 min until adjustment of parameter
(5)	1	Wail (induced by ordinary conversation)	none	Postoperative 1 month (newly activated)	During programming	Med-off	5 min until adjustment of parameter
	2	Wail (induced by ordinary conversation)			During programming	Med-off	7 min
	3	Wail (induced by talking about the past)			During programming	Med-on	5 min
(6)	1	Hypomania (losing temper to wife)	33	Postoperative 26 months	At home, after programming	Med-on	Improved after 10 min
	2	Hypomania (kicking roadside cars)			At home, after programming	Med-on	2 min, improved 1 min after deactivation
(7)	1	Inexplicable euphoria (laughing foolishly)	20	Postoperative 3 months (during programming)	During programming	1 h after intake	10 h
	2	Inexplicable euphoria (laughing foolishly)			During programming	1.5 h after intake	3 min
(8)	1	Hypomania (lost temper and smashed objects)	34	Postoperative 3 months (during programming)	The 2nd day after hospital discharge	Med-on	2 h
	2	Hypomania (flight of ideas and fidgeting)			The 2nd day after getting home	Med-on	2 h
(9)	1	Hypomania (emotional and quarreling)	34	Postoperative 14 months	Day 6 after hospital discharge; 20 min after raising the voltage of 0.5 V with programming by patients	Med-on 1.5 h	1.5 h. Family members restored the stimulation parameter originally set by doctors

TABLE 2: Continued.

Number	Times	Description of episode		Interval between episode and operation	Time of occurrence	Relationship with medication	Duration
		Chief complaints and symptoms	YMRS				
(10)	1	Abnormal sense of spatial orientation (unaware of his location when out of clinic)	none	Postoperative 3.5 months (during programming)	During programming	Med-off	10 min, returned clinic for readjustment of parameters
	2	Abnormal sense of spatial orientation			During programming	Med-off	15 min, improved 2 min after parameter adjustment
(11)	1	Hypomania (shouting and fidgeting)	29	Postoperative 2.5 months (during programming)	In the car on his way home after programming	Med-on	1.5 h, improved after readjustment of parameters in the clinic

TABLE 3: The stimulation parameters and STPS.

Number of PD Patients	Status	STPS times	Chief complaints and symptoms of STPS	Stimulation pattern	CV/CC	Intensity (V/mA)	Pulse width (μs)	Frequency (Hz)	Left/right	Cathode	Anode	IPG	Electrode	Active contact location	UPDRS-III score (med off/IPG-on)
(1)	Pre-STPS			IPG-off								Activa RC	3389	Medial STN	
	STPS	1	Inexplicable euphoria	Monopolar	CV	2.5	60	160	Left	1	Case				None*
	STPS	2	Inexplicable euphoria	Monopolar	CV	2.2	60	160	Left	1	Case				14
	Final			Monopolar	CV	1.9	70	160	Left	1	Case				14
(2)	Pre-STPS			Monopolar	CV	2.3	80	140	Left	1	Case	Activa RC	3389	Medial part of STN	
				Monopolar	CV	2.5	90	140	Right	9	Case				
	STPS	1	Wail	Monopolar	CV	2.5	90	140	Left	1	Case				13
	Final			Bipolar	CV	2.6	90	140	Left	1	2				13
(3)	Pre-STPS			Monopolar	CV	2.5	60	150	Right	9	Case	Activa RC	3389	Medial Inferior part of STN	
				Monopolar		2.3	60	150	Left	2	Case				
	STPS	1	Hallucination	Monopolar	CV	2.9	70	150	Right	9	Case				25
	STPS	2	Hallucination	Monopolar		2.6	90	130	Right	9	Case				23
	Final			Interleaving	CV	2.5	90	125	Right	2	Case				23
						1.8	70	125		3					
(4)	Pre-STPS			Monopolar	CV	2.3	100	90	Left	1	Case	Activa RC	3389	Inferior part of STN/substantia nigra	
				Monopolar	CV	2.5	110	90	Right	10	Case				
	STPS	1	Hypomania	Double polar	CV	2.4	100	90	Left	0,1	Case				25
	STPS	2	Hypomania	Double polar	CV	2.2	110	85	Left	0,1	Case				25
	Final			Interleaving	CV	2.0	100	90	Left	0	Case				25
						2.3	100	90		1					
(5)	Pre-STPS						IPG off					Activa PC	3389	Lateral part of STN/Close to Zona incerta	
	STPS	1	Wail	Monopolar	CC	1.9	60	140	Right	10	Case				None*
	STPS	2	Wail	Monopolar	CC	1.7	60	130	Right	10	Case				13
	STPS	3	Wail	Bipolar	CC	1.8	60	130	Right	10	11				13
	Final			Monopolar	CC	1.9	60	130	Right	11	Case				13
(6)	Pre-STPS			Double-polar	CV	2.5	60	160	Left	0,1	Case	Activa RC	3389	Inferior part of STN/Close to substantia nigra	
				Monopolar	CV	2.7	70	160	Right	9	Case				
	STPS	1	Hypomania	Double polar	CV	2.8	60	160	Left	0,1	Case				40
	STPS	2	Hypomania	Interleaving	CV	2.5	80	125	Left	0	Case				39
						2.8	80	125		1	Case				
	Final			Interleaving	CV	2.5	70	125	Left	0	Case				41
						2.7	80	125		1,2	Case				
(7)	Pre-STPS			Monopolar	CC	2.1	60	145	Left	3	Case	Activa RC	3389	Lateral part of STN/Close to Internal capsule	
				Monopolar	CC	2.0	70	145	Right	10	Case				
	STPS	1	Inexplicable euphoria	Monopolar	CC	2.1	60	145	Left	3	Case				40
	STPS	2	Inexplicable euphoria	Monopolar	CC	1.9	70	145	Left	3	Case				38
	Final			Bipolar	CV	2.3	70	145	Left	3	2				38

TABLE 3: Continued.

Number of PD Patients	Status	STPS times	Chief complaints and symptoms of STPS	Stimulation pattern	CV/CC	Intensity (V/mA)	Pulse width (μs)	Frequency (Hz)	Left/right	Cathode	Anode	IPG	Electrode	Active contact location	UPDRS-III score (med off/IPG-on)
(8)	Pre-STPS			Monopolar	CV	2.6	60	150	Left	1	Case				
	Pre-STPS			Monopolar	CV	2.5	60	150	Right	10	Case				
	STPS	1	Hypomania	Monopolar	CV	3.1	60	150	Left	1	Case	Activa RC	3389	Medial part of STN	40
	STPS	2	Hypomania	Monopolar	CV	2.8	70	145	Left	1	Case				40
	Final			Monopolar	CV	3	60	140	Left	2	case				40
(9)	Pre-STPS			Monopolar	CV	2.7	90	160	Right	9	Case				
	STPS	1	Hypomania	Double-polar	CV	2.5	80	160	Left	2,3	Case	Activa RC	3389	Lateral part of STN	25
	Final			Monopolar	CV	3.2	90	160	Right	9	Case				24
				Monopolar	CV	2.9	110	130	Right	9	Case				
(10)	Pre-STPS			Monopolar	CC	2.0	60	160	Right	9	Case				
	Pre-STPS			Monopolar	CC	2.2	60	160	Left	2	Case				
	STPS	1	Abnormal spatial orientation	Monopolar	CC	2.2	60	160	Right	9	Case	Activa PC	3389	Medial part of STN	26
	STPS	2	Abnormal spatial orientation	Monopolar	CC	2.0	70	140	Right	9	Case				25
	Final			Interleaving	CV	2.8	60	125	Right	9	Case				25
						2.1	60	125		10	Case				
(11)	Pre-STPS			Monopolar	CV	2.8	70	135	Left	2	Case				
	Pre-STPS			Monopolar	CV	2.5	60	135	Right	10	Case				
	STPS	1	Hypomania	Monopolar	CV	3.0	70	135	Left	2	Case	Activa RC	3389	Lateral part of STN	34
	Final			Monopolar	CV	2.7	80	135	Left	2	Case				34

CV, constant voltage; CC, constant current. *The patients with no UPDRS-III score (med-off/IPG-on) because they were in the first programming and have not been evaluated with UPDRS-III score yet.

TABLE 4: Programming procedure of patient number 6.

	Pattern	Voltage (V)	Pulse width (µs)	Frequency (Hz)	Cathode	Anode	UPDRS-III score (med-off/IPG-on)	Chief complaints
Pre-programming	Double polar	2.5	60	160	0,1	Case	41	Spastic pain in the right shoulder
(1)	Double polar	2.8	80	160	0,1	Case	40	STPS occurred
(2)	Interleaving	2.5	80	125	0	Case	39	STPS occurred with hat-like constriction surrounding the head
		2.8	80	125	1	Case		
(3)	Interleaving	2.5	70	125	0	Case	40	Rigidity of neck and posterior extension
		2.8	90	125	1	Case		
(4)	Interleaving	2.5	70	125	0	Case	39	Dizziness and palpitation
		3.1	80	125	1	Case		
(5)	Double polar	2.5	70	130	0,1	Case	40	Fidgeting, feel like preliminary appearance of STPS
(6)	Interleaving	2.5	70	125	0	Case	40	Dizzy and palpitation
		2.7	100	125	1	Case		
(7)	Interleaving	2.5	70	125	0	Case	42	Rigidity of neck and posterior extension with pain in the right shoulder.
		2.8	80	125	1	2		
(8)*	Interleaving	2.5	70	125	0	Case	41	Pain in shoulders improved, with no newly developed symptoms
		2.7	80	125	1,2	Case		
(9)	Interleaving	2.5	70	125	0	Case	41	Dizziness
		2.8	80	125	1,2	Case		

*The patient chose the 8th programming parameters.

could reach to 3 mm. As a result, the limbic part of STN could easily be affected and cause STPS. (3) Thirdly, even in the most experienced PD treatment center could not guarantee that both anticipated contacts location and curative stimulation effect could be satisfied. Meanwhile, STPS could be easily induced when increasing stimulation intensity or testing side effects.

China has the largest number of patients with PD in the world. In recent years, there have been more than 100 centers which carry out STN-DBS surgery for the treatment of PD. As a result, there is a strong likelihood of an increasing number of PD patients suffering STPS after STN-DBS programming. It is therefore very important to rapidly diagnose, locate contacts, and program parameters to eliminate STPS. It is also paramount to maintain the PD patient's optimal motor function according to algorithms set by programming doctors at different levels.

4.2. Confirmation of STPS and the Impact Factors. Psychiatric disorders are one of the symptoms manifested in PD patients. However, antiparkinsonism medications also manifest similar symptoms as drug side effects. Levodopa and dopaminergic drugs could induce dopamine dysregulation syndrome, hallucinations and psychosis, mania and hypomania, and impulse control disorders, which were similar to STPS [16]. The treatment of psychiatric symptoms induced by the above drugs is in the reduction of medication in most times. STPS is known to manifest similarly. Therefore the diagnosis of psychiatric symptoms induced by drug side effects or PD should not be misinterpreted for STPS. The diagnosis of STPS should only be made upon confirmation.

Patients in our study had neither any preexisting psychiatric symptoms nor their PD medication altered for than one month. Although preoperative LEDD given to our patients on average was more than the reported average dose before DBS surgery in previous studies [17, 18], the subsequent doses would reduce more than 50% similar to that reported by Jiang and colleagues [17]. Levodopa withdrawal symptoms mainly include apathy and depression. In our study, all 11 patients had no symptoms of apathy and depression. Moreover in the first three-month follow-up after STPS programming, except for the two patients who had STPS at IPG initiation, there was no change in the LEDD in the other patients (Table 1). We, therefore, deduced that the antiparkinsonism medication is not the main factor inducing psychiatric symptoms. Otherwise, some psychiatric symptoms may have reoccurred within the first 3 months of follow-up.

To avoid drugs side effect interference during DBS effect evaluation, all the patients were programming in the state of "off time." Patients were given daily doses of anti-Parkinson's disease drugs after the final stimulation parameters were set. To achieve the satisfactory therapeutic effects, the motor complications were evaluated during "on time" state. However, the interesting point is that 70% (14/20) STPS occurred in "on time" state or over 1 hour after taking medications (though some patients had not felt medicine effect already); see Table 2. Whether medications for PD work with electrical stimulation to cause psychiatric symptoms or not needs further study. We excluded the effect of PD drugs by maintaining

the same dosage that was given on the first occurrence of STPS. So we believe the electrical stimulation should be the main factor of psychiatric symptoms.

To improve the diagnosis of STPS, we developed the algorithm (Figure 2). The causative active contact of patients with acute symptoms of STPS could be easily identified using the flow chart. However, the causative active contact in patients with transient STPS symptoms was more difficult to identify. In the process of locating suspicious contacts in such patients, we do not recommend increasing stimulation intensity to induce STPS to identify contacts. The reason is that (1), theoretically, increasing stimulation intensity of any contact to a certain threshold, the volume of tissue activated (VTA) may affect limbic part of STN and induce STPS. So it may mislead the doctor to regard the contacts which were not the initial responsible contacts. The doctor may even locate wrong responsible electrodes and contacts. (2) If there are multiple active contacts (double polar, interleaving mode) on one side of the electrode, the adjacent contacts have a higher chance to induce STPS (although the ventral contacts are with a higher chance). If randomly increasing stimulation intensity of random contacts to induce STPS, it can also lead to wrong contact. (3) Intentionally induced STPS might cause patients extra distress, leading them to distrust doctors, increased complaints, and decreased satisfaction. Therefore, we recommend the utilization of the algorithm (Figure 2) to locate the contacts carefully and accurately. In our study, the active contacts which induced STPS were identified by using an algorithm (Figure 2) and eliminated by programming in all the 11 patients.

The clinical significance incidence rate of STPS which necessitated programming was about 2%. This was significantly lower as compared to 28.6% in previous studies [14]. This difference may be attributed to the stimulation intensity used and the exclusion criteria we used to enroll patients with STPS symptoms in this study. In this study, the stimulating voltage was rarely more than 3.0 V. However, the stimulating voltage did not exceed 3.3 V.

We noted that time interval for the occurrence STPS fell within 48 hours after new settings of stimulation parameters. Therefore, the psychiatric and psychological status of patients should be thoroughly assessed in MED-ON/STIM-ON after each programming session before patients were discharged. It is also necessary to instruct the family to timely identify the occurrence of STPS, since some symptoms may not be recognized by patients themselves [19].

4.3. Principles of STPS Programming. We observed that STPS is likely to develop when programming clinicians increase the voltage or pulse width of the active contact. The increase in active contact voltage or pulse width gives patients a brief false sense of relief masked by improvement in motor functions. Even though the improvement of motor functions are most often minor (1 or 2 point differences in UPDRS-III), STPS set in as residual effects of the increase in voltage. Patients usually find themselves in a quagmire on whether to maintain improved motor functions or settle for removal of STPS and have less appealing motor functions. However, few reports were mentioning how to maintain the optimal improvement for motor functions while avoiding STPS at the same time.

We conducted a literature review using PubMed database of earlier authors who encountered and managed STPS while maintaining optimal motor functions. We designed a programming procedure and protocol to determine the active contacts that induce STPS to rapidly alleviate patients' psychiatric symptoms and maintain improved motor functions.

Previous reports [20] suggest that STPS was associated with high level of voltage. This suggests that the VTA might impact the limbic neuronal networks that induce STPS. They further reported that various programming methods decrease or change the VTA enabling eliminating STPS. These methods include (1) reducing voltage [20], (2) switching to bipolar stimulation [19], and (3) changing dorsal active contacts [9, 21, 22].

Although there are many ways to improve STPS through programming, the order of choice must not be random but with precise principles and in chronological order (Figure 3). These principles include that (1) the solutions for eliminating STPS must be rapid; (2) simple and replicable; (3) and with minimal or no STPS reoccurrence and (4) must preserve optimal motor functions.

There are six methods to adjust the stimulation parameter: (1) bipolar stimulation, (2) reducing voltage by 0.3 V–0.5 V until SITNPS disappears; (3) decreasing of voltage and increasing the pulse width; (4) declining voltage and frequency and increasing pulse width; (5) interleaving of original and dorsal contacts; (6) changing the active contacts to dorsal the position.

4.3.1. Bipolar Stimulation.
The first option is bipolar stimulation. We choose to select bipolar stimulation to easily set stimulation parameters and quickly narrow the sphere VTA (Figure 3). This could promote STPS regression and reduce recurrence. However, due to the rapid narrowing of VTA, it often leads to the aggravation of motor functions.

4.3.2. Reducing Voltage.
We reduced the voltage on the basis of initial stimulation parameter (with STPS). This adjustment can also quickly reduce the VTA and intensity of the activation domain.

4.3.3. Decreasing of Voltage and Increasing the Pulse Width.
The adjustment of programming parameters mentioned above may reduce activation domain [23] while in the meantime declining the stimulating intensity of motor functions-related neural pathways [24]. Therefore a slight increase in the pulse width to maintain stimulation intensity in the narrowed VTA might be needed when the voltage is decreased. Some inexperienced programming physicians may conceive that it is hard to modulate pulse width appropriately. It will be easier to operate according to the formula of total electrical energy delivered (TEED) to calculate how to increase the pulse width according to the voltage reduced (new TEED should be not more than the original one with STPS).

4.3.4. Declining Voltage and Frequency and Increasing Pulse Width.
If necessary, we can even adjust the frequency (+5–10 Hz) to fit the change of the voltage and pulse width, to achieve the appropriate stimulation intensity to eliminate STPS while maintaining the improvement of motor functions. In addition to reducing the stimulation frequency to reduce intensity, interleaving technology could be used when adjusting the voltage.

4.3.5. Interleaving of Original and Dorsal Contacts.
The adjustment of the pulse width is critical in improving patient's optimal movement symptom after the frequency has reduced to 125 Hz. In the case where the active contact responsible for inducing STPS was ventrally positioned, stimulation parameters remain unaltered. Subsequently, the dorsally located contacts are activated into interleaving stimulation mode. This adjustment has proven to maintain optimal motor function.

4.3.6. Changing the Active Contacts to Dorsal the Position.
In isolated patients, motor functions reacted better to stimulation frequency than the later adjustment. As reported, the contacts located anterior, medial, and inferior to STN were easier to precipitate STPS [14]; thus if using the above-mentioned scheme cannot eliminate STPS and achieve optimal improvement of motor functions at the same time, we change the active contact to more dorsal position to acquire a larger range in the adjustment of stimulation parameters. If the inactive contacts were suspended for a long time, curative and side effects might change from previous stimulation record and need retitration which is time-consuming. Also, after the inactivated contacts have been activated, the contact impedance may change with time causing instability of symptom control among patients [25]. We recommend that the interleaving mode generates two isolated VTA: the ventral and dorsal contact. The ventral contact maintains the previous stimulation parameters before the occurrence of STPS. We activate the dorsal contact by gradually increasing the voltage and pulse width to archive optimal motor function [26]. In contrast to the COMPARE trial [27], we have put in consideration preserving patient's motor function while eliminating STPS. Therefore the use of interleaving stimulation was our priority than changing the active contact to dorsal one.

4.4. Patient Follow-Up.
The impedance of the active contacts reduces over time [25]. Therefore, after STPS programming, patients needed to be followed up for a period to ensure no appearance of similar psychiatric symptoms. STPS was considered eliminated after clinical programming at three (03) months. In the event there was a need to adjust the intensity of stimulation upwards, increasing the width of pulse was given priority. This is because the expansion of the activated domain was not as significant as that of the voltage [28].

4.5. Limitations.
The limitations of the study are inadequate sample size and limited categories of STPS. Additionally, the flow diagrams adopted in this study are limited to Medtronic Activa PC and RC models. This was a single center study.

5. Conclusion

The stimulation contacts in STPS could be determined with use of flow diagram. Appropriate programming could remove STPS while maintaining optimal improvement of motor functions for most patients.

Additional Points

Recommendations. The flow diagrams for patients with other models of IPG should be adjusted accordingly. A meta-analysis could increase the sample size and attain statistical significance.

Disclosure

This work was presented as a poster at the 2017 Chinese Medical Association of Nerve Regulation Professional Committee Annual Meeting and the 8th Session of the Chinese Nerve Regulation Conference. Xi Wu and Yiqing Qiu are co-first authors.

References

[1] A. Castrioto, A. M. Lozano, Y.-Y. Poon, A. E. Lang, M. Fallis, and E. Moro, "Ten-year outcome of subthalamic stimulation in Parkinson disease: A blinded evaluation," *Archives of Neurology*, vol. 68, no. 12, pp. 1550–1556, 2011.

[2] M. G. Rizzone, A. Fasano, A. Daniele et al., "Long-term outcome of subthalamic nucleus DBS in Parkinson's disease: from the advanced phase towards the late stage of the disease?" *Parkinsonism and Related Disorders*, vol. 20, no. 4, pp. 376–381, 2014.

[3] M. L. Janssen, A. A. Duits, A. M. Tourai et al., "Subthalamic Nucleus High-Frequency Stimulation for Advanced Parkinson's Disease: Motor and Neuropsychological Outcome after 10 Years," *Stereotactic and Functional Neurosurgery*, vol. 92, no. 6, pp. 381–387, 2014.

[4] P. J. Rossi, A. Gunduz, and M. S. Okun, "The Subthalamic Nucleus, Limbic Function, and Impulse Control," *Neuropsychology Review*, vol. 25, no. 4, pp. 398–410, 2015.

[5] A. Funkiewiez, C. Ardouin, E. Caputo et al., "Long term effects of bilateral subthalamic nucleus stimulation on cognitive function, mood, and behaviour in Parkinson's disease," *Journal of Neurology, Neurosurgery & Psychiatry*, vol. 75, no. 6, pp. 834–839, 2004.

[6] H. J. Kim, B. S. Jeon, and S. H. Paek, "Nonmotor functions and Subthalamic Deep Brain Stimulation in Parkinson's Disease," *Journal of Movement Disorders*, vol. 8, no. 2, pp. 38–91, 2015.

[7] D. Drapier, S. Drapier, P. Sauleau et al., "Does subthalamic nucleus stimulation induce apathy in Parkinson's disease?" *Journal of Neurology*, vol. 253, no. 8, pp. 1083–1091, 2006.

[8] M. Sensi, R. Eleopra, M. A. Cavallo et al., "Explosive-aggressive behavior related to bilateral subthalamic stimulation," *Parkinsonism and Related Disorders*, vol. 10, no. 4, pp. 247–251, 2004.

[9] D. Raucher-Chéné, C.-L. Charrel, A. D. de Maindreville, and F. Limosin, "Manic episode with psychotic symptoms in a patient with Parkinson's disease treated by subthalamic nucleus stimulation: Improvement on switching the target," *Journal of the Neurological Sciences*, vol. 273, no. 1-2, pp. 116-117, 2008.

[10] P. Krack, R. Kumar, C. Ardouin et al., "Mirthful laughter induced by subthalamic nucleus stimulation," *Movement Disorders*, vol. 16, no. 5, pp. 867–875, 2001.

[11] J. Volkmann, C. Daniels, and K. Witt, "Neuropsychiatric effects of subthalamic neurostimulation in Parkinson disease," *Nature Reviews Neurology*, vol. 6, no. 9, pp. 487–498, 2010.

[12] D. Floden, S. E. Cooper, S. D. Griffith, and A. G. Machado, "Predicting quality of life outcomes after subthalamic nucleus deep brain stimulation," *Neurology*, vol. 83, no. 18, pp. 1627–1633, 2014.

[13] R. C. Young, J. T. Biggs, V. E. Ziegler, and D. A. Meyer, "A rating scale for mania: reliability, validity and sensitivity," *The British Journal of Psychiatry*, vol. 133, pp. 429–435, 1978.

[14] O. A. Abulseoud, A. Kasasbeh, H.-K. Min et al., "Stimulation-induced transient nonmotor psychiatric symptoms following subthalamic deep brain stimulation in patients with Parkinson's disease: Association with clinical outcomes and neuroanatomical correlates," *Stereotactic and Functional Neurosurgery*, vol. 94, no. 2, pp. 93–101, 2016.

[15] P. Justin Rossi, C. Peden, O. Castellanos et al., "The human subthalamic nucleus and globus pallidus internus differentially encode reward during action control," *Human Brain Mapping*, vol. 38, no. 4, pp. 1952–1964, 2017.

[16] I. Beaulieu-Boire and A. E. Lang, "Behavioral effects of levodopa," *Movement Disorders*, vol. 30, no. 1, pp. 90–102, 2015.

[17] L.-L. Jiang, J.-L. Liu, X.-L. Fu et al., "Long-term efficacy of subthalamic nucleus deep brain stimulation in parkinson's disease: A 5-year follow-up study in China," *Chinese Medical Journal*, vol. 128, no. 18, pp. 2433–2438, 2015.

[18] J. Li, Y. Zhang, and Y. Li, "Long-term follow-up of bilateral subthalamic nucleus stimulation in Chinese Parkinson's disease patients," *British Journal of Neurosurgery*, vol. 29, no. 3, pp. 329–333, 2015.

[19] T. S. Mandat, T. Hurwitz, and C. R. Honey, "Hypomania as an adverse effect of subthalamic nucleus stimulation: Report of two cases," *Acta Neurochirurgica*, vol. 148, no. 8, pp. 895–898, 2006.

[20] A. Chopra, S. J. Tye, K. H. Lee et al., "Voltage-dependent mania after subthalamic nucleus deep brain stimulation in Parkinson's disease: A case report," *Biological Psychiatry*, vol. 70, no. 2, pp. e5–e7, 2011.

[21] T. T. Ugurlu, G. Acar, F. Karadag, and F. Acar, "Manic episode following deep brain stimulation of the subthalamic nucleus for Parkinson's disease: A case report," *Turkish Neurosurgery*, vol. 24, no. 1, pp. 94–97, 2014.

[22] L. Mallet, M. Schüpbach, K. N'Diaye et al., "Stimulation of subterritories of the subthalamic nucleus reveals its role in the integration of the emotional and motor aspects of behavior," *Proceedings of the National Academy of Sciences of the United States of America*, vol. 104, no. 25, pp. 10661–10666, 2007.

[23] B. Mädler and V. A. Coenen, "Explaining clinical effects of deep brain stimulation through simplified target-specific modeling of the volume of activated tissue," *American Journal of Neuroradiology*, vol. 33, no. 6, pp. 1072–1080, 2012.

[24] N. Yousif, R. Bayford, P. G. Bain, and X. Liu, "The peri-electrode space is a significant element of the electrode-brain interface in deep brain stimulation: A computational study," *Brain Research Bulletin*, vol. 74, no. 5, pp. 361–368, 2007.

[25] C. J. Hartmann, L. Wojtecki, J. Vesper et al., "Long-term evaluation of impedance levels and clinical development in subthalamic deep brain stimulation for Parkinson's disease," *Parkinsonism and Related Disorders*, vol. 21, no. 10, article no. 2753, pp. 1247–1250, 2015.

[26] S. Miocinovic, P. Khemani, R. Whiddon et al., "Outcomes, management, and potential mechanisms of interleaving deep brain stimulation settings," *Parkinsonism and Related Disorders*, vol. 20, no. 12, pp. 1434–1437, 2014.

[27] M. S. Okun, H. H. Fernandez, W. u. SS et al., "Cognition and mood in Parkinson's disease in subthalamic nucleus versus globus pallidus interna deep brain stimulation: the COMPARE trial," *Annals of Neurology*, vol. 65, no. 5, pp. 586–595, 2009.

[28] A. Chaturvedi, J. L. Luján, and C. C. McIntyre, "Artificial neural network based characterization of the volume of tissue activated during deep brain stimulation," *Journal of Neural Engineering*, vol. 10, no. 5, Article ID 056023, 2013.

Genetic Variations and mRNA Expression of NRF2 in Parkinson's Disease

Caroline Ran,[1] **Karin Wirdefeldt,**[2,3] **Lovisa Brodin,**[2] **Mehrafarin Ramezani,**[1]
Marie Westerlund,[4] **Fengqing Xiang,**[5] **Anna Anvret,**[1] **Thomas Willows,**[2] **Olof Sydow,**[2]
Anders Johansson,[2] **Dagmar Galter,**[1] **Per Svenningsson,**[2] **and Andrea Carmine Belin**[1]

[1]*Department of Neuroscience, Karolinska Institutet, 17177 Stockholm, Sweden*
[2]*Department of Clinical Neuroscience, Karolinska Institutet, 17177 Stockholm, Sweden*
[3]*Department of Medical Epidemiology and Biostatistics, Karolinska Institutet, 17177 Stockholm, Sweden*
[4]*Department of Neurobiology, Care Sciences and Society, Karolinska Institutet, 14183 Huddinge, Sweden*
[5]*Department of Women's and Children's Health, Karolinska Institutet, 17176 Stockholm, Sweden*

Correspondence should be addressed to Caroline Ran; caroline.ran@ki.se

Academic Editor: Hélio Teive

Nuclear factor erythroid 2-like 2 *(NRF2)* encodes a transcription factor regulating mechanisms of cellular protection and is activated by oxidative stress. *NRF2* has therefore been hypothesized to confer protection against Parkinson's disease and so far an *NRF2* haplotype has been reported to decrease the risk of developing disease and delay disease onset. Also *NRF2* adopts a nuclear localization in Parkinson's disease, which is indicative of increased *NRF2* activity. We have investigated the association between *NRF2* and Parkinson's disease in a Swedish case-control material and whether *NRF2* expression levels correlate with *NRF2* genetic variants, disease, or disease onset. Using pyrosequencing, we genotyped one intronic and three promoter variants in 504 patients and 509 control subjects from Stockholm. Further, we quantified *NRF2* mRNA expression in EBV transfected human lymphocytes from patients and controls using quantitative real-time reverse transcription PCR. We found that one of the promoter variants, rs35652124, was associated with age of disease onset (X^2 = 14.19, *p* value = 0.0067). *NRF2* mRNA expression levels however did not correlate with the rs35652124 genotype, Parkinson's disease, or age of onset in our material. More detailed studies on *NRF2* are needed in order to elucidate how this gene affects pathophysiology of Parkinson's disease.

1. Introduction

Parkinson's disease (PD) is the second most common neurodegenerative disorder in the aging population; approximately 20,000 people are affected by PD in Sweden which has a population around 9.6 million. PD is characterized by degeneration of dopamine (DA) neurons in substantia nigra (SN), but there is degeneration of other neurons as well. Although there is a relatively large body of knowledge on the pathology of PD, there is little understanding of the etiology. The existing treatment for PD today, for example, replacing DA, improving the effect of DA, or inhibiting the breakdown of DA, does not cure the disease but only reduces the symptoms. In order to develop better ways of combating

PD or better still prevent clinical symptoms altogether, one must decipher the causes of disease.

Typically, candidate genes for PD do not specifically relate to the DA system. Instead, they tend to serve general cellular purposes, such as to protect against reactive molecules or participate in mitochondrial function [1]. One gene that has been suggested to confer protection against PD is the nuclear factor erythroid 2-like 2 *(NRF2)* (OMIM 600492), on chromosome 2q31. It belongs to a family of genes together with *NFE2* (OMIM 601490) and *NFE2L1* (OMIM 163260), encoding basic leucine zipper (bZIP) transcription factors [2]. In normal conditions, NRF2 is not active; it resides in the cytoplasm bound to KEAP1 (kelch-like ECH association protein 1), a ubiquitin E3 ligase complex, which mediates

TABLE 1: Demographics of the study population.

TABLE 1: Demographics of the study population.

	Participants, n	Females, n (%)	Mean age at enrolment, years	Mean age at diagnosis, years	Heredity, n (%)
Controls	509	290 (57.3)	71*	NA	NA
PD	501	184 (36.7)	67.2	59.5	88 (28.5)**

PD: Parkinson's disease; NA: not applicable; *age was unknown for 95 blood donors; **estimation based on 319 individuals for which this information was known.

NRF2 degradation by the proteasome. In response to oxidative stress, NRF2 is released from KEAP1 and translocated from the cytoplasm into the nucleus where it transactivates expression of genes with antioxidant activity, detoxifying enzymes, cell survival, and anti-inflammatory factors [3]. Expression of Nrf2, the rat orthologue of NRF2, decreases with increasing age and is accompanied by a drop in activity of phase II antioxidant enzymes, which are upregulated by NRF2 [4–6]. Subsequently, the decrease in NRF2 expression results in increased sensitivity to oxidative damage.

In PD, nuclear localization of NRF2 has been reported to be strongly induced in nigral neurons, but this response may be insufficient to protect neurons from degeneration [7]. Five genetic association studies have been published on NRF2 in relation to PD with variable results [8–12]. In 2010, von Otter et al. performed a genetic study in a Swedish and a Polish PD material and identified a haplotype including three promoter single nucleotide polymorphisms (SNPs) and five tag SNPs that was associated with decreased risk of PD as well as later age of onset of PD [11]. The association with delayed disease onset was later replicated in an extended study comprising more than 1000 PD patients [12]. Another replication study on a subset of these SNPs in a Taiwanese PD population could not confirm these findings [8]. The importance of NRF2 SNPs has also been assessed in a Chinese PD population in which an association was discovered with two exonic SNPs but not with the promoter SNPs suggested by von Otter et al. [9, 11]. Yet another SNP was found to be associated with PD risk in an Australian sample and, in this study, several SNPs and haplotypes were also found to affect the age of onset [10]. What is more, haplotype association has also been reported between NRF2 and Alzheimer's disease (AD) as well as with age-related cataract and amyotrophic lateral sclerosis (ALS) [13, 14]. Overall it seems likely that genetic variants in NRF2 affect both the risk of developing neurodegenerative disorders such as PD and the age of onset, but as different sets of SNPs were included in these studies, as well as the differential distribution of haplotypes in populations with different ethnicity, it is difficult to pinpoint what combination of SNPs is responsible for the reported associations.

NRF2 may play an important role in cellular protection in neurodegenerative diseases as well as being a viable therapeutic target in the future. As described above, there are several indications supporting the involvement of NRF2 in neurodegenerative disorders. In the present study, we investigated four genetic variants in NRF2, rs35652124 (A>G), rs6706649 (G>A), rs6721961 (C>A), and rs2001350 (A>G), and their possible association with PD in our large homogenous Swedish case-control material in order to expand on

the knowledge on NRF2 genetic variations as a risk factor in PD. The SNPs included in our study have previously been reported to be associated with PD in a Caucasian material consisting of Swedish and Polish individuals [11]. We additionally wanted to examine whether the NRF2 gene is differently expressed in patients and controls or affecting age of onset and if genetic variants identified to be associated with PD in this study affected expression in vivo.

2. Materials and Methods

2.1. Patients and Controls. PD patients were recruited to the study during routine outpatient visits to the Neurology clinic at Karolinska University Hospital, Stockholm, Sweden. Patients ($n = 504$) were unrelated of Swedish origin, mean age was 67.2 years, age at diagnosis was 59.4 years, and 36.7% were females (Table 1). All patients fulfilled the "UK Parkinson's Disease Society's Brain Bank Clinical Diagnostic Criteria" for idiopathic PD except that 28.2% reported one or more first, second, or third-degree relative diagnosed with PD [15]. Early onset (EO) was defined as being less than or equal to 50 years of age at diagnosis and late onset (LO) was defined as 51 years or more at diagnosis. As controls ($n = 509$) we included neurologically healthy individuals visiting the Neurology Clinic, spouses of PD patients, anonymous blood donors, and individuals from the SNAC-K project (The Swedish National Study on Aging and Care in Kungsholmen, http://www.snac-k.se/), mean age was 71.8 years, and 57.3% were females (Table 1). Samples from patients and controls were collected after informed consent and approval of the local ethics committee Stockholm. DNA was obtained from blood samples using standard protocols. Blood from patients and control individuals randomly selected from the individuals recruited at the Neurology Clinic was used for Epstein-Barr virus (EBV) transfection of B-lymphocytes, EO patients ($n = 10$), LO patients ($n = 10$), and controls ($n = 10$). All investigations on human subjects were carried out following the rules of the Declaration of Helsinki of 1975, revised in 2008. A subset of the patients ($n = 330$) and controls ($n = 317$) was previously genotyped in a preliminary study published in a doctoral thesis [16].

2.2. Genotyping by Pyrosequencing and qPCR. We genotyped four SNPs in NRF2: rs35652124, rs6706649, rs6721961 in the promoter, and rs2001350. Genotyping of the three promoter SNPs was performed by pyrosequencing [17]. Rs2001350 was genotyped by TaqMan® quantitative real-time PCR (qPCR). For pyrosequencing, a PCR was run using Taq polymerase enzyme and two oligonucleotide primers in order to isolate a sequence of 209 base pairs containing the three promoter SNPs; forward primer, 5′-GAATGGAGACACGTGGGAGT-3′; and reverse primer, 5′-ACTTTACCGCCCGAGAATG-3′ (Thermo Fisher Scientific, Hägersten, Sweden). The forward primer was biotinylated at the 5′ end. The PCR was programmed as follows: denaturation, at 95°C for 5 minutes, 45 cycles of amplification at 95°C for 20 sec, 57°C for 20 sec, and 72°C for 30 sec, and terminal elongation at 72°C for 7 minutes. The forward strand of the PCR product was captured and isolated on streptavidin coated sepharose beads and then purified according to manufacturer's instructions using a filter-probe vacuum prep-tool. The single stranded DNA fragment was incubated with a sequencing primer and annealed for 2 min at 80°C. SNPs rs35652124 and rs6706649 could be sequenced with the same sequence primer, 5′-TCACCCTGAACGC-3′, and rs6721961 was sequenced with sequencing primer 5′-GGAGATGTGGACA-3′. Sequences were analyzed using a pyrosequencing PSQ 96MA system (BIOTAGE AB, Uppsala, Sweden) using PyroMark Gold Q96 Reagents (QIAGEN Nordic, Sollentuna, Sweden). Rs2001350 was analyzed with TaqMan Fast 7500 qPCR. Rs2001350 was genotyped with a premade SNP genotyping assay, assay ID number C__11634985_10. We used a standard cycling program: pre-PCR reading at 60°C for one minute, polymerase activation at 95°C for 10 minutes, 55 cycles comprising denaturation at 92°C for 15 seconds and annealing/extension at 60°C for 1 minute, and last post-PCR reading at 60°C for 1 minute. TaqMan genotyping mix and assays were purchased from Applied Biosystems/Life Technologies (Life Technologies Europe BV, Stockholm, Sweden).

2.3. EBV Transfection of Lymphocytes. B-Lymphocytes were isolated from full blood using Ficoll-Paque according to manufacturer's instructions (GE Healthcare Bio-Sciences Corp., Piscataway, NJ, USA). Lymphocytes were cultivated in RPMI 1640 medium (SIGMA, St. Louis, MO, USA) with 20% fetal calf serum, L-glutamine (200 mM), penicillin-streptomycin (5000 μg/mL) (Invitrogen, Carlsbad, CA, USA), and cyclosporine (1 μL/mL, Apoteket, Stockholm, Sweden). Transfection was achieved by adding and filtering supernatant of Epstein-Barr virus (EBV) infected B95-8 cells to the medium. When immortalized, cells were frozen and kept at −140°C until use [18].

2.4. Reverse Transcription qPCR (qRT-PCR). EBV transfected B-lymphocytes were thawed, reseeded, and harvested when cell count reached around 5 million cells and kept in −130°C. RNA was extracted from frozen cells using RNeasy Mini Kit according to manufacturer's instructions (QIAGEN Nordic, Sollentuna, Sweden). RNA concentration was measured and DNA contamination was eliminated. In order to avoid sample degradation, stable cDNA was synthesized from the RNA using a QuantiTect Reverse Transcription Kit (QIAGEN Nordic). The cDNA template was used for quantifying gene expression of *NRF2* in PD patients and controls by qRT-PCR. Gene specific primers were designed

for exon four of *NRF2*, which is present in all mRNA transcripts: forward primer 5′-CTTTTGGCGCAGACATTCC-3′ and reverse primer 5′-AAGACTGGGCTCTCGATGTG-3′. *GAPDH* was used as housekeeping gene: forward primer 5′-AGCCACATCGCTCAGACA-3′ and reverse primer 5′-GCCCAATACGACCAAATCC-3′ (Thermo Fisher Scientific). *NRF2* primer pair gave an R^2 value of 0.9507 and *GAPDH* primes gave an R^2 value of 0.9809. The qRT-PCR reaction was performed according to standard protocols, using triplicates of each sample and SYBR green qRT-PCR mastermix from Applied Biosystems (Applied Biosystems, Life Technologies Europe BV, Stockholm, Sweden). The cycler was programmed as follows: holding stage for pre-PCR read and enzyme activation: 50°C for 2 min and 95°C for 10 min, amplification for 45 cycles: 95°C for 15 sec, 60°C for 1 min, and last melting curve and post-PCR read: 95°C for 15 sec, 60°C for 1 min, 95°C for 30 sec, and 60°C for 15 sec.

2.5. Statistical Analysis and Image Analysis. Genotype and allele frequencies were compared between PD patients and controls. Association for genotypes was evaluated with Chi square (X^2) test and allele association was analyzed using Fisher's exact test. We used GraphPad Prism 5.03 (GraphPad Software Inc., La Jolla, CA, USA) for the analysis, significance level of 5% and two-sided p values. Bonferroni correction was used to correct for multiple testing. To control for the skewed gender distribution in the patient group (males = 63.3%), genotype analysis was verified using a logistic regression with gender as cofactor; analysis was run in PLINK v1.07 [19]. Hardy-Weinberg equilibrium was evaluated using a free online software through a X^2 based test [20]. Haplotype analysis was run using the software Haploview4.2 [21]. qRT-PCR data was analyzed in qBase 1.3.3, a software used for automated analysis of real-time quantitative PCR data [22], and evaluated with a student's t-test or a one-way ANOVA using GraphPad Prism 5.03.

3. Results

3.1. Genotyping by Pyrosequencing and qPCR. We have genotyped four common SNPs in the *NRF2* gene in 504 PD patients from the Stockholm area of Sweden and 509 geographically matched control individuals. One genetic variation, rs2001350, lies in the large second intron of the gene; the three other SNPs, rs35652124, rs6706649, and rs6721961, are promoter SNPs. Results for the genotype and allele analysis can be found in Table 2. Genotype and allele association analysis revealed no significant associations with PD. All four SNPs were in Hardy-Weinberg equilibrium (data not shown). The logistic regression, which included gender as a covariate, was run under a genotypic model with 2 degrees of freedom confirming the results from the genotype association analysis (supplementary table 1 in Supplementary Material available online at https://doi.org/10.1155/2017/4020198), verifying that there was no bias introduced by the skewed gender distributions in the patient and control group. In order to analyze the combined effect of several SNPs in *NRF2*, we further ran a haplotype analysis, which did not reveal any association between these four SNPs and PD (supplementary table 2).

TABLE 2: Results from genotype and allele analysis.

	Controls% (n)	PD% (n)	X² (DF)	OR (95% CI)	p value
rs35652124					
AA	47.7 (230)	45.0 (215)	0.79 (2)		0.68
AG	43.6 (210)	45.4 (217)			
GG	8.7 (42)	9.6 (46)			
A	69.5 (670)	67.7 (647)		1.09 (0.90–1.32)	0.40
G	30.5 (294)	32.3 (309)			
rs6706649					
GG	80.0 (387)	80.2 (385)	0.011 (2)		0.99
GA	18.6 (90)	18.3 (88)			
AA	1.4 (7)	1.5 (7)			
G	89.3 (864)	89.4 (858)		0.99 (0.74–1.32)	0.94
A	10.7 (104)	10.6 (102)			
rs6721961					
CC	74.8 (365)	77.4 (370)	2.39 (2)		0.30
CA	24.6 (120)	21.3 (102)			
AA	0.6 (3)	1.3 (6)			
C	87.1 (850)	88.1 (842)		0.91 (0.70–1.20)	0.54
A	12.9 (126)	11.9 (114)			
rs2001350					
AA	80.5 (388)	79.5 (387)	2.66 (2)		0.26
AG	19.3 (93)	19.5 (95)			
GG	0.2 (1)	1.0 (5)			
A	90.1 (869)	89.2 (869)		1.12 (0.82–1.48)	0.55
G	9.9 (95)	10.8 (105)			

n: number of individuals; PD: Parkinson's disease; X²: chi square; DF: degrees of freedom; OR: odds ratio; 95% CI: 95% confidence interval.

TABLE 3: Results from age stratified genotype and allele analysis for rs35652124.

rs35652124	Controls% (n)	LO PD% (n)	EO PD% (n)	X² (DF)	p value
AA	47.7 (230)	41.9 (163)	58.4 (52)	14.19 (4)	0.0067
AG	43.6 (210)	49.4 (192)	28.1 (25)		
GG	8.7 (42)	8.7 (34)	13.5 (12)		
A	69.5 (670)	66.6 (518)	72.5 (129)	3.82 (2)	0.15
G	30.5 (294)	33.4 (260)	27.5 (49)		

n: number of individuals; PD: Parkinson's disease; LO: late onset; EO: early onset; X²: chi square; DF: degrees of freedom.

When patients were stratified in groups of EO or LO, genotype association analysis showed that one of the promoter SNPs, rs35652124, was significantly associated with EO PD when compared to controls (X² = 14.19 p = 0.0067), (Table 3); both the WT genotype AA and the mutated genotype GG of rs35652124 were observed more frequently in PD patients with EO than in individuals in the two other groups, while EO heterozygous carriers were significantly fewer. The significance remained after correction for multiple testing, p = 0.027. The association was dissected further, which showed that the significance was dependent on the group of patients with early onset. The significance remained when comparing controls to EO patients only (p = 0.019) and when comparing LO patients to EO patients (p = 0.0013), but not when comparing controls to LO patients (p = 0.20). An additional analysis comparing patients with EO PD against

LO PD and controls under a recessive model (AA + GA versus GG) and a dominant model (AA versus GA + GG), respectively, confirmed the association under a dominant model (X² = 6.68, p = 0.013) and enabled us to establish the causality between the absence of G alleles and EO PD. Allele frequencies for rs35652124 were not associated with age at diagnosis (p = 0.15), nor did genotype or allele for rs6706649, rs6721961, and rs200350 (supplementary table 3).

3.2. mRNA Expression Analysis. Since promoter SNPs in *NRF2* have been suggested to influence gene expression in vitro, we further wanted to investigate whether gene expression correlated with the rs35652124 genotype [23]. We performed qRT-PCR on a subset of the patients included in our genetic study; mRNA levels were normalized to *GAPDH* expression and to a reference sample consisting of mixed

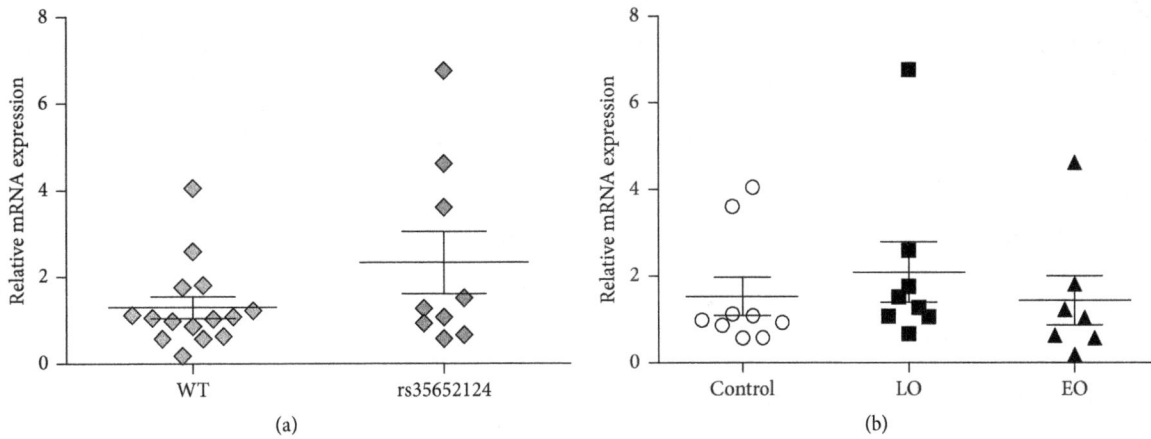

FIGURE 1: *rs35652124 genotype and age of onset do not correlate with NRF2 mRNA expression. NRF2* mRNA expression in EBV transfected human lymphocytes. Values were normalized to *GAPDH* mRNA and to a reference sample consisting of cDNA from all control individuals; groups were compared using a *t*-test (a) or one-way ANOVA (b) analysis. Error bars: standard error of mean. In (a) mRNA expression of all subjects was divided into two groups depending on their genotype for the promoter SNPs rs35652124. WT: subjects wild type for rs35652124 and rs35652124; subjects heterozygous ($n = 8$) and homozygous ($n = 1$) for rs35652124, $p = 0.121$. In (b) mRNA levels are analyzed according to disease status; LO: late onset PD; EO: early onset PD; $p = 0.695$.

cDNA from all control individuals. mRNA expression in wild-type (WT) carriers of the promoter SNP rs35652124 ($n = 15$) was compared to individuals carrying one ($n = 8$) or two ($n = 1$) mutated alleles at this position. We found no significant difference between the carriers and noncarriers, (Student's *t*-test, $p = 0.121$) (Figure 1(a)). It is noteworthy that the individual with the highest relative *NRF2* expression (6.76) was homozygous GG for rs35652124 but carried the WT allele of the three other SNPs; exact mRNA levels and genotypes are found in supplementary table 4. We additionally compared *NRF2* mRNA levels in healthy controls ($n = 9$) and PD patients ($n = 15$) and found no significant difference ($p = 0.712$, supplementary table 4). Also when stratifying the material into two patient groups with LO PD ($n = 8$) or EO PD ($n = 7$) expression levels were similar in all three groups ($p = 0.695$) (Figure 1(b), supplementary table 4). *NRF2* mRNA levels in these individuals were quite variable, displaying a few higher expressing individuals in all groups. Last we analyzed the expression data with respect to age using linear regression (Figure 2, supplementary table 4). We found no correlation between expression levels of *NRF2* and age either when analyzing the entire sample regardless of disease status ($p = 0.799$) or in controls alone ($p = 0.429$).

4. Discussion

We have found a genotype association of rs35652124 with EO PD. Genotype frequencies for this SNP were difficult to interpret, as the EO patients were more often homozygous for both the wild-type and mutant allele. This could possibly mean that the mode of penetrance of this genetic variation is unlikely to be additive or multiplicative. When combining the genotypes, we found that both genotypes comprising the mutated allele, heterozygous GA or homozygous GG, were more common in the control group and PD patients with late onset, which is consistent with the minor allele G being

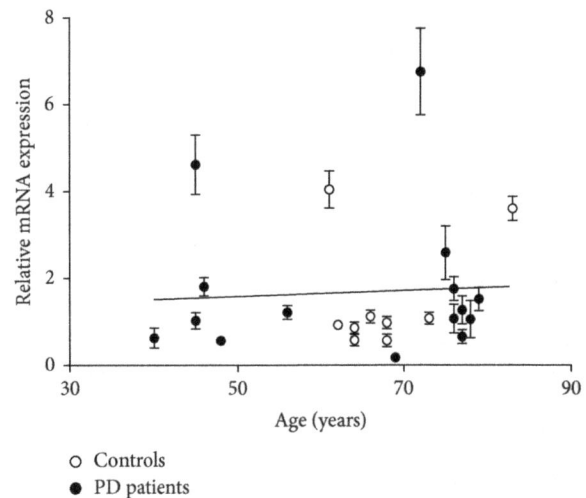

FIGURE 2: *mRNA levels do not correlate with age. NRF2* mRNA expression in EBV transfected lymphocytes from individuals of different age spanning from 40 years to 80; PD patients are represented in black and controls in white. Each data point corresponds to the mean value of triplicates normalized to *GAPDH* and to a reference sample consisting of cDNA from all control individuals; error bars: standard error of mean. Correlation between age and expression of *NRF2* was evaluated using linear regression and was found nonsignificant (slope = 0.0068, $p = 0.799$) when the entire material was analyzed regardless of disease and when controls were analyzed separately (regression line not shown, slope = 0.060, $p = 0.429$).

rarer in the early onset population. Analyzing the material under a dominant model confirmed the association between the absence of G alleles and earlier disease onset. We therefore stipulate that the G allele confers some protection against PD by delaying the onset of symptoms. von Otter et al. previously reported a promoter haplotype consisting of the wild-type alleles of rs35652124, rs6706649, and rs6721961 associated with later age of onset and less risk of developing disease [11]. Together, these datasets point to a disease modifying role for promoter SNPs, in particular rs35652124.

In vitro data indicate that the promoter SNPs analyzed by us could influence the transcriptional activity of *NRF2* [23, 24]. The mutated allele of rs6706649 and rs6721961 has been reported to cause a drastic decrease of *NRF2* gene transcription in transfected cells, while decrease is less pronounced when the mutated allele of rs35652124 is combined with the mutated allele of rs6706649. This information, together with the results from our genetic analysis, prompted us to investigate the functional implication of the rs35652421 SNP in human tissue [23, 24]. *NRF2* mRNA expression was quantified using qRT-PCR in patient specific cell-lines. Although qRT-PCR analysis showed no significant differences in mRNA levels when subjects were stratified according to genotype, quantification also revealed that *NRF2* expression levels were quite variable in both groups, and the standard error of mean in these groups was consequently large. Further analysis of gene expression data did not reveal any difference between control individuals and PD patients or between groups of patients receiving a diagnosis before and after the age of 50 years. There was still great variability between individuals within all groups. Furthermore, the variable expression levels did not correlate with the age of the study participants (spanning from 40 to 83 years), which is surprising considering previous reports of Nrf2 decreasing with increasing age [4, 6]. The marked divergence in expression levels within the different groups in our study indicates that there is a regulatory parameter not included in our analysis. We might therefore hypothesize that there are more regulatory *NRF2* SNPs which could influence the gene expression of *NRF2*, independently or in concert with rs35652421.

5. Conclusions

We have found a genotype association of rs35652124 with EO PD, a finding which supports the involvement of *NRF2* in PD. Our results indicate that *NRF2* has a disease modifying effect rather than affecting disease risk, but more detailed studies of the *NRF2* gene in larger populations are warranted. Quantification of mRNA in human blood cells showed that *NRF2* expression in control subjects and that of PD patients were similar and that the promoter SNP rs35652124 does not have a consistent effect on mRNA levels. Thus far, there is sparse functional evidence available to illuminate the role of genetic variants in *NRF2* in PD. Therefore it is also important to expand the knowledge on the function of *NRF2* in pathophysiology in order to conclude on the importance of this gene in PD.

Acknowledgments

The authors would like to thank Laura Fratiglioni for providing them with control samples from the SNAC-K project. Postmortem human tissue was provided by the Netherlands Brain Bank (Amsterdam, Netherlands). This study was supported by the Swedish Brain Power, the Swedish Research Council, the Swedish Parkinson Foundation, the Swedish Brain Foundation, Åke Wibergs Stiftelse, and Karolinska Institutet Funds.

References

[1] C. Ran and A. C. Belin, "The genetics of Parkinson's disease: review of current and emerging candidates," *Journal of Parkinsonism and Restless Legs Syndrome*, vol. 2014, no. 4, pp. 63–75, 2014.

[2] P. Moi, K. Chan, I. Asunis, A. Cao, and Y. W. Kan, "Isolation of NF-E2-related factor 2 (Nrf2), a NF-E2-like basic leucine zipper transcriptional activator that binds to the tandem NF-E2/AP1 repeat of the β-globin locus control region," *Proceedings of the National Academy of Sciences of the United States of America*, vol. 91, no. 21, pp. 9926–9930, 1994.

[3] T. W. Kensler, N. Wakabayashi, and S. Biswal, "Cell survival responses to environmental stresses via the Keap1-Nrf2-ARE pathway," *Annual Review of Pharmacology and Toxicology*, vol. 47, pp. 89–116, 2007.

[4] P.-H. Shih and G.-C. Yen, "Differential expressions of antioxidant status in aging rats: the role of transcriptional factor Nrf2 and MAPK signaling pathway," *Biogerontology*, vol. 8, no. 2, pp. 71–80, 2007.

[5] K. Itoh, T. Chiba, S. Takahashi et al., "An Nrf2/small Maf heterodimer mediates the induction of phase II detoxifying enzyme genes through antioxidant response elements," *Biochemical and Biophysical Research Communications*, vol. 236, no. 2, pp. 313–322, 1997.

[6] J. H. Suh, S. V. Shenvi, B. M. Dixon et al., "Decline in transcriptional activity of Nrf2 causes age-related loss of glutathione synthesis, which is reversible with lipoic acid," *Proceedings of the National Academy of Sciences of the United States of America*, vol. 101, no. 10, pp. 3381–3386, 2004.

[7] C. P. Ramsey, C. A. Glass, M. B. Montgomery et al., "Expression of Nrf2 in neurodegenerative diseases," *Journal of Neuropathology and Experimental Neurology*, vol. 66, no. 1, pp. 75–85, 2007.

[8] Y.-C. Chen, Y.-R. Wu, Y.-C. Wu, G.-J. Lee-Chen, and C.-M. Chen, "Genetic analysis of NFE2L2 promoter variation in Taiwanese Parkinson's disease," *Parkinsonism and Related Disorders*, vol. 19, no. 2, pp. 247–250, 2013.

[9] Y. Gui, L. Zhang, W. Lv, W. Zhang, J. Zhao, and X. Hu, "NFE2L2 variations reduce antioxidant response in patients with Parkinson disease," *Oncotarget*, vol. 7, no. 10, pp. 10756–10764, 2016.

[10] M. Todorovic, J. R. B. Newman, J. Shan et al., "Comprehensive assessment of genetic sequence variants in the antioxidant 'master regulator' Nrf2 in idiopathic parkinson's disease," *PLoS ONE*, vol. 10, no. 5, Article ID e0128030, 2015.

[11] M. von Otter, S. Landgren, S. Nilsson et al., "Association of Nrf2-encoding NFE2L2 haplotypes with Parkinson's disease," *BMC Medical Genetics*, vol. 11, no. 1, article 36, 2010.

[12] M. von Otter, P. Bergström, A. Quattrone et al., "Genetic associations of Nrf2-encoding variants with Parkinson's disease — a multicenter study," *BMC Medical Genetics*, vol. 15, no. 1, article 131, 2014.

[13] M. von Otter, S. Landgren, S. Nilsson et al., "Nrf2-encoding NFE2L2 haplotypes influence disease progression but not risk in Alzheimer's disease and age-related cataract," *Mechanisms of Ageing and Development*, vol. 131, no. 2, pp. 105–110, 2010.

[14] P. Bergström, M. Von Otter, S. Nilsson et al., "Association of NFE2L2 and KEAP1 haplotypes with amyotrophic lateral sclerosis," *Amyotrophic Lateral Sclerosis and Frontotemporal Degeneration*, vol. 15, no. 1-2, pp. 130–137, 2014.

[15] S. E. Daniel and A. J. Lees, "Parkinson's Disease Society Brain Bank, London: overview and research," *Journal of Neural Transmission. Supplementa*, vol. 39, pp. 165–172, 1993.

[16] C. Ran, *On Genes Involved in Common Neurological Disorders: Focus on Parkinson's Disease. Karolinska Institutet*, Sweden, Stockholm, 2014.

[17] M. Ronaghi, M. Uhlén, and P. Nyrén, "A sequencing method based on real-time pyrophosphate," *Science*, vol. 281, no. 5375, pp. 363–365, 1998.

[18] E. V. Walls, M. G. Doyle, K. K. Patel, M. J. Allday, D. Catovsky, and D. H. Crawford, "Activation and immortalization of leukaemic B cells by Epstein-Barr virus," *International Journal of Cancer*, vol. 44, no. 5, pp. 846–853, 1989.

[19] S. Purcell, B. Neale, K. Todd-Brown et al., "PLINK: a tool set for whole-genome association and population-based linkage analyses," *American Journal of Human Genetics*, vol. 81, no. 3, pp. 559–575, 2007.

[20] S. Rodriguez, T. R. Gaunt, and I. N. M. Day, "Hardy-Weinberg equilibrium testing of biological ascertainment for Mendelian randomization studies," *American Journal of Epidemiology*, vol. 169, no. 4, pp. 505–514, 2009.

[21] J. C. Barrett, B. Fry, J. Maller, and M. J. Daly, "Haploview: analysis and visualization of LD and haplotype maps," *Bioinformatics*, vol. 21, no. 2, pp. 263–265, 2005.

[22] J. Hellemans, G. Mortier, A. de Paepe, F. Speleman, and J. Vandesompele, "qBase relative quantification framework and software for management and automated analysis of real-time quantitative PCR data," *Genome Biology*, vol. 8, no. 2, p. R19, 2007.

[23] J. M. Marzec, J. D. Christie, S. P. Reddy et al., "Functional polymorphisms in the transcription factor NRF2 in humans increase the risk of acute lung injury," *FASEB Journal*, vol. 21, no. 9, pp. 2237–2246, 2007.

[24] C.-C. Hua, L.-C. Chang, J.-C. Tseng, C.-M. Chu, Y.-C. Liu, and W.-B. Shieh, "Functional haplotypes in the promoter region of transcription factor Nrf2 in chronic obstructive pulmonary disease," *Disease Markers*, vol. 28, no. 3, pp. 185–193, 2010.

Crossing Virtual Doors: A New Method to Study Gait Impairments and Freezing of Gait in Parkinson's Disease

Luis I. Gómez-Jordana ⓘ,[1] James Stafford,[2] C. (Lieke) E. Peper,[1] and Cathy M. Craig ⓘ[2,3]

[1]*Department of Human Movement Sciences, Faculty of Behavioural and Movement Sciences, Vrije Universiteit Amsterdam, Amsterdam Movement Sciences, Amsterdam, Netherlands*
[2]*School of Psychology, Queens University Belfast, David Kier Building, 18-30 Malone Road, Belfast BT7 1NN, UK*
[3]*INCISIV Ltd., Ormeu Avenue, Belfast, UK*

Correspondence should be addressed to Cathy M. Craig; cathy@incisiv.tech

Academic Editor: Hélio Teive

Studying freezing of gait (FOG) in the lab has proven problematic. This has primarily been due to the difficulty in designing experimental setups that maintain high levels of ecological validity whilst also permitting sufficient levels of experimental control. To help overcome these challenges, we have developed a virtual reality (VR) environment with virtual doorways, a situation known to illicit FOG in real life. To examine the validity of this VR environment, an experiment was conducted, and the results were compared to a previous "real-world" experiment. A group of healthy controls ($N = 10$) and a group of idiopathic Parkinson disease (PD) patients without any FOG episodes ($N = 6$) and with a history of freezing (PD-f, $N = 4$) walked under three different virtual conditions (no door, narrow doorway (100% of shoulder width) and standard doorway (125% of shoulder width)). The results were similar to those obtained in the real-world setting. Virtual doorways reduced step length and velocity while increasing general gait variability. The PD-f group always walked slower, with a smaller step length, and showed the largest increases in gait variability. The narrow doorway induced FOG in 66% of the trials, while the standard doorway caused FOG in 29% of the trials. Our results closely mirrored those obtained with real doors. In short, this methodology provides a safe, personalized yet adequately controlled means to examine FOG in Parkinson's patients, along with possible interventions.

1. Introduction

Parkinson's disease (PD) is a degenerative disease that is characterized, in part, by the loss of dopamine-generating cells in the basal ganglia [1]. This lack of dopamine can cause bradykinesia (movement slowness), hypokinesia (reduced movement amplitude), akinesia (problems initiating movement), tremor, rigidity, and postural instability [2–4]. Approximately half of the patients with advanced stages of PD experience freezing of gait (FOG; [5]), a symptom where walking is interrupted by a brief, episodic absence, or marked reduction, of forward progression despite the intention to continue walking [3]. This debilitating symptom severely impairs mobility, hampers independence, and increases the risk of falling [3, 4].

Although the causes of FOG episodes are multifaceted, they often occur in response to certain environmental triggers (e.g., doorways) that may or may not require some kind of gait adaptation (e.g., turning or slowing down [6–10]). In this study, we aim to show how immersive, interactive virtual reality (VR) technology can offer a new methodological framework for studying FOG in people with Parkinson's. We will examine how well this technology can allow us to manipulate the visual context to induce changes in gait characterics in PD patients who have and have not experienced FOG episodes. Moreover, the use of an immersive, interactive VR environment can allow us to determine the extent to which different visual scenes (e.g., doorways) can induce FOG and impact gait performance.

Previous FOG-inducing protocols with a high level of experimental control are very different to how PD patients normally experience episodes of FOG in real life (e.g., [11, 12]) and as a result have low ecological validity [13]. In contrast, protocols that examine FOG in ecologically valid situations (e.g., in the patient's home [14]) usually suffer from limited experimental control, compromising analytic rigor and the subsequent interpretation of the data. A notable exception to this is a study by Cowie et al. [15, 16], who asked their participants to cross real doorways constructed and presented in a laboratory setting and that were scaled to an individual participant's shoulder width. This paradigm not only induced episodes of FOG but ensured that a high level of ecological validity and experimental control was maintained. In this study, we will attempt to recreate this real-doorway paradigm in an immersive, interactive virtual reality environment that not only preserves ecological validity [17] but offers enhanced possibilities for experimental manipulation and control. Moreover, this technology also allows for the quick and personalized manipulation of the information delivered to each participant [18], yet offering reproducibility across trials.

The objective of this study was to see if a virtual environment with virtual doorways can induce FOG episodes in Parkinson's patients in the same way as real doorways [15, 16]. To examine the effectiveness of the virtual doorway manipulation, we followed Cowie et al.'s protocol [15, 16] and presented both narrow and standard doorways, comparing gait characteristics of PD patients with and without a history of FOG to those of healthy controls. We expected to find similar results to Cowie et al. [15, 16], namely, reduced step velocity, step length, and increased gait variability in Parkinson's patients, with the effects being larger for patients who have a history of FOG. It is also predicted that the FOG group will experience more freezing episodes in conditions with narrow doorways.

2. Methods

2.1. Participants. Three groups of participants were recruited: one group of healthy controls (HC; $N = 10$; mean age = 63.0 yr.; SD = 8.6 yr; 6 females), one group of idiopathic PD patients (PD; $N = 6$; mean age = 62.7 yr.; SD = 8.9 yr; 3 females), and a group of PD patients all of whom had a history of FOG (PD-f; $N = 4$; mean age = 67.5 yr.; SD = 7.0; 2 females). Motor disability was assessed using part III of the MDS-UPDRS questionnaire [19]. "The freezing of gait questionnaire" (FOGQ [20]) was used to assess if participants had experienced FOG consistently in the week prior to the experiment. A mean score >2 indicated that this was the case. The results of these tests are presented in Table 1, along with demographic information about the PD participants. The study was approved by the university's ethics committee.

2.2. Immersive, Interactive Virtual Reality. A virtual representation of a hallway was presented to participants using an Oculus Rift DK2 stereoscopic head-mounted display (Oculus VR, Irvine, California, USA). The screen had a resolution of 1920 × 1080, was updated 75 times per second, and had a field of view of 100°. To allow participants the freedom to walk up and down the virtual hallway, the Intersense IS900 (InterSense Inc., Bedford, Massachusetts, USA) tracking system was used

instead of the Oculus tracking (see Figure 1(a) for image of a participant performing a trial). Both head position and orientation were tracked and updated in the virtual environment at 120 Hz. The tracked space was 12 m long by 5 m wide.

The virtual environment was constructed using the games engine software Unity (version 5.4.1f1). The environment consisted of a virtual hallway 20 m long and 2.5 m high. In order to increase the realism of the environment, a clay texture was added to the walls and ceiling. Furthermore, to make the floor look as realistic as possible a texture was also added to make it look like a white carpet (Figure 2(a)).

The width of the hallway was personalized for each participant and was equivalent to 5 shoulder widths. Likewise, the width of the virtual doorways was also designed so that they were directly related to the participant's shoulder width (Figure 2(b)). Shoulder width was a parameter that was inputted at the start of each block of trials. The participants had to walk along the hallway between a red and a yellow line which were positioned 6.5 meters apart.

2.3. Walking Metrics. To capture gait performance data, participants had a rigid body containing three reflective markers attached to the back of each shoe (Figure 1(b)). The movement of these reflective markers was recorded at 100 Hz using 12 Qualisys infrared motion capture cameras (Qualisys Ltd., Göteborg, Sweden). In order to allow participants to see their own feet in the virtual environment, data were streamed in real-time from the infrared motion capture system into the virtual environment (Qualisys Unity SDK), 30 times a second. The position of the two rigid bodies was used to control the position and orientation of two cuboids that were used to virtually represent the position of the feet (Figure 2(c)).

2.4. Procedure. Before the start of the experiment, the participant's shoulder width was measured and entered into Unity to scale the width of the virtual doorway and the hallway to the participant's own bodily proportions. The experiment was carried out by two experimenters. One experimenter controlled the virtual environment and the motion capture system while the other walked next to the participant, holding the cable that connects the headset to the computer, to ensure the participant's safety. In accordance with Cowie et al. [16], three conditions were created: no virtual doorway (no door (ND)); a virtual doorway with a width that corresponded to the participant's own shoulder width (narrow door (NaD)) or to 125% of the participant's shoulder width (standard door (StaD)).(Note that the large door condition (150% shoulder width) that was included in Cowie's experiment was omitted from our study. It was found not to induce any changes in gait characteristics nor any FOG episodes in patients with an FOG history.) Supplementary Video 1 of the supplementary material includes an example of what a healthy control saw in the VR environment while completing each of the three conditions. Supplementary Video 2 includes an example of a healthy control completing one trial in each of the three conditions.

TABLE 1: Demographic information about the PD participants.

Participant	Age (years)	Gender	Years from diagnosis	Clinical state	UPDRS part III	FOG-Q
PD1	61	Female	7	On	10	0.33 (0.51)
PD2	77	Male	6	Off	29	0.66 (1.06)
PD3	64	Female	2	On	18	0.33 (0.52)
PD4	66	Female	4	On	37	0.5 (0.55)
PD5	50	Male	2	On	23	0.66 (1.03)
PD6	58	Male	7	On	27	0.66(1.03)
PD-f1	68	Female	6	Off	35	3.00 (0.63)
PD-f2	76	Male	5	On	28	3.16 (0.43)
PD-f3	59	Female	4	On	36	2.66 (0.81)
PD-f4	69	Male	6	Off	41	3.33 (0.51)

The clinical state is related to the effect of the medication: on = responding well to medication; off = not responding to medication. The results of the FOGQ are presented as the mean (SD) of all the results in the test. Participants PD1-6 = idiopathic PD group; PD-f1–f4 = PD participants that have experienced freezing in the past.

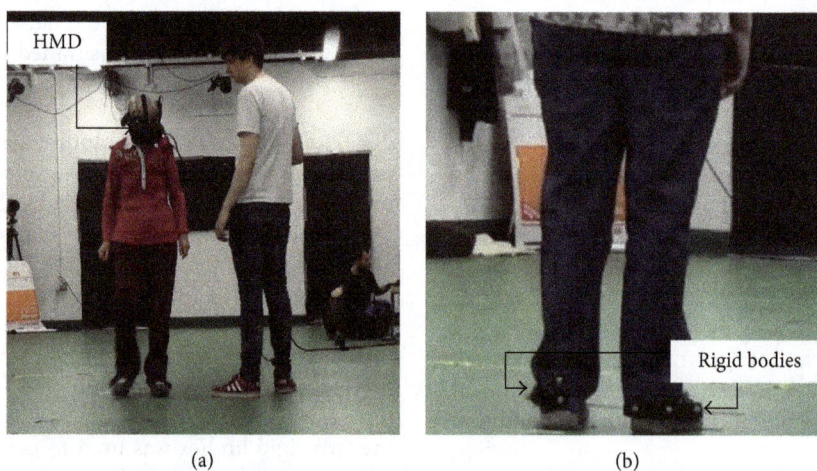

(a)   (b)

FIGURE 1: (a) A participant performing a trial. The participant wore a head-mounted display (HMD). Two experimenters are present, one to ensure the safety of the participant and another one to control the computer. (b) The two rigid bodies attached to the back of the shoes were used to track the position of the feet.

The three experimental conditions (ND, NaD, and StaD) were randomly presented six times giving a total of 18 trials. Before the start of the experiment, participants were given a familiarisation phase, where they walked up and down the virtual hallway eight times. Each time they were confronted with doors with slightly different widths to the ones used in the experimental trials.

In the conditions where a doorway was present, it was placed 4 meters in front of the participant with the red or yellow line indicating the end of the trial, positioned a further 2.5 m beyond the doorway. In all conditions, the participants were instructed to pass through the virtual doorway as they would normally pass through a doorway in real life and walk towards the yellow or red line in front of them. Once they reached the line indicating the end of the trial, the trial automatically ended and participants, with the help of the experimenter, were asked to turn around and face the opposite direction ready for the next trial. After each block of six trials, the participants were allowed to rest for 2 minutes to again minimise fatigue. The procedure lasted about 20 minutes.

2.5. Gait Analysis. For the conditions that involved a doorway, the gait parameter analysis (step length, cadence, and step velocity) was restricted to the area around the doorway (3.5 m before the doorway to 1 m beyond the doorway). For the no door (ND) condition, the same location was used to ensure the walking distance analysed was similar in all three conditions. The Qualisys data were analysed using custom-made Matlab (Matlab 2016b; Mathworks, Inc, Natick, Massachusetts, USA) routines. After low-pass filtering the gait data (recursive Butterworth; 2nd order; cutoff frequency: 10 Hz), heel strikes were marked automatically based on the moments at which the marker nearest to the heel reached zero velocity in a vertical direction. Step length was defined as the distance between two successive heel strikes in the walking direction. Step cadence was formalized as the number of steps taken each second. Step velocity was calculated by dividing step length by the time it took to complete that step. For each trial, the mean and coefficient of variation (CV; i.e., the ratio between the standard deviation and the mean) was calculated.

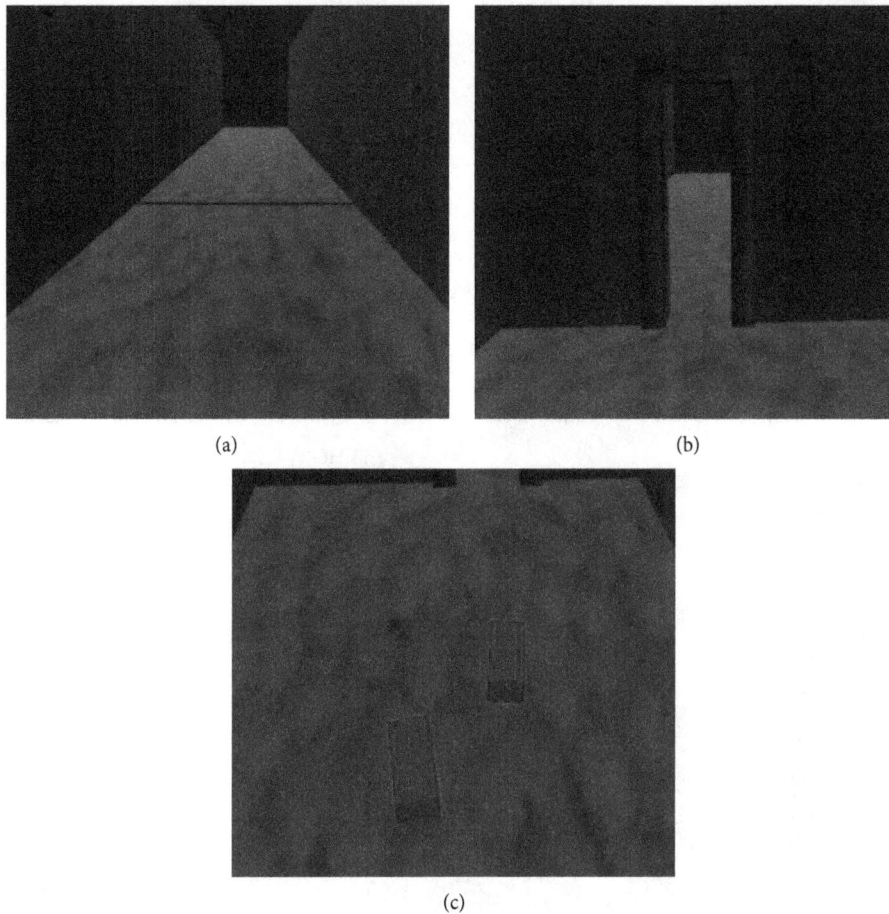

(a)

(b)

(c)

FIGURE 2: (a) The no doorway (ND) condition along with the red line indicating the end of the trial in that direction, (b) the narrow doorway (NaD) condition, and (c) a visual representation of the two cuboids that represent the placement of the participant's feet in the virtual environment (note that the image is captured from behind the participant).

To determine whether FOG was induced in the PD-f group, we followed the analysis of Cowie et al. [16] which is based solely on step velocity. According to this method, FOG episodes were defined as sections of a trial where step velocity dropped below 10% of the mean velocity obtained for the same participant in the ND condition. If there were fewer than three strides between two identified FOG episodes, these two episodes were considered to reflect a single FOG episode. For each PD-f participant, we determined the percentage of trials in which FOG episodes were detected, as well as the mean duration of these episodes and the respective standard deviation.

2.6. Statistical Analysis. All statistical analyses were conducted using RStudio (RStudio 1.138; RStudio, Inc., Boston, MA). Two-way mixed ANOVAs with the between-subjects factor being group (HC, PD, and PD-f) and the within-subjects factor being door (ND, NaD, and StaD) were carried out on the means and CVs of the three gait parameters. The results were considered significant if p was less than 0.05. Post hoc comparisons were based on simple effects analysis [21] and (if required) pairwise t-tests with Bonferroni correction were used. The size of the effect was also presented using the ω_p^2 that is believed to be a better

estimate of the size of the effect than η_p^2 [22]. This statistic can take values from 0 to 1, higher values indicating a higher effect size.

Kruskal–Wallis tests with a within-subject factor door (ND, NaD, and StaD) were conducted on the percentage of FOG episodes in the PD-f group. The results were considered significant if p was less than 0.05. If needed, post hoc Dunn tests with Bonferroni corrections were carried out to test for significant main effects. Mean durations of these episodes and respective standard deviations were not submitted for statistical analysis.

3. Results

3.1. Gait Parameters

3.1.1. Mean Gait Parameter Values. The ANOVA results for step length (Figure 3(a)) and step velocity were similar. In both cases, the main effect of door was significant (step length: $F_{(2,34)} = 68.34$, $p < 0.001$, $\omega_p^2 = 0.180$; step velocity: $F_{(2,34)} = 67.45$, $p < 0.001$, $\omega_p^2 = 0.178$). Post hoc analyses revealed a significantly smaller step length and lower step velocity in the NaD condition compared to the ND condition (Figure 3(c)). For both gait parameters, the effect of group was also significant (step length: $F_{(2,17)} = 5.08$,

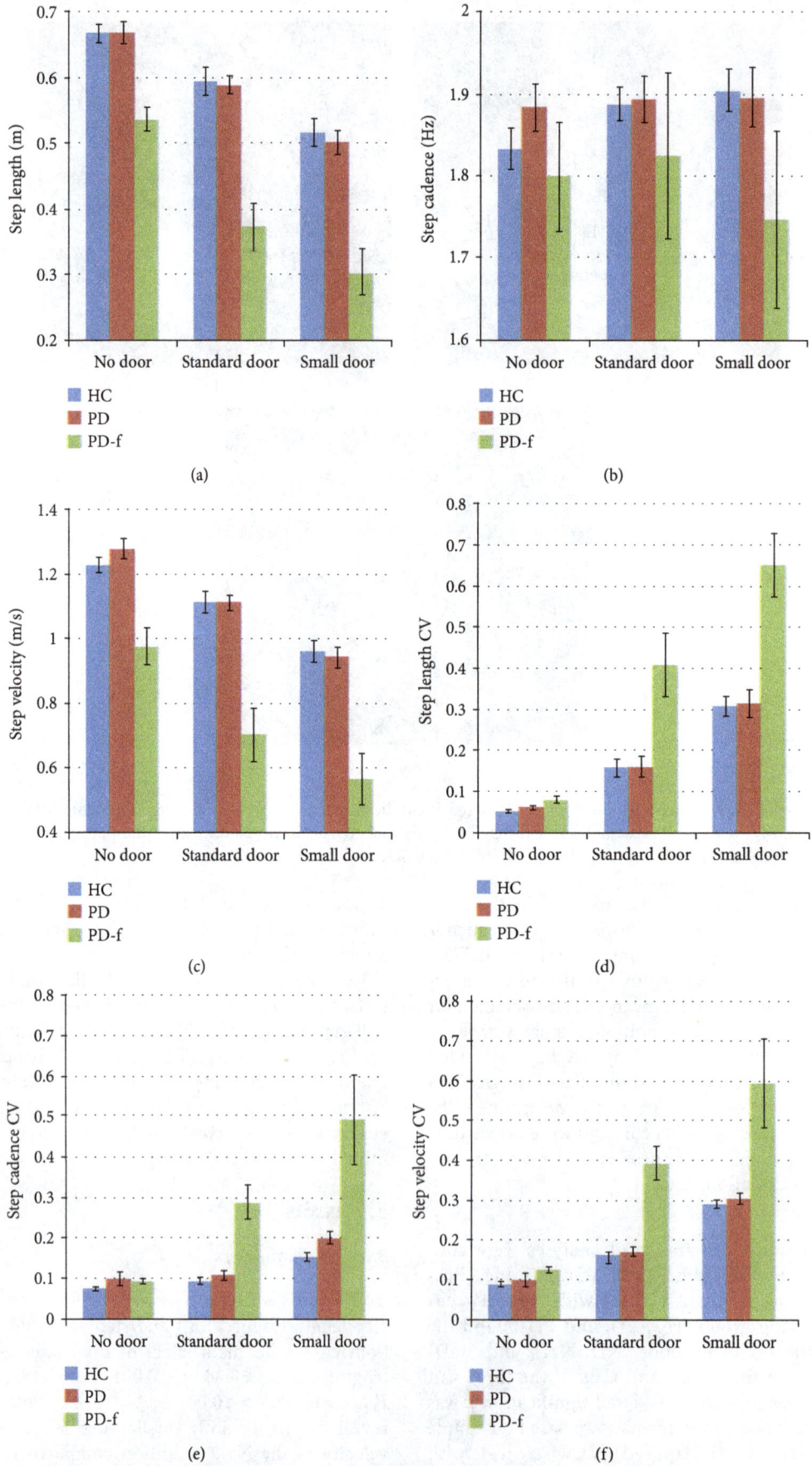

FIGURE 3: Results for step length (a), step cadence (b), step velocity (c), step length CV (d), step cadence CV (e), and step velocity CV (f) for the three groups, for the three different door conditions. The data for step length are presented in meters. The data of step cadence are presented in hertz that can be understood as the number of steps per second. Finally, the data for the step velocity are presented in meters per second (m/s). The error bars represent the standard error of the mean.

TABLE 2: Characteristics of induced FOG episodes for each participant in the PD-f group as a function of door condition.

Participants	Door condition	% trials with an FOG episode	Mean duration of an FOG episode	Max duration of an FOG episode	Min duration of an FOG episode
PD-f1	No door	0	NA	NA	NA
	Standard door	33	5.64 s ± 4.07 s	8.972 s	0.51 s
	Narrow door	100	7.64 s ± 5.26 s	17.93 s	1.00 s
PD-f2	No door	0	NA	NA	NA
	Standard door	0	NA	NA	NA
	Narrow door	16	1.00 s ± 0.00 s	1.00 s	1.00 s
PD-f3	No door	0	NA	NA	NA
	Standard door	0	NA	NA	NA
	Narrow door	50	0.61 s ± 0.23 s	0.87 s	0.45 s
PD-f4	No door	16	0.85 s ± 0.00 s	0.85 s	0.85 s
	Standard door	83	2.85 s ± 3.71 s	9.45 s	0.85 s
	Narrow door	100	3.1 s ± 1.68 s	6.35 s	1.97 s

The results include percentage of trials in which patients experienced FOG; mean duration of these episodes (including standard deviation); and maximum and minimum duration of the episodes. NA indicates that no FOG episode was observed.

$p = 0.018$, $\omega_p^2 = 0.026$; step velocity: $F_{(2,17)} = 5.51$, $p = 0.014$, $\omega_p^2 = 0.028$), with post hoc analyses showing that both parameters were significantly smaller in the PD-f group than in the two other groups. For step cadence (Figure 3(b)), no significant effects were obtained.

3.1.2. Variability (CV) of the Gait Parameters. The results of the three ANOVAs that were conducted on the gait parameter CVs also showed close correspondence. In all cases, main effects were obtained for door (step length CV: $F_{(2,34)} = 36.87$, $p < 0.001$, $\omega_p^2 = 0.105$; step cadence: $F_{(2,34)} = 10.20$, $p < 0.001$, $\omega_p^2 = 0.044$; step velocity: $F_{(2,34)} = 34.51$ $p < 0.001$, $\omega_p^2 = 0.099$) and group ($F_{(2,17)} = 4.07$, $p = 0.036$, $\omega_p^2 = 0.020$; $F_{(2,17)} = 5.65$, $p = 0.013$, $\omega_p^2 = 0.029$; $F_{(2,17)} = 5.26$ $p = 0.017$, $\omega_p^2 = 0.028$, resp.),while the interaction between these two factors was also significant ($F_{(4,37)} = 3.08$, $p = 0.029$, $\omega_p^2 = 0.015$; $F_{(4,37)} = 3.48$, $p = 0.017$; $\omega_p^2 = 0.017$; $F_{(4,37)} = 3.13$, $p = 0.027$; $\omega_p^2 = 0.015$, resp.). For step length CV (Figure 3(d)) and step velocity CV (Figure 3(f)), post hoc analysis of the effect of door revealed that variability was larger in the NaD condition compared to the other two conditions. For step cadence CV (Figure 3(e)), variability in the NaD condition was larger than in the ND condition. The group effect was similar for all three CVs, showing higher variability for the PD-f group than for the other two groups. The door x group interaction was also similar for all three CVs, indicating that in the PD-f group, all door conditions differed significantly from one another, while in the other two groups the difference was significant only between the NaD and ND conditions. The analysis indicated that there was no significant difference between groups in the ND condition, but the difference between the PD-f group and the other groups was significant for both the NaD and the StaD doorways.

3.2. Freezing Episodes. Table 2 presents, per condition, the percentage of trials in which FOG episodes were detected for the individual participants who made up the PD-f group, along with information regarding the durations of these FOG episodes. The NaD condition induced at least one FOG episode in all four patients, with FOG occurring in all of the

NaD trials for two of the participants (PD-f1 and PD-f4). The StaD condition was less effective in this regard, but still induced FOG in 83% of the trials in PD-f4 and 33% of the trials in PD-f1. The Kruskal–Wallis test yielded a significant effect for the factor door ($\chi^2 = 24.32$ $p < 0.001$). Post hoc analysis revealed that the three door conditions were significantly different, with the NaD condition (66%) inducing more FOG episodes than the StaD condition (29%) which in turn caused more FOG episodes than the ND condition (4%). Supplementary Video 3 shows PD-f1 completing a trial in each doorway condition and illustrates how both doorway conditions cause her to experience a FOG episode.

4. Discussion

We developed an immersive, interactive VR environment that was used to manipulate the visual context within which participants control their walking along a virtual hallway. The technology not only allows us to systematically examine how environmental changes such as the presence of virtual doorways of different widths influences various gait characteristics, but also how these visual changes influence the number of FOG episodes participants with Parkinson's disease experience. By using the power of VR to recreate real-life situations commonly known to induce FOG (namely narrow doorways), we were able to measure the effects these doorways had on a participant's gait. Overall, the results obtained in our VR environment were very similar to those found in the studies conducted by Almeida and Lebold [23] and Cowie et al. [15] who used real-life stimuli. In sum, the PD-f group walked slower with smaller steps and demonstrated a higher degree of gait variability than the other two groups. When confronted with narrow doorways, all groups reduced speed and step length, compared to the condition in which no doorway was presented.

A further validation of our method was the fact that the narrow doorway elicited higher degrees of gait variability for *all* groups of participants compared to the condition without a door. Moreover, our virtual doorways induced freezing-like episodes in the majority of our PD-f patients. These episodes ranged from 1 s to 18 s, with a median of around 8 s. All of these participants had more freezing episodes when presented with the narrow doorway compared to the standard doorway. These findings clearly demonstrate how the visual information presented in the virtual environment influences gait in the same way as real doorways [16].

The close correspondence between our current results and those obtained in experiments using real doorways, speaks to the high levels of behavioural realism and ecological validity induced by the VR environment. What is interesting about this technology is that it can be easily used to examine gait in Parkinson's disease but also be used to successfully induce FOG episodes in a patient population. Moreover, VR environments can not only be used to assess the symptoms of PD, but also to test the effects potential interventions may have on improving quality of life in a safe and systematic way. For instance, the effectiveness of specific forms of visual cueing [24], to reduce FOG and improve Parkinsonian gait, may be readily examined in a VR environment. This also holds true for testing visual cueing techniques that use augmented reality glasses [25–27] which may ultimately offer a more practical application for adding virtual cues to real-life conditions. Other lines of research may also focus on the development of ecologically valid, immersive VR environments that are representative of other problematic situations for PD patients (like initiating gait or turning) and test potential intervention strategies that can be personalized to meet the needs of the individual participant.

In conclusion, immersive, interactive virtual reality is an exciting methodology that allows for the preservation of the perception/action loop. By controlling the presentation of sensory information (e.g., visual context), we can systematically and accurately measure the effects on different movement behaviours.

References

[1] J. Jankovic, "Parkinson's disease: clinical features and diagnosis," *Journal of Neurology, Neurosurgery and Psychiatry*, vol. 79, no. 4, pp. 368–376, 2008.

[2] O. Blin, A. M. Ferrandez, J. Pailhous, and G. Serratrice, "Dopa-sensitive and dopa-resistant gait parameters in Parkinson's disease," *Journal of the Neurological Sciences*, vol. 103, no. 1, pp. 51–54, 1991.

[3] B. R. Bloem, J. M. Hausdorff, J. E. Visser, and N. Giladi, "Falls and freezing of gait in Parkinson's disease: a review of two interconnected, episodic phenomena," *Movement Disorders*, vol. 19, no. 8, pp. 871–884, 2004.

[4] J. D. Schaafsma, Y. Balash, T. Gurevich, A. L. Bartels, J. M. Hausdorff, and N. Giladi, "Characterization of freezing of gait subtypes and the response of each to levodopa in Parkinson's disease," *European Journal of Neurology*, vol. 10, no. 4, pp. 391–398, 2003.

[5] N. Giladi, T. A. Treves, E. S. Simon et al., "Freezing of gait in patients with advanced Parkinson's disease," *Journal of Neural Transmission*, vol. 108, no. 1, pp. 53–61, 2001.

[6] N. Giladi, D. McMahon, S. Przedborski et al., "Motor blocks in Parkinson's disease," *Neurology*, vol. 42, no. 2, pp. 333–339, 1992.

[7] S. Fahn, "The Freezing Phenomenon in Parkinsonism," in *Negative Motor Phenomena: Advances in Neurology*, S. Fahn, M. Hallett, H. O. Luders, and C. D. Marsden, Eds., vol. 67, pp. 53–63, Lippincott-Raven Publishers, Philadelphia, PA, USA, 1995.

[8] P. Lamberti, S. Armenise, V. Castaldo et al., "Freezing gait in Parkinson's Disease," *European Journal of Neurology*, vol. 38, no. 4, pp. 297–301, 1997.

[9] A. P. Denny and M. Behari, "Motor fluctuations in Parkinson's disease," *Journal of Neurological Science*, vol. 165, no. 1, pp. 18–23, 1999.

[10] N. Giladi, Y. Balash, and J. M. Hausdorff, "Gait Disturbances in Parkinson's Disease," in *Mapping the Progress of Alzheimer's and Parkinson's Disease*, Y. Mizuno, A. Fisher, and I. Hanin, Eds., pp. 329–335, Kluwer Academic/Plenum Publishers, New York, NY, USA, 2002.

[11] J. Nantel, C. de Solages, and H. Bronte-Stewart, "Repetitive stepping in place identifies and measures freezing episodes in subjects with Parkinson's disease," *Gait Posture*, vol. 34, no. 3, pp. 329–333, 2011.

[12] W. R. Young, L. Shreve, E. J. Quinn, C. Craig, and H. Bronte-Stewart, "Auditory cueing in Parkinson's patients with freezing of gait. What matters most: action-relevance or cue-continuity?," *Neuropsychologia*, vol. 87, pp. 54–62, 2016.

[13] E. Brunswik, "Representative design and probabilistic theory in a functional psychology," *Psychological Review*, vol. 62, no. 3, pp. 193–217, 1955.

[14] M. Bachlin, M. Plotnik, D. Roggen et al., "Wearable assistant for Parkinson's disease patients with the freezing of gait symptom," *IEEE Transactions on Information Technology in Biomedicine*, vol. 14, no. 2, pp. 436–446, 2010.

[15] D. Cowie, P. Limousin, A. Peters, and B. L. Day, "Insights into the neural control of locomotion from walking through doorways in Parkinson's disease," *Neuropsychologia*, vol. 48, no. 9, pp. 2750–2757, 2010.

[16] D. Cowie, P. Limousin, A. Peters, M. Hariz, and B. L. Day, "Doorway-provoked freezing of gait in Parkinson's disease," *Movement Disorders*, vol. 27, no. 4, pp. 492–499, 2012.

[17] C. Craig, "Understanding perception and action in sport: how can virtual reality technology help?," *Sports Technology*, vol. 6, no. 4, pp. 161–169, 2014.

[18] M. T. Schultheis and A. A. Rizzo, "The application of virtual reality technology in rehabilitation," *Rehabilitation Psychology*, vol. 46, no. 3, pp. 296–312, 2001.

[19] CG Goetz, BC Tilley, SR Shaftman et al., "Movement disorder society-sponsored revision of the unified Parkinson's disease rating scale (MDS-UPDRS): scale presentation and clinimetric testing results," *Movement Disorders*, vol. 23, no. 15, pp. 2129–2170, 2008.

[20] N. Giladi, H. Shabtai, E. S. Simon, S. Biran, J. Tal, and A. D. Korczyn, "Construction of freezing of gait questionnaire for patients with Parkinsonism," *Parkinsonism and Related Disorders*, vol. 6, no. 3, pp. 165–170, 2000.

[21] G. Keppel and S. Zedeck, *Data Analysis for Research Designs*, Freeman, New York, NY, USA, 1989.

[22] K. Okada, "Is omega squared less biased? A comparison of three major effect size indices in one-way ANOVA," *Behaviormetrika*, vol. 40, no. 2, pp. 129–147, 2013.

[23] Q. J. Almeida and C. A. Lebold, "Freezing of gait in Par-

kinson's disease: a perceptual cause for a motor impairment?," *Journal of Neurology, Neurosurgery*, vol. 81, no. 5, pp. 513–518, 2010.

[24] J. P. Azulay, S. Mesure, and O. Blin, "Influence of visual cues on gait in Parkinson's disease: contribution to attention or sensory dependence?," *Journal of the Neurological Sciences*, vol. 248, no. 1, pp. 192–195, 2006.

[25] H. J. Griffin, R. Greenlaw, P. Limousin, K. Bhatia, N. P. Quinn, and M. Jahanshahi, "The effect of real and virtual visual cues on walking in Parkinson's disease," *Journal of neurology*, vol. 258, no. 6, pp. 991–1000, 2011.

[26] S. Janssen, B. Bolte, J. Nonnekes et al., "Usability of three-dimensional augmented visual cues delivered by smart glasses on (freezing of) gait in Parkinson's disease," *Frontiers in Neurology*, vol. 8, pp. 279–289, 2017.

[27] J. H. McAuley, P. M. Daly, and C. R. Curtis, "A preliminary investigation of a novel design of visual cue glasses that aid gait in Parkinson's disease," *Clinical Rehabilitation*, vol. 23, no. 8, pp. 687–695, 2009.

Cognitive Training and Transcranial Direct Current Stimulation for Mild Cognitive Impairment in Parkinson's Disease: A Randomized Controlled Trial

Blake J. Lawrence [ID],[1,2,3,4] Natalie Gasson,[1,2] Andrew R. Johnson,[1,2] Leon Booth,[1,2] and Andrea M. Loftus[1,2]

[1]Curtin Neuroscience Laboratory, School of Psychology and Speech Pathology, Curtin University, Bentley, WA 6102, Australia
[2]ParkC Collaborative Research Group, Curtin University, Bentley, WA 6102, Australia
[3]Ear Science Institute Australia, Subiaco, WA, Australia
[4]Ear Sciences Centre, School of Surgery, The University of Western Australia, Crawley, WA, Australia

Correspondence should be addressed to Blake J. Lawrence; blake.lawrence@earscience.org.au

Academic Editor: HaiBo Chen

This study examined whether standard cognitive training, tailored cognitive training, transcranial direct current stimulation (tDCS), standard cognitive training + tDCS, or tailored cognitive training + tDCS improved cognitive function and functional outcomes in participants with PD and mild cognitive impairment (PD-MCI). Forty-two participants with PD-MCI were randomized to one of six groups: (1) standard cognitive training, (2) tailored cognitive training, (3) tDCS, (4) standard cognitive training + tDCS, (5) tailored cognitive training + tDCS, or (6) a control group. Interventions lasted 4 weeks, with cognitive and functional outcomes measured at baseline, post-intervention, and follow-up. The trial was registered with the Australian New Zealand Clinical Trials Registry (ANZCTR: 12614001039673). While controlling for moderator variables, Generalized Linear Mixed Models (GLMMs) showed that when compared to the control group, the intervention groups demonstrated variable statistically significant improvements across executive function, attention/working memory, memory, language, activities of daily living (ADL), and quality of life (QOL; Hedge's g range = 0.01 to 1.75). More outcomes improved for the groups that received standard or tailored cognitive training combined with tDCS. Participants with PD-MCI receiving cognitive training (standard or tailored) or tDCS demonstrated significant improvements on cognitive and functional outcomes, and combining these interventions provided greater therapeutic effects.

1. Introduction

There is a growing body of research examining mild cognitive impairment in Parkinson's disease (PD-MCI) and the potential of nonpharmacological interventions (e.g., cognitive training and noninvasive brain stimulation) for improving cognitive function in PD and PD-MCI [1].

There are two frequently used methods of computer-based cognitive training: standard or tailored. Standard cognitive training involves cognitive tasks that are not customised to the individual's cognitive deficits, whereas tailored cognitive training is deficit specific. Recent studies report improved cognition following standard and tailored cognitive training in PD. París et al. [2] examined whether standard multimedia and paper/pencil cognitive training improved cognitive functioning, quality of life (QOL), and activities of daily living (ADL) in PD. Compared to the control group, the trained group improved across all cognitive domains except language, but no improvement was found for QOL and ADL [2]. In a randomized controlled trial, Edwards et al. [3] examined whether standard computer-based cognitive training improved speed of processing in PD. There were significant improvements in speed of processing for those with mild/moderate PD [3]. For tailored cognitive training, Naismith et al. [4] examined the effect of two-hour sessions twice a week, which involved psychoeducation and tailored computer-based tasks. Episodic memory and learning retention significantly improved posttraining [4]. Cerasa et al. [5] examined neurofunctional correlates between trained cognitive domains and synaptic plasticity of those domains in PD. Participants completed 12 hours of computer-based cognitive training tailored to their pretraining cognitive impairment(s). Compared to the control group, the training group demonstrated attentional improvements which increased neural resting state (fMRI) activity in the superior parietal and prefrontal dorsolateral cortices [5]. There is increasing evidence supporting standard and tailored cognitive training for cognition in PD, but it remains unclear which modality has greater therapeutic potential [6].

Transcranial direct current stimulation (tDCS) modulates neuronal activity by delivering low-intensity electrical currents to specific cortical regions [7]. Initial studies report improved cognition following tDCS in PD. Boggio et al. [8] demonstrated that 2 mA tDCS over left DLPFC improved working memory in PD, whereas 1 mA and sham tDCS provided no beneficial effects for cognition. Pereira et al. [9] examined whether 20 minutes of counterbalanced 2 mA tDCS over left DLPFC and left temporoparietal cortices immediately improved executive functions. In a randomized controlled trial of tDCS in PD, Doruk et al. [10] compared 2 mA tDCS applied over left (group one) or right (group two) DLPFC with sham stimulation (control group) for executive function. Compared to the control group, significant improvements in the Trail Making Test (Part B) were found for both tDCS groups immediately following the two-week intervention and at one-month follow-up [10]. These studies provide preliminary evidence that tDCS may improve cognitive function in PD, but more standardised clinical trials are required to substantiate these findings.

One recent study [11] combined cognitive training with tDCS simultaneously and reported a trend towards significant improvement in memory, but the lack of a control group limits interpretation of intervention effects. It remains unclear whether combining cognitive training with tDCS provides optimal conditions (stimulation and compensation) to elicit neuronal plasticity and improve cognition in PD and PD-MCI. The present study examined whether standard cognitive training, tailored cognitive training, tDCS, standard cognitive training + tDCS, and tailored cognitive training + tDCS improved cognitive function and practical outcomes in PD-MCI.

2. Methods

2.1. Study Design. This study was a parallel, randomized controlled trial conducted in accordance with CONSORT requirements (see Supplementary Table S1) [12]. Participants were randomized to one of six groups (5 intervention and 1 control) by a computer generated list using block randomization at a ratio of 1 : 1. Blinding is difficult to achieve in nonpharmacological trials, and so participants and researchers were not blinded to the interventions.

Participants in the standard or tailored cognitive training groups completed computer-based training for 45 minutes, 3 times per week for 4 weeks. Cognitive training was completed using the website version of Smartbrain Pro™ (http://www.smartbrain.net) in participants' homes. Participants in a tDCS group completed 20 minutes of stimulation, once a week for 4 weeks. Each session of tDCS was completed at Curtin University. All participants completed the same neuropsychological tests at baseline (week 0), post-intervention (week 5), and follow-up (week 12).

Curtin University's Ethics Committee provided approval (approval number: HR 189/2014), and this study was registered with the Australian New Zealand Clinical Trials Registry (ANZCTR: 12614001039673). All participants provided informed consent, and participation was completed during participants' "ON" stage of medication.

2.2. Study Population. Participant recruitment and neuropsychological assessments were completed at Curtin University, Western Australia, in 2015. The following inclusion criteria applied: (1) participants diagnosed with idiopathic PD in accordance with the UK PD Brain Bank criteria, (2) presence of MCI in accordance with the Movement Disorder Society (MDS) PD-MCI Level II diagnostic criteria [13], (3) a stable response to antiparkinsonian medication at pre-intervention and during the course of the intervention, and (4) cognitive deficits that did not interfere with functional independence (i.e., UPDRS-II score less than 3). The following exclusion criteria applied: (1) presence of PD-Dementia, (2) recent history of brain surgery, (3) Deep Brain Stimulation (DBS) implant, (4) active skin disease on the scalp, (5) history of migraine or epilepsy, and (6) metal implants in the head/brain. 70 participants completed baseline neuropsychological assessments, with 42 meeting inclusion criteria (Figure 1). All participants completed their intervention and post-intervention neuropsychological assessments. Four participants (9.5%) did not complete follow-up assessments due to inability to travel due to disease progression ($N = 2$) and lack of time ($N = 2$).

2.3. Cognitive Training. Smartbrain Pro is an interactive computer-based training program designed to train each cognitive domain. Smartbrain Pro has been used in trials which have demonstrated improvements in cognitive functioning in Alzheimer's disease and PD [2, 14]. Smartbrain Pro was streamed directly from the Internet onto participants' home computers or onto Acer™ Aspire E3-112 portable computers via Optus™ E5251 Mini Wifi Modems (provided by the researcher). Performance was automatically monitored by the program to adjust individual difficultly levels for each activity. Participants in the standard cognitive training and standard cognitive training + tDCS groups completed a predetermined program comprising 10 activities, two activities per cognitive domain (see Supplementary Table S2). Participants in the tailored cognitive training and tailored cognitive training + tDCS groups completed activities which were individualized to their baseline neuropsychological test results. For example, a participant who demonstrated memory and executive function impairment at baseline completed only memory and executive function activities during cognitive training.

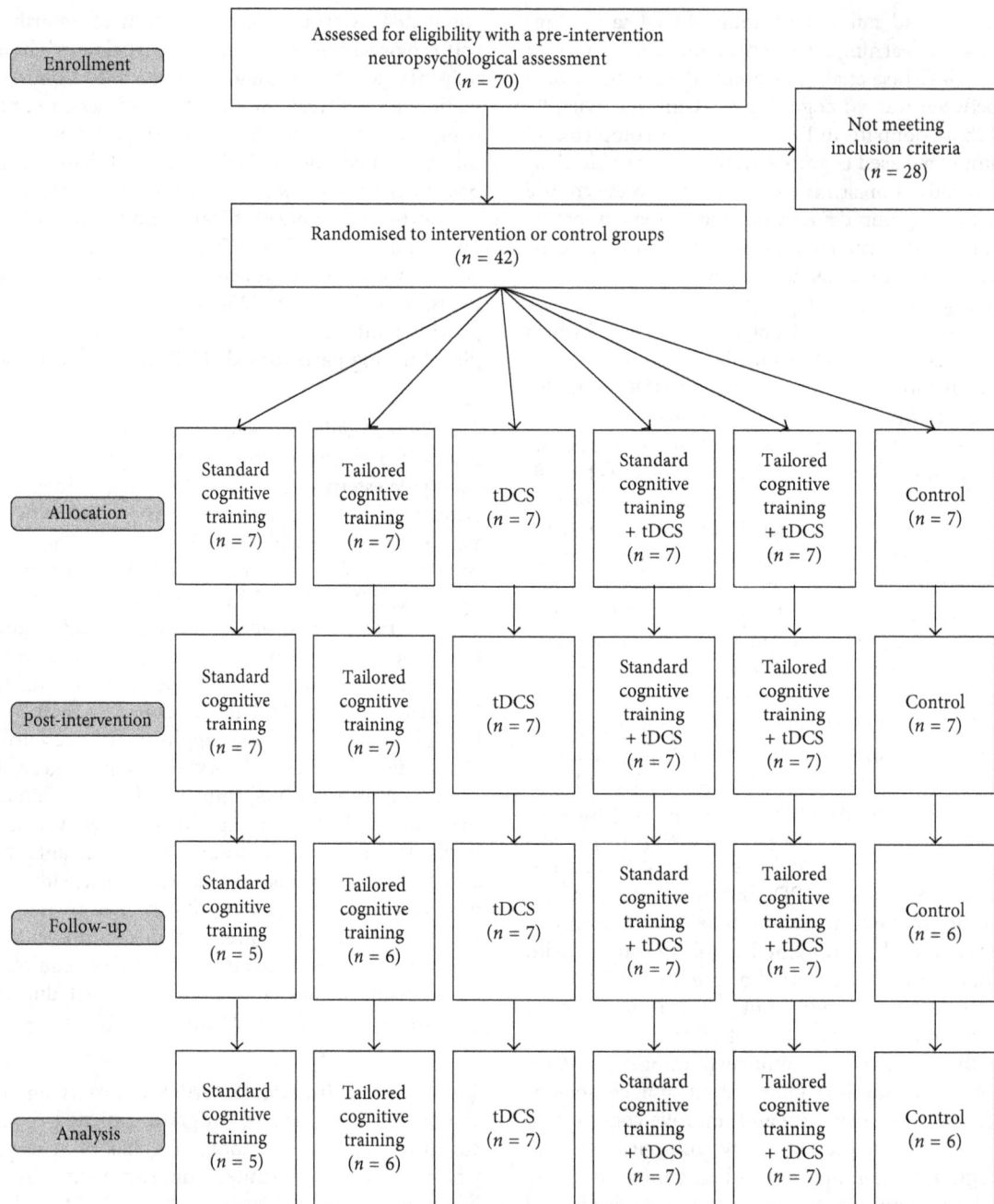

Figure 1: CONSORT flow diagram.

The activities themselves were the same as for the standard cognitive training, and normative data were used to define each participant's degree of cognitive impairment, as described in earlier work [15].

2.4. Brain Stimulation. tDCS is a noninvasive brain stimulation procedure delivering low-intensity electrical currents to specific cortical areas. For participants in the tDCS, standard cognitive training + tDCS, and tailored cognitive training + tDCS groups, stimulation sessions were scheduled for the same day and time each week for 4 weeks. During each session, participants received 20 minutes of constant

current 1.5 mA stimulation over left dorsal lateral prefrontal cortex (LDPFC). tDCS was delivered using the TCT™ tDCS stimulator (http://www.trans-cranial.com/) and administered with two $50 \times 70 \, mm^2$ sponge electrodes soaked in saline solution. The anode electrode was placed over F3 according to the 10–20 international system, and the cathode electrode was placed above the left eye. Executive function and attention/working memory are most frequently impaired cognitive domains in PD [15, 16] and associated with cortical activation of the left DLPFC [5]. Previous studies demonstrate improved cognitive functioning following tDCS over left DLPFC in PD [8, 9]. Left DLPFC was therefore targeted for tDCS in this study.

2.5. Control Group. Participants in the control group completed baseline, post-intervention, and 12-week follow-up neuropsychological assessments, but did not complete cognitive training or tDCS.

2.6. Neuropsychological Assessment. Neuropsychological assessments were conducted by doctoral researchers with extensive training and experience in administration, scoring, and interpretation of neuropsychological tests in PD. The following tests were selected in accordance with MDS Task Force [13] recommendations: (1) *executive function* was assessed using the Stockings of Cambridge (SOC) subtest from CANTAB™ and the Controlled Oral Word Association Task (COWAT) [17], (2) *attention and working memory* was assessed using the Letter-Number Sequencing (LNS) [18] and the Stroop (Colour-Word Interference) Test [19], (3) *memory* was assessed using the Hopkins Verbal Learning Test-Revised (HVLT-R) immediate recall subtest [20] and the Paragraph Recall test [21], (4) *visuospatial abilities* were assessed with the Judgement of Line Orientation (JLO) test [22] and the Hooper Visual Organisation Test (HVOT) [23], and (5) language was assessed using the Boston Naming Test-Short Form (BNT) [24] and the Similarities test [18]. Global cognition was assessed using the Parkinson's Disease—Cognitive Rating Scale (PD-CRS) [25] and the Mini-Mental State Examination (MMSE) [26]. Premorbid intelligence was assessed using the Australian version of the National Adult Reading Test (AUSNART) [27]. PD-MCI was classified as less than one standard deviation (SD) below normative scores on two or more neuropsychological tests [13]. Please refer to our earlier work [15] for a detailed description of our application of the MDS Task Force criteria for classification of PD-MCI in this study's sample of participants.

Activities of daily living (ADL) and quality of life (QOL) are impacted by cognitive impairment in PD, but few non-pharmacological trials have included these outcomes. ADL and QOL were assessed by the Unified Parkinson's Disease Rating Scale (Section II) [28] and the Parkinson's Disease Questionnaire-39 (PDQ-39) [29], respectively. Depression was included as a potential covariate and assessed using the Depression, Anxiety, and Stress Scale-21 (DASS-21) [30].

2.7. Data Analysis. Generalized linear mixed models (GLMMs) analysed outcome variables [31] in SPSS version 22.0. Separate GLMMs were run for each outcome variable to optimise the likelihood of convergence. To control the Type 1 error rate and conserve statistical power, outcome variables were grouped by cognitive domain (e.g., executive function and memory) and a more stringent alpha level was applied ($p < 0.025$) to interaction effects. Each GLMM was assessed for statistically significant Group × Time interaction effects, main effects of Time (per group), and pairwise contrasts. Statistically significant simple main effects of Group were not of interest for this study. Significant simple main effects of Group indicate a significant difference between group outcome scores at either pre-intervention, post-intervention, or follow-up time intervals. However, this study investigated whether there was a significantly different degree of *change* (over time) on outcome variables, between groups. Therefore, pre-intervention, post-intervention, or follow-up group differences provided no statistical evidence to support the effect of interventions (or no effect of the control group) on outcome variables. Effect sizes (Hedge's g) were calculated using the change score method and represent a comparison between each corresponding intervention group and the control group. Sample size was determined using G*Power 3. París et al. [2] and Naismith et al. [4] found moderate to large effect sizes for cognitive outcomes. To detect a moderate effect (power = 0.80 and $\alpha = 0.05$), 54 participants were required (9 per group).

3. Results

No data were missing at baseline. Little's Missing Completely at Random (MCAR) test showed data missing at post-intervention ($\chi = 23.80$, $p = 0.64$) and follow-up ($\chi = 40.34$, $p = 0.07$) were not systematically linked to included variables. Given that GLMMs account for missing data, means and standard deviations at post-intervention and follow-up assessments were slightly adjusted by each model and do not reflect the raw data at those time points. Refer to Supplementary Tables S3, S4, and S5 for raw neuropsychological test results.

Age significantly correlated with the HVLT ($r = -0.43$, $p = 0.004$), MMSE ($r = -0.43$, $p = 0.01$), and PD-CRS ($r = -0.37$, $p = 0.02$). Gender significantly correlated with the Stroop test ($r = 0.35$, $p = 0.03$). Years of education significantly correlated with Similarities ($r = 0.31$, $p = 0.04$) and MMSE ($r = 0.34$, $p = 0.03$). Premorbid IQ significantly correlated with Similarities ($r = 0.44$, $p = 0.003$), JLO ($r = 0.33$, $p = 0.03$), and MMSE ($r = 0.38$, $p = 0.01$). Disease duration significantly correlated with the HVOT ($r = -0.32$, $p = 0.04$). LED significantly correlated with Similarities ($r = 0.33$, $p = 0.03$). Depression significantly correlated with Similarities ($r = -0.39$, $p = 0.01$) and the PDQ-39 ($r = 0.59$, $p < 0.001$). Variables with significant correlations at baseline were included as covariates in corresponding GLMMs. An analysis of variance (ANOVA) of baseline demographic statistics indicated no statistically significant differences between groups (Table 1).

A significant interaction effect was observed for SOC, indicating a differential rate of improvement in executive function between groups ($F = 3.82$, $p < 0.001$). Significant improvements were identified for the standard cognitive training + tDCS group ($F = 10.73$, $p < 0.001$) and tailored cognitive training + tDCS group ($F = 12.00$, $p < 0.001$). No other groups improved on SOC, and no groups improved on the COWAT. Refer to Tables 2–4 for pairwise comparison statistics, effect sizes, and group baseline, post-intervention, and follow-up results.

For attention/working memory, a significant interaction effect was observed for the Stroop test ($F = 2.91$, $p = 0.003$). Significant improvements were identified for the tDCS group ($F = 4.06$, $p = 0.02$) and standard cognitive training + tDCS group ($F = 35.05$, $p < 0.001$). No other groups improved on the Stroop test. A significant interaction effect was observed for LNS ($F = 4.53$, $p < 0.001$). Significant improvement was identified for the tailored cognitive training group ($F = 6.62$, $p = 0.002$)

TABLE 1: Baseline demographic information for the intervention and control groups.

Outcome	Standard CT		Tailored CT		tDCS		Standard CT+tDCS		Standard CT+tDCS		Control		Group differences	
	M	SD	M	SD	M	SD	M	SD	M	SD	M	SD	F	p
Gender (%, ♀)	43% (N = 3)		57% (N = 4)		71% (N = 5)		71% (N = 5)		71% (N = 5)		57% (N = 4)		0.36	0.87
Age[++]	68.14	8.69	65.57	5.20	72	6.45	63.57	15.68	67.43	6.37	72.29	6.21	0.80	0.56
Education[++]	13.57	2.64	12.21	2.83	13.57	3.69	15.50	3.35	15.86	1.35	11.71	2.98	2.34	0.06
Premorbid IQ	103.29	6.96	107.21	12	108.21	5.83	111.96	4.37	111.08	3.59	103.64	7.53	1.76	0.15
Disease Duration[++]	5.29	4.23	5.79	4.97	5.50	5.66	6.79	4.60	4.43	2.70	5.36	4.14	0.20	0.96
LED	295	313.40	383	178.62	573.29	586.25	350.71	322.37	464.29	358.78	292.88	274.51	0.64	0.68
DASS-D	2.29	2.56	1.29	1.50	3	2	3	5.07	3.29	4.11	2.71	3.15	0.34	0.89

M = mean; SD = standard deviation; F = ANOVA; p = level of statistical significance; N = number of participants; LED = levodopa equivalent dose; DASS-D = Depression, Anxiety, and Stress Scale (Depression subscale); IQ = intelligence quotient; CT = cognitive training; tDCS = transcranial direct current stimulation; ♀ = male gender; ++ = years.

TABLE 2: Standard cognitive training and tailored cognitive training group cognitive performance at baseline, post-intervention, and follow-up.

Standard cognitive training

Outcome	Baseline		Post-intervention		Follow-up		Pairwise comparison statistics					
							Baseline to post-intervention			Baseline to follow-up		
	M	SD	M	SD	M	SD	t	p	g^a	t	p	g^a
COWAT	38.86	13.89	44.14	11.40	42.20	13.60	1.81	0.07	0.70	1.31	0.19	-0.16
SOC	8.17	0.64	6.43	2.52	7.69	2.33	-1.90	0.06	-1.19	-0.51	0.61	-0.70
LNS	18.73	2.54	19.02	4.77	17.14	3.97	0.24	0.81	-0.04	-1.26	0.21	-0.42
Stroop test	33.83	6.20	36.11	6.76	36.16	5.31	0.82	0.42	0.35	1.67	0.10	-0.31
HVLT	22.08	5.41	26.94	5.35	27.44	2.33	3	0.003[b]	0.46	2.76	0.01[b]	0.44
Paragraph Recall	5	2.20	6.36	2.28	7.09	2.71	1.36	0.18	0.62	3.16	0.002*	0.93
BNT	14.14	1.72	13.86	0.98	13.60	1.17	-0.73	0.43	-0.55	-0.79	0.43	0.01
Similarities	22.14	3.05	23.71	3.31	21.89	1.17	1.51	0.25	0.28	-0.30	0.76	-0.70
JLO	25.61	3.39	24.90	4.35	20.61	3.42	-0.71	0.48	-0.08	-2.94	0.004*	-1.19
HVOT	24.49	3.76	25.21	3.45	26.07	2.96	0.84	0.40	0.06	1.38	0.17	0.36
MMSE	26.95	2.09	26.80	1.78	28.19	2.24	-0.19	0.85	0.41	0.86	0.39	-0.09
PD-CRS	89.42	10.28	96.13	9.12	100.09	8.94	1.42	0.16	0.44	2.29	0.02[b]	0.28
PDQ-39	24.20	10.07	20.68	10.76	25.60	9.95	-3.05	0.003*	0.24	0.71	0.48	0.06
UPDRS-II	0.96	0.77	0.73	0.74	0.85	0.74	-4.60	0.001**	0.33	-1.55	0.13	0.36

Tailored cognitive training

Outcome	Baseline		Post-intervention		Follow-up		Pairwise comparison statistics					
							Baseline to post-intervention			Baseline to follow-up		
	M	SD	M	SD	M	SD	t	p	g^a	t	p	g^a
COWAT	32.43	16.59	34.71	12.19	37.17	21.27	0.56	0.58	0.42	0.96	0.34	-0.07
SOC	6.43	2.33	6.55	2.07	5.26	2.84	0.14	0.89	-0.51	-0.98	0.33	-0.85
LNS	17.39	4.43	18.87	3.10	19.81	2.70	1.95	0.06	0.19	3.30	0.001*	0.30
Stroop test	31.89	9.01	35.17	10.65	31.83	9.49	1.42	0.16	0.34	-0.03	0.98	-0.51
HVLT	22.15	5.35	24.58	6.15	26.52	6.36	2.41	0.02[b]	0.05	2.93	0.004[b]	0.27
Paragraph Recall	5.64	2.20	7.36	3.50	7.23	3.21	2.21	0.03[b]	0.58	1.35	0.18	0.74
BNT	13.14	1.25	13.86	1.25	13.78	1.05	1.48	0.14	0.09	1.14	0.26	0.66
Similarities	22.11	2.47	23.71	3.31	22.72	1.52	-0.03	0.98	-0.36	0.51	0.61	-0.54
JLO	20.25	3.55	22.97	4.32	22.32	3.87	2.13	0.04[b]	0.49	1.94	0.06	-0.06
HVOT	20.37	3.76	23.22	3.45	23.19	5.35	3.35	0.001[b]	0.61	2.62	0.01[b]	0.65
MMSE	25.49	2.44	26.92	2.54	25.85	1.20	-2.70	0.01[b]	0.98	0.55	0.59	-0.45
PD-CRS	86.58	12.72	95.29	21.44	98.61	18.28	2.31	0.02[b]	0.39	3.64	0.001[b]	0.35
PDQ-39	21.41	7.39	18.09	5.19	18.21	8.65	-2.46	0.02*	0.26	-2.44	0.02*	0.30
UPDRS-II	0.68	0.32	0.80	0.40	0.71	0.27	0.88	0.38	-0.06	0.17	0.87	-0.24

M = mean; SD = standard deviation; t = t statistic; a = effect size computed using change scores with the control group; positive effect favours corresponding intervention group; b = not statistically significant due to nonsignificant main effect; * = $p < 0.05$; ** = $p < 0.001$; tDCS = transcranial direct current stimulation; COWAT = Controlled Oral Word Association Test; SOC = Stockings of Cambridge; LNS = Letter-Number Sequencing; HVLT = Hopkin's Verbal Learning Test; BNT = Boston Naming Test; JLO = Judgement of Line Orientation; HVOT = Hooper's Visual Orientation Test; MMSE = Mini-Mental State Examination; PD-CRS = Parkinson's Disease—Cognitive Rating Scale; UPDRS-II = Unified Parkinson's Disease Rating Scale—Section II (ADL); PDQ-39 = Parkinson's Disease Questionnaire-39.

TABLE 3: tDCS and standard cognitive training + tDCS group cognitive performance at baseline, pos-tintervention, and follow-up.

tDCS

Outcome	Baseline M	Baseline SD	Post-intervention M	Post-intervention SD	Follow-up M	Follow-up SD	B to post t	p	g[a]	B to follow-up t	p	g[a]
COWAT	30.86	16.14	36	15.11	30.57	17.57	1.86	0.06	0.58	-0.17	0.86	-0.30
SOC	5.50	1.35	6.50	1.62	7	1.88	2.12	0.04[b]	-0.13	1.94	0.06	0.14
LNS	14.82	5.99	16.11	6.39	16.18	4.74	1.70	0.09	0.12	1.15	0.25	0.13
Stroop test	21.38	6.76	27.66	10.41	26.52	7.47	2.09	0.04*	0.65	2.41	0.02*	0.01
HVLT	20.33	8.27	25.33	6.28	23.33	7.45	4.45	0.001[b]	0.45	3.71	0.001[b]	0.03
Paragraph Recall	4	2.23	6.29	2.05	4.36	1.72	4.73	0.001**	1.11	0.70	0.49	0.28
BNT	12.57	1.06	13.71	1.83	13.29	1.67	2.23	0.03[b]	0.30	1.63	0.11	0.65
Similarities	22.37	2.68	23.42	2.41	21.38	1.67	1.29	0.20	0.13	-0.76	0.45	-1.25
JLO	21.30	7.90	22.44	5.51	24.59	4.80	0.80	0.43	0.24	2.31	0.02[b]	0.18
HVOT	20.99	3.76	22.42	3.45	20.99	3.26	1.68	0.10	0.24	0.00	1	-0.01
MMSE	24.31	1.54	26.02	1.64	25.45	2.43	2.29	0.02[b]	1.36	1.84	0.07	0.55
PD-CRS	74.76	17.57	85.04	18.10	79.04	20.59	5.10	0.001[b]	0.53	1.51	0.14	-0.06
PDQ-39	23.04	8.45	18.09	5.19	18.21	8.65	-0.96	0.34	0.22	-1.11	0.27	0.37
UPDRS-II	1.27	0.56	1.06	0.66	1.23	0.66	-2.25	0.03[b]	0.32	-0.48	0.63	0.24

Standard cognitive training + tDCS

Outcome	Baseline M	Baseline SD	Post-intervention M	Post-intervention SD	Follow-up M	Follow-up SD	B to post t	p	g[a]	B to follow-up t	p	g[a]
COWAT	37.71	9.88	46.14	4.85	39.86	11.26	3.23	0.002[b]	1.33	0.44	0.66	-0.22
SOC	7.43	1.41	9.57	1.64	9.14	2.09	4.62	0.001**	0.41	2.29	0.02*	0.23
LNS	18.54	2.17	18.87	2.47	18.56	2.60	0.34	0.73	-0.04	0.01	0.99	-0.14
Stroop test	24.52	9.30	30.52	8.29	33.81	9.01	2.23	0.03*	0.60	5.76	0.001**	0.24
HVLT	26.51	4.08	28.51	5.10	29.94	4.85	1.43	0.16	-0.03	2.59	0.01[b]	0.09
Paragraph Recall	6	2.07	8.21	1.38	6.43	2.23	2.30	0.02[b]	1.29	3.25	0.002[b]	0.57
BNT	13.29	1.59	14.43	0.74	14	0.93	1.75	0.08	0.39	1.83	0.07	0.77
Similarities	21.59	2.49	23.51	1.72	21.02	2.31	2.70	0.01*	0.59	2.02	0.06	-0.95
JLO	22.83	5.43	24.55	4.74	22.98	7	1.58	0.12	0.37	0.11	0.91	-0.23
HVOT	23.82	3.79	25.11	3.45	24.11	3.29	1.51	0.14	0.21	1.03	0.78	0.05
MMSE	27.02	1.72	26.87	1.30	27.73	1.33	-0.20	0.84	0.46	1.36	0.18	0.50
PD-CRS	87.08	16.93	98.79	13.03	94.94	18.02	5.30	0.001[b]	0.71	2.69	0.01[b]	0.10
PDQ-39	20.05	11.74	16.33	7.84	19.48	10.87	-1.82	0.07	0.27	-0.30	0.77	-0.09
UPDRS-II	1	0.48	0.62	0.53	0.77	0.32	-2.51	0.01*	0.55	-1.74	0.08	0.51

M = mean; SD = standard deviation; t = t statistic; a = effect size computed using change scores with the control group, positive effect favours corresponding intervention group; b = not statistically significant due to nonsignificant main effect; * = $p < 0.05$; ** = $p < 0.001$; tDCS = transcranial direct current stimulation; COWAT = Controlled Oral Word Association Test; SOC = Stockings of Cambridge; LNS = Letter-Number Sequencing; HVLT = Hopkins Verbal Learning Test; BNT = Boston Naming Test; JLO = Judgement of Line Orientation; HVOT = Hooper's Visual Orientation Test; MMSE = Mini-Mental State Examination; PD-CRS = Parkinson's Disease—Cognitive Rating Scale; UPDRS-II = Unified Parkinson's Disease Rating Scale—section II (ADL); PDQ-39 = Parkinson's Disease Questionnaire-39.

TABLE 4: Tailored cognitive training + tDCS and control group cognitive performance at baseline, post-intervention, and follow-up.

Outcome	Tailored cognitive training + tDCS						Pairwise comparison statistics					
	Baseline		Post-intervention		Follow-up		Baseline to post-intervention			Baseline to follow-up		
	M	SD	M	SD	M	SD	t	p	g^a	t	p	g^a
COWAT	32.14	9.22	36.29	8.45	35.86	11.50	1.74	0.08	0.70	1.77	0.08	-0.12
SOC	5.29	1.03	7	2.07	8.57	2.20	2.29	0.02*	0.19	3.86	0.001**	0.92
LNS	17.63	2.54	18.25	1.99	19.24	1.96	0.72	0.47	0.02	2.21	0.03*	0.22
Stroop test	29.95	11.50	30.66	6.97	32.38	7.10	0.18	0.86	0.14	0.87	0.39	-0.17
HVLT	21.04	2.70	24.90	2.28	25.19	5.30	5.21	0.001^b	0.37	2.78	0.01^b	0.22
Paragraph Recall	3.21	1.43	5.71	1.64	6.43	2.23	4.60	0.001**	1.36	3.25	0.002*	1.75
BNT	14	1.43	14.29	1.03	14.57	0.50	0.86	0.39	-0.18	-0.42	0.68	0.73
Similarities	22.89	3.18	26.03	2.25	20.75	2.20	3.73	0.001**	1.06	-2.15	0.03*	-1.58
JLO	22.33	7.71	22.47	6.31	22.04	7.13	0.12	0.91	0.06	-0.55	0.59	-0.28
HVOT	21.51	3.79	24.08	3.71	24.37	3.29	3.02	0.003^b	0.54	2.76	0.01^b	0.62
MMSE	26.37	1.99	26.51	1.38	26.37	1.54	0.21	0.84	0.61	0.00	1	0.19
PD-CRS	85.56	12.91	93.84	11.69	90.99	8.98	2.41	0.02^b	0.51	2.66	0.01^b	-0.02
PDQ-39	25.62	14.63	27.25	10.52	20.44	11.32	0.53	0.60	-0.14	-1.64	0.11	0.27
UPDRS-II	1.17	0.56	0.97	0.48	1.16	0.48	-1.47	0.14	0.34	-0.01	0.99	0.22

Outcome	Control						Pairwise comparison statistics					
	Baseline		Post-intervention		Follow-up		Baseline to post-intervention			Baseline to follow-up		
	M	SD	M	SD	M	SD	t	p	g^a	t	p	g^a
COWAT	30.14	15.45	27.43	9.94	36	19.16	-0.87	0.39	—	1.81	0.07	—
SOC	6	2.84	7.28	2.27	7.21	1.84	1.89	0.06	—	1.75	0.08	—
LNS	14.30	6.07	14.82	5.78	14.97	5.02	0.77	0.44	—	1.04	0.30	—
Stroop test	19.03	10.07	18.60	9.38	24.24	20.56	-0.34	0.74	—	0.86	0.39	—
HVLT	21.26	5.51	23.40	5.75	24.04	5.71	1.49	0.14	—	2.84	0.01^b	—
Paragraph Recall	4.07	2.41	4.07	1.80	3.81	1.30	0.00	1	—	-0.36	0.72	—
BNT	12.43	1.99	13	1.76	11.87	1.84	3.06	0.003^b	—	-0.87	0.39	—
Similarities	18.80	1.99	19.55	1.96	20.70	2.43	1.06	0.29	—	1.85	0.07	—
JLO	21.10	6.92	20.82	7.55	23.56	8.18	-0.37	0.71	—	1.38	0.17	—
HVOT	23.60	4.06	24.10	3.71	23.66	3.38	0.54	0.59	—	0.05	0.96	—
MMSE	24.38	2.07	24.38	2.16	25.82	2.31	-1.37	0.17	—	0.71	0.48	—
PD-CRS	76.50	19.35	77.50	14.81	82.22	20.21	0.33	0.74	—	3.21	0.002^b	—
PDQ-39	24.02	14.52	23.76	14.92	24.59	11.81	-0.35	0.73	—	0.39	0.70	—
UPDRS-II	1.18	0.69	1.25	0.94	1.35	0.93	0.71	0.48	—	1.04	0.30	—

M = mean; SD = standard deviation; t = t statistic; a = effect size computed using change scores with the control group, positive effect favours corresponding intervention group; b = not statistically significant due to nonsignificant main effect; * = $p < 0.05$; ** = $p < 0.001$; tDCS = transcranial direct current stimulation; COWAT = Controlled Oral Word Association Test; SOC = Stockings of Cambridge; LNS = Letter-Number Sequencing; HVLT = Hopkin's Verbal Learning Test; BNT = Boston Naming Test; JLO = Judgement of Line Orientation; HVOT = Hooper's Visual Orientation Test; MMSE = Mini-Mental State Examination; PD-CRS = Parkinson's Disease—Cognitive Rating Scale; UPDRS-II = Unified Parkinson's Disease Rating Scale—section II (ADL); PDQ-39 = Parkinson's Disease Questionnaire-39.

and tailored cognitive training + tDCS group ($F = 5.11$, $p = 0.01$). No other groups improved on the LNS.

For memory, a significant interaction effect was observed for Paragraph Recall ($F = 2.51$, $p = 0.01$). Significant improvements were identified for the standard cognitive training group, ($F = 5.24$, $p = 0.01$), tDCS group, ($F = 17.82$, $p < 0.001$), and tailored cognitive training + tDCS group ($F = 12.09$, $p < 0.001$). No other groups improved on Paragraph Recall, and no groups improved on HVLT.

For language, a significant interaction effect was observed for the Similarities test ($F = 3.25$, $p = 0.001$). Significant improvements were identified for the standard cognitive training + tDCS group ($F = 5.23$, $p = 0.01$) and tailored cognitive training + tDCS group ($F = 17.43$, $p < 0.001$). No other groups improved on the Similarities test, and no groups improved on the BNT.

For visuospatial abilities, a significant interaction effect was observed for JLO ($F = 3.76$, $p < 0.001$). However, a significant decline was identified for the standard cognitive training group ($F = 6.57$, $p = 0.002$). Therefore, no groups improved on JLO, and no groups improved on HVOT.

No groups improved on measures of global cognition (MMSE and PD-CRS).

For QOL, a significant interaction effect was observed for the PDQ-39 ($F = 2.96$, $p = 0.003$). Significant improvements were identified for the standard cognitive training group ($F = 7.21$, $p = 0.001$) and tailored cognitive training group ($F = 12.48$, $p < 0.001$). No other groups improved on QOL.

For ADL, a significant interaction effect was observed for the UPDRS-II ($F = 1.96$, $p = 0.04$). Significant improvements were identified for the standard cognitive training group ($F = 11.29$, $p < 0.001$) and standard cognitive training + tDCS group ($F = 3.40$, $p = 0.04$). No other groups improved on ADL.

4. Discussion

In support of the therapeutic potential of cognitive training and tDCS, differential rates of improvements in cognition, ADL, and QOL were observed across intervention groups. The control group did not improve on any outcome measures.

The standard cognitive training group improved on memory, ADL, and QOL. Previous standard cognitive training studies report improved memory [2] and ADL in PD [32], but this study is the first to report improvement in QOL. París et al. [2] used the same computer-based cognitive training program (Smartbrain Pro) and the same QOL outcome measure (PDQ-39), but their participants did not improve. This may reflect a ceiling effect as half the participants in París et al.'s [2] cognitive training group were identified as having normal cognition. Nonetheless, ADL and QOL are frequently impaired in PD and associated with cognitive decline [33, 34]. The current findings indicate that standard cognitive training improves ADL and QOL for those with PD.

The tailored cognitive training group improved on attention/working memory and QOL. One tailored cognitive training study has reported "attentional improvements," evidenced by increased neural resting state activity (measured by fMRI) in the superior parietal and prefrontal dorsolateral

cortices following training [5]. The current study is the first to report improvements in QOL following tailored cognitive training in participants with PD or PD-MCI. Despite limited evidence in PD, a Cochrane review of cognitive training for people with mild to moderate dementia reported positive effects of cognitive training for QOL (and cognitive function) [35]. The positive results in dementia and in the current study indicate that future studies should explore the potential of tailored cognitive training to improve QOL in PD-MCI.

The tDCS group improved on attention/working memory and memory. Recent studies report significant improvements in attention/working memory in PD [8] and attentional/executive abilities [9, 10]. The current study is the first to demonstrate memory improvement following tDCS in PD-MCI. In accordance with the "dual syndrome hypothesis" [36], if participants in the current study had the APOE allelic genetic abnormality associated with memory deficits in the posterior cortex, the Scaffolding Theory of Ageing and Cognition [37] suggests that their impaired posterior cortical function may have led to compensatory activation of the prefrontal cortices (i.e., left DLPFC) to account for increased cognitive demand during complex tasks (i.e., neuropsychological assessments). Anodal tDCS may have therefore enhanced compensatory activation of the left DLPFC, leading to increased neural activity of frontal functions that were associated with improved memory performance in PD-MCI.

The standard cognitive training + tDCS group improved on executive function, attention/working memory, and ADL. Multiple uncontrolled studies combined standard cognitive training with tDCS, but the results vary. Biundo et al. [11] reported a decline in executive skills and improved attention and memory. Conversely, research in Alzheimer's disease paired repetitive transcranial magnetic stimulation (rTMS) with standard cognitive training and reported improved global cognition [38]. However, different methods of non-invasive stimulation, both anodal tDCS and high-frequency rTMS, increase cortical excitability to improve cognitive functioning [7]. In accordance with Mowszowski et al. [39], combining standard cognitive training with tDCS in the current study may have resulted in "positive plasticity" to alleviate cognitive deficits. Standard cognitive training may have stimulated and strengthened existing neural connections (synaptogenesis), while tDCS provided compensatory activation of a cortical region (left DLPFC) associated with higher-order cognition and functional improvement in ADL.

This is the first standard cognitive training and tDCS study to report language improvements in PD. Improved language abilities may be explained by the overlap between the language skills needed to complete the Similarities outcome test and those needed to complete the cognitive training program. During the language activities, participants finished sentences by selecting an appropriate word and determining the relationship between a group of words by applying a semantic category to those words. Successful completion of the Similarities test also involves application of semantic word categories to describe the most appropriate relationship between a set of words [18]. Participants in the standard cognitive training + tDCS group may have therefore trained and improved language skills that were most beneficial for successful performance on the Similarities language test. There is mounting evidence indicating that some people with PD demonstrate language impairment [16, 40], and the current study suggests that combining standard cognitive training with tDCS may alleviate this deficit.

The tailored cognitive training + tDCS group improved on executive function, attention/working memory, and memory. Among studies that have examined these interventions independently, several reports improved executive function and attention/working memory in PD [5, 9]. The current study is the first to report memory improvements following tailored cognitive training and tDCS in PD. Memory impairment is common in PD and may predict progression to PD-Dementia [41]. Future clinical trials of tDCS and tailored cognitive training need to include standardised memory outcomes and interventions targeting memory impairment in PD.

The current study is also the first to report improved language abilities following tailored cognitive training and tDCS in PD. For the tailored cognitive training + tDCS group, language improvements were observed on the Similarities test, but not the BNT. The MDS Task Force classifies the Similarities test as a measure of language abilities [13]. However, the Similarities test is a subtest of the verbal IQ index of the WAIS battery and involves abstract reasoning [18]. Abstract reasoning is a higher-order cognitive ability associated with executive function and involves ordering, comparing, analysing, and synthesizing information [42]. When completing the Similarities test, participants need to describe in what ways are two concepts/words alike, which requires the use of abstract reasoning (an executive skill) to synthesise information related to both concepts/words. As a task requiring executive function, completing the Similarities test may involve increased activation of left DLPFC, which was also the target of tDCS for this group. Participants in this group also demonstrated impaired executive function (lowest baseline SOC score) and completed cognitive training tasks tailored to executive function skills. Pairing this form of tailored cognitive training with tDCS applied to left DLPFC may have increased cortical activity associated with improved performance on SOC *and* Similarities, tasks involving executive *and* language abilities. According to the theoretical model proposed by Kim and Kim [43], combining a stimulation and compensation-focussed intervention (tailored cognitive training) with another compensation-focussed intervention (tDCS) may have provided optimal conditions for neuronal plasticity, which led to improved performance across several cognitive domains.

There are limitations to the current study. Several outcomes did not improve across intervention groups, which may be due to a number of reasons. Despite selecting outcomes in accordance with MDS Task Force recommendations [13], a lack of sensitivity of some cognitive tests for detecting change in PD may have contributed to nonsignificant improvement for those tests (e.g., HVLT, BNT, and MMSE). [42] Researchers should consult compendiums of neuropsychological tests [42] to ensure that sensitive outcomes are included in future clinical trials. The cognitive training and tDCS parameters used in this study may have also impacted nonsignificant results. No improvements were observed for visuospatial abilities as measured by HVOT and JLO. These tests involve perceptual organisation (HVOT) and estimation of angled lines (JLO), but the visuospatial activities in the cognitive training interventions involved different visuospatial skills (e.g., identifying coordinates and time ranges on an analog clock). Furthermore, the tDCS in this study stimulated a cortical region (left DLPFC) that is not associated with visuospatial performance. Several studies report more dominant involvement of the right posterior hemisphere during completion of HVOT and JLO [44, 45]. It is therefore likely that the cognitive training tasks and site of tDCS were not conducive to improved visuospatial abilities. It is also important to note that two participants in the standard cognitive training group with high JLO scores at pre-intervention dropped out of the study preceding the follow-up assessment, which may account for this group's significant decline in JLO performance at follow-up. This study was also somewhat underpowered, which may have impacted nonsignificant outcome effects. Lastly, exposure was not matched between intervention groups. Participants allocated to the cognitive training groups (standard or tailored) completed 12 sessions of training. Whereas, participants in the cognitive training + tDCS groups completed 12 sessions of cognitive training *and* 4 sessions of tDCS. Completing both interventions exposed participants to a greater number of therapeutic sessions designed to improve cognition, which may have produced additive beneficial effects on neuropsychological outcomes. Future studies should account for these methodological parameters when exploring the therapeutic potential of cognitive training and tDCS in PD and PD-MCI.

5. Conclusions

This study provides evidence in support of cognitive training, tDCS, and cognitive training combined with tDCS for PD-MCI. The rate of participant attrition was low (<10%), and cognitive performance was measured in line with MDS Task Force recommendations for Level II diagnostic criteria of PD-MCI [13]. Overall, a greater number of outcomes improved for the groups that received standard or tailored cognitive training combined with tDCS. These findings suggest that cognitive training combined with tDCS may provide optimal conditions for neuronal plasticity, leading to improvements in cognition and functional outcomes for those with PD-MCI.

Acknowledgments

The authors thank the participants for giving up their time to take part in the research and Parkinson's Western Australia Inc. for providing funding to support this research.

References

[1] J. G. Goldman and D. Weintraub, "Advances in the treatment of cognitive impairment in Parkinson's disease," *Movement Disorders*, vol. 30, no. 11, pp. 1471–1489, 2015.

[2] A. P. París, H. G. Saleta, M. de la Cruz Crespo Maraver et al., "Blind randomized controlled study of the efficacy of cognitive training in Parkinson's disease," *Movement Disorders*, vol. 26, no. 7, pp. 1251–1258, 2011.

[3] J. D. Edwards, R. A. Hauser, M. L. O'Connor, E. G. Valdés, T. A. Zesiewicz, and E. Y. Uc, "Randomized trial of cognitive speed of processing training in Parkinson disease," *Neurology*, vol. 81, no. 15, pp. 1284–1290, 2013.

[4] S. L. Naismith, L. Mowszowski, K. Diamond, and S. J. Lewis, "Improving memory in Parkinson's disease: a healthy brain ageing cognitive training program," *Movement Disorders*, vol. 28, no. 8, pp. 1097–1103, 2013.

[5] A. Cerasa, M. C. Gioia, M. Salsone et al., "Neurofunctional correlates of attention rehabilitation in Parkinson's disease: an explorative study," *Neurological Sciences*, vol. 35, no. 8, pp. 1173–1180, 2014.

[6] B. J. Lawrence, N. Gasson, R. S. Bucks, L. Troeung, and A. M. Loftus, "Cognitive training and noninvasive brain stimulation for cognition in Parkinson's disease: a meta-analysis," *Neurorehabilitation and Neural Repair*, vol. 31, no. 7, pp. 597–608, 2017.

[7] R. Nardone, J. Bergmann, M. Christova et al., "Effect of transcranial brain stimulation for the treatment of Alzheimer disease: a review," *International Journal of Alzheimer's Disease*, vol. 2012, Article ID 687909, 5 pages, 2012.

[8] P. S. Boggio, R. Ferrucci, S. P. Rigonatti et al., "Effects of transcranial direct current stimulation on working memory in patients with Parkinson's disease," *Journal of the Neurological Sciences*, vol. 249, no. 1, pp. 31–38, 2006.

[9] J. B. Pereira, C. Junqué, D. Bartrés-Faz et al., "Modulation of verbal fluency networks by transcranial direct current stimulation (tDCS) in Parkinson's disease," *Brain Stimulation*, vol. 6, no. 1, pp. 16–24, 2013.

[10] D. Doruk, Z. Gray, G. L. Bravo, A. Pascual-Leone, and F. Fregni, "Effects of tDCS on executive function in Parkinson's disease," *Neuroscience Letters*, vol. 582, pp. 27–31, 2014.

[11] R. Biundo, L. Weis, E. Fiorenzato et al., "Double-blind randomized trial of t-DCS versus sham in Parkinson patients with mild cognitive impairment receiving cognitive training," *Brain Stimulation*, vol. 8, no. 6, pp. 1223–1240, 2015.

[12] I. Boutron, D. Moher, D. G. Altman, K. F. Schulz, and P. Ravaud, "Extending the CONSORT statement to randomized trials of nonpharmacologic treatment: explanation and elaboration," *Annals of Internal Medicine*, vol. 148, no. 4, pp. 295–309, 2008.

[13] I. Litvan, J. G. Goldman, A. I. Tröster et al., "Diagnostic criteria for mild cognitive impairment in Parkinson's disease: Movement Disorder Society Task Force guidelines," *Movement Disorders*, vol. 27, pp. 349–356, 2012.

[14] L. Tárraga, M. Boada, G. Modinos et al., "A randomised pilot study to assess the efficacy of an interactive, multimedia tool of cognitive stimulation in Alzheimer's disease," *Journal of Neurology, Neurosurgery & Psychiatry*, vol. 77, no. 10, pp. 1116–1121, 2006.

[15] B. J. Lawrence, N. Gasson, and A. M. Loftus, "Prevalence and subtypes of mild cognitive impairment in Parkinson's disease," *Scientific Reports*, vol. 6, no. 1, p. 33929, 2016.

[16] B. A. Cholerton, C. P. Zabetian, J. Y. Wan et al., "Evaluation of mild cognitive impairment subtypes in Parkinson's disease," *Movement Disorders*, vol. 29, no. 6, pp. 756–764, 2014.

[17] A. L. Benton, "Differential behavioral effects in frontal lobe disease," *Neuropsychologia*, vol. 6, no. 1, pp. 53–60, 1968.

[18] D. Wechsler, *Wechsler Adult Intelligence Scale–Fourth Edition (WAIS–IV)*, NCS Pearson, San Antonio, TX, USA, 2008.

[19] C. J. Golden and S. Freshwater, *Stroop Colour and Word Test: Revised Examiner's Manual*, Stoelting Co., Wood dale, IL, USA, 2002.

[20] J. Brandt and R. H. Benedict, *Hopkins Verbal Learning Test-Revised: Professional Manual*, Psychological Assessment Resources, Lutz, FL, USA, 2001.

[21] B. Wilson, J. Cockburn, A. Baddeley, and R. Hiorns, "The development and validation of a test battery for detecting and monitoring everyday memory problems," *Journal of Clinical and Experimental Neuropsychology*, vol. 11, no. 6, pp. 855–870, 1989.

[22] A. L. Benton, K. D. Hamsher, and A. B. Sivan, *Multilingual Aphasia Examination: Manual of Instructions*, AJA, Iowa City, IA, USA, 1994.

[23] H. Hooper, *Hooper Visual Organisation Test: Manual*, Western Psychological Services, Los Angeles, CA, USA, 1983.

[24] E. Kaplan, H. Goodglass, and S. Weintraub, *Boston Naming Test*, Pro-Ed, Austin, TX, USA, 2001.

[25] J. Pagonabarraga, J. Kulisevsky, G. Llebaria, C. García-Sánchez, B. Pascual-Sedano, and A. Gironell, "Parkinson's disease-cognitive rating scale: a new cognitive scale specific for Parkinson's disease," *Movement Disorders*, vol. 23, no. 7, pp. 998–1005, 2008.

[26] M. F. Folstein, S. E. Folstein, and P. R. McHugh, ""Mini-mental state": a practical method for grading the cognitive state of patients for the clinician," *Journal of Psychiatric Research*, vol. 12, pp. 189–198, 1975.

[27] M. Hennessy and B. Mackenzie,, "AUSNART: The development of an Australian version of the NART," in *Proceedings of the 18th Annual Brain Impairment Conference*, pp. 183–188, Hobart, Australia, June 1995.

[28] C. G. Goetz, B. C. Tilley, S. R. Shaftman et al., "Movement Disorder Society-sponsored revision of the Unified Parkinson's Disease Rating Scale (MDS-UPDRS): scale presentation and clinimetric testing results," *Movement Disorders*, vol. 23, no. 15, pp. 2129–2170, 2008.

[29] V. Peto, C. Jenkinson, and R. Fitzpatrick, "PDQ-39: a review of the development, validation and application of a Parkinson's disease quality of life questionnaire and its associated measures," *Journal of Neurology*, vol. 245, pp. 10–14, 1998.

[30] P. F. Lovibond and S. H. Lovibond, "The structure of negative emotional states: comparison of the Depression Anxiety Stress Scales (DASS) with the Beck Depression and Anxiety Inventories," *Behaviour Research and Therapy*, vol. 33, no. 3, pp. 335–343, 1995.

[31] M. Borenstein, L. V. Hedges, J. Higgins, and H. R. Rothstein, "A basic introduction to fixed-effect and random-effects models for meta-analysis," *Research Synthesis Methods*, vol. 1, no. 2, pp. 97–111, 2010.

[32] J. E. Pompeu, F. A. Mendes, K. G. Silva et al., "Effect of Nintendo Wii™-based motor and cognitive training on activities of daily living in patients with Parkinson's disease: a randomised clinical trial," *Physiotherapy*, vol. 98, no. 3, pp. 196–204, 2012.

[33] B. J. Lawrence, N. Gasson, R. Kane, R. S. Bucks, and A. M. Loftus, "Activities of daily living, depression, and

quality of life in Parkinson's disease," *PloS One*, vol. 9, no. 7, article e102294, 2014.

[34] D. Muslimović, B. Post, J. D. Speelman, B. Schmand, R. J. de Haan, and CARPA Study Group, "Determinants of disability and quality of life in mild to moderate Parkinson disease," *Neurology*, vol. 70, no. 23, pp. 2241–2247, 2008.

[35] B. Woods, E. Aguirre, A. E. Spector, and M. Orrell, "Cognitive stimulation to improve cognitive functioning in people with dementia," *Cochrane Database of Systematic Reviews*, no. 2, p. CD005562, 2012.

[36] C. Nombela, J. B. Rowe, S. E. Winder-Rhodes et al., "Genetic impact on cognition and brain function in newly diagnosed Parkinson's disease: ICICLE-PD study," *Brain*, vol. 137, no. 10, pp. 2743–2758, 2014.

[37] J. O. Goh and D. C. Park, "Neuroplasticity and cognitive aging: the scaffolding theory of aging and cognition," *Restorative Neurology and Neuroscience*, vol. 27, pp. 391–403, 2009.

[38] J. M. Rabey, E. Dobronevsky, S. Aichenbaum, O. Gonen, R. G. Marton, and M. Khaigrekht, "Repetitive transcranial magnetic stimulation combined with cognitive training is a safe and effective modality for the treatment of Alzheimer's disease: a randomized, double-blind study," *Journal of Neural Transmission*, vol. 120, no. 5, pp. 813–819, 2013.

[39] L. Mowszowski, J. Batchelor, and S. L. Naismith, "Early intervention for cognitive decline: can cognitive training be used as a selective prevention technique?," *International Psychogeriatrics*, vol. 22, no. 4, pp. 537–548, 2010.

[40] J. G. Goldman, S. Holden, B. Bernard, B. Ouyang, C. G. Goetz, and G. T. Stebbins, "Defining optimal cutoff scores for cognitive impairment using Movement Disorder Society Task Force criteria for mild cognitive impairment in Parkinson's disease," *Movement Disorders*, vol. 28, no. 14, pp. 1972–1979, 2013.

[41] D. Muslimovic, B. Schmand, J. D. Speelman, and R. J. De Haan, "Course of cognitive decline in Parkinson's disease: a meta-analysis," *Journal of the International Neuropsychological Society*, vol. 13, no. 6, pp. 920–932, 2007.

[42] M. Lezak, D. Howieson, and D. Loring, *Neuropsychological Assessment*, Oxford University Press, Oxford, UK, 2012.

[43] E. Y. Kim and K. W. Kim, "A theoretical framework for cognitive and non-cognitive interventions for older adults: stimulation versus compensation," *Aging & Mental Health*, vol. 18, no. 3, pp. 304–315, 2014.

[44] J. D. Nadler, J. Grace, D. A. White, M. A. Butters, and P. F. Malloy, "Laterality differences in quantitative and qualitative Hooper performance," *Archives of Clinical Neuropsychology*, vol. 11, no. 3, pp. 223–229, 1996.

[45] V. Ng, E. T. Bullmore, G. De Zubicaray, A. Cooper, J. Suckling, and S. C. Williams, "Identifying rate-limiting nodes in large-scale cortical networks for visuospatial processing: an illustration using fMRI," *Journal of Cognitive Neuroscience*, vol. 13, no. 4, pp. 537–545, 2001.

Association between Objectively Measured Physical Activity and Gait Patterns in People with Parkinson's Disease: Results from a 3-Month Monitoring

Micaela Porta,[1] **Giuseppina Pilloni,**[1] **Roberta Pili,**[2] **Carlo Casula,**[2] **Mauro Murgia,**[3] **Giovanni Cossu,**[2] **and Massimiliano Pau** [1]

[1]*Department of Mechanical, Chemical and Materials Engineering, University of Cagliari, Cagliari, Italy*
[2]*A.O.B. "G. Brotzu" General Hospital, Cagliari, Italy*
[3]*Department of Life Sciences, University of Trieste, Trieste, Italy*

Correspondence should be addressed to Massimiliano Pau; massimiliano.pau@dimcm.unica.it

Academic Editor: Hélio Teive

Background. Although physical activity (PA) is known to be beneficial in improving motor symptoms of people with Parkinson's disease (pwPD), little is known about the relationship between gait patterns and features of PA performed during daily life. *Objective.* To verify the existence of possible relationships between spatiotemporal and kinematic parameters of gait and amount/intensity of PA, both instrumentally assessed. *Methods.* Eighteen individuals affected by PD (10F and 8M, age 68.0 ± 10.8 years, 1.5 ≤ Hoehn and Yahr (H&Y) < 3) were required to wear a triaxial accelerometer 24 h/day for 3 consecutive months. They also underwent a 3D computerized gait analysis at the beginning and end of the PA assessment period. The number of daily steps and PA intensity were calculated on the whole day, and the period from 6:00 to 24:00 was grouped into 3 time slots, using 3 different cut-point sets previously validated in the case of both pwPD and healthy older adults. 3D gait analysis provided spatiotemporal and kinematic parameters of gait, including summary indexes of quality (Gait Profile Score (GPS) and Gait Variable Score (GVS)). *Results.* The analysis of hourly trends of PA revealed the existence of two peaks located in the morning (approximately at 10) and in the early evening (between 18 and 19). However, during the morning time slot (06:00–12:00), pwPD performed significantly higher amounts of steps (4313 vs. 3437 in the 12:00–18:00 time slot, $p < 0.001$, and vs. 2889 in the 18:00–24:00 time slot, $p = 0.021$) and of moderate-to-vigorous PA (43.2% vs. 36.3% in the 12:00–18:00 time slot, $p = 0.002$, and vs. 31.4% in the 18:00–24:00 time slot, $p = 0.049$). The correlation analysis shows that several PA intensity parameters are significantly associated with swing-phase duration (rho = −0.675 for sedentary intensity, rho = 0.717 for moderate-to-vigorous intensity, $p < 0.001$), cadence (rho = 0.509 for sedentary intensity, rho = −0.575 for moderate-to-vigorous intensity, $p < 0.05$), and overall gait pattern quality as expressed by GPS (rho = −0.498 to −0.606 for moderate intensity, $p < 0.05$) and GVS of knee flexion-extension (rho = −0.536 for moderate intensity, $p < 0.05$). *Conclusions.* Long-term monitoring of PA integrated by the quantitative assessment of spatiotemporal and kinematic parameters of gait may represent a useful tool in supporting a better-targeted prescription of PA and rehabilitative treatments in pwPD.

1. Introduction

In people with Parkinson's disease (pwPD), walking dysfunctions represent a very common and disabling feature which is typically expressed by a gait pattern characterized by short stride length, increased cadence, and reduced velocity [1]. Such issues tend to further deteriorate with the progression of the disease [2], thus limiting the ability of the affected individual to perform daily activities and severely reducing the quality of life [3].

Although physical activity (PA) has been found to be beneficial in improving mobility in pwPD [4, 5], they may be reluctant to engage in structured or unstructured PA programs, owing to their increased motor difficulties which tend to favor a sedentary lifestyle. This originates a vicious circle since physical inactivity further negatively affects several clinical domains of PD [6, 7]. Thus, a detailed assessment of both the amount and intensity of PA performed represents a critical issue in evaluating the effectiveness of programs and trials aimed to improve mobility in pwPD. To this end, several studies have attempted to employ objective measurements (e.g., using pedometers or accelerometers) [8] to replace or integrate self-reported data collected using questionnaires [9], which may not adequately reflect the actual activity carried out by pwPD [10]. The availability of continuous quantitative data on mobility has made it possible to precisely identify what aspects of the disease are most involved in PA levels [11, 12], their relationship to history of falls [13], and cognition, depression, and quality of life [14, 15]. However, data collection is usually limited to few days or a week, while long-term monitoring appears to be infrequent, probably owing to compliance issues.

While there is a certain consensus on the fact that PA contributes to improving gait and mobility [5, 16], it is noteworthy that most studies that consider gait parameters as the primary outcome only consider few aspects of them (usually gait speed and cadence) mainly assessed using timed tests. In contrast, few data are available on the whole kinematics of the gait pattern (i.e., spatiotemporal parameters, kinematics, and range of motion during gait of hip, knee, and ankle joints), acquired with state-of-the-art technologies such as motion-capture systems or inertial sensors. Such information would be of interest to better understand the complex pathophysiology of gait disturbance in PD [17] and to assess the effects of neurosurgical, pharmacological, and rehabilitative treatments [18]. Summarizing, the main drawbacks of the study performed to date to investigate the effects of PA on gait in pwPD are the following: the limited period of PA monitoring and the limited number of gait parameters assessed to relate PA to mobility.

To partly overcome such limits, this study aims firstly to describe the patterns of PA in a cohort of pwPD based on a 3-month monitoring. Then, during the same period, quantitative data on the quality of gait patterns, by means of spatiotemporal and kinematic parameters, were also collected and correlated with PA indicators. The hypothesis to verify is that individuals who exhibit better gait features are characterized by higher and more intense PA during their daily lives.

2. Methods

2.1. Participants. The study was performed in the period March–December 2017 and involved 18 outpatients with PD (10 females and 8 males) followed up at the Neurology Department of the G. Brotzu General Hospital (Cagliari, Italy) who were enrolled on a voluntary basis. Their demographic and clinical characteristics are shown in Table 1.

All participants met the following criteria: diagnosis of PD according to the UK Brain Bank criteria [19]; ability to walk independently; absence of significant cognitive impairment (i.e., Mini-Mental Status Examination (MMSE) > 24; Frontal Assessment Battery (FAB) > 13); absence of

psychiatric or severe systemic illnesses; and mild-to-moderate disability assessed by means of the modified Hoehn and Yahr (H&Y) staging scale ($1.5 \leq$ H&Y < 3). At the time of enrollment, the pharmacologic treatment included levodopa for all participants and MAO-B inhibitors for 11 of them ($n = 8$ had rasigiline and $n = 3$ had safinamide). The study was carried out in compliance with the ethical principles for research involving human subjects expressed in the Declaration of Helsinki and was approved by the local ethics committee (Prot. PG/2014/19654). All participants signed an informed consent form after a detailed explanation of the purposes of the study and the methodology used in the experimental tests.

2.2. Data Collection and Processing: Physical Activity. Data on PA were collected using a triaxial accelerometer (ActiGraph GT3X; Acticorp Co., Pensacola, FL, USA) previously employed in similar studies carried out on individuals with PD [20–22]. During the first meeting with participants, their anthropometric data required to initialize the device (i.e., stature and body mass) were recorded using an ultrasonic digital height meter (Soehnle 5003; Soehnle, Germany) and a digital scale (RE310; Wunder, Italy). Each participant was then asked to wear the accelerometer on the nondominant wrist for 3 months 24 h/day and instructed to remove it only for showering, bathing, and any other water-based activities (i.e., swimming). The choice of the wrist as the site of placement was made to increase wear time compliance and provide data on sleep [23–25]. The devices were set to collect data using 60 s epochs and 30 Hz frequency and were usually operative for at least 30 days before the battery ran out of charge. At that point, the participants came back to the laboratory to download the acquired data and charge the accelerometer. At the end of the third month, raw data were processed using ActiLife® software v6.13.3 to perform step counts and PA classification based on the cut-points defined by Hildebrand et al. [26], Wallén et al. [20], and Nero et al. [21] for the acceleration vector magnitude (VM) defined as follows:

$$VM = \sqrt{x^2 + y^2 + z^2}, \qquad (1)$$

where x, y, and z are the accelerations recorded by the device in each of the three directions.

The use of 3 different processing procedures, although all based on the same device and the same physical variable (i.e., VM), was suggested by the fact that, to date, a validated set of cut-points for wrist placement of the accelerometer in individuals with PD is unavailable. Thus, the algorithm of Hildebrand et al. [26] was chosen because it is the only one available for wrist-worn data acquisition on elderly people, while the algorithms of Wallén et al. [20] and Nero et al. [21] were previously validated for individuals with PD but in the case of hip placement. In particular, the Nero algorithm provides a set of cut-points for different walking speeds. All the PA parameters were then grouped by considering the following three time slots, namely, 6:00–12:00 (TS 1, morning), 12:00–18:00 (TS 2, afternoon), and 18:00–24:00

TABLE 1: Anthropometric and demographic aspects of participants.

Variable		Mean ± SD	Range (min–max)
Age (years)		68.0 ± 10.8	53–83
Height (cm)		165.6 ± 7.9	150–178
Body mass (kg)		69.2 ± 9.4	50–81
PD duration (years)		9.9 ± 6.0	4–27
Hoehn and Yahr (H&Y)		1.9 ± 0.4	1.5–2.5
Unified Parkinson's Disease Rating Scale	Overall score	17.8 ± 9.6	5–32
(UPDRS III)	Axial subscore (items 27–30)	2.8 ± 1.5	1–5

Values are expressed as mean ± SD.

(TS 3, evening). The acquired data were considered valid if wear time amounted to at least 16 h/day, by considering nonwear time as a time interval of at least 60 consecutive minutes of zero accelerometric counts.

2.3. Data Collection and Processing: 3D Gait Analysis.

A 3D computerized gait analysis was performed at the beginning (T0) and at the end (T3) of the 3-month evaluation period to calculate both spatiotemporal and kinematic gait parameters using an optoelectronic system composed of 8 infrared cameras (Smart-D; BTS Bioengineering, Italy) set at a frequency of 120 Hz. After anthropometric data collection, 22 spherical retroreflective passive markers (14 mm in diameter) were placed on the skin of the individual's lower limbs and trunk at specific landmarks, following the protocol described by Davis et al. [27]. Participants were then asked to walk barefoot at a self-selected comfortable speed in the most natural manner possible on a 10 m walkway for at least six times, allowing suitable rest times between the trials. The raw data were then processed with the Smart Analyzer (BTS Bioengineering, Italy) dedicated software to calculate the following:

(i) Five spatiotemporal parameters (gait speed, cadence, stride length, stance, and swing-phase duration)

(ii) Nine kinematic parameters, namely, pelvic tilt, rotation, and obliquity, hip flexion-extension, adduction-abduction, and rotation, knee flexion-extension, ankle dorsi-plantarflexion, and foot progression (i.e., the angle between the axis of the foot and the walking direction)

(iii) Dynamic range of motion (ROM) for hip and knee flexion-extension and ankle dorsi-plantarflexion calculated during the whole gait cycle as the difference between the maximum and minimum values of each angle recorded during a trial

Kinematic data were summarized using the Gait Variable Score (GVS) and the Gait Profile Score (GPS), which are concise measures of gait quality proposed by Baker et al. [28]. Although originally proposed for children with cerebral palsy, this approach was found to be effective in characterizing gait alterations in individuals with PD [29, 30]. Specifically, the GVS represents the root mean square (RMS) difference between the tested subject's curve for a certain movement of the nine previously listed parameters (e.g., knee flexion-extension) and a reference curve calculated as the mean value of tests performed on the unaffected subjects. The GPS combines the nine GVS values in a single score, which indicates the degree of deviation from a hypothetical "normal" gait (i.e., the larger the GPS, the less physiological the gait pattern); values for healthy individuals lie in the range 5-6° [31]. In the present study, the reference data were obtained from a database of healthy individuals of the same age range of the subjects tested here, available from the Smart Analyzer software.

2.4. Statistical Analyses.

The possible differences in PA levels associated with each time slot were assessed using the one-way analysis of variance for repeated measures (RM-ANOVA) considering as the independent variable the time slot and as dependent variables the PA parameters. The level of significance was set at $p < 0.05$, and effect sizes were assessed using the eta-squared coefficient (η^2). Influence of time on spatiotemporal and kinematic parameters of gait was assessed using one-way RM-ANOVA considering time (T0, T3) as the independent variable and the previously listed gait parameters as dependent variables. All analyses were performed using the IBM SPSS Statistics v.20 software (IBM, Armonk, NY, USA). Finally, the relationship between PA and gait parameters was explored using Spearman's rank correlation coefficient, again by setting the level of significance at $p < 0.05$.

3. Results

The hourly trends of step count and VM and the mean values of PA classified as a function of its intensity calculated on the 3 selected time slots are illustrated in Figures 1 and 2, while Table 2 shows the classification of PA parameters according to the cut-points defined by the 3 algorithms previously described.

ANOVA revealed a significant main effect of the time slot for both step counts ($F(2,17) = 9.81$, $p < 0.001$, $\eta^2 = 0.11$) and VM counts ($F(2,17) = 9.76$, $p < 0.001$, $\eta^2 = 0.01$). The highest values for both variables were observed in the 6:00–12:00 time slot, while participants appeared to be less active in the evening.

The results of the classification of PA intensity with the three algorithms employed show similar results. For the Hildebrand algorithm, the effect of time slots was significant for percentage of time spent in sedentary activity ($F(2,17) = 8.22$, $p < 0.001$, $\eta^2 = 0.07$), low intensity ($F(2,17) = 4.73$,

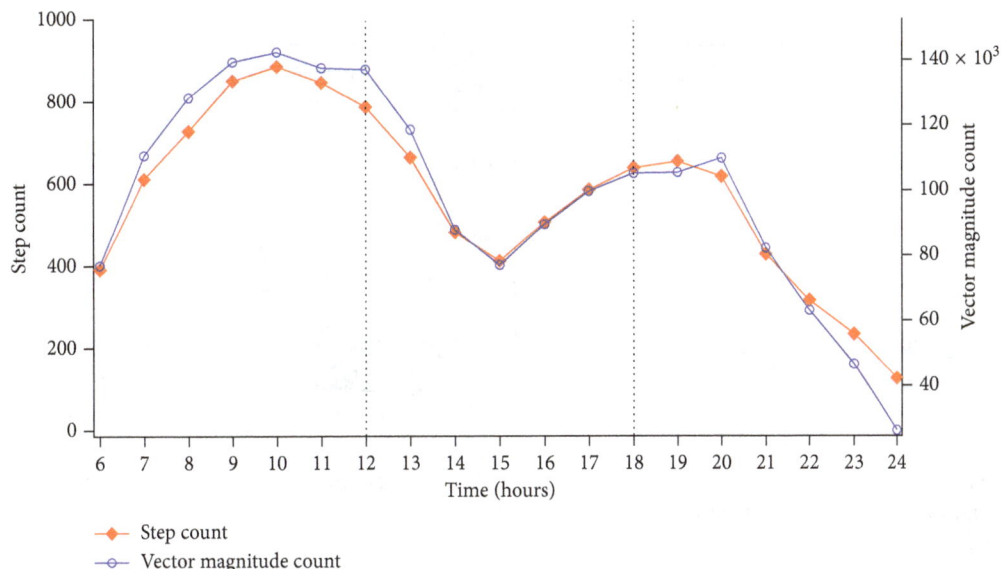

FIGURE 1: Hourly trend (average value of 3 months) of step counts and vector magnitude counts.

$p = 0.015$, $\eta^2 = 0.05$), and moderate-to-vigorous intensity (MVPA) ($F(2,17) = 6.57$, $p = 0.004$, $\eta^2 = 0.06$), with sedentary behavior being reduced in the morning and increased in the evening (59.1% vs. 70.9%, $p < 0.001$) and, conversely, higher MVPA in the morning (40.9% vs. 29.9%, $p = 0.003$). The Wallén algorithm yielded a significant effect of time for all the intensity levels: sedentary ($F(2,17) = 4.67$, $p = 0.017$, $\eta^2 = 0.05$), low intensity ($F(2,17) = 3.43$, $p = 0.044$, $\eta^2 = 0.05$), moderate intensity ($F(2,17) = 4.16$, $p = 0.024$, $\eta^2 = 0.05$), and MVPA ($F(2,17) = 7.42$, $p = 0.002$, $\eta^2 = 0.05$). Finally, for the Nero algorithm, which classifies PA intensity in terms of gait speed, time was found to significantly influence the percentage of time spent at speeds below 1.04 m/s ($F(2,17) = 7.55$, $p = 0.002$, $\eta^2 = 0.06$), at speeds in the range 1.05–1.30 m/s ($F(2,17) = 3.79$, $p = 0.033$, $\eta^2 = 0.05$), and at speeds above 1.31 m/s ($F(2,17) = 5.36$, $p = 0.009$, $\eta^2 = 0.04$). Even in this case, the morning represents the time of day characterized by higher percentages of time spent at the higher gait speed (14.6% vs. 8.7% in the evening, $p = 0.008$).

Spatiotemporal and kinematic parameters of gait did not vary significantly between the beginning and the end of the 3-month period, except for the GVS of pelvic tilt, as visible from data in Tables 3 and 4.

To conclude, Tables 5 and 6 show the results of the correlations between PA and gait variables.

Duration of the swing phase and cadence were found to be the gait variables significantly correlated with a larger number of PA parameters regardless of the algorithm considered (11 to 14 significant correlations out of 15 possible). Stride length was found to be significantly correlated only with step counts (rho = 0.59) and percentage of sedentary activity (rho = −0.48) calculated according to Wallén, while no significant correlations were found for gait speed. As regards the kinematic variables, the GPS was found to be significantly correlated negatively with the percentage of moderate activity as calculated by the Wallén (rho = −0.61) and Hildebrand (rho = −0.50) algorithms. The

GVS associated with knee flexion-extension was also found to be negatively correlated with the percentage of moderate activity according to Wallén (rho = −0.54) and with the percentage of time spent at walking speed between 1.05 and 1.30 m/s (Nero algorithm, rho = −0.53). Dynamic ROM of the knee was negatively correlated with sedentary activity (Wallén algorithm, rho = −0.47) and positively correlated with vigorous activity (Hildebrand algorithm, rho = 0.49). Finally, step count was found to be positively correlated with both dynamic ROMs of the hip and knee (rho = 0.50 and 0.57, respectively).

4. Discussion

4.1. Hourly Trends of PA. The aim of the present study was to perform long-term monitoring of PA in pwPD and investigate the existence of possible correlations between PA and gait parameters, with these being objectively assessed using the gold standard for quantitative analysis of human motion, namely, the motion capture system. Our results detected a pattern for PA of pwPD with low-mild disability. They clearly show the existence of two peaks of PA, one in the morning (approximately hour 10) and another in the evening located between 6 and 7 PM. Unfortunately, a direct comparison with previous studies is difficult because even though several of these continuously monitored PA, they mostly report only examples of the curves of variation of PA parameters (usually the number of steps) during the day [31, 32]. To our knowledge, only the recent study by Cai et al. [12] calculated a mean curve of variation for step counts calculated for a sample of 21 pwPD, but their data appear not to suggest the existence of a well-defined pattern. However, our results do appear to be partly consistent with those reported in two studies performed on healthy older adults [33, 34], both of which observed a marked peak in PA (expressed in terms of either steps or accelerometric counts) approximately at 10. Sartini et al. [33] detected a second peak

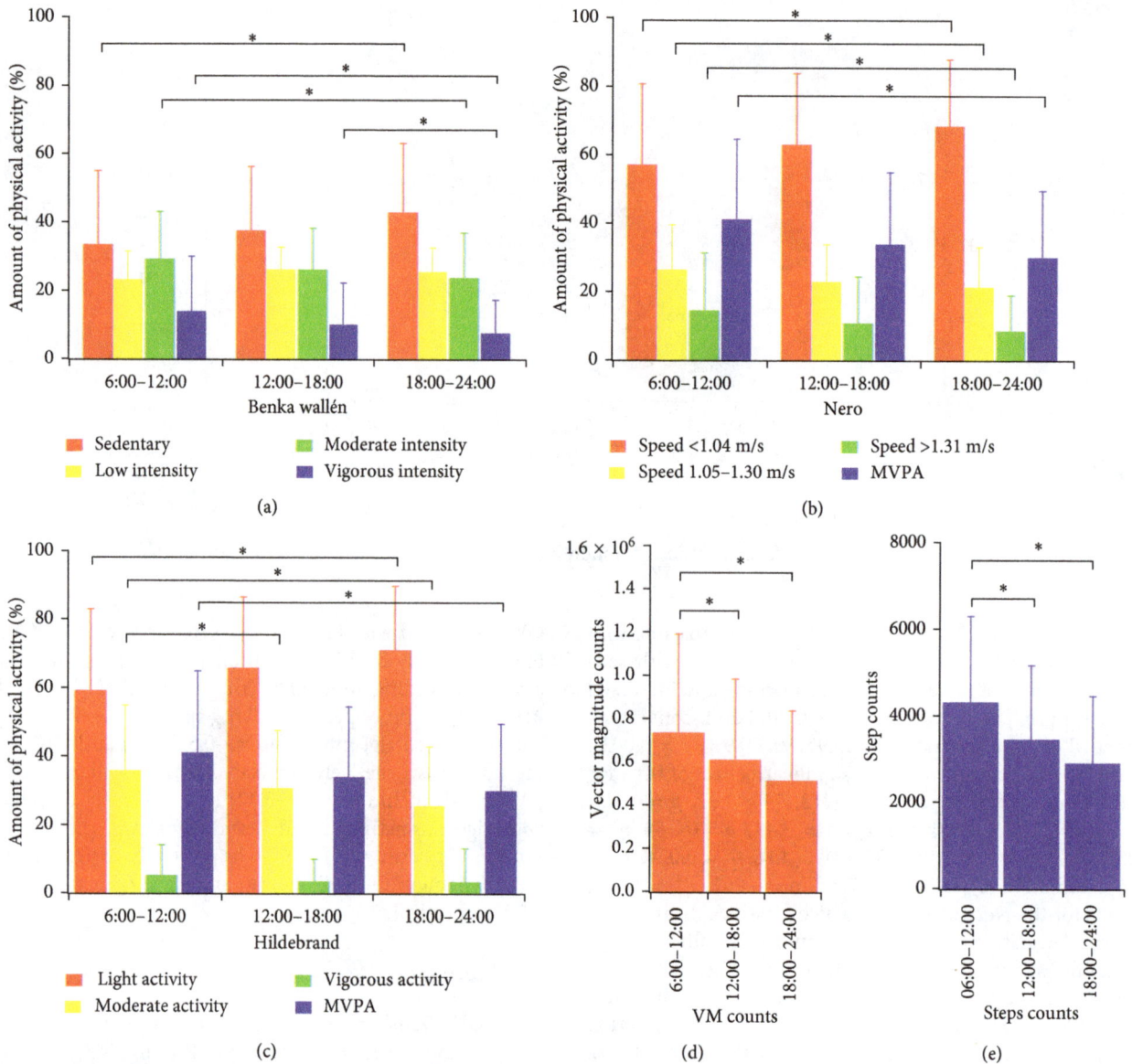

FIGURE 2: Physical activity amount classified as a function of intensity for the 3 time slots. (MVPA = moderate-to-vigorous physical activity; VM = vector magnitude).

located approximately at 14-15, while in the study by Valenti et al. [34], activity appears to monotonically decrease from 10 until night. As previously mentioned, in the present study, a second relevant PA peak was found between 18 and 19 and thus later in the day with respect to Sartini et al. [33]. Such differences can probably be explained by the fact that, in our case, PA was mostly monitored during months characterized by favorable environmental conditions (Cagliari has a mild climate for most of the year) which probably encouraged participants to walk or spend time outdoor in the evening as well. In any case, it must be noted that when PA is analyzed on the basis of the 3 defined time slots, our results appear to be fully consistent also with those of Valenti et al. [34] who also detected a significant reduction in PA in the evening time slots.

4.2. Comparison between Different Algorithms for PA Intensity Classification. One of the purposes of our study was to compare different algorithms previously validated for use in pwPD [20, 21] but designed for waist placement of the accelerometer and one calibrated on older adults [26] in the case of nondominant wrist placement. The results show that, despite the different cut-points and the correction applied by the ActiLife® software for wrist placement with algorithms designed for waist placement, the hourly trend for the different intensities appears to be very similar. For example, Figure 3 shows a comparison between the hourly trends for the lowest PA intensity (i.e., <3 MET), namely, sedentary/light intensity [20], walking speed <1.04 m/s [21], and light intensity [26], which demonstrates the good agreement of the 3 algorithms.

TABLE 2: Physical activity patterns for the morning, afternoon, and evening time slots calculated as means of the 3-month monitoring period.

		Physical activity patterns		
		TS 1 (hours 6–12)	TS 2 (hours 12–18)	TS 3 (hours 18–24)
Wallén et al. [20]	Sedentary behavior (%)	33.41 ± 21.66	37.62 ± 18.70	42.78 ± 21.28[a]
	Low intensity (%)	23.09 ± 8.55	26.01 ± 6.72	25.59 ± 6.91
	Moderate intensity (%)	29.32 ± 13.85	26.21 ± 12.03	23.79 ± 13.05[a]
	Vigorous intensity (%)	13.93 ± 16.06	10.08 ± 12.21[a]	7.66 ± 9.70[a]
	MVPA* (%)	43.25 ± 20.31	36.29 ± 18.50[a]	31.45 ± 16.53[a]
Nero et al. [21]	Speed ≤ 1.04 m/s (%)	57.08 ± 26.65	62.99 ± 20.81	68.39 ± 19.62[a]
	Speed 1.05–1.30 m/s (%)	26.53 ± 13.00	23.00 ± 10.86	21.38 ± 11.60[a]
	Speed ≥ 1.31 m/s (%)	14.65 ± 16.82	10.96 ±13.42	8.68 ± 10.39[a]
	MVPA (%)	41.18 ± 23.47	33.96 ± 21.10	30.07 ± 19.56[a]
Hildebrand et al. [26]	Light intensity (%)	59.05 ± 23.93	65.97 ± 20.41[a]	70.87 ± 18.75[a]
	Moderate intensity (%)	35.77 ± 19.10	30.58 ± 16.87	25.54 ±17.25[a]
	Vigorous intensity (%)	5.18 ± 8.91	3.44 ± 6.54	3.22 ± 9.86
	MVPA** (%)	40.95 ± 23.93	34.03 ± 20.41	29.91 ± 19.59[a]
	Steps counts (daily steps)	4313 ± 1973	3437 ± 1719[a]	2889 ± 1557[a]
	Vector magnitude (counts per day)	735639 ± 452680	610262 ± 372729[a]	512835 ± 323037[a,b]

Values are expressed as mean ± SD. MVPA: moderate-to-vigorous physical activity; TS: time slot; [a]significant difference vs. TS 1; [b]significant difference vs. TS 2; *sum of moderate and vigorous intensity; **sum of light and moderate intensity.

TABLE 3: Values of the spatiotemporal parameters of gait at the beginning and end of the 3-month observation period.

Spatiotemporal parameters of gait			
	T0	T3	p value
Step length (m)	0.59 ± 0.10	0.59 ± 0.01	0.824
Gait speed (m/s)	1.18 ± 0.23	1.18 ± 0.19	0.980
Cadence (steps/min)	120.39 ± 11.18	120.88 ± 9.09	0.819
Stance-phase duration (s)	0.60 ± 0.07	0.60 ± 0.05	0.754
Swing-phase duration (s)	0.40 ± 0.04	0.39 ± 0.03	0.522

Values are expressed as mean ± SD.

TABLE 4: Values of the kinematic parameters of gait at the beginning and end of the 3-month observation period.

Kinematic parameters of gait				
		T0	T3	p value
GVS (°)	GPS (°)	7.31 ± 1.61	7.84 ± 2.44	0.637
	Pelvic tilt	5.51 ± 3.90	7.64 ± 5.10	0.042
	Pelvic rotation	3.80 ± 1.30	4.29 ± 1.79	0.285
	Pelvic obliquity	2.47 ± 1.18	2.67 ± 1.13	0.481
	Hip flexion-extension	8.30 ± 4.09	10.41 ± 6.22	0.059
	Hip abduction-adduction	3.96 ± 1.59	4.15 ± 1.50	0.564
	Hip rotation	8.59 ± 2.70	8.14 ± 2.99	0.641
	Knee flexion-extension	9.17 ± 3.64	9.37 ± 4.13	0.157
	Ankle dorsi-plantarflexion	7.17 ± 2.48	6.22 ± 2.28	0.319
	Foot progression	7.80 ± 3.77	7.89 ± 4.14	0.828
ROM (°)	Hip flexion-extension	42.15 ± 7.45	43.27 ± 7.23	0.197
	Knee flexion-extension	57.39 ± 4.23	57.72 ± 5.28	0.479
	Ankle dorsi-plantarflexion	25.22 ± 6.70	26.47 ± 6.82	0.129

Values are expressed as mean ± SD.

4.3. Correlation between PA and Gait Parameters. The most innovative aspect of the present study is represented by the search for possible correlations between PA and gait patterns, with the latter being investigated using 3D computerized gait analysis, which represents the gold standard for human movement analysis. The results show that cadence and swing-phase duration exhibit the highest number of significant correlations with amount and intensity of PA performed. Individuals who spent less time in sedentary behavior and more time in moderate-to-vigorous activity are likely to exhibit a gait pattern characterized by reduced cadence and increased swing phase. Instead, the relationship of PA intensity with both stride length and stance-phase duration appears to be less generalized.

The reduction in swing-phase duration, which is a physiologic sign of gait deterioration associated with aging [35] and further worsened in pwPD [30], is a cofactor involved in the risk of falls [36]. However, it has been demonstrated that exercise (for healthy older adults [37]) or specific gait training integrated with rhythmic auditory stimulation (for pwPD [38]) can partly reverse this negative trend. In this context, our data suggest that pwPD engaged in higher and more intense levels of PA are characterized by increased swing-phase duration and thus, indirectly, probably exposed to a lower risk of falls.

Cadence has been recognized as one of the gait parameters most suitable for representing ambulatory activity in free living, and in young healthy individuals, it has been found to be strongly correlated with PA intensity [39]. Our results suggest that, in our cohort of pwPD, participants with higher baseline cadence tend to spend more time in sedentary/low-intensity behavior, while those characterized by lower baseline cadence are more likely to engage in moderate-to-vigorous activity. Although there is no specific evidence about the role of cadence in preventing/promoting PA engagement, it is possible to hypothesize that individuals with higher (e.g., above normality) cadence are also those

TABLE 5: Spearman's correlation analysis between physical activity intensity and spatiotemporal parameters of gait.

		Gait speed	Stride length	Cadence	Stance phase	Swing phase
		\multicolumn{5}{c}{Correlation between physical activity and spatiotemporal parameters of gait}				
Wallén et al. [20]	Sedentary behavior (%)	−0.088	−0.482*	0.509*	−0.430	−0.675**
	Low intensity (%)	0.060	−0.049	0.309	−0.153	−0.361
	Moderate intensity (%)	−0.105	0.159	−0.451	0.374	0.612**
	Vigorous intensity (%)	0.067	0.423	−0.531*	0.427	0.674**
	MVPA*	0.007	0.378	−0.575*	0.457	0.717**
Nero et al. [21]	Speed ≤ 1.04 m/s (%)	−0.009	−0.356	0.591**	−0.503*	−0.687**
	Speed 1.05–1.30 m/s (%)	−0.104	0.169	−0.534*	0.444	0.683**
	Speed ≥ 1.31 m/s (%)	0.024	0.367	−0.544*	0.412	0.669**
	MVPA (%)	−0.025	0.325	−0.591**	0.495*	0.690**
Hildebrand et al. [26]	Light intensity (%)	0.007	−0.358	0.575*	−0.467	−0.704**
	Moderate intensity (%)	−0.072	0.291	−0.575*	0.474	0.734**
	Vigorous intensity (%)	0.206	0.514*	−0.437	0.313	0.604**
	MVPA (%)	0.007	0.378	−0.575*	0.456	0.717**
	Step count	0.343	0.586*	−0.375	0.239	0.588*
	Vector magnitude count	−0.001	0.360	−0.577*	0.469*	0.704**

$^*p < 0.05$; $^{**}p < 0.001$.

TABLE 6: Correlation analysis between physical activity intensity and kinematic parameters of gait.

		GPS	GVS hip FE	GVS knee FE	GVS ankle DP	ROM hip	ROM knee	ROM ankle
		\multicolumn{7}{c}{Correlation between physical activity and kinematic parameters of gait}						
Wallén et al. [20]	Sedentary behavior (%)	0.310	0.019	0.203	−0.106	−0.346	−0.474*	−0.424
	Low intensity (%)	0.123	0.239	−0.181	−0.465	−0.038	−0.007	−0.267
	Moderate intensity (%)	−0.606**	−0.380	−0.536*	0.63	0.143	0.276	0.246
	Vigorous intensity (%)	−0.334	−0.099	−0.168	0.205	0.315	0.397	0.329
	MVPA*	−0.336	−0.164	−0.135	0.276	0.286	0.373	0.341
Nero et al. [21]	Speed ≤ 1.04 m/s (%)	0.326	0.216	0.143	−0.244	−0.315	−0.381	−0.307
	Speed 1.05–1.30 m/s (%)	−0.576*	−0.394	−0.527*	0.018	0.195	0.377	0.212
	Speed ≥ 1.31 m/s (%)	−0.275	−0.107	−0.100	0.265	0.282	0.383	0.304
	MVPA (%)	−0.306	−0.217	−0.115	0.272	−0.275	0.370	0.298
Hildebrand et al. [26]	Light intensity (%)	0.327	0.182	0.143	−0.265	−0.276	−0.356	−0.328
	Moderate intensity (%)	−0.498*	−0.279	−0.307	0.216	0.207	0.313	0.266
	Vigorous intensity (%)	−0.308	−0.094	−0.156	0.112	0.424	0.490*	0.402
	MVPA (%)	−0.336	−0.164	−0.135	0.276	0.286	0.373	0.341
	Step count	−0.184	−0.106	−0.001	0.108	0.503*	0.575*	0.336
	Vector magnitude count	−0.323	−0.170	−0.150	0.261	0.282	0.362	0.320

$^*p < 0.05$; $^{**}p < 0.001$.

who experience increased difficulties in optimally managing the stride length-cadence relationship [40] and thus are more likely to exhibit a disturbed gait which somehow discourages them from being active. This may also partly explain why we also detected more marked sedentary behavior (at least with the Wallén approach) in pwPD with shorter steps. In brief, individuals who walk with shorter steps/higher cadence appear to be characterized by prevalent sedentary/low-intensity PA.

Finally, the overall quality of the gait pattern, as expressed by GPS, appears to be moderately correlated with the percentage of time spent in moderate-intensity PA, consistent in all the tested approaches; in particular, the alterations at the knee joint level appear to be the most involved in this process. Previous studies highlighted the existence of alterations of knee flexion-extension during gait,

especially in terms of inadequate extension in the stance phase [30]. This is probably due to reduced muscle strength in the knee extensors, a phenomenon commonly observed in pwPD [41, 42], which can also be the result of impairment of dynamic stability [43]. Such results suggest that a detailed analysis of the role of walking abilities in PA features cannot be based solely on the study of spatiotemporal parameters but should also take into account possible kinematic alterations.

Some limitations of the study are to be acknowledged. Firstly, the participants were all volunteers, as the particular nature of the study (i.e., long-term use of a wearable device 24 h/day) required high levels of compliance to achieve reliable results [44]. Secondly, the tested sample was composed of a very homogeneous group of highly motivated individuals (as shown by their good PA performance) with

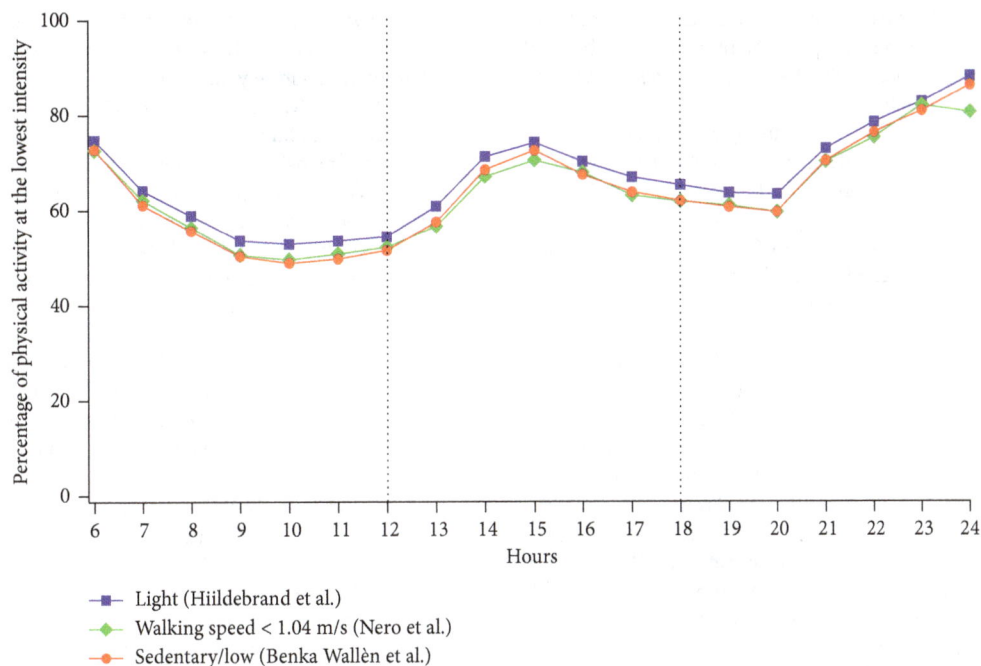

FIGURE 3: Hourly trends for lowest-intensity physical activity (<3 MET) as calculated using 3 different cut-point sets.

low-mild disability living in an inner city residential area. Such biases make it difficult to generalize our results [45] particularly to different geographic and socioeconomic contexts and to individuals with PD more severely impaired. Also, it should be considered that the gait parameters were acquired in the laboratory with participants undressed and barefoot, while PA was assessed under daily living conditions; thus, the measurement conditions are obviously quite different.

5. Conclusion

This study investigated the relationship between amount and intensity of PA performed by individuals affected by PD with low-mild disability (objectively assessed using wrist-worn triaxial accelerometers) and the kinematic features of their gait patterns provided by computerized 3D gait analysis. PA parameters were estimated using different sets of cut-points for the accelerometric counts previously validated on pwPD and healthy older adults. The results show a daily trend, described similarly by all the approaches tested, characterized by two distinct peaks of activity, located in the morning and early evening. The main hypothesis of the study, namely, the existence of a relationship between the quality of the gait pattern and amount/intensity of performed PA, was substantially confirmed by the results of the correlation analysis. In particular, higher and more intense activity appears to be related to swing-phase duration and cadence, while the percentage of time spent in moderate activity also appears to be associated with the overall quality of gait kinematics (expressed by means of the GPS summary index) and with the alteration of flexion-extension of the knee joint.

Although further studies on larger cohorts are necessary to better elucidate the influence of the disability level, gender, and socioeconomic status, the findings of the present study suggest that the continuous monitoring of PA in pwPD may represent a useful tool in predicting possible changes in the gait pattern and verify the effectiveness of rehabilitative treatments and PA programs.

Authors' Contributions

MPa, MM, CC, and RP planned the study. GC, CC, and RP recruited participants and performed neurologic and clinical assessments. MPa, MPo, and GP acquired and analyzed the data. MPa and MPo wrote and corrected the manuscript.

Acknowledgments

The authors wish to thank the Sardinian Association of Patients with Parkinson's Disease (ASAMPA) and in particular the chairperson Prof. Carlo Anchisi, for their valuable support. This study was funded by the Autonomous Region of Sardinia (grant CRP-78543 L.R. 7/2007) and by the Fondazione di Sardegna.

References

[1] M. E. Morris, F. Huxham, I. McGinley, K. Dodd, and R. Iansek, "The biomechanics and motor control of gait in Parkinson's disease," *Clinical Biomechanics*, vol. 16, no. 6, pp. 459–470, 2001.

[2] O. Blin, A. M. Ferrandez, and G. Serratrice, "Quantitative analysis of gait in Parkinson patients: increased variability of stride length," *Journal of the Neurological Sciences*, vol. 98, no. 1, pp. 91–97, 1990.

[3] S. E. Soh, J. L. McGinley, J. J. Watts et al., "Determinants of health-related quality of life in people with Parkinson's disease: a path analysis," *Quality of Life Research*, vol. 22, no. 7, pp. 1543–1553, 2013.

[4] S. C. LaHue, C. L. Comella, and C. M. Tanner, "The best medicine? the influence of physical activity and inactivity on Parkinson's disease," *Movement Disorders*, vol. 31, no. 10, pp. 1444–1454, 2016.

[5] M. Lauzè, J. F. Daneault, and C. Duval, "The effects of physical activity in Parkinson's disease: a review," *Journal of Parkinsons Disease*, vol. 6, no. 4, pp. 685–698, 2016.

[6] A. D. Speelman, B. P. van der Warrenburg, M. van Nimwegen, G. M. Petzinger, M. Munneke, and B. R. Bloem, "How might physical activity benefit patients with Parkinson's disease?," *Nature Reviews Neurology*, vol. 7, no. 9, pp. 528–534, 2011.

[7] J. Snider, M. L. Müller, V. Kotagal et al., "Non-exercise physical activity attenuates motor symptoms in Parkinson's disease independent from nigrostriatal degeneration," *Parkinsonism and Related Disorders*, vol. 21, no. 10, pp. 1227–1231, 2015.

[8] W. Maetzler, J. Domingos, K. Srulijes, J. J. Ferreira, and B. R. Bloem, "Quantitative wearable sensors for objective assessment of Parkinson's disease," *Movement Disorders*, vol. 28, no. 12, pp. 1628–1637, 2013.

[9] M. van Nimwegen, A. D. Speelman, S. Overeem et al., "Promotion of physical activity and fitness in sedentary patients with Parkinson's disease: randomised controlled trial," *BMJ*, vol. 346, p. f576, 2013.

[10] C. A. Jones, M. Wieler, J. Carvajal, L. Lawrence, and R. Haennel, "Physical activity in persons with Parkinson's disease: a feasibility study," *Health*, vol. 4, no. 11, pp. 1145–1152, 2012.

[11] H. Nero, M. B. Wallén, E. Franzén, D. Conradsson, A. Ståhle, and M. Hagströmer, "Objectively assessed physical activity and its association with balance, physical function and dyskinesia in Parkinson's disease," *Journal of Parkinson's Disease*, vol. 6, no. 4, pp. 833–840, 2016.

[12] G. Cai, Y. Huang, S. Luo, Z. Lin, H. Dai, and Q. Ye, "Continuous quantitative monitoring of physical activity in Parkinson's disease patients by using wearable devices: a case-control study," *Neurological Sciences*, vol. 38, no. 9, pp. 1657–1663, 2017.

[13] Y. H. Hiorth, J. P. Larsen, K. Lode et al., "Impact of falls on physical activity in people with Parkinson's disease," *Journal of Parkinson's Disease*, vol. 6, no. 1, pp. 175–182, 2016.

[14] P. D. Loprinzi, M. M. Danzl, E. Ulanowski, and C. Paydo, "A pilot study evaluating the association between physical activity and cognition among individuals with Parkinson's disease," *Disability and Health Journal*, vol. 11, no. 1, pp. 165–168, 2018.

[15] J. M. T. van Uem, B. Cerff, M. Kampmeyer et al., "The association between objectively measured physical activity, depression, cognition, and health-related quality of life in Parkinson's disease," *Parkinsonism and Related Disorders*, vol. 48, pp. 74–81, 2018.

[16] P. Borrione, E. Tranchita, P. Sansone, and A. Parisi, "Effects of physical activity in Parkinson's disease: a new tool for rehabilitation," *World Journal of Methodology*, vol. 4, no. 3, pp. 133–143, 2014.

[17] A. Peppe, C. Chiavalon, P. Pasquetti, D. Crovato, and C. Caltagirone, "Does gait analysis quantify motor rehabilitation efficacy in Parkinson's disease patients?," *Gait and Posture*, vol. 26, no. 3, pp. 452–462, 2007.

[18] M. Morris, R. Iansek, J. McGinley, T. Matyas, and F. Huxham, "Three-dimensional gait biomechanics in Parkinson's disease: evidence for a centrally mediated amplitude regulation disorder," *Movement Disorders*, vol. 20, no. 1, pp. 40–50, 2005.

[19] W. R. Gibb and A. J. Lees, "The relevance of the lewy body to the pathogenesis of idiopathic Parkinson's disease," *Journal of Neurology, Neurosurgery, and Psychiatry*, vol. 51, no. 6, pp. 745–752, 1998.

[20] M. Wallén, E. Franzen, H. Nero, and M. Hagströmer, "Levels and patterns of physical activity and sedentary behavior in elderly people with mild to moderate Parkinson disease," *Physical Therapy*, vol. 95, no. 8, pp. 1135–1141, 2015.

[21] H. Nero, M. B. Wallén, E. Franzén, A. Ståhle, and M. Hagströmer, "Accelerometer cut points for physical activity assessment of older adults with Parkinson's disease," *PLoS One*, vol. 10, no. 9, Article ID e0135899, 2015.

[22] C. Christiansen, C. Moore, M. Schenkman et al., "Factors associated with ambulatory activity in de Novo Parkinson's disease," *Journal of Neurologic Physical Therapy*, vol. 41, no. 2, pp. 93–100, 2017.

[23] R. Troiano, J. J. McClain, R. Brychta, and K. Y. Chen, "Evolution of accelerometer methods for physical activity research," *British Journal of Sports Medicine*, vol. 48, no. 13, pp. 1019–1023, 2014.

[24] A. V. Rowlands, T. S. Olds, M. Hillsdon et al., "Assessing sedentary behavior with the GENEActiv: introducing the sedentary sphere," *Medicine and Science in Sports and Exercise*, vol. 46, no. 6, pp. 1235–1247, 2014.

[25] J. A. Schrack, R. Cooper, A. Koster et al., "Assessing daily physical activity in older adults: unraveling the complexity of monitors, measures, and methods," *Journals of Gerontology, Series A: Biological Sciences and Medical Sciences*, vol. 71, no. 8, pp. 1039–1048, 2016.

[26] M. Hildebrand, V. T. van Hees, B. H. Hansen, and U. Ekelund, "Age group comparability of raw accelerometer output from wrist- and hip-worn monitors," *Medicine and Science in Sports and Exercise*, vol. 46, no. 9, pp. 1816–1824, 2014.

[27] R. B. Davis, S. Ounpuu, D. Tyburki, and J. R. Gage, "A gait analysis data collection and reduction technique," *Human Movement Science*, vol. 10, no. 5, pp. 575–587, 1991.

[28] R. Baker, J. L. McGinley, M. H. Schwartz et al., "The gait profile score and movement analysis profile," *Gait and Posture*, vol. 30, no. 3, pp. 265–269, 2009.

[29] D. D. Speciali, J. C. F. Corrêa, N. M. Luna et al., "Validation of GDI, GPS and GVS for use in Parkinson's disease through evaluation of effects of subthalamic deep brain stimulation and levodopa," *Gait and Posture*, vol. 39, no. 4, pp. 1142–1145, 2014.

[30] F. Corona, M. Pau, M. Guicciardi, M. Murgia, R. Pili, and C. Casula, "Quantitative assessment of gait in elderly people affected by Parkinson's disease," in *Proceedings of IEEE International Symposium on Medical Measurements and Applications (MeMeA)*, Benevento, Italy, May 2016.

[31] M. P. Ford, L. A. Malone, H. C. Walker, I. Nyikos, R. Yelisetty, and C. S. Bickel, "Step activity in persons with Parkinson's disease," *Journal of Physical Activity and Health*, vol. 7, no. 6, pp. 724–729, 2010.

[32] J. T. Cavanaugh, T. D. Ellis, G. M. Earhart, M. P. Ford, K. B. Foreman, and L. E. Dibble, "Capturing ambulatory

activity decline in Parkinson's disease," *Journal of Neurologic Physical Therapy*, vol. 36, no. 2, pp. 51–57, 2012.

[33] C. Sartini, S. G. Wannamethee, S. Iliffe et al., "Diurnal patterns of objectively measured physical activity and sedentary behaviour in older men," *BMC Public Health*, vol. 15, no. 1, p. 609, 2015.

[34] G. Valenti, A. G. Bonomi, and K. R. Westerterp, "Diurnal patterns of physical activity in relation to activity induced energy expenditure in 52 to 83 year-old adults," *PLoS One*, vol. 11, no. 12, Article ID e0167824, 2016.

[35] P. DeVita and T. Hortobagyi, "Age causes a redistribution of joint torques and powers during gait," *Journal of Applied Physiology*, vol. 88, no. 5, pp. 1804–1811, 2000.

[36] J. Verghese, R. Holtzer, R. B. Lipton, and C. Wang, "Quantitative gait markers and incident fall risk in older adults," *The Journals of Gerontology, Series A: Biological Sciences and Medical Sciences*, vol. 64, no. 8, pp. 896–901, 2009.

[37] M. Pau, B. Leban, G. Collu, and G. M. Migliaccio, "Effect of light and vigorous physical activity on balance and gait of older adults," *Archives of Gerontology and Geriatrics*, vol. 59, no. 3, pp. 568–573, 2014.

[38] M. Pau, F. Corona, R. Pili et al., "Effects of physical rehabilitation integrated with rhythmic auditory stimulation on spatio-temporal and kinematic parameters of gait in Parkinson's disease," *Frontiers in Neurology*, vol. 7, p. 126, 2016.

[39] C. Tudor-Locke and D. A. Rowe, "Using cadence to study free-living ambulatory behaviour," *Sports Medicine*, vol. 42, no. 5, pp. 381–398, 2012.

[40] M. Morris, R. Iansek, T. Matyas, and J. Summers, "Abnormalities in the stride length-cadence relation in Parkinsonian gait," *Movement Disorders*, vol. 13, no. 1, pp. 61–69, 1998.

[41] L. M. Inkster, J. J. Eng, D. L. MacIntyre, and A. J. Stoessl, "Leg muscle strength is reduced in Parkinson's disease and relates to the ability to rise from a chair," *Movement Disorders*, vol. 18, no. 2, pp. 157–162, 2003.

[42] E. D. Borges, M. S. Silva, M. Bottaro, R. M. Lima, N. Allam, and R. J. de Oliveira, "Isokinetic muscle strength of knee extensors in individuals with Parkinson's disease," *Fisioterapia em Movimento*, vol. 26, no. 4, pp. 803–811, 2013.

[43] J. R. Nocera, T. Buckley, D. Waddell, M. S. Okun, and C. J. Hass, "knee extensor strength, dynamic stability, and functional ambulation: are they related in Parkinson's disease?," *Archives of Physical Medicine and Rehabilitation*, vol. 91, no. 4, pp. 589–595, 2010.

[44] R. D. Remington, H. L. Taylor, and E. R. Buskirk, "A method for assessing volunteer bias and its application to a cardiovascular disease prevention programme involving physical activity," *Journal of Epidemiology and Community Health*, vol. 32, no. 4, pp. 250–255, 1978.

[45] M. Ganguli, M. E. Lytle, M. D. Reynolds, and H. H. Dodge, "Random versus volunteer selection for a community-based study," *Journal of Gerontology series A Biological Sciences and Medical Sciences*, vol. 53, no. 1, pp. M39–M46, 1998.

Predictors of Functional and Quality of Life Outcomes following Deep Brain Stimulation Surgery in Parkinson's Disease Patients: Disease, Patient, and Surgical Factors

Hesham Abboud,[1,2,3] Gencer Genc,[1] Nicolas R. Thompson,[4,5] Srivadee Oravivattanakul,[1] Faisal Alsallom,[2] Dennys Reyes,[6] Kathy Wilson,[1] Russell Cerejo,[1] Xin Xin Yu,[1] Darlene Floden,[1] Anwar Ahmed,[1] Michal Gostkowski,[1] Ayman Ezzeldin,[3] Hazem Marouf,[3] Ossama Y. Mansour,[3] Andre Machado,[1] and Hubert H. Fernandez[1]

[1]Center for Neurological Restoration, Cleveland Clinic, 9500 Euclid Avenue, Mail Code U2, Cleveland, OH 44195, USA
[2]Case Western Reserve University, University Hospitals of Cleveland, 11100 Euclid Avenue, Cleveland, OH 44106, USA
[3]Department of Neurology, Alexandria University, El Hadara University Hospital, El Hadara Kebly, Alexandria, Egypt
[4]Department of Quantitative Health Sciences, Cleveland Clinic, 9500 Euclid Avenue, Mail Code JJN3-01, Cleveland, OH 44195, USA
[5]Neurological Institute, Center for Outcomes Research and Evaluation, Cleveland Clinic, 9500 Euclid Avenue, Cleveland, OH 44195, USA
[6]Department of Neurology, Cleveland Clinic Florida, 2950 Cleveland Clinic Blvd, Fl 3, Weston, FL 33331, USA

Correspondence should be addressed to Hesham Abboud; hesham.abboud@uhhospitals.org

Academic Editor: Jan Aasly

Objective. The primary objective was to evaluate predictors of quality of life (QOL) and functional outcomes following deep brain stimulation (DBS) in Parkinson's disease (PD) patients. The secondary objective was to identify predictors of global improvement. *Methods.* PD patients who underwent DBS at our Center from 2006 to 2011 were evaluated by chart review and email/phone survey. Postoperative UPDRS II and EQ-5D were analyzed using simple linear regression adjusting for preoperative score. For global outcomes, we utilized the Patient Global Impression of Change Scale (PGIS) and the Clinician Global Impression of Change Scale (CGIS). *Results.* There were 130 patients in the dataset. Preoperative and postoperative UPDRS II and EQ-5D were available for 45 patients, PGIS for 67 patients, and CGIS for 116 patients. Patients with falls/postural instability had 6-month functional scores and 1-year QOL scores that were significantly worse than patients without falls/postural instability. For every 1-point increase in preoperative UPDRS III and for every 1-unit increase in body mass index (BMI), the 6-month functional scores significantly worsened. Patients with tremors, without dyskinesia, and without gait-freezing were more likely to have "much" or "very much" improved CGIS. *Conclusions.* Presence of postural instability, high BMI, and worse baseline motor scores were the greatest predictors of poorer functional and QOL outcomes after DBS.

1. Introduction

Although deep brain stimulation surgery (DBS) has been established as a superior treatment option for advanced Parkinson's disease (PD) [1], there has been a discrepancy between motor and functional/quality of life (QOL) outcomes after surgery [2, 3]. While motor outcomes are believed to improve significantly in the majority of patients following

DBS compared to medical therapy alone [2], QOL outcomes are not as consistent with only about 50% of patients showing some improvement in QOL after surgery [3]. This has led to a recent shift of focus in DBS research from motor outcomes to functional and QOL outcomes. In recent years, an increasing number of studies attempted to find new clinical predictors of these outcomes to complement or replace traditional motor predictors with the goal of ultimately translating into better selection of surgical candidates [4–7]. In addition to commonly studied factors such as age and disease duration, our group and others explored less conventional outcome predictors like socioeconomic status [8], mood and psychosocial factors [3, 9], and preoperative cognitive patterns [10]. In this study, we look at the effect of several disease, patient, and surgical factors on QOL, functional, and global measures.

2. Methods

We performed a retrospective review of consecutive PD patients who underwent DBS implantation (subthalamic or internal globus pallidus) at our center from 2006 to 2011 and had near-complete charting. We collected two health status measures (HSM), the European Quality of Life 5-Dimension Questionnaire (EQ-5D) and the Unified Parkinson's Disease Rating Scale, part 2: activities of daily living (UPDRS II) [the Movement Disorders Society-Unified Parkinson's Disease Rating Scale or MDS-UPDRS II was used for visits after 2008], for the following time points when available: latest preoperatively (within one month prior to surgery), 6 months postoperatively (range: 3–9 months), and 12 months postoperatively (range: 9–15 months). The EQ-5D is a standardized instrument for measuring health-related QOL in terms of five dimensions (5D), mobility, self-care, usual activities, pain/discomfort, and anxiety/depression, producing a single index value for overall health status. In addition, we also conducted a one-item Patient Global Impression of Change Scale (PGIS) via phone/email survey using an IRB-approved phone/email script for all study subjects to provide additional long-term global outcome specific for this study. The PGIS aims at determining the patient's global impression of his/her current state compared to the state prior to DBS surgery with the following possible answers: very much improved, much improved, minimally improved, no change, minimally worse, much worse, or very much worse. The PGIS survey was distributed in mid-2011 (1 to 5 years from date of first surgery). To match our patient-perceived outcomes to clinicians' perception of overall outcome after surgery, we also conducted a one-item Clinician's Global Impression of Change Scale (CGIS) survey for study subjects. The CGIS aims at determining the clinician's impression of the overall clinical change in each patient after surgery using the same 7-point anchor as the PGIS. The CGIS scores were retrospectively determined based on the full information derived from patients' medical records and postoperative office visits during the same time periods when the PGIS was obtained.

The following potential clinical predictors were collected for all patients from their preoperative visits and operative reports:

(i) Disease factors: disease duration, dopaminergic burden (based on levodopa equivalent daily dose [LEDD] conversion), preoperative UPDRS part III motor subscale (MDS-UPDRS part III after 2008) in the ON state, presence of tremors, dyskinesia, freezing of gait (FOG), and falls/balance dysfunction. Clinical symptoms were based on the patients' major complaints when presenting for DBS evaluation. Although these complaints were matched to their UPDRS III/MDS-UPDRS III subscores on exam, no formal score cutoffs were used for quantification. This was based, in part, on the difficulty of developing unified cutoff scores for the two different versions of the motor scale. More importantly, since this study was geared towards patients' experience, we meant to put more emphasis on patient-reported symptoms rather than motor subscores as potential predictors of QOL and functional outcomes

(ii) Patient factors: age, marital status, and body mass index (BMI)

(iii) Surgical factors: surgery type (i.e., unilateral, staged bilateral, or simultaneous bilateral) and number of intraoperative microelectrode passes

2.1. Statistical Analysis. To determine short-term and intermediate predictors of improved functional state and QOL, we created simple linear regression models where the 6-month and 12-month postoperative UPDRS II/MDS-UPDRS II score or EQ-5D index was the dependent variable. For each of these models, we adjusted for the preoperative score by including it in the model as a covariate. For each of the clinical predictors listed in Methods, we created a separate model where that predictor was the independent variable. The effect of each predictor on outcome is provided through estimated beta coefficients and associated 95% confidence intervals. Patients with missing data for certain time point were not included in the analysis for that time point.

To determine predictors of global outcomes based on patient's and clinician's perceptions, we dichotomized the responses in the PGIS and CGIS into "much improved" or "very much improved" versus all other responses. For categorical predictors, we computed the proportion and percent of patients with PGIS or CGIS of "much improved" or "very much improved." Fisher's exact tests were used to determine statistical significance. For continuous predictors, we created logistic regression models. We estimated odds ratios and computed 95% confidence intervals for each. Due to the exploratory nature of this study, we did not correct for multiple comparisons.

All analyses were conducted using R, version 3.0.1, and P values less than 0.05 were considered statistically significant. This study was approved by Cleveland Clinic's institutional review board.

3. Results

3.1. Predictors of Functional and QOL Outcomes. There were 130 patients in the dataset. Overall, patients had an average age at time of surgery of 63.0 (±9.1) years, had PD for 10.7 (±5.1) years, had an average BMI of 27.5 (±5.2) kg/m^2, and had an average LEDD of 1190 (±666). The cohort was more predominantly male (70.8%), white (86.9%), and married (66.9%). Of the 130 patients, 55 (42.3%) had unilateral surgery, 50 (38.4%) had bilateral staged surgery, and 25 (19.2%) had bilateral unstaged surgery. Most patients were implanted in the STN, 124 (95.3%).

TABLE 1: Beta estimates for health status measures collected at 2 follow-ups.

			6 months postop.			1 year postop.	
		N	Estimate (95% CI)	P value	N	Estimate (95% CI)	P value
UPDRS II	Age	39	−0.05 (−0.34, 0.23)	0.7058	32	0.03 (−0.3, 0.36)	0.8438
	Disease duration	38	−0.45 (−1.00, 0.11)	0.1127	31	0.21 (−0.56, 0.97)	0.5859
	BMI	37	0.49 (0.04, 0.94)	**0.0332**	32	0.68 (−0.002, 1.37)	0.0507
	Laterality (versus unilateral)						
	Staged bilateral	39	1.16 (−4.58, 6.89)	0.6849	32	0.53 (−6.75, 7.82)	0.8819
	Simultaneous bilateral	39	−3.68 (−12.69, 5.32)	0.4118	32	−5.46 (−14.34, 3.42)	0.2179
	Electrode passes (right)	29	2.09 (−0.41, 4.60)	0.0978	24	1.96 (−1.77, 5.69)	0.2876
	Electrode passes (left)	35	−1.21 (−4.29, 1.87)	0.4300	30	−2.18 (−6.14, 1.78)	0.2681
	Electrode passes (total)	36	0.31 (−1.15, 1.76)	0.6731	30	0.00 (−1.96, 1.97)	0.9963
	% equivalent levodopa dose	37	1.83 (−3.93, 7.58)	0.5233	30	0.89 (−6.15, 7.94)	0.7967
	On UPDRS III	39	0.09 (−0.21, 0.38)	0.5535	31	0.22 (−0.10, 0.54)	0.1709
	Tremor	39	−0.95 (−5.78, 3.88)	0.6909	32	1.35 (−4.41, 7.12)	0.6345
	Dyskinesia	39	−2.46 (−7.28, 2.36)	0.3072	32	−2.06 (−7.86, 3.74)	0.4736
	Freezing	39	2.32 (−2.97, 7.62)	0.3792	32	3.85 (−2.55, 10.26)	0.2284
	Falls/balance	39	6.48 (1.11, 11.84)	**0.0193**	32	6.45 (−0.38, 13.28)	0.0634
	Marital status	38	−1.86 (−7.35, 3.63)	0.4958	31	2.74 (−3.88, 9.36)	0.4041
EQ-5D index	Age	45	0.00 (−0.01, 0.00)	0.3403	36	0.00 (−0.01, 0.01)	0.9897
	Disease duration	43	0.01 (0.00, 0.02)	0.1810	35	−0.01 (−0.02, 0.00)	0.0696
	BMI	45	0.001 (−0.009, 0.011)	0.8450	36	−0.002 (−0.014, 0.011)	0.7983
	Laterality (versus unilateral)						
	Staged bilateral	44	0.08 (−0.02, 0.19)	0.1252	36	−0.01 (−0.14, 0.12)	0.9127
	Simultaneous bilateral	44	0.13 (−0.04, 0.29)	0.1351	36	0.003 (−0.15, 0.16)	0.9654
	Electrode passes (right)	33	−0.02 (−0.06, 0.02)	0.3494	28	−0.03 (−0.09, 0.04)	0.3837
	Electrode passes (left)	38	0.04 (−0.02, 0.11)	0.2006	32	0.07 (0.00, 0.14)	0.0508
	Electrode passes (total)	41	0.02 (−0.01, 0.05)	0.2458	34	0.01 (−0.03, 0.04)	0.6988
	Equivalent levodopa dose	42	−0.07 (−0.19, 0.04)	0.2000	34	0.06 (−0.06, 0.19)	0.3138
	On UPDRS III	44	−0.01 (−0.01, 0.00)	**0.0050**	35	0.00 (−0.01, 0.00)	0.6310
	Tremor	44	0.03 (−0.07, 0.13)	0.5516	36	0.07 (−0.03, 0.17)	0.1602
	Dyskinesia	44	−0.01 (−0.11, 0.09)	0.8448	36	0.02 (−0.09, 0.12)	0.7197
	Freezing	44	−0.03 (−0.13, 0.08)	0.5955	36	−0.09 (−0.19, 0.01)	0.0762
	Falls/balance	44	−0.06 (−0.17, 0.05)	0.269	36	−0.12 (−0.23, −0.02)	**0.0191**
	Marital status	44	−0.04 (−0.15, 0.08)	0.4992	35	−0.04 (−0.16, 0.07)	0.4668

Forty-five patients had both preoperative and postoperative data at 6 months and at 12 months. This group had mostly similar characteristics to the group with incomplete data except for having a younger average age (60.4 years, P = 0.019). Of these 45 patients, 29 patients (64.4%) had bilateral surgery. At 6 months, statistically significant improvement was seen for both the mean EQ-5D index (P = 0.03) and the average UPDRS II/MDS-UPDRS II score (P = 0.002). However, one year after surgery, no significant improvement or worsening was found for either scale.

There were 116 patients for which the CGIS could be completed from the available records. Of these, 19 (16.4%) were rated as "very much improved," 63 (54.3%) as "much improved," 23 (19.8%) as "minimally improved," 6 (5.2%) as "no change," 3 (2.6%) as "minimally worsened," and 2 (1.7%) as "much worsened."

There were 67 patients that completed the PGIS. Of these 67 patients, 29 (43.3%) reported "very much improved,"

25 (37.3%) reported "much improved," 10 (14.9%) reported "minimally improved," 2 (3.0%) reported "much worse," and 1 (1.5%) reported "very much worse."

Table 1 displays results of the simple linear regression models relating different predictors to approximate 6-month and 1-year HSM. Patients that had falls/balance-dysfunction had 6-month mean UPDRS II/MDS-UPDRS II scores that were 6.48 points worse than patients that did not have falls/balance-dysfunction (P = 0.019). A similar estimated effect of falls/balance-dysfunction was found at the 1-year UPDRS II/MDS-UPDRS II scores, but statistical significance was not achieved (Estimated effect = 6.45; P = 0.0634). Similarly, patients that had falls/balance dysfunction at baseline had 1-year mean EQ-5D index scores that were 0.12 points lower than patients who did not have falls/balance dysfunction (P = 0.019) but this effect was not significant at 6 months (P = 0.2690). After adjusting for preoperative EQ-5D index, for every one-point increase in the preoperative

TABLE 2: Patient Global Impression of Change Scale (PGIS) and Clinician's Global Impression of Change Scale (CGIS) results by various categorical predictors.

	% PGIS much improved or very much improved (proportion)	P value	% CGIS much improved or very much improved (proportion)	P value
Tremor	76.9% (20/26)	0.7566	84.0% (42/50)	**0.0075**
No tremor	82.1% (32/39)		60.0% (42/70)	
Dyskinesia	83.7% (36/43)	0.5167	64.2% (52/81)	**0.0380**
No dyskinesia	75.0% (18/24)		83.7% (36/43)	
Freezing	78.8% (26/33)	0.7591	61.9% (39/63)	**0.0315**
No freezing	82.4% (28/34)		80.3% (49/61)	
Falls/balance	75.0% (21/28)	0.3688	66.1% (41/62)	0.3218
No falls/balance	84.6% (33/39)		75.8% (47/62)	
Left unilateral	75.0% (6/8)	1.0000	63.6% (7/11)	1.0000
Right unilateral	77.8% (14/18)		67.6% (23/34)	
Unilateral	76.9% (20/26)		66.7% (30/45)	
Two-stage bilateral	81.5% (22/27)	0.7906	73.1% (38/52)	0.7741
Unstaged bilateral	85.7% (12/14)		73.1% (19/26)	

UPDRS III/MDS-UPDRS III score in the ON state, the 6-month EQ-5D index worsened by 0.01 units ($P = 0.005$). However, no relationship between UPDRS III/MDS-UPDRS III score in the ON state and the EQ-5D index was seen at 1 year. Moreover, no relationship was found between the UPDRS III/MDS-UPDRS III and the UPDRS II/MDS-UPDRS II scores at either 6 months or 1 year.

The BMI distribution in the patient group was as follows: underweight, 0 patients; normal weight, 12 patients; overweight, 16 patients; and obese, 15 patients. After excluding 2 outliers, the estimated effect of BMI on 6-month UPDRS II/MDS-UPDRS II score was significant ($P = 0.033$). For every one-unit increase in BMI, the UPDRS II/MDS-UPDRS II score at 6 months worsened by 0.49 points on average. There was also evidence of a similar but weaker association at 1 year ($P = 0.0507$). However, at both six months and one year after surgery, no significant associations were found between BMI and EQ-5D index.

3.2. Predictors of Global Outcomes. Table 2 displays the results relating categorical predictors to the PGIS and CGIS. While the majority of the patients in our cohort were rated to be "very much" or "much" improved in the PGIS and CGIS, of patients that had tremor, 84.0% showed "much" or "very much" improvement on the CGIS, whereas only 60.0% of patients without tremor showed "much" or "very much" improvement ($P = 0.0075$). Patients without dyskinesia and patients without freezing were more likely to show "much" or "very much" improvement on the CGIS ($P = 0.038$ and $P = 0.0315$, resp.). There were no statistically significant results when correlating continuous predictors to the CGIS and the PGIS. There was also no correlation between global outcomes and the cognitive and mood predictors included in our previously reported cognitive study [10].

3.3. Noninfluential Factors. There was no significant association between QOL, functional, or global outcomes and

patients' age, disease duration, laterality of surgery (unilateral versus bilateral), number of intraoperative electrode passes, LEDD, or marital status. However, some interesting trends were observed including a trend between shorter disease duration and more improvement in EQ-5D index at 1 year ($P = 0.0696$) and a PGIS of "much" or "very much improvement" ($P = 0.0683$). There was also a trend between higher number of intraoperative microelectrode passes on the left and less improvement of EQ-5D index at 1 year ($P = 0.0508$).

4. Discussion

In this study, we looked at predictors of functional and QOL outcomes of DBS in a cohort of PD patients who underwent DBS under a standardized protocol. We explored a large number of potential predictors including several disease, patient, and surgical factors. We have previously reported the socioeconomic and cognitive data of the same cohort [8, 10]. In the current study, we found that the baseline presence of falls/balance dysfunction was associated with worse 6-month functional outcome after DBS with a trend towards a similar poor outcome at 1 year after surgery. Falls/balance dysfunction were also predictive of poor QOL outcome at 1 year. In addition, the presence of FOG and absence of tremors, other indicators of predominantly axial disease, predicted poorer CGIS. These relationships are in agreement with findings by Welter and colleagues who reported poor functional outcomes 6 months after surgery in patients with axial motor symptoms preoperatively [4]. On the same note, Maier and colleagues reported an association between higher axial motor score and worse subjective perceived outcome after DBS [11]. Patients with predominantly axial disease are known to attain less motoric benefit from DBS [12] and our results suggest that this might extend into functional, QOL, and global outcomes after surgery.

The presence of dyskinesia preoperatively was associated with somewhat poorer long-term global outcome in our study as represented by the CGIS. In 2011, Daniels and colleagues reported similar findings showing that patients with lower preoperative dyskinesia scores did better on QOL measures after surgery as represented by the Parkinson's Disease Questionnaire-39 (PD-Q39) and the 36-Item Short Form Health Survey (SF-36) [5]. Although the presence of dyskinesia is considered a classical indication for DBS and patients often experience reduction of dyskinesia after surgery especially when the dose of levodopa is successfully reduced [13], this does not necessarily translate into improvement in QOL or global perceivable outcome [5]. It is well known that, in many occasions, dyskinesia is more bothersome to patients' families than the patients themselves and is not detrimental to the QOL of PD patients [14]; in addition, the loss of levodopa peak-dose euphoria after dose reduction postoperatively may explain why patients with preoperative dyskinesia report less improvement in QOL after surgery when their dyskinesia improves as suggested by Daniels and colleagues [5]. Other possible explanations include the fact that the presence of dyskinesia, in general, indicates more advanced disease and that some patients may rarely experience worsening dyskinesia with stimulation [15].

Our results agreed with both Welter's and Daniels' studies in confirming a role for preoperative UPDRS III motor score in predicting functional/QOL outcomes following DBS, with higher scores indicating worse outcomes, perhaps as a general indication of more advanced disease [4, 5]. Soulas and colleagues confirmed the finding by Welter which demonstrates that age and disease duration are predictors of poorer outcome after surgery [6], but these factors were noninfluential in our study, although longer disease duration showed a weak trend towards poorer EQ-5D and PGIS in our group. In a study by Floden and colleagues from our group utilizing a different QOL scale (PDQ-39), preoperative episodic memory, depression, and bilateral surgery were the most influential predictors [3]. Table 3 displays a summary of the studies that looked at predictors of functional, QOL, and global DBS outcomes since the early 2000s.

In addition to disease characteristics, our study suggests that certain patient characteristics, regardless of disease severity, may also influence functional and QOL outcomes after DBS. In addition to the impact of socioeconomic status, which we previously reported [8], BMI seems to have a similar effect on DBS outcomes. Higher preoperative BMI predicted worse functional outcomes at 6 months and, to a lesser extent, at 1 year after surgery. This finding could be another reflection of poorer socioeconomic status where obesity is more prevalent [16] but it may also be related to further weight gain incurred after surgery. Weight gain after DBS has been frequently reported in literature and is thought to be secondary to reduction in the metabolic rate after resolution of tremor/dyskinesia and/or a direct stimulation effect on appetite centers [17–20]. Adding more weight after DBS in patients who are already overweight or obese can translate into patient perception of a suboptimal functional outcome. A post hoc analysis of our patient group revealed that the BMI increased in 55% of the patients at 1 year after surgery with an increment higher than $1 \, \text{kg/m}^2$ in 35% and higher than $2 \, \text{kg/m}^2$ in 17%. In a recent study, preoperative obesity

was associated with poor axial and cognitive outcomes after DBS [21] but our study is the first to test the effect of BMI on functional and QOL outcomes. This is an important area that warrants further study. Exploring the role of dieting and/or exercise prior to DBS on motor and nonmotor outcomes may be of value.

There are several limitations to our study. In addition to the retrospective nature of the study, the sample size was fairly small for the number of comparisons and the study may have been underpowered, especially for the functional and QOL outcomes. Nonetheless, the demographic features of the subset of patients with complete data versus the entire cohort showed largely similar demographics; therefore, we believe that this subset still represented the PD population who underwent DBS surgery. The slight difference in age between the two groups is probably attributed to the fact that younger patients are more familiar with technology and therefore more likely to complete computer-based surveys and assessment scales. Further studies utilizing larger patient cohorts are needed to better study predictors of functional and QOL outcomes following DBS. We did not look into other QOL measures that are more specific for PD such as the PDQ-39 due to limited availability of data in this cohort; however, PDQ-39 data were available in a more recent patient cohort and were recently published by our group in a separate paper as discussed earlier [3]. Also we did not study functional/QOL outcomes beyond 1 year after surgery which, although consistent with other similar studies, does not account for how the benefit from surgery holds up against disease progression over the years. The absence of statistically significant difference in QOL and functional scores one year after surgery compared to preoperative scores was inconsistent with the results of previous DBS randomized trials [22]. However, the majority of our patients rated their overall global outcome as much or very much improved on the PGIS survey that was distributed to the patients 1 to 5 years after the date of surgery. This indicates that DBS still exerted a very positive impact on patients' global outcome many years after surgery even if not reflected on the EQ-5D and UPDRS II scores. In addition, there was also no significant worsening of the QOL and functional scores one year after surgery despite the progressive nature of the disease. This means that DBS still had a relative positive impact on QOL and functional outcomes one year after surgery in this real-life patient cohort though understandably less pronounced than what was seen in the more carefully selected cohorts in randomized trials. Although the CGIS was completed for most of the patients, the scoring was done retrospectively by our investigators exploiting data from patients' charts. The scoring system relied on documentation made by the first-hand clinicians, a method that has not been validated in other studies. The effect on caregiver burden was also not addressed. Finally, we did not correct for multiple comparisons due to the exploratory nature of the study and since we were looking at predetermined predictors prior to data collection [23]. Still, the relatively large number of comparisons in absence of such correction may have confounded the results to some degree; therefore the results of our study should be interpreted with caution in view of the limitations related to sample size

TABLE 3: Studies of functional, QOL, and global impression outcomes after DBS in PD.

Study	Functional, QOL, or global impression scale	Significant predictors	Number of patients	Time lapse since surgery
Welter et al., 2002	UPDRS II	(i) Age (ii) Disease duration (iii) UPDRS III (iv) Axial motor score (v) LED	41	6 months
Daniels et al., 2011	PD-Q39 SF-36	(i) Daily off time (+ve) (ii) Lower dyskinesia score (+ve) (iii) Improvement in UPDRS III (+ve) (iv) Improvement in psychiatric scales (+ve) (v) Reduction of dyskinesia (−ve)	61	6 months
Soulas et al., 2011	PD-Q39 SF-36	(i) Age (ii) Disease duration (iii) Depression (iv) Less use of social support coping	41	6 months and 12 months
Smeding et al., 2011	PDQL	(i) L-dopa response at baseline (+ve)	105	12 months
Maier et al., 2013	Subjective perceived outcome	(i) Depression (ii) Apathy	30	3 months
Floden et al., 2014	PD-Q39	(i) Depression (ii) Single-trial learning (episodic memory) (iii) Preoperative PD-Q39 score (iv) Bilateral surgery (+ve)	85	8 months (average)
Genc et al., 2016	MDS-UPDRS II EQ-5D CGIS	(i) Household median income	125 (43 for MDS-UPDRS II and EQ-5D)	6 months and 12 months
Maier et al., 2016	Subjective perceived outcome	(i) Apathy (ii) Axial motor score	28	12 months
Abboud et al.	MDS-UPDRS II EQ-5D PGIS CGIS	(i) Falls/balance dysfunction (ii) Dyskinesia (iii) Absence of tremors (iv) Freezing (v) UPDRS III (vi) Preoperative BMI	130 (45 FOR MDS-UPDRS II and EQ-5D)	6 months and 12 months

UPDRS II: Unified Parkinson's Disease Rating Scale, part 2: activities of daily living; LED: L-dopa equivalent dose; PD-Q39: Parkinson's Disease Questionnaire-39; SF-36: 36-Item Short Form Health Survey; PDQL: Parkinson's Disease Quality of Life Questionnaire; MDS-UPDRS II: Movement Disorders Society-Unified Parkinson's Disease Rating Scale, part 2: motor experience of daily living; EQ-5D: European Quality of Life 5-dimension Questionnaire; CGIS: Clinician's Global Impression of Change Scale; PGIS: Patient Global Impression of Change Scale.

and methodology. Overall, the majority of the significant predictors in our study conform to prior DBS literature which increases the confidence in those results. Our novel significant predictors like BMI will need validation in other cohorts.

In conclusion, our study suggests that certain disease characteristics may influence outcomes after DBS. While the majority of the patients in our cohort were globally rated as significantly improved on global scales, falls and balance dysfunction, absence of tremors, presence of dyskinesia, freezing of gait, and preoperative motor severity as represented by UPDRS III/MDS-UPDRS III were the most influential predictors of poorer outcome. In addition, some previously underrecognized patient characteristics may also influence DBS outcomes such as higher preoperative BMI and lower socioeconomic status. By confirming known DBS outcome predictors and identifying new factors, we hope to provide new insights into the process of patient selection and risk stratification prior to DBS. Further prospective studies utilizing higher number of patients and combining both objective and subjective outcome measures should be performed to confirm or refute the results of our study.

Disclosure

This study was presented as an abstract at the 2015 International Parkinson's and Movement Disorders Congress and at the 2016 American Academy of Neurology Annual Meeting.

Conflicts of Interest

Gencer Genc, Nicolas R. Thompson, Srivadee Oravivat-tanakul, Faisal Alsallom, Dennys Reyes, Kathy Wilson, Russell Cerejo, Xin Xin Yu, Darlene Floden, Ayman Ezzeldin, Hazem Marouf, Ossama Y. Mansour, Anwar Ahmed, and Michal Gostkowski report no conflicts of interest. Dr. Hesham Abboud is a consultant for Biogen, Genentech, and Genzyme. Dr. Andre Machado received personal compensation from IntElect Medical/Boston Scientific, ATI, Cardionomics, and Monteris for consulting services and is a consultant for Functional Neuromodulation, Spinal Modulation, and Icahn. He holds distribution rights from intellectual property in ATI, Cardionomic, and Enspire; fellowship support from Medtronic; and research funding from the National Institutes of Health. Dr. Hubert H. Fernandez has received honoraria from Advanced Health Media, Cleveland Clinic CME, Medical Communications Media, Movement Disorders Society, and Vindico Medical Education, as a speaker in CME events. Hubert H. Fernandez has received honoraria from Ipsen, Merz Pharmaceuticals, Pfizer, Teva Neuroscience, and Zambon Pharmaceuticals, as a speaker and/or consultant. Hubert H. Fernandez has received personal compensation for serving as Co-Medical Editor of the Movement Disorders Society Website. Hubert H. Fernandez has received royalty payments from Demos Publishing and Manson Ltd. for serving as a book author/editor. Hubert H. Fernandez has received research support from Abbott, Acadia, Biotie Therapies, EMD Serono, Huntington Study Group, Merck, Michael J. Fox Foundation, Movement Disorders Society, National Parkinson Foundation, NIH/NINDS, Novartis, Parkinson Study Group, Synosia, and Teva but has no owner interest in any pharmaceutical company.

Authors' Contributions

Dr. Hesham Abboud was responsible for conception and design of the study, acquisition of data, interpretation of data, literature search, writing of the first draft, and revising the manuscript. Dr. Gencer Genc was responsible for acquisition of data, interpretation of data, literature search, and reviewing/revising the manuscript. Mr. Nicolas R. Thompson performed the statistical analysis and contributed to writing of the statistical methods and results. Drs. Srivadee Oravivattanakul, Faisal Alsallom, and Xin Xin Yu were responsible for acquisition and interpretation of data. Drs Dennys Reyes, Russell Cerejo, and Kathy Wilson designed the body mass index analysis and analyzed and interpreted the data. Drs. Darlene Floden, Michal Gostkowski, Anwar Ahmed, Ayman Ezzeldin, Hazem Marouf, Ossama Y. Mansour, and Andre Machado critiqued, reviewed, and revised the manuscript. Dr. Hubert H. Fernandez was responsible for the conception and design of the study and review, revision, and final approval of the manuscript. All persons who meet authorship criteria are listed as authors, and all authors certify that they have participated sufficiently in the work to take public responsibility for the content. Each author confirms that all authors have read the manuscript.

References

[1] J. M. Bronstein, M. Tagliati, R. L. Alterman et al., "Deep brain stimulation for Parkinson disease an expert consensus and review of key issues," *Archives of Neurology*, vol. 68, no. 2, pp. 165–171, 2011.

[2] J. A. Obeso, C. W. Olanow, M. C. Rodriguez-Oroz, P. Krack, R. Kumar, and A. E. Lang, "Deep-brain stimulation of the subthalamic nucleus or the pars interna of the globus pallidus in Parkinson's disease," *New England Journal of Medicine*, vol. 345, no. 13, pp. 956–963, 2001.

[3] D. Floden, S. E. Cooper, S. D. Griffith, and A. G. Machado, "Predicting quality of life outcomes after subthalamic nucleus deep brain stimulation," *Neurology*, vol. 83, no. 18, pp. 1627–1633, 2014.

[4] M. L. Welter, J. L. Houeto, S. Tezenas du Montcel et al., "Clinical predictive factors of subthalamic stimulation in Parkinson's disease," *Brain*, vol. 125, no. 3, pp. 575–583, 2002.

[5] C. Daniels, P. Krack, J. Volkmann et al., "Is improvement in the quality of life after subthalamic nucleus stimulation in Parkinson's disease predictable?" *Movement Disorders*, vol. 26, no. 14, pp. 2516–2521, 2011.

[6] T. Soulas, S. Sultan, J.-M. Gurruchaga, S. Palfi, and G. Fnelon, "Depression and coping as predictors of change after deep brain stimulation in Parkinson's disease," *World Neurosurgery*, vol. 75, no. 3-4, pp. 525–532, 2011.

[7] H. M. M. Smeding, J. D. Speelman, H. M. Huizenga, P. R. Schuurman, and B. Schmand, "Predictors of cognitive and psychosocial outcome after STN DBS in Parkinson's disease," *Journal of Neurology, Neurosurgery and Psychiatry*, vol. 82, no. 7, pp. 754–760, 2011.

[8] G. Genc, H. Abboud, S. Oravivattanakul et al., "Socioeconomic status may impact functional outcome of deep brain stimulation surgery in Parkinson's disease," *Neuromodulation*, vol. 19, no. 1, pp. 25–29, 2016.

[9] F. Maier, C. J. Lewis, N. Horstkoetter et al., "Patients' expectations of deep brain stimulation, and subjective perceived outcome related to clinical measures in Parkinson's disease: A mixed-method approach," *Journal of Neurology, Neurosurgery and Psychiatry*, vol. 84, no. 11, pp. 1273–1281, 2013.

[10] H. Abboud, D. Floden, N. R. Thompson et al., "Impact of mild cognitive impairment on outcome following deep brain stimulation surgery for Parkinson's disease," *Parkinsonism and Related Disorders*, vol. 21, no. 3, pp. 249–253, 2015.

[11] F. Maier, C. J. Lewis, N. Horstkoetter et al., "Subjective perceived outcome of subthalamic deep brain stimulation in Parkinson's disease one year after surgery," *Parkinsonism and Related Disorders*, vol. 24, pp. 41–47, 2016.

[12] A. Fasano, C. C. Aquino, J. K. Krauss, C. R. Honey, and B. R. Bloem, "Axial disability and deep brain stimulation in patients with Parkinson disease," *Nature Reviews Neurology*, vol. 11, no. 2, pp. 98–110, 2015.

[13] G. Oyama, K. D. Foote, C. E. Jacobson et al., "GPi and STN deep brain stimulation can suppress dyskinesia in Parkinson's disease," *Parkinsonism and Related Disorders*, vol. 18, no. 7, pp. 814–818, 2012.

[14] M. C. Hechtner, T. Vogt, Y. Zöllner et al., "Quality of life in Parkinson's disease patients with motor fluctuations and dyskinesias in five European countries," *Parkinsonism and Related Disorders*, vol. 20, no. 9, pp. 969–974, 2014.

[15] Z. Zheng, Y. Li, J. Li, Y. Zhang, X. Zhang, and P. Zhuang, "Stimulation-induced dyskinesia in the early stage after subthalamic deep brain stimulation," *Stereotactic and Functional Neurosurgery*, vol. 88, no. 1, pp. 29–34, 2010.

[16] A. W. Watts, S. M. Mason, K. Loth, N. Larson, and D. Neumark-Sztainer, "Socioeconomic differences in overweight and weight-related behaviors across adolescence and young adulthood: 10-year longitudinal findings from Project EAT," *Preventive Medicine*, vol. 87, pp. 194–199, 2016.

[17] K. A. Mills, R. Scherzer, P. A. Starr, and J. L. Ostrem, "Weight change after globus pallidus internus or subthalamic nucleus deep brain stimulation in Parkinson's disease and dystonia," *Stereotactic and Functional Neurosurgery*, vol. 90, no. 6, pp. 386–393, 2012.

[18] P. Sauleau, E. Leray, T. Rouaud et al., "Comparison of weight gain and energy intake after subthalamic versus pallidal stimulation in Parkinson's disease," *Movement Disorders*, vol. 24, no. 14, pp. 2149–2155, 2009.

[19] M. Barichella, A. M. Marczewska, C. Mariani, A. Landi, A. Vairo, and G. Pezzoli, "Body weight gain rate in patients with Parkinson's disease and deep brain stimulation," *Movement Disorders*, vol. 18, no. 11, pp. 1337–1340, 2003.

[20] E. Markaki, J. Ellul, Z. Kefalopoulou et al., "The role of ghrelin, neuropeptide y and leptin peptides in weight gain after deep brain stimulation for Parkinson's disease," *Stereotactic and Functional Neurosurgery*, vol. 90, no. 2, pp. 104–112, 2012.

[21] A. Rouillé, S. Derrey, R. Lefaucheur et al., "Pre-operative obesity may influence subthalamic stimulation outcome in Parkinson's disease," *Journal of the Neurological Sciences*, vol. 359, no. 1-2, pp. 260–265, 2015.

[22] A. Williams, S. Gill, T. Varma et al., "Deep brain stimulation plus best medical therapy versus best medical therapy alone for advanced Parkinson's disease (PD SURG trial): a randomised, open-label trial," *The Lancet Neurology*, vol. 9, no. 6, pp. 581–591, 2010.

[23] K. J. Rothman, "No adjustments are needed for multiple comparisons," *Epidemiology*, vol. 1, no. 1, pp. 43–46, 1990.

Should Skin Biopsies Be Performed in Patients Suspected of Having Parkinson's Disease?

Timo Siepmann,[1] Ana Isabel Penzlin,[2] Ben Min-Woo Illigens,[3] and Heinz Reichmann[1]

[1]*Department of Neurology, University Hospital Carl Gustav Carus, Technische Universitaet Dresden, Dresden, Germany*
[2]*Department of Neurology and Rehabilitation, Klinik Bavaria Kreischa, Kreischa, Germany*
[3]*Department of Neurology, Beth Israel Deaconess Medical Center, Harvard Medical School, Boston, MA, USA*

Correspondence should be addressed to Timo Siepmann; timo.siepmann@uniklinikum-dresden.de

Academic Editor: Hélio Teive

In patients with Parkinson's disease (PD), the molecularly misfolded form of α-synuclein was recently identified in cutaneous autonomic nerve fibers which displayed increased accumulation even in early disease stages. However, the underlying mechanisms of synucleinopathic nerve damage and its implication for brain pathology in later life remain to be elucidated. To date, specific diagnostic tools to evaluate small fiber pathology and to discriminate neurodegenerative proteinopathies are rare. Recently, research has indicated that deposition of α-synuclein in cutaneous nerve fibers quantified via immunohistochemistry in superficial skin biopsies might be a valid marker of PD which could facilitate early diagnosis and monitoring of disease progression. However, lack of standardization of techniques to quantify neural α-synuclein deposition limits their utility in clinical practice. Additional challenges include the identification of potential distinct morphological patterns of intraneural α-synuclein deposition among synucleinopathies to facilitate diagnostic discrimination and determining the degree to which structural damage relates to dysfunction of nerve fibers targeted by α-synuclein. Answering these questions might improve our understanding of the pathophysiological role of small fiber neuropathy in Parkinson's disease, help identify new treatment targets, and facilitate assessment of response to neuroprotective treatment.

1. Introduction

Clinical management of Parkinson's disease (PD) has undergone substantial innovations that comprise both diagnostic assessment and pharmacotherapy. However, the disease still poses a clinical challenge due its high prevalence and our restricted understanding of its underlying pathology. The latter explains why, to date, no causative treatment is available. Moreover, the range of tools to detect early and premotor pathology is limited. This may prevent timely initiation of dopaminergic treatment and thereby improvement of quality of life [1]. In order to provide individualized treatment, it is also important to differentiate PD from atypical Parkinsonism syndromes, a problem which is difficult to solve in clinical practice, particularly in early and prodromal disease stages. In an effort to address these challenges research has focused on identifying reliable disease markers. The molecularly misfolded form of the protein α-synuclein has

recently been identified in autonomic nerve fibers of the skin. In these small lightly myelinated and unmyelinated nerve fibers, α-synuclein deposits are present even in the early stages of PD as demonstrated by an analysis of skin biopsies immunohistochemically costained for α-synuclein and nerve fibers [2]. This technique has enabled, for the first time, assessment of synucleinopathic changes in the peripheral nervous system and has been reproduced or modified in several research studies in patients with PD [3–5]. However, the mechanisms whereby synucleinopathic nerve damage relates to central neurodegeneration in later life and how it might play a causative role in PD remain unknown.

Immunohistochemical detection of intraneural α-synuclein deposition in epidermal structures innervated by autonomic small fibers offers a novel tool to study pathology in PD and might provide a valid biomarker of PD as suggested by a number of well-designed experimental studies [2, 6, 7]. We reviewed the current literature on detection of α-synuclein in skin biopsies in order to approach the question whether this technique might be a useful supplement to other clinical diagnostic tests in patients with possible Parkinson's disease.

2. Synucleinopathic Small Fiber Neuropathy: What Do We Know?

The epidermal layer of the skin is innervated by small fibers, which comprise unmyelinated C-fibers and thinly myelinated A-delta fibers [8]. A structural analysis of cutaneous denervation in a population of PD patients has displayed a link between α-synuclein deposition in autonomic small fibers and severity of clinical symptoms related to autonomic dysregulation such as orthostatic hypotension or sweating disturbances, indicating the usefulness of skin pathology as potentially valid disease marker [2]. Additional analyses within the same cohort have shown that, in patients with PD, the amount of α-synuclein positive nerve fibers normalized to total intraepidermal nerve fiber density (α-synuclein ratio) is enhanced in both sympathetic cholinergic (sweat gland innervating) and sympathetic adrenergic (pilomotor muscle innervating) nerve fibers. Interestingly, higher α-synuclein ratios were also associated with higher severity of motor symptoms in this study. However, if and to what degree this positive correlation might point to a direct causative association between peripheral autonomic and central motor pathology remains unknown. An indirect indication toward such an association has been provided by the similar morphology of misfolded α-synuclein accumulation in cutaneous small fibers and in neurites in the substantia nigra. In both structures, α-synuclein staining showed an irregular line following the course of the neural structure (small fiber and neurite, resp.) [6].

Subsequent investigations have corroborated these observations and provided Class III evidence. An analysis of skin biopsies detected α-synuclein aggregation in skin samples from all 21 patients with PD but no aggregation in any of the samples from the 20 individuals with Parkinsonism syndromes (i.e., vascular Parkinsonism, tauopathies, and pathogenic Parkin mutations) [9]. The study was limited by the lack of quantitative analysis of intraneural α-synuclein load and the absence of normalization to intraepidermal nerve fiber loss. Its strength, however, was the use of an antibody targeting the presumably pathogenic misfolded (phosphorylated) form of α-synuclein. Another study used skin biopsies with quantification of α-synuclein deposition in pilomotor and sudomotor nerve fibers normalized to the overall intraepidermal nerve fiber density. This analysis demonstrated >90% sensitivity and >90% specificity to distinguish PD patients from control individuals via α-synuclein ratios in a prospective longitudinal study [7].

3. Cutaneous α-Synuclein in Prodromal Disease Stages/Possible PD

Since phosphorylated α-synuclein is present in patients in PD even in the early stages of the disease (Hoehn and Yahr I

and II), research has recently addressed the question whether this pathology might also be present in the premotor stages. Skin nerve pathology was assessed in individuals with REM sleep behaviour disorder (RBD) as these patients display a substantially increased risk of developing PD in later life. The likelihood of developing PD was further determined based on additional predictors such as reduced dopamine transporter binding in FP-CIT-SPECT and anosmia. Consistent associations between α-synuclein deposition and presence of RBD, dopamine transporter insufficiency, and olfactory dysfunction were observed [10]. In line with this observation, a recent study in 12 patients with polysomnographically confirmed RBD and 55 sex- and age-matched healthy controls has provided Class III evidence that intraneural deposition of phosphorylated α-synuclein is present in patients with RBD [11].

These findings indicate that cutaneous phosphorylated α-synuclein might help to identify individuals with prodromal Parkinson's disease which might be particularly important in the development of novel disease modifying strategies. Although promising, these results need to be considered with care since only 18 patients with RBD were included in the analyses. Longitudinal data is warranted to assess whether phosphorylated α-synuclein might indeed predict conversion from RBD into PD. Additionally, experiments need to be repeated in a larger study population to allow evaluation of external validity.

4. Distinguishing Synucleinopathies and Nonsynucleinopathic Neurodegenerative Disorders

Among the potential clinical applications of cutaneous α-synuclein assessment, its capacity to differentiate patients with PD from patients with other synucleinopathies based on distinct patterns of neural skin pathology has been discussed. In a cross-sectional investigation, 62% of skin biopsies from PD patients showed cutaneous α-synuclein, whereas only 7% of skin biopsies from patients with atypical Parkinson syndrome were positive for α-synuclein. However, this study considered α-synuclein inclusions in the epidermis and in pilosebaceous units but did not specifically assess intraneural accumulation [12]. Further limitations include a relative small sample size (34 subjects with PD, 33 patients with atypical Parkinson syndrome, and 20 control individuals) and heterogeneity within the group of atypical Parkinson syndrome which included synucleinopathies, such as dementia with Lewy bodies (DLB), multisystem atrophy (MSA), and tauopathies such as Alzheimer's disease (AD) and progressive supranuclear palsy (PSP), possibly jeopardizing interpretability.

Synucleinopathic neurodegenerative disorders have been hypothesized to display distinct patterns of α-synuclein aggregates in the central and the peripheral nervous system. Contrarily to PD, MSA has been described as isolated disorder of the central nerve system with accumulation of phosphorylated α-synuclein limited to brain tissue and preganglionic neurons [13]. In line with this assumption, the examination of cutaneous autonomic adrenergic nerve fibers revealed no deposition of phosphorylated α-synuclein in MSA patients [14]. However, an immunohistochemical analysis of cutaneous somatosensory fibers has unexpectedly revealed enhanced α-synuclein deposition in sensory fibers in 67% of MSA patients, whereas a similar fraction of PD patients showed α-synuclein aggregation in autonomic small fibers [15]. In line with this observation, sudomotor denervation has been reported in patients with MSA indicating postganglionic impairment of the sympathetic nervous system which may contribute alongside degeneration of central autonomic structures to dysautonomia in these patients [16]. These observations modify the current conception of MSA as a solely or predominant disease of the central nervous system.

Further insights into the pathophysiology of synucleinopathies have been provided by Donadio et al. who found length-dependent somatic and autonomic small fiber damage, both in patients with PD and in those with pure autonomic failure (PAF). The degree of cutaneous denervation was associated with the amount of α-synuclein accumulation [17]. Interestingly, differences in patterns of cutaneous denervation and α-synuclein accumulation appear not to be related to patterns of autonomic dysfunction including cardiovascular dysfunction detected by head-up tilt-test and sympathetic nerve dysfunction characterized by microneurography [18]. These discrepancies between structural and functional changes of the autonomic nervous system among synucleinopathies underscore our still limited understanding of the underlying pathophysiological mechanisms [19]. However, it also implies that defining disease specific patterns of α-synuclein pathology might improve early diagnosis, help monitoring synucleinopathies in clinical practice, and facilitate assessment of response to disease modifying treatment. In order to improve our understanding of the direct effects of α-synuclein on skin nerves, to what extent structural changes of these nerves are related to their functional impairment of these fibers ought to be investigated. This highlights the need for detailed characterization of skin denervation patterns, including quantitative examinations of intraneural α-synuclein deposition beyond autonomic fibers in following investigations. Further research is needed to provide a detailed characterization of α-synuclein accumulation patterns among somatic and autonomic small nerve fibers in large populations of affected patients with synucleinopathies such as PD and MSA. This should also include longitudinal studies to characterize progression of neuropathy.

5. How to Obtain and Handle Skin Biopsies

The structural assessment of autonomic skin innervation is still on an experimental level. Both techniques to obtain and handle biopsies and procedures to process and analyze specimens require standardization. Proposed protocols include immunohistochemical analysis of phosphorylated α-synuclein or the α-synuclein/PGP-ratio in skin punch biopsies obtained from varying skin areas such as the dorsal forearms or the lower legs. Commonly, three-millimeter biopsies are obtained following local anesthesia with lidocaine (see Figure 1).

Biopsy specimens are then fixed (e.g., in Zamboni solution) and cryoprotected. Frozen tissue blocks are cut into

sections using a microtome. Parameters and techniques vary among published protocols. Multiple costains with α-synuclein, phosphorylated α-synuclein, protein gene product (PGP) 9.5 (nonspecific nerve fiber marker), tyrosine hydroxylase (TH, adrenergic fiber marker), and vasoactive peptide (VIP, cholinergic fiber marker) allow analyses of α-synuclein deposits in different types of small fibers. To determine intraepidermal nerve fiber density PGP 9.5-positive fibers in skin biopsies should be counted in blinded fashion with results expressed as number of fibers crossing the dermal-epidermal junction per millimeter. Sweat glands and pilomotor muscles can be imaged and nerve fiber densities quantified, preferably in a blinded fashion. In sweat glands, the number of nerve fibers intersecting the circles within the area of interest is counted and reported as the percentage of circles with nerve fiber crossing. Similarly, in pilomotor muscles, the average number of nerve fibers intersecting horizontal lines across the width of the pilomotor muscle in 3 μm thick confocal images is reported in fibers/mm. Techniques to assess α-synuclein deposition in vasomotor fibers are still being designed. Alpha-synuclein/nerve fiber density ratios can then be calculated for (a) epidermis, (b) sweat glands, and (c) pilomotor muscles [2, 7, 17]. Other approaches include advanced morphological qualitative analyses of α-synuclein deposition [6, 10].

6. Functional Assessment of Cutaneous Autonomic Denervation

Dysfunction of autonomic small fibers is of clinical relevance. In general, autonomic neuropathies constitute a group of conditions in which the small, unmyelinated, and lightly myelinated autonomic nerve fibers display structural and functional impairment. Autonomic symptoms involve the cardiovascular, urogenital, gastrointestinal, sudomotor, and pupillomotor systems. Clinical manifestations range from bladder dysfunction over orthostatic hypotension to dyshidrosis, erectile dysfunction, and obstipation. Although diabetes is the most prevalent cause of autonomic fiber dysfunction in more developed countries, targeted fiber damage can also occur in various systemic diseases such as amyloidosis, paraneoplastic syndromes, and infectious diseases and has been shown to be targeted by peripheral synucleinopathies such as PD [3, 18–20].

While structural assessment of α-synuclein pathology in skin biopsies is the most direct test of cutaneous α-synuclein pathology, evaluation of small fiber dysfunction resulting from intraneural α-synuclein deposition might be of additional diagnostic value. This rationale is indirectly supported by a strong correlation between α-synuclein load in cutaneous small fibers and measures of cardiovascular sympathetic and parasympathetic function, although these tests are composite measures of central and peripheral autonomic function and do not specifically capture small fiber integrity [2]. On these composite assessments, cutaneous α-synuclein deposits can be present even in PD patients without autonomic dysfunction. This raises the question if more specific tests of functional integrity of small autonomic fibers might be necessary in the assessment of cutaneous autonomic

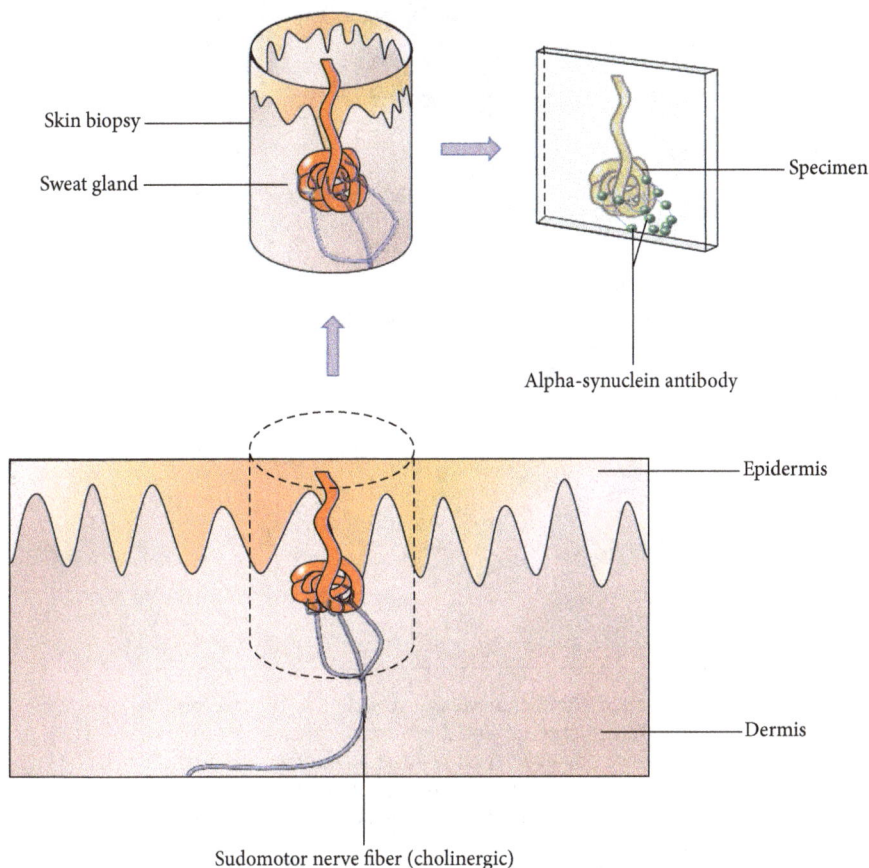

FIGURE 1: Obtaining a skin biopsy containing a sweat gland and staining of sudomotor nerve fibers. A punch biopsy is obtained and stained using immunohistochemical antibodies for α-synuclein (e.g., anti-phosphorylated α-synuclein antibody) and nerve fibers (anti-protein gene product 9.5 antibody). Additional costaining with the cholinergic marker vasoactive intestinal peptide can be performed to specifically identify α-synuclein deposits in cholinergic sudomotor fibers. Figure designed by Dr. Siepmann and Dr. Illigens.

denervation compared to current cardiovascular tests. In fact, functional evaluation of autonomic cutaneous small fibers is of growing importance in the assessment of autonomic neuropathy [20]. A recent study has shown that pilomotor nerve fibers display functional impairment in early stages of PD which correlated with severity of autonomic symptoms [21]. However, skin biopsies have not been obtained in this study. Therefore, it remains speculative whether pilomotor dysfunction relates to α-synuclein deposition in these nerve fibers. It is however noteworthy that, among types of autonomic small fibers, pilomotor nerves displayed the highest concentration of intraneural α-synuclein, supporting the potential usefulness of pilomotor function assessment in the detection of early disease related changes [2].

Assessment of autonomic cutaneous small fiber function is based on quantification of axon reflex responses. Autonomic skin nerve fibers respond to mechanical, physical, and chemical stimuli with an axon reflex-mediated response. Local stimulation of the cutaneous vasomotor (blood vessel innervating) fibers by iontophoretic application of acetylcholine evokes orthodromic conduction of an action potential which then reaches an axon branch point. From this branch point, the potential is conducted antidromically to adjacent cutaneous blood vessels. These vessels are located in an "indirect" area surrounding the skin area where the axon reflex inducing stimulus is applied. There, activated vasomotor small fibers release vasoactive substances such as substance P and calcitonin gene related peptide to cause vasodilation and plasma extravasation [22] (Figure 2). This response can be quantified by laser Doppler assessment of blood flow increase in the indirect skin region [23, 24]. Similarly, functional integrity of sudomotor nerve fibers can be examined via imaging-based quantification of axon reflex responsivity to cholinergic stimulation (adrenergic stimulation in pilomotor fibers, resp.) [22, 25]. In addition to pilomotor dysfunction, sudomotor axon reflex responsiveness was shown to be reduced in PD [26]. Nevertheless, the degree of association between functional impairment and structural deterioration of the cutaneous small fibers has not yet been elucidated. Forthcoming such considerations, the reproducibility and external validity of quantitative tests of autonomic sudomotor and pilomotor functions in the evaluation of PD patients and its association with the α-synuclein load are currently being investigated in an ongoing longitudinal controlled multicenter trial [19].

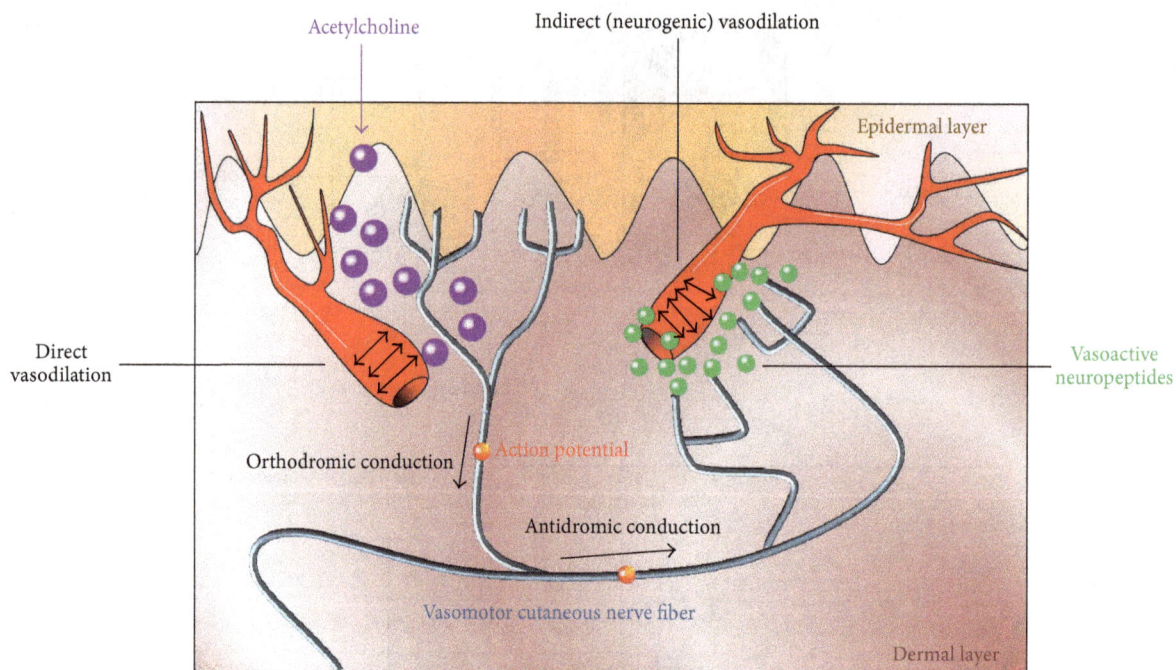

FIGURE 2: Illustration of the vasomotor axon reflex. Iontophoresis of acetylcholine induces vasodilation in the "direct" skin region of application via receptor activation. Consequently, an action potential emerges in the afferent nerve innervating this vessel. This potential travels in an orthodromic fashion to an axonal branch point where it switches to another vasomotor fiber. Upon antidromic conduction, the action potential reaches terminal nerve endings adjacent to a neighboring population of blood vessels. From these terminals, vasoactive substances are released to cause "indirect" vasodilation in a skin region which is surrounding the region of iontophoresis. Consecutive enhancement of blood flow relates to functional integrity of the stimulated vasomotor nerve fiber. Similarly, the axon reflex can be evoked in sympathetic adrenergic pilomotor and sympathetic cholinergic sudomotor fibers. Figure designed by Dr. Siepmann and Dr. Illigens.

7. Limitations and Challenges

While growing evidence emphasizes the diagnostic value of the assessment of α-synuclein pathology in PD, most of the available data is restricted to the detection of α-synuclein positive skin nerve fibers. Only few studies provide quantitative data on the extent of α-synuclein accumulation in sudomotor and pilomotor nerve fibers [2, 4]. Additionally, most of the available date is originated from single center studies and lack independent blinded evaluation.

Alpha-synuclein load in cutaneous small fibers might be a valid biomarker for PD. However, several limitations will have to be addressed to allow its broad clinical application. First, consensus on the most accurate method of immunohistochemical staining and evaluation is needed in order to provide uniform data and determine clinical standards. Heterogeneous methods have been described including (1) the α-synuclein ratio: normalization of the total α-synuclein load to loss of intraepidermal nerve fibers, controlling for neural damage due to other causes, (2) employment of an antibody selective for the assumed pathological form of α-synuclein (phosphorylated α-synuclein), and (3) quantification of native α-synuclein without specificity for the pathological form or normalization to fiber loss [2, 7, 14]. While normalization to loss of intraepidermal nerve fibers and use of phosphorylated α-synuclein specific antibodies seem superior over native α-synuclein quantification, the optimal evaluation method remains to be determined. Second,

α-synuclein aggregates were reported in distinct subtypes of skin autonomic fibers, comprising pilomotor and sudomotor fibers. However, which fiber type represents the most accurate diagnostic target needs to be answered and potential pathology in vasomotor fibers needs to be unveiled. Although two investigations assessing α-synuclein damage normalized to intraepidermal nerve fiber density reported most pronounced damage in pilomotor nerve fibers, potentially indicating high diagnostic value of this type of autonomic small fibers, independent replication of these observations is still warranted [2, 7]. Third, longitudinal multicenter studies in PD and other synucleinopathies that relate cumulative nerve fiber damage over time to progression of clinical symptoms are still lacking. Such studies are also necessary to confirm external validity of the applied techniques. Fourth, the influence of dopaminergic and neuroprotective treatment on the progression of autonomic synucleinopathic neuropathy needs to be elucidated [27]. Lastly, while immunohistochemical quantification of α-synuclein burden in small fibers reflects structural pathology, its implication on functional nerve fiber integrity is unknown.

8. Conclusion

Accumulating evidence supports an important pathogenic role of deposition of α-synuclein in cutaneous small nerve fibers in PD which seems to contribute even to development of the disease in its premotor stages. Quantitative analysis of this pathology in skin biopsies might facilitate early diagnostic discrimination among synucleinopathies, disease monitoring, and evaluation of response to neuroprotective treatment. Further research is needed to standardize evaluation techniques, characterize progression of pathology, and unveil the relation between functional and structural damage to small nerve fibers caused by α-synuclein accumulation, which might eventually answer the question whether we should perform skin biopsies routinely in patients suspected of having PD.

Acknowledgments

Dr. Timo Siepmann's research is supported by grants from the Michael J. Fox Foundation, Prothena Biosciences, and the German Parkinson's Disease Foundation (Deutsche Parkinson Gesellschaft). The authors thank Professor Roy Freeman and Professor Chirstopher Gibbons for their general support.

References

[1] D. Kremens, R. A. Hauser, and E. R. Dorsey, "An update on Parkinson's disease: improving patient outcomes," *American Journal of Medicine*, vol. 127, no. 1, article S3, 2014.

[2] N. Wang, C. H. Gibbons, J. Lafo, and B. S. R. Freeman, "α-synuclein in cutaneous autonomic nerves," *Neurology*, vol. 81, no. 18, pp. 1604–1610, 2013.

[3] T. Siepmann, B. M.-W. Illigens, and K. Barlinn, "Alpha-synuclein in cutaneous small nerve fibers," *Neuropsychiatric Disease and Treatment*, vol. 12, pp. 2731–2735, 2016.

[4] J. M. Lee, P. Derkinderen, J. H. Kordower et al., "The search for a peripheral biopsy indicator of α-synuclein pathology for parkinson disease," *Journal of Neuropathology & Experimental Neurology*, vol. 76, no. 1, pp. 2–15, 2017.

[5] S. A. Schneider, M. Boettner, A. Alexoudi, D. Zorenkov, G. Deuschl, and T. Wedel, "Can we use peripheral tissue biopsies to diagnose Parkinson's disease? A review of the literature," *European Journal of Neurology*, vol. 23, no. 2, pp. 247–261, 2016.

[6] K. Doppler, S. Ebert, N. Üçeyler et al., "Cutaneous neuropathy in Parkinson's disease: a window into brain pathology," *Acta Neuropathologica*, vol. 128, no. 1, pp. 99–109, 2014.

[7] C. H. Gibbons, J. Garcia, N. Wang, L. C. Shih, and R. Freeman, "The diagnostic discrimination of cutaneous α-synuclein deposition in Parkinson disease," *Neurology*, vol. 87, no. 5, pp. 505–512, 2016.

[8] J. Dineen and R. Freeman, "Autonomic Neuropathy," *Seminars in Neurology*, vol. 35, no. 4, pp. 458–468, 2015.

[9] V. Donadio, A. Incensi, V. Leta et al., "Skin nerve α-synuclein deposits: a biomarker for idiopathic Parkinson diseasee," *Neurology*, vol. 82, no. 15, pp. 1362–1369, 2014.

[10] K. Doppler, H.-M. Jentschke, L. Schulmeyer et al., "Dermal phospho-alpha-synuclein deposits confirm REM sleep behaviour disorder as prodromal Parkinson's disease," *Acta Neuropathologica*, vol. 133, no. 4, pp. 535–545, 2017.

[11] E. Antelmi, V. Donadio, A. Incensi, G. Plazzi, and R. Liguori, "Skin nerve phosphorylated α-synuclein deposits in idiopathic

[12] I. Rodríguez-Leyva, A. L. Calderón-Garcidueñas, M. E. Jiménez-Capdeville et al., "α-Synuclein inclusions in the skin of Parkinson's disease and parkinsonism," *Annals of Clinical and Translational Neurology*, vol. 1, no. 7, pp. 471–478, 2014.

[13] T. Peerally, "Multiple system atrophy," *Seminars in Neurology*, vol. 34, no. 2, pp. 174–181, 2014.

[14] L. Zange, C. Noack, K. Hahn, W. Stenzel, and A. Lipp, "Phosphorylated α-synuclein in skin nerve fibres differentiates Parkinson's disease from multiple system atrophy," *Brain*, vol. 138, no. 8, pp. 2310–2321, 2015.

[15] K. Doppler, J. Weis, K. Karl et al., "Distinctive distribution of phospho-alpha-synuclein in dermal nerves in multiple system atrophy," *Movement Disorders*, vol. 30, no. 12, pp. 1688–1692, 2015.

[16] V. Provitera, M. Nolano, G. Caporaso et al., "Postganglionic sudomotor denervation in patients with multiple system atrophy," *Neurology*, vol. 82, no. 24, pp. 2223–2229, 2014.

[17] V. Donadio, A. Incensi, C. Piccinini et al., "Skin nerve misfolded α-synuclein in pure autonomic failure and Parkinson disease," *Annals of Neurology*, vol. 79, no. 2, pp. 306–316, 2016.

[18] V. Donadio, P. Cortelli, M. Elam et al., "Autonomic innervation in multiple system atrophy and pure autonomic failure," *Journal of Neurology, Neurosurgery & Psychiatry*, vol. 81, no. 12, pp. 1327–1335, 2010.

[19] T. Siepmann, A. Pintér, S. J. Buchmann et al., "Cutaneous autonomic pilomotor testing to unveil the role of neuropathy progression in early parkinson's disease (CAPTURE PD): protocol for a multicenter study," *Frontiers in Neurology*, vol. 8, article 212, 2017.

[20] R. Freeman, "Autonomic peripheral neuropathy," *The Lancet*, vol. 365, no. 9466, pp. 1259–1270, 2005.

[21] T. Siepmann, E. Frenz, A. I. Penzlin et al., "Pilomotor function is impaired in patients with Parkinson's disease: A study of the adrenergic axon-reflex response and autonomic functions," *Parkinsonism & Related Disorders*, vol. 31, pp. 129–134, 2016.

[22] M. Berghoff, M. Kathpal, S. Kilo, M. J. Hilz, and R. Freeman, "Vascular and neural mechanisms of ACh-mediated vasodilation in the forearm cutaneous microcirculation," *Journal of Applied Physiology*, vol. 92, no. 2, pp. 780–788, 2002.

[23] B. M. W. Illigens and C. H. Gibbons, "Sweat testing to evaluate autonomic function," *Clinical Autonomic Research*, vol. 19, no. 2, pp. 79–87, 2009.

[24] T. Siepmann, C. H. Gibbons, B. M. Illigens, J. A. Lafo, C. M. Brown, and R. Freeman, "Quantitative pilomotor axon reflex test: A novel test of pilomotor function," *JAMA Neurology*, vol. 69, no. 11, pp. 1488–1492, 2012.

[25] B. M. W. Illigens, T. Siepmann, J. Roofeh, and C. H. Gibbons, "Laser Doppler imaging in the detection of peripheral neuropathy," *Autonomic Neuroscience: Basic and Clinical*, vol. 177, no. 2, pp. 286–290, 2013.

[26] J. B. Kim, B.-J. Kim, S.-B. Koh, and K.-W. Park, "Autonomic dysfunction according to disease progression in Parkinson's disease," *Parkinsonism & Related Disorders*, vol. 20, no. 3, pp. 303–307, 2014.

[27] M. Nolano, V. Provitera, F. Manganelli et al., "Loss of cutaneous large and small fibers in naive and l-dopa–treated PD patients," *Neurology*, vol. 89, no. 8, pp. 776–784, 2017.

21

The Cognition of Maximal Reach Distance in Parkinson's Disease

Satoru Otsuki[1,2] and Masanori Nagaoka[2]

[1]Department of Rehabilitation, Juntendo University Nerima Hospital, 3-1-10 Takanodai, Nerima-ku, Tokyo 177-8521, Japan
[2]Department of Rehabilitation Medicine, Juntendo University Graduate School, 2-1-1 Hongo, Bunkyo-ku, Tokyo 113-8421, Japan

Correspondence should be addressed to Satoru Otsuki; sootsuki@juntendo.ac.jp

Academic Editor: Cristine Alves da Costa

This study aimed to investigate whether the cognition of spatial distance in reaching movements was decreased in patients with Parkinson's disease (PD) and whether this cognition was associated with various symptoms of PD. Estimated and actual maximal reaching distances were measured in three directions in PD patients and healthy elderly volunteers. Differences between estimated and actual measurements were compared within each group. In the PD patients, the associations between "error in cognition" of reaching distance and "clinical findings" were also examined. The results showed that no differences were observed in any values regardless of dominance of hand and severity of symptoms. The differences between the estimated and actual measurements were negatively deviated in the PD patients, indicating that they tended to underestimate reaching distance. "Error in cognition" of reaching distance correlated with the items of posture in the motor section of the Unified Parkinson's Disease Rating Scale. This suggests that, in PD patients, postural deviation and postural instability might affect the cognition of the distance from a target object.

1. Introduction

In daily life, we frequently perform movements such as extending a hand toward an object. Such movements are expressed as reaching movements. The reaching movement is composed of postural control and transport of the upper limbs and hands. These elements are considered to be automatic processes. Regarding the association between the reaching movement and postural control, the functional reach test developed by Duncan et al. [1] determines the maximal reaching distance and uses postural stability as an indicator. Before the reaching movement is actually performed, there is also an essential cognitive process in which people visually perceive a target object and decide how to reach it. Presumably, people estimate how far they can spatially reach on the basis of information from the visual, auditory, and somatic senses and their past experiences and then start movement on the basis of this estimation [2, 3]. The distances that study participants estimate to be reachable through this cognitive process can be measured, and there are several reports on this subject [4–10].

This reaching movement is limited by diseases affecting the movement of the upper limbs and postural control. The reaching movement of patients with Parkinson's disease (PD) has also been described in many reports, and the reported characteristics of their reaching movement include the delay of the start of movement [11], slow speed of movement [12], and impaired coordination between the arm and the trunk [13]. Moreover, in PD patients, the reaching distance determined by the functional reach test is shorter in those with a history of falls than in those without [10, 14, 15], and the reaching distance is suggested to be associated with decreased postural stability and falls. It is assumed that, in PD patients, reaching movement is limited by decreased movement of the upper limbs due to akinesia or bradykinesia, decreased flexibility due to rigidity of the four limbs and trunk, and the impairment of postural reflexes associated with these decreases. Moreover, it has been reported that PD patients experience disorders in eye movement [16–18] and coordination between the eyes and head with reaching movements [19–21]. Presumably, decreased motility of the eyes, head, and neck due to PD may affect the ability to detect the accurate position of a target object in space.

Regarding the estimated reaching distance, in studies on PD patients, Kamata et al. [9] reported that overestimation of reaching distance due to progression of symptoms is associated with falls. On the other hand, some reports showed PD patients tend to underestimate spatial distance [10, 22, 23]. Factors affecting the cognition of spatial distance have considered physical factors and environment factors [4–6]. Ehgoetz Martens et al. [24] reported that the cognition of spatial distance differs in experimental conditions in PD patients. But the association with detailed motor symptoms of PD has not yet been clarified. These issues of underestimation or overestimation are related factors that need more investigation and are still open to discuss. The difference in the right and left sides of the spatial cognition has been discussed in PD patients [22, 23, 25, 26]. In PD patients, although estimated reaching distance was analyzed only front reach [9, 10], the differences in the right and left sides need more investigation. Thus, regarding the distance estimated in reaching movement by PD patients, we evaluated distance cognition in a more spatial manner by measuring estimated and actual maximal reaching distance in the right and left directions, in addition to the front direction. Furthermore, the association with the symptoms of PD was also investigated.

While various terms are used to indicate estimated reaching distance, we use the term estimated reaching distance (ED) in the present study. Correspondingly, the term actual reaching distance (AD) is used to indicate the actually reachable distance.

2. Subjects and Methods

2.1. Subjects. The subjects were 27 PD patients (8 men and 19 women; mean age ± standard deviation (SD): 71.9 ± 5.3 years, mean height ± SD: 155.5 ± 7.6 cm) and a control group of 28 healthy elderly volunteers matched for age and height (10 men and 18 women with a mean age ± SD: 73.6 ± 5.2 years and mean height ± SD: 157.1 ± 8.7 cm). All participants were right-handed. In the case of PD patients, those who provided consent for the objectives and contents of the study were included if they could remain standing for long enough to perform the tasks and had cognitive function sufficient to understand the tasks (24 or higher on the Mini-Mental State Exam [MMSE]). The present study was conducted with the approval of the ethics committee of our institution (Ethics Approval Number 13-29).

2.2. Methods. In the PD patients, the following data were collected: disease duration, Hoehn-Yahr scale, the motor section of the Unified Parkinson's Disease Rating Scale (UPDRS3), and history of falls. Moreover, the medications that the PD patients were receiving were identified. All patients were treated with levodopa and measurements were taken under the effects of the medications (on-stage). No patients showed dyskinesia during measurement.

In the experiments, both ED and AD were measured by the following method. Regarding the AD measurement,

functional reach test was verified as reliable [1]. The reliability of ED measurement was verified by Robinovitch and Cronin [7] but was not sufficient. The measurement of ED was performed three times and an Intraclass Correlation Coefficient (ICC) was used for the intrarater reliability. According to the method developed by Fischer [5], ED was measured under the following conditions. The participants estimated the range in which they could grasp a 3 cm square wooden block on a plate at the level of the shoulder in the standing position without taking a step, in the front, right, and left directions. In order to investigate differences in spatial cognition due to directional effects, ED was measured in not only the front direction but also the right and left directions. During measurement, the participants were prohibited from extending their arms or tilting their bodies and measured the distance only by sight. For estimation of the front reaching distance, the participants stood in front of the block placed at the level of their right acromion. This position was regarded as the starting position. They were instructed to slowly step backward in a straight line from any point where they could grasp the block with certainty and to stop at the farthest point where they decided that they could grasp it with both feet touching the floor. The point at the tip of the right big toe was marked, and the distance from the intersection point between the vertical line from the block and the floor to the marked point was measured and regarded as the front ED (Figure 1(a)). For estimation of the right reaching distance, the participants stood in a way that the block placed at the same position as in estimation of the front ED was positioned immediately lateral to the right acromion. This position was regarded as the starting position. They were instructed to slowly step leftward in straight line from any point where they could grasp the block with certainty and to stop at the farthest point where they decided that they could grasp it with both feet touching the floor. The point at the distal end of the right fifth metatarsal bone was marked, and the distance from the intersection point between the vertical line from the block and the floor to the marked point was measured and regarded as the right ED. Estimation of the left reaching distance was performed in the same manner, and the results were regarded as the left ED.

After ED was measured in the three directions, the farthest range in which the participants could actually grasp the block was measured in the three directions in the order of the front, right, and left directions by the following method based on the multidirectional reach test, which Newton [27] had developed by modifying the functional reach test for multidirectional measurement. The participants were instructed to stand at the points marked during measurement of ED and to grasp the block without moving their feet (Figure 1(b)). The block was moved by 1 cm at a time away when they could grasp it or closer when they could not until the farthest point where they could grasp it without stepping out was determined. In this manner, AD was measured in the front direction (front AD), the right direction (right AD), and the left direction (left AD).

2.3. Data Analysis. The measurements obtained from the functional reach test have been shown to correlate with

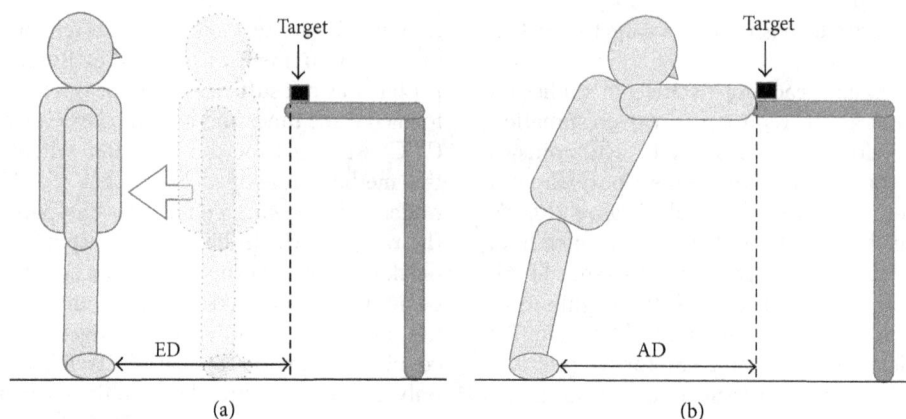

FIGURE 1: (a) Measurement of front ED. Participants stood on the starting position (dotted line). They stepped backward and stopped at the farthest point where they decided that they could grasp target (solid line). The distance from target to stopping point was regarded as ED. (b) Measurement of front AD. Participants reach out and grasp the target. The distance from target to farthest standing position was regarded as AD.

body height [1]. Thus, in data analysis, each measurement (i.e., ED and AD) was divided by body height, and values were adjusted for individual differences in body constitution. In order to analyze the differences between estimated and actual measurements, the differences between ED and AD (ED–AD) were calculated. In the present study, these differences are expressed as the difference between ED and AD (DEA). Absolute values of DEA were used for analysis to assess the degree of the differences between ED and AD.

In the control group, the right and left sides were regarded as the dominant and nondominant sides, respectively, to perform data analysis. In the PD patients, the symptomatically milder side (MS) and severer side (SS) were determined according to the total scores obtained from the scores on the items of UPDRS3 for the right and left sides. When the total scores were the same, the affected side at the time of onset was determined as the SS. Each measurement (i.e., right ED, left ED, right AD, and left AD) was classified by MS and SS into MS-ED, SS-ED, MS-AD, and SS-AD.

In order to assess the association between each measurement and its directionality, Pearson correlation coefficients were calculated for each measurement obtained from the dominant and nondominant sides in the control group and the MS and SS in the PD patients (p values were corrected by the Bonferroni correction, $p < 0.012$). Moreover, a one-way analysis of variance (ANOVA) was performed with ED, AD, DEA, and absolute values of DEA in each direction (the Bonferroni correction was used for the post hoc test).

In both groups, total values of measurement in the three directions were calculated for ED (total ED) and AD (total AD), and their mean values were compared between the two groups by unpaired t-test. In order to evaluate errors in cognition, the mean value was compared between total ED and total AD within each group by paired t-test. Initial significance level was set at 0.05 (p values were corrected by the Bonferroni correction, $p < 0.012$).

As for PD patients, a stepwise linear regression analysis was performed to identify clinical symptoms associated with errors in cognition. Total DEA obtained from DEA in the

three directions and absolute values of total DEA were used as target variables. The following items were used as explanatory variables: MMSE, disease duration, Hoehn-Yahr scale, history of falls, UPDRS3 total score, and individual items of UPDRS3 (tremor: 20, 21; rigidity: 22; diadochokinesis: 23–26; posture: 28, 30; walking: 29; and akinesia: 31). Significance level was set at 0.05.

For all statistical analyses, SPSS version 21 was used.

3. Results

3.1. Characteristics of PD. Mean and standard deviation (SD) of each item were 27.6 ± 1.8 for MMSE, 5.9 ± 3.3 years for disease duration, 2.6±0.7 for Hoehn-Yahr scale, and 16.0±9.5 for UPDRS3. The number of falling subjects was 12 and the number of nonfalling subjects was 15.

3.2. Reliability of ED Measurement. A result of the reliability verification of ED measurement showed ICC (1,3) = 0.953; therefore it is considered as reliable method.

3.3. Validity of the Methods and Measurements. In the control group, the correlation coefficients for each value obtained from the dominant and nondominant sides were $r = 0.907$ ($p < 0.001$) for ED, $r = 0.620$ ($p < 0.001$) for AD, $r = 0.930$ ($p < 0.001$) for DEA, and $r = 0.792$ ($p < 0.001$) for the absolute values of DEA. All variables showed significantly positive correlation. The PD group included 9 patients with SS at the right side and MS at the left side and 18 patients with SS at the left side and MS at the right side. In the PD group, the correlation coefficients for each value obtained at the MS and SS sides were $r = 0.820$ ($p < 0.001$) for ED, $r = 0.704$ ($p < 0.001$) for AD, $r = 0.860$ ($p < 0.001$) for DEA, and $r = 0.695$ ($p < 0.001$) for the absolute values of DEA. All variables showed significantly positive correlation (Figure 2). According to directions, no significant differences in ED, AD, and DEA or in the absolute values of DEA were observed either between the dominant and nondominant sides in the

TABLE 1: Means and standard deviations of ED, AD, DEA, and absolute value of DEA in each direction.

(a)

		Front	Dominant	Nondominant	
Healthy elderly $n = 28$	ED cm/cm	0.51 ± 0.05	0.52 ± 0.06	0.52 ± 0.06	n.s.
	AD cm/cm	0.53 ± 0.03	0.52 ± 0.03	0.52 ± 0.02	n.s.
	DEA cm/cm	-0.02 ± 0.04	0.00 ± 0.05	-0.01 ± 0.06	n.s.
	|DEA| cm/cm	0.04 ± 0.03	0.04 ± 0.03	0.05 ± 0.03	n.s.

(b)

		Front	Milder side: MS	Severer side: SS	
PD $n = 27$	ED cm/cm	0.47 ± 0.08	0.47 ± 0.08	0.47 ± 0.09	n.s.
	AD cm/cm	0.50 ± 0.03	0.50 ± 0.03	0.50 ± 0.03	n.s.
	DEA cm/cm	-0.04 ± 0.06	-0.04 ± 0.07	-0.04 ± 0.07	n.s.
	|DEA| cm/cm	0.07 ± 0.05	0.06 ± 0.05	0.07 ± 0.05	n.s.

Mean ± SD [cm/cm].
The one-way ANOVA was performed with each item.
ED: estimated distance, AD: actual distance, DEA: difference between ED and AD, |DEA|: absolute value of DEA, and n.s.: not significant.

control group or between the MS and SS sides in the PD group. Moreover, the values obtained from measurement in the front direction did not significantly differ from those obtained from measurement in the right and left directions (Table 1).

3.4. Relationship between the AD and the ED in the Two Groups. The mean total AD (1.57 ± 0.07 cm/cm in the control group and 1.50 ± 0.09 cm/cm in the PD group) showed a significant difference between the two groups (total AD: $t(53)$ = 3.246, $p = 0.002$) (Figure 3(a)). The mean total ED (1.55 ± 0.17 cm/cm in the control group and 1.39 ± 0.20 cm/cm in the PD group) showed a significant difference between the two groups (total ED: $t(53) = 3.337$, $p = 0.002$) (Figure 3(a)). No significant differences between the total AD and the total ED were observed in control group ($t(27) = 0.722$, $p = 0.476$) (Figure 3(b)). A significant difference between the total AD and the total ED was observed in PD group ($t(26) = 3.165$, $p = 0.004$) (Figure 3(b)).

3.5. Association with Clinical Symptoms of PD. Although clinical features associated with total DEA were investigated, all items were not included as significant factors for the total DEA in the PD group. On the other hand, the result of the stepwise multiple regression analysis for the absolute value of total DEA, posture, was shown to be the only significant factor ($R^2 = 0.268$, $\beta = 0.518$, $p = 0.006$). A relationship between the posture and the absolute value of total DEA is shown in Figure 4. MMSE, disease duration, Hoehn-Yahr scale, history of falls, UPDRS3 total score, tremor, rigidity, diadochokinesis, walking, and akinesia were not included as significant factors for the absolute value of total DEA.

4. Discussion

4.1. What Does DEA Indicate? To evaluate distance cognition in a more actual milieu, we measured ED and AD in three directions. ED and DEA are values determined through cognitive processing and may be affected by hand dominance and the order of measurement. Thus, we first measured ED and AD in not only the front direction but also the right and left directions. Then, we examined whether there was any variance in the measurements with the dominant hand, nondominant hand, severity of symptoms, and order of measurement. All values obtained in each reaching direction showed correlations between the right and left sides (Figure 2), and no difference was observed in the mean values of each variable (Table 1). Thus, ED and DEA are assumed to be free from the effects of reaching direction and hand dominance. In the PD patients, these values were not affected by the differences in the severity of motor dysfunction between the right and left sides. This result may support the report that spatial distance was not affected by the difference between right and left symptoms [22, 25]. Furthermore, as Table 1 shows that the values obtained in the front direction do not differ from those obtained in the right or left directions (the dominant and nondominant sides in the controls and the symptomatically milder and severer sides in the PD patients [right SS : left SS = 9 : 18]), the values are also assumed to be free from the effects of the order of measurement. ED, which is considered to be determined on the basis of sensory information and past experience, is affected by environmental factors, such as position of a target object, and physical factors, such as postural stability, body constitution, and flexibility [4–6]. While information on the spatial and positional relationship based on interactions between the environment and the motor system of the body is stored in the brain, this spatial and positional information is considered to be necessary for reaching movement [3]. ED indicates perception of such spatial and positional relationships, and it is assumed that the accuracy of perception can be determined by DEA and absolute value of DEA. Thus, as described in the following section, the characteristics of the PD patients were assessed with regard to cognition of spatial distance.

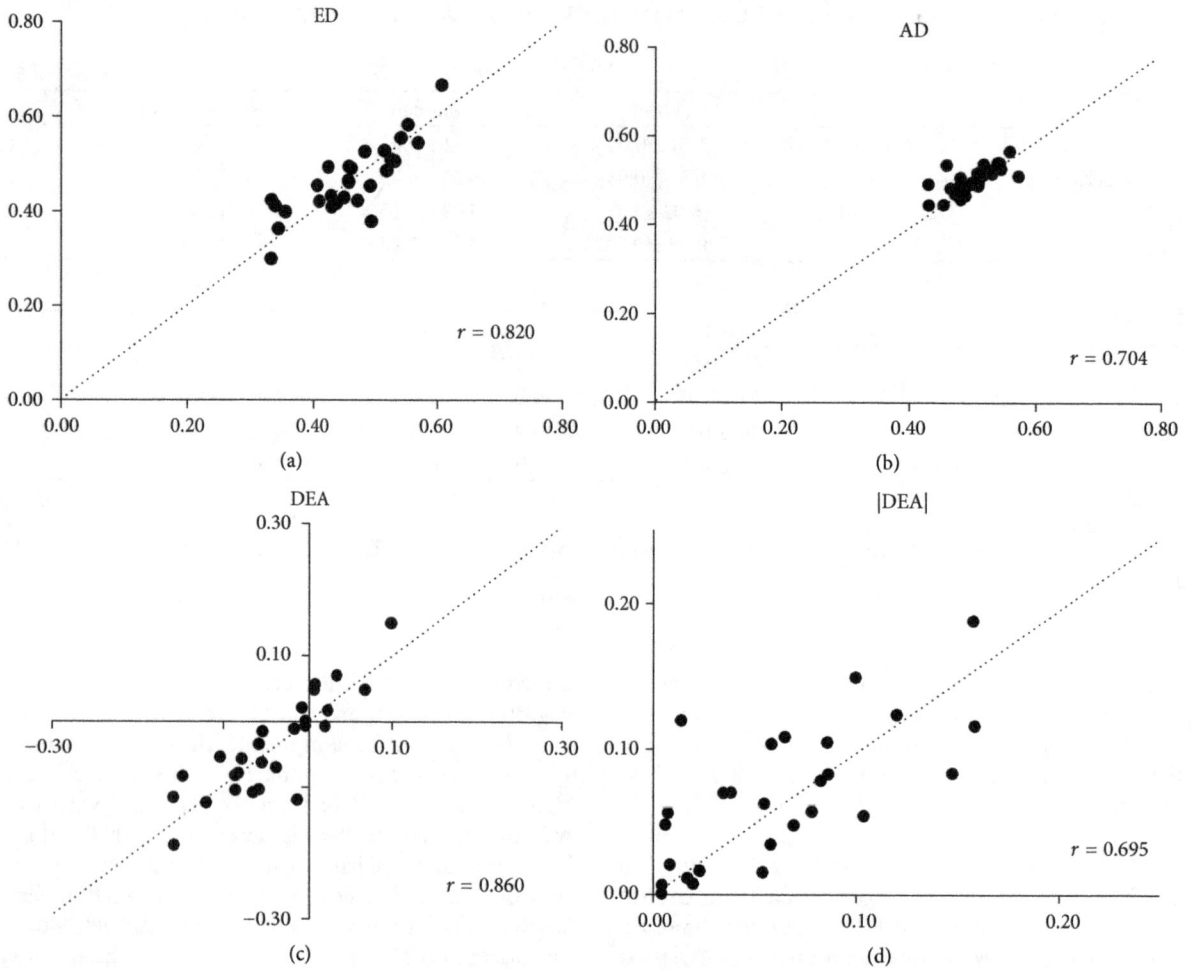

FIGURE 2: Distribution of each value in PD. The vertical axis shows severer side (SS) [cm/cm], and the horizontal axis shows milder side (MS) [cm/cm]. Dotted line shows $x = y$ line. The value distributed on the top left (above $x = y$ line) shows SS is larger than MS. In contrast, the value distributed on the bottom right (below $x = y$ line) shows MS is larger than SS.

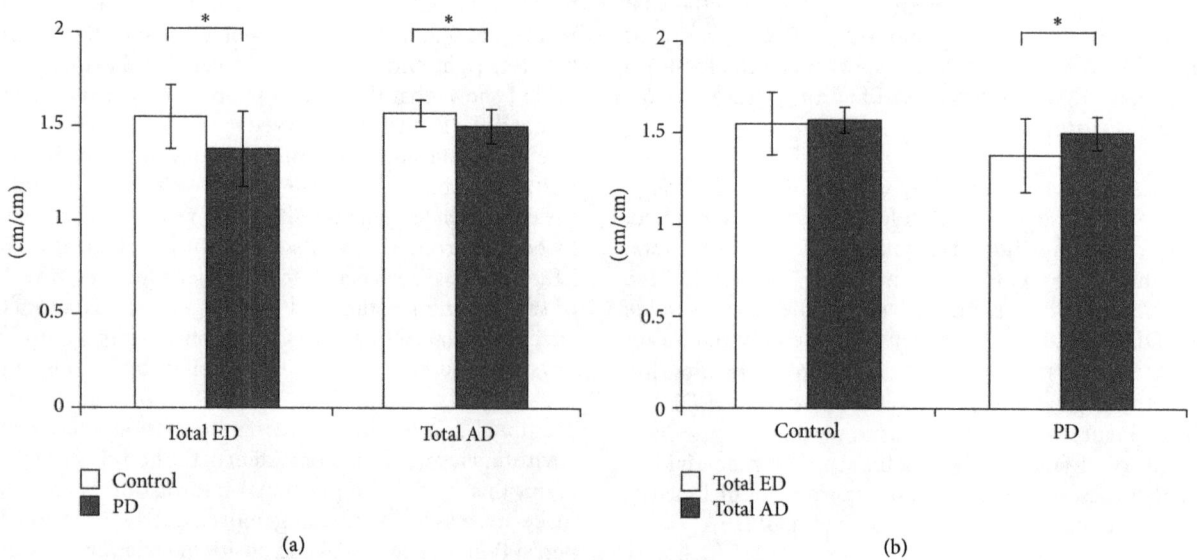

FIGURE 3: (a) Means and standard deviations demonstrated by each group during total ED and total AD. The PD group showed small value compared with control in both total ED and total AD. (b) Comparison between total ED and total AD within each group is shown. Only the PD group showed a significant difference ($^{*}p < 0.012$).

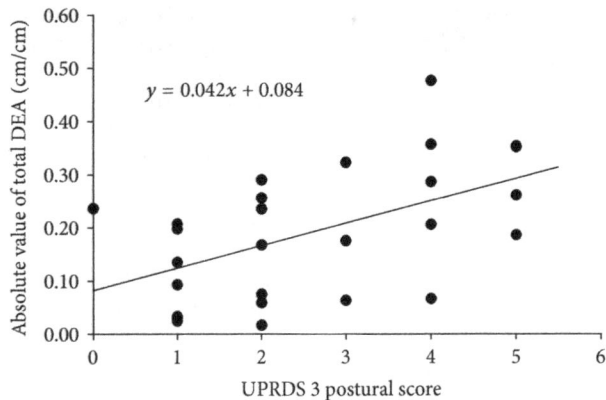

FIGURE 4: This figure indicates a regression line obtained by multiple regression analysis for the absolute value of total DEA. Postural score was shown to be the only significant factor ($p = 0.006$).

4.2. Stability Limits and Cognition of the Limits in the PD Patients.

According to comparisons of total AD, the reaching distance is shorter in the PD patients than in the controls, and the range where the point vertically projected from the center of gravity can be kept within the base of support (stability limit) is shown to be small in the PD patients. This result is consistent with the results reported in many studies [10, 28–30]. In PD, it is considered that the stability limit becomes smaller because of mobility being reduced by rigidity, impaired postural reaction, impaired motion perception, and so forth [28–30].

Moreover, total ED was also smaller in the PD patients than in the controls, showing that the range of stability limit recognized by the PD patients was small. As described above, it is assumed that ED is affected by environmental and physical factors. However, the present study focused on the differences in ED due to physical factors while the environmental factors, such as direction of reaching movement and height of a target object, were kept constant. In the present study, the physical factors include the cognitive process in which people perceive the distance to a target object, compare this distance to their physical status, and determine whether they can reach the target object. ED obtained in the present study might have been affected by the physical characteristics of the participants under these conditions. It can be assumed that the range of stability limit recognized by PD patients on the basis of their physical characteristics is small.

4.3. Do PD Patients Underestimate Spatial Distance?

In the PD group, if both AD and ED have decreased equally, it can be assumed that there is no error in cognition of distance. In order to evaluate error in cognition, AD and ED were compared within each group. The results showed that ED tended to be negative compared to AD in the PD group, in other words, showing that the PD group tended to underestimate reaching distance. While people presumably estimate reaching distance on the basis of information from the visual, auditory, and somatic senses and their past experiences in the cognitive process before executing reaching movement

[2, 3], PD patients underestimate reaching distance in this process. In PD patients, because it has been reported that their perception of the range of motion of the upper limbs [31] and joint motion angle [32] is lower than the actual values, underestimation of motion perception may affect estimation of spatial distance. Moreover, other studies [33, 34] reported that the decreased range of motion in PD patients is attributable to the lack of perception of their limited motion. Underestimation by the PD group as observed in the present study suggests that PD patients cannot perceive that the distance recognized by them is smaller than actual distance.

Regarding the error in cognition of reaching distance that has been described above, Kamata et al. [9] reported that PD patients tend to overestimate reaching distance. Their result contradicts that of the present study. The reasons for this may be the following 2 factors. One factor is the differences in patient groups. Our results show that although some PD patients overall underestimated the reaching distance, some patients overestimated it. Distribution of MS-DEA and SS-DEA shows the same tendency (Figure 2; DEA, underestimation: the third quadrant, overestimation: the first quadrant). Similarly, the results obtained by Kamata et al. also included overestimation and underestimation values. Depending on the distribution of patients participating in a study, results may show either tendency. The other possible factor is the differences in methods to measure ED. A major difference involves whether the target object is moved or whether participants move during measurement of ED. Ehgoetz Martens et al. [24] investigated the differences in perception of spatial distance by PD patients between the static condition in which they perceived distance from only visual information without moving and the dynamic condition in which they moved to perceive distance. On the basis of these results, Ehgoetz Martens et al. reported that distance is more likely to be underestimated under the dynamic condition than under the static condition. Similarly, Kabasakalian et al. [22] reported hypometric estimates of distance under the dynamic condition. Although the static condition is used in many studies [4–10] including that of Kamata et al., the dynamic condition was used in the present study. This difference in the conditions may cause an underestimation of the reaching distance. Because reaching movements performed in daily life are based on the dynamic condition, the present study may provide important findings with regard to risk factors for falls.

4.4. Error in Cognition of Reaching Distance in PD Patients and Causes of the Error.

We investigated the factors affecting impaired cognition of distance in PD patients. Because UPDRS3 total scores or Hoehn-Yahr scale were not included as significant factors for both DEA and absolute values of DEA, impaired cognition of reaching distance is not assumed to be necessarily associated with progression of the disease, because all items were not included as significant factors for DEA, which means the factors that affect underestimation of spatial distance were not identified. The tendency of underestimation seems to be affected by the conditions discussed in the previous section rather than clinical symptoms of PD. Meanwhile, it was suggested that postural factors (i.e., posture and postural stability) greatly contributed to the large absolute values of DEA. In PD patients, it has been reported that their perception of body axis is impaired [35, 36]. Moreover the other study reported that impaired spatial cognition correlates with postural factors of UPDRS [37]. Changes in the body axis due to the abnormally flexed posture of PD patients may affect errors in cognition of distance. Moreover, one of the reported factors affecting error in cognition of reaching distance is postural stability. It has been reported that, without the certainty of a stable posture, the error increases [4, 5, 38]. Thus, abnormal posture and impaired postural stability in PD patients appear to be associated with perception of spatial information on the position of their bodies and affect their decisions regarding distance.

In this study, measurements were taken only in on-stage. Levodopa may have affected the results of this study because levodopa improves motor functions of PD [35, 39, 40]. Moreover, some researchers reported that levodopa affects perception of movement and space [24, 41–43]. The results of this study showed that spatial cognition of PD patients was impaired even under the effects of levodopa.

4.5. Limitations. While the participants in the present study appear to be adequately distributed between mild and moderate severity of PD, the inclusion criteria have been set to ensure the reliability and validity of measurement methods. Although the clinical symptoms of the PD patients widely varied, it was difficult to examine all symptoms and their severity in the present study. Thus, the abnormal cognition of reaching distance observed in the present study may not be applicable to all PD patients.

Disclosure

The present affiliation of Satoru Otsuki is as follows: Department of Rehabilitation, Juntendo Tokyo Koto Geriatric Medical Center, 3-3-20 Shinsuna, Koto-ku, Tokyo 136-0075, Japan.

Acknowledgments

The authors want to thank members of the Department of Neurology and the Department of Rehabilitation in Juntendo University Nerima Hospital for their assistance with the present study.

References

[1] P. W. Duncan, D. K. Weiner, J. Chandler, and S. Studenski, "Functional reach: a new clinical measure of balance," *Journals of Gerontology*, vol. 45, no. 6, pp. M192–M197, 1990.

[2] R. A. Andersen and C. A. Buneo, "Intentional maps in posterior parietal cortex," *Annual Review of Neuroscience*, vol. 25, pp. 189–220, 2002.

[3] A. Shumway-Cook and M. Woollacott, "Normal reach, grasp, and manipulation," in *Motor Control*, pp. 443–467, Lippincott Williams & Wilkins, Philadelphia, Pa, USA, 3rd edition, 2007.

[4] C. Carello, A. Grosofsky, F. D. Reichel, H. Y. Solomon, and M. T. Turvey, "Visually perceiving what is reachable," *Ecological Psychology*, vol. 1, no. 1, pp. 27–54, 1989.

[5] M. H. Fischer, "Estimating reachability: whole body engagement or postural stability?" *Human Movement Science*, vol. 19, no. 3, pp. 297–318, 2000.

[6] S. N. Robinovitch, "Perception of postural limits during reaching," *Journal of Motor Behavior*, vol. 30, no. 4, pp. 352–358, 1998.

[7] S. N. Robinovitch and T. Cronin, "Perception of postural limits in elderly nursing home and day care participants," *Journal of Gerontology, Biological Sciences A*, vol. 54, no. 3, pp. B124–B130, 1999.

[8] C. Gabbard, D. Ammar, and S. Lee, "Perceived reachability in single- and multiple-degree-of-freedom workspaces," *Journal of Motor Behavior*, vol. 38, no. 6, pp. 423–429, 2006.

[9] N. Kamata, Y. Matsuo, T. Yoneda, H. Shinohara, S. Inoue, and K. Abe, "Overestimation of stability limits leads to a high frequency of falls in patients with Parkinson's disease," *Clinical Rehabilitation*, vol. 21, no. 4, pp. 357–361, 2007.

[10] G. Ryckewaert, M. Luyat, M. Rambour et al., "Self-perceived and actual ability in the functional reach test in patients with Parkinson's disease," *Neuroscience Letters*, vol. 589, pp. 181–184, 2015.

[11] U. Castiello, G. E. Stelmach, and A. N. Lieberman, "Temporal dissociation of the prehension pattern in Parkinson's disease," *Neuropsychologia*, vol. 31, no. 4, pp. 395–402, 1993.

[12] T. Flash, R. Inzelberg, E. Schechtman, and A. D. Korczyn, "Kinematic analysis of upper limb trajectories in Parkinson's disease," *Experimental Neurology*, vol. 118, no. 2, pp. 215–226, 1992.

[13] H. Poizner, A. G. Feldman, M. F. Levin et al., "The timing of arm-trunk coordination is deficient and vision-dependent in Parkinson's patients during reaching movements," *Experimental Brain Research*, vol. 133, no. 3, pp. 279–292, 2000.

[14] A. L. Behrman, K. E. Light, S. M. Flynn, and M. T. Thigpen, "Is the functional reach test useful for identifying falls risk among individuals with Parkinson's disease?" *Archives of Physical Medicine and Rehabilitation*, vol. 83, no. 4, pp. 538–542, 2002.

[15] F. Smithson, M. E. Morris, and R. Iansek, "Performance on clinical tests of balance in Parkinson's disease," *Physical Therapy*, vol. 78, no. 6, pp. 577–592, 1998.

[16] R. A. Armstrong, "Visual symptoms in Parkinson's Disease," *Parkinson's Disease*, vol. 2011, Article ID 908306, 9 pages, 2011.

[17] H. Matsumoto, Y. Terao, T. Furubayashi et al., "Small saccades restrict visual scanning area in Parkinson's disease," *Movement Disorders*, vol. 26, no. 9, pp. 1619–1626, 2011.

[18] V. Goyal, M. Behari, A. Srivastava, S. K. Sood, G. Shukla, and R. Sharma, "Saccadic eye movements in Parkinson's disease," *Indian Journal of Ophthalmology*, vol. 62, no. 5, pp. 538–544, 2014.

[19] B. K. Baziyan, L. A. Chigaleichik, E. L. Teslenko, and D. R. Lachinova, "Analysis of trajectories of eye, head, and hand movements for early diagnosis of Parkinson's disease," *Bulletin of Experimental Biology and Medicine*, vol. 143, no. 5, pp. 553–555, 2007.

[20] J. A. Waterston, G. R. Barnes, M. A. Grealy, and S. Collins, "Abnormalities of smooth eye and head movement control in Parkinson's disease," *Annals of Neurology*, vol. 39, no. 6, pp. 749–760, 1996.

[21] K. Srulijes, D. J. Mack, J. Klenk et al., "Association between vestibulo-ocular reflex suppression, balance, gait, and fall risk in ageing and neurodegenerative disease: protocol of a one-year prospective follow-up study," *BMC Neurology*, vol. 15, no. 1, article 192, 2015.

[22] A. Kabasakalian, T. Kesayan, J. B. Williamson et al., "Hypometric allocentric and egocentric distance estimates in parkinson disease," *Cognitive and Behavioral Neurology*, vol. 26, no. 3, pp. 133–139, 2013.

[23] F. M. Skidmore, V. Drago, B. Pav, P. S. Foster, C. Mackman, and K. M. Heilman, "Conceptual hypometria? An evaluation of conceptual mapping of space in Parkinson's disease," *Neurocase*, vol. 15, no. 2, pp. 119–125, 2009.

[24] K. A. Ehgoetz Martens, C. G. Ellard, and Q. J. Almeida, "Dopaminergic contributions to distance estimation in Parkinson's disease: a sensory-perceptual deficit?" *Neuropsychologia*, vol. 51, no. 8, pp. 1426–1434, 2013.

[25] N. Verreyt, G. M. S. Nys, P. Santens, and G. Vingerhoets, "Cognitive differences between patients with left-sided and right-sided Parkinson's disease. A review," *Neuropsychology Review*, vol. 21, no. 4, pp. 405–424, 2011.

[26] K. Karádi, T. Lucza, P. Ács et al., "Visuospatial impairment in Parkinson's disease: the role of laterality," *Laterality*, vol. 20, no. 1, pp. 112–127, 2015.

[27] R. A. Newton, "Validity of the multi-directional reach test: a practical measure for limits of stability in older adults," *Journals of Gerontology—Series: A Biological Sciences and Medical Sciences*, vol. 56, no. 4, pp. M248–M252, 2001.

[28] F. B. Horak, J. G. Nutt, and L. M. Nashner, "Postural inflexibility in parkinsonian subjects," *Journal of the Neurological Sciences*, vol. 111, no. 1, pp. 46–58, 1992.

[29] M. Mancini, L. Rocchi, F. B. Horak, and L. Chiari, "Effects of Parkinson's disease and levodopa on functional limits of stability," *Clinical Biomechanics*, vol. 23, no. 4, pp. 450–458, 2008.

[30] F. B. Horak, D. Dimitrova, and J. G. Nutt, "Direction-specific postural instability in subjects with Parkinson's disease," *Experimental Neurology*, vol. 193, no. 2, pp. 504–521, 2005.

[31] T. Klockgether, M. Borutta, H. Rapp, S. Spieker, and J. Dichgans, "A defect of kinesthesia in Parkinson's disease," *Movement Disorders*, vol. 10, no. 4, pp. 460–465, 1995.

[32] S. Zia, F. Cody, and D. O'Boyle, "Joint position sense is impaired by Parkinson's disease," *Annals of Neurology*, vol. 47, no. 2, pp. 218–228, 2000.

[33] B. G. Farley and G. F. Koshland, "Training BIG to move faster: the application of the speed-amplitude relation as a rehabilitation strategy for people with Parkinson's disease," *Experimental Brain Research*, vol. 167, no. 3, pp. 462–467, 2005.

[34] C. Fox, G. Ebersbach, L. Ramig, and S. Sapir, "LSVT LOUD and LSVT BIG: Behavioral treatment programs for speech and body movement in Parkinson disease," *Parkinson's Disease*, vol. 2012, Article ID 391946, 12 pages, 2012.

[35] W. G. Wright, V. S. Gurfinkel, L. A. King, J. G. Nutt, P. J. Cordo, and F. B. Horak, "Axial kinesthesia is impaired in Parkinson's disease: effects of levodopa," *Experimental Neurology*, vol. 225, no. 1, pp. 202–209, 2010.

[36] J. Konczak, D. M. Corcos, F. Horak et al., "Proprioception and motor control in Parkinson's disease," *Journal of Motor Behavior*, vol. 41, no. 6, pp. 543–552, 2009.

[37] H. Murakami, Y. Owan, Y. Mori et al., "Correlation between motor and cognitive functions in the progressive course of Parkinson's disease," *Neurology and Clinical Neuroscience*, vol. 1, no. 5, pp. 172–176, 2013.

[38] C. Gabbard, A. Cordova, and S. Lee, "Examining the effects of postural constraints on estimating reach," *Journal of Motor Behavior*, vol. 39, no. 4, pp. 242–246, 2007.

[39] Parkinson Study Group, "Pramipexole vs levodopa as initial treatment for Parkinson disease," *The Journal of the American Medical Association*, vol. 284, no. 15, pp. 1931–1938, 2000.

[40] Parkinson Study Group, "Pramipexole vs Levodopa as initial treatment for Parkinson disease: a 4-year randomized controlled trial," *Archives of Neurology*, vol. 61, no. 7, pp. 1044–1053, 2004.

[41] M. Barnett-Cowan, R. T. Dyde, S. H. Fox, E. Moro, W. D. Hutchison, and L. R. Harris, "Multisensory determinants of orientation perception in Parkinson's disease," *Neuroscience*, vol. 167, no. 4, pp. 1138–1150, 2010.

[42] J. Konczak, K. Krawczewski, P. Tuite, and M. Maschke, "The perception of passive motion in Parkinson's disease," *Journal of Neurology*, vol. 254, no. 5, pp. 655–663, 2007.

[43] M. Maschke, C. M. Gomez, P. J. Tuite, and J. Konczak, "Dysfunction of the basal ganglia, but not the cerebellum, impairs kinaesthesia," *Brain*, vol. 126, no. 10, pp. 2312–2322, 2003.

22

Standardised Neuropsychological Assessment for the Selection of Patients Undergoing DBS for Parkinson's Disease

Jennifer A. Foley [ID],[1,2] **Tom Foltynie,**[1,2] **Patricia Limousin,**[1,2] **and Lisa Cipolotti** [ID][1,3]

[1]*National Hospital for Neurology and Neurosurgery, Queen Square, London, UK*
[2]*UCL Institute of Neurology, Queen Square, London, UK*
[3]*Dipartimento di Scienze Psicologiche, Pedagogiche e della Formazione, Università degli Studi di Palermo, Palermo, Italy*

Correspondence should be addressed to Jennifer A. Foley; jennifer.foley@uclh.nhs.uk

Academic Editor: Jan Aasly

DBS is an increasingly offered advanced treatment for Parkinson's disease (PD). Neuropsychological assessment is considered to be an important part of the screening for selection of candidates for this treatment. However, no standardised screening procedure currently exists. In this study, we examined the use of our standardised neuropsychological assessment for the evaluation of surgical candidates and to identify risk factors for subsequent decline in cognition and mood. A total of 40 patients were assessed before and after DBS. Evaluation of mood and case notes review was also undertaken. Before DBS, patients with PD demonstrated frequent impairments in intellectual functioning, memory, attention, and executive function, as well as high rates of mood disorder. Post-DBS, there was a general decline in verbal fluency only, and in one patient, we documented an immediate and irreversible global cognitive decline, which was associated with older age and more encompassing cognitive deficits at baseline. Case note review revealed that a high proportion of patients developed mood disorder, which was associated with higher levels of depression at baseline and greater reduction in levodopa medication. We conclude that our neuropsychological assessment is suitable for the screening of candidates and can identify baseline risk factors, which requires careful consideration before and after surgery.

1. Introduction

Drug therapies for advanced Parkinson's disease (PD) can be unsatisfactory, with unwanted side effects, and/or insufficient control of disabling motor symptoms. Thus, there has been resurgence in interest in surgical treatments, with deep brain stimulation (DBS) now increasingly offered as an option. DBS is the chronic, high-frequency electrical stimulation of most usually the subthalamic nucleus (STN) or internal segment of the globus pallidus (GPi) [1], which is thought to alter the pattern of neural activity, with resulting beneficial effects upon motor function [2]. Its success relies heavily upon appropriate selection of candidates, which in turn relies in part upon neuropsychological screening [3, 4]. However, no standardised screening procedure currently exists, and it remains unclear what level of cognitive dysfunction precludes

successful surgery. In this study, we discuss the limitations of existing presurgical protocols and evaluate the use of standardised neuropsychological assessment in a sample of patients undergoing DBS for PD. We describe patients' performance on this neuropsychological assessment before and after DBS and identify potential baseline predictors of after DBS decline, which warrant further investigation.

DBS has been shown to be relatively safe, with few negative events occurring during or following surgery, when performed on appropriate candidates [5]. However, STN DBS is thought to result in better improvements in motor control; there is some evidence to suggest that it also poses a greater risk of negatively affecting speech articulation, impulsive behaviours, and/or mood [6–10], and therefore, GPi DBS may be preferred for patients presenting with these difficulties. However, marked global cognitive deterioration has also been reported [11, 12], and mild decline in verbal fluency has frequently been documented [13–30].

Decline in cognitive functioning following DBS has been found to be more common in patients who are older, especially above 70 years [29, 31], particularly affecting frontal executive functions [28]. Yet others have cautioned against a strict age criterion, as many people older than 70 can demonstrate good outcomes [32, 33]. Indeed, it has been reported that other factors, particularly cognitive performance, may be more useful as predictors of postoperative decline [3, 29, 34, 35]. Several studies have suggested that lower cognitive functioning at baseline is predictive of poorer cognitive outcome following surgery [36], perhaps because of lower "cognitive reserve" [35]. It has even been suggested that the presence of any cognitive deficits at baseline, particularly in executive function and memory, should serve as exclusion [36, 37]. However, PD is usually accompanied by at least mild cognitive deficits, particularly in executive function, and the evolution of a dementia is rather insidious, without any clear boundary features. Thus, it remains unclear what level of impairment should constitute a contraindication to surgery.

Despite the widespread agreement on the importance of appropriate screening and careful selection of surgery candidates, to the best of our knowledge no standardised neuropsychological assessment procedure currently exists. The Consensus on DBS for PD [38] published guidance on presurgical screening and selection of patients but did not provide a presurgical neuropsychological protocol. Rather, they listed an extensive range of neuropsychological domains to be assessed and tests commonly used. The tests listed ranged from very brief screens (including the MMSE) to very long and extensive batteries (such as the Wechsler Memory Scales and Delis–Kaplan Executive Functioning System). They stated that tests chosen should be reliable and valid, with adequate normative data for referencing performance. However, without any guidance on how to choose between the vast range of tests, nor how to interpret scores when deciding on suitability for surgery, it remains unclear how to use neuropsychological assessments to identify candidates suitable for DBS. Indeed, defining what constitutes unacceptable cognitive dysfunction remains the most controversial aspect of patient selection [2].

Moreover, there is scant official guidance. The British Psychological Society [39] recommends that candidates undergo presurgery neuropsychological evaluation but does not describe what this should consist of. The Australian guidelines [40] simply recommend that patients should be able to give a good account of themselves and capable of giving informed consent. Of course, even marked cognitive impairment may be masked by higher levels of cognitive reserve and/or fluctuating levels of attention and vice versa; gross physical and speech disability may mask intact cognition. Thus, the absence of any firm guidelines for the assessment and interpretation of cognitive performance clearly poses a significant hurdle for the appropriate selection of candidates for DBS.

In lieu of such guidance, several studies have relied upon brief cognitive screens only, such as the Mini-Mental State Examination (MMSE) [41]. This may be criticised for a number of reasons. Firstly, the MMSE comprises very few subtests that are sensitive to the typical cognitive dysfunction displayed in PD, namely, executive dysfunction [42–48] and cognitive slowing [49–52] and thus is insufficient for detecting cognitive impairment [53, 54]. Secondly, the MMSE suffers from significant ceiling and floor effects [55], so cannot capture very mild nor very severe cognitive dysfunction. Thirdly, MMSE scores are affected by age and education [56, 57], so that a low score in an older person with minimal formal schooling may present a false positive for dementia. Fourthly, an individual may attain a low MMSE score for a number of noncognitive reasons, including poor speech intelligibility, high levels of anxiety, fatigue, and distracting dyskinesia. Therefore, a low score on this test should not necessarily be used to preclude surgery.

Moreover, such brief screening tools do not permit scrutiny of the wider cognitive profile, important for confirming diagnosis. Many cases of "failed" DBS have been later found to have atypical Parkinsonian syndromes, known not to benefit from DBS [58]. Thus, there is a need to identify a suitable presurgical neuropsychological protocol, which is sufficiently sensitive to both the typical cognitive dysfunction displayed in PD and atypical cognitive decline, as seen in other Parkinsonian disorders and has clear guidelines for its interpretation.

In addition to changes in cognition, there are also a few reports of dramatic deterioration in mood and greatly increased apathy following DBS [22, 59–61], with an associated elevated risk of suicide despite successful reduction of motor symptoms [62, 63]. As such deterioration can clearly negate any potential benefits [64], it is essential that candidates at high risk of such postoperative decline are identified at baseline. Specifically, postoperative risk of suicide has been associated with higher levels of mood disorder, apathy, and/or family or social stress at baseline [65, 66]. This may not only reflect the additional stressor of surgery [67, 68] but also the direct effects of the stimulation itself [69] and any reductions in dopaminergic medication [70, 71]. As mood disorder is so prevalent in PD and may reduce with improvements in motor symptoms following surgery [35], it remains unclear what level of mood disorder should act as an absolute contraindication for DBS.

Thus, the aims of this study were to evaluate the use of our standardised neuropsychological protocol in the evaluation of patients undergoing DBS for PD in order to identify any contraindication for surgery and to be sensitive to changes following DBS.

2. Methods

2.1. Participants. A total of 40 patients (29 male, 11 female) who underwent DBS took part in this study. All patients had had a diagnosis of idiopathic PD for at least five years (according to Queen Square Brain Bank criteria), were younger than 70 years, and suffered from disabling motor complications despite optimal treatment. Each patient underwent multidisciplinary evaluation to decide on suitability for DBS. Formal levodopa challenge confirmed dopaminergic drug responsiveness. A structural MRI was obtained to exclude surgical contraindications, such as advanced brain atrophy, white matter changes, or any other abnormality contraindicating surgery. Detailed neuropsychological and neuropsychiatric assessments excluded patients with significant cognitive impairment and/or psychiatric comorbidities. Contraindications for STN DBS included the presence of clinically relevant speech difficulties and cognitive impairment. The final decision regarding suitability for DBS and appropriate target for each patient was taken during a joint meeting of patient, immediate family, neurologist(s), and neurosurgeon(s).

Motor status was evaluated using part III of the Unified Parkinson's Disease Rating Scale (UPDRS-III). Prior to surgery, patients were assessed in the practically defined "off state" after overnight withdrawal of anti-Parkinsonian drugs and the "on state," following a levodopa challenge using a suprathreshold dose of oral levodopa. After DBS, motor assessments were sequentially performed under the following conditions, in open fashion: off medication/on stimulation (with stimulation switched on after 12 h medication withdrawal) and on medication/on stimulation (1 h after the administration of a routine dose of levodopa while stimulation was reintroduced). All medications before and after surgery were recorded, noting any dopamine agonist treatment, and levodopa-equivalent dosage was calculated (www.parkinsonsmeasurement.org). History of impulse control disorder was recorded by reviewing the medical notes and noting any mention of compulsive gambling, eating, shopping, or sexual behaviour before or after DBS.

All patients underwent assessment of neuropsychological and mood functioning before and after surgery, under optimal conditions. Thus, preoperatively, this was in the on medication and postoperatively on stimulation/on medication. The postoperative assessment was performed a mean of 19.60 months after surgery (range = 1–54; SD = 11.56). This broad range reflected the early recall of one patient following concern about cognition immediately following DBS, as well as later routine follow-up of cognitively intact patients after surgery.

The most appropriate DBS target was chosen on clinical grounds based on patient motor phenotype, imaging, and preoperative cognitive assessment. Twenty-eight patients underwent bilateral STN DBS and twelve bilateral GPi DBS.

2.2. *Neuropsychological Assessment.* The tests included general screening and IQ measures, as well as tests of specific cognitive functions. This was to enable both the quantification of any intellectual deficit and the elucidation of specific cognitive profiles. Thus, the measures included tests of general cognitive functioning, memory, language, visuoperceptual ability, attention, executive functions, and speed of processing. The tests chosen were considered to have acceptable test validity and reliability, as described below. The assessments took around two hours to complete and were as follows:

(1) The MMSE was used as a screening test of global cognitive functioning [41]. It is not sufficient as a measure of cognition in Parkinson's disease [53],

but as the "gold standard" screening instrument, it permits easy comparison between studies.

(2) Vocabulary, similarities, arithmetic, and digit span subtest scores from the Wechsler Adult Intelligence Scale-Third Edition (WAIS-III) [72] were prorated to generate verbal IQ (VIQ). Picture Completion and Matrix Reasoning subtest scores were prorated to generate scores for nonverbal IQ (PIQ). The WAIS-III has been found to have good sensitivity and specificity for cognitive disorders [73] and good reliability for Parkinson's disease [74].

(3) The National Adult Reading Test-Revised (NART-R) [75] was used to estimate the premorbid level of intellectual functioning, by generating each patient's Predicted Full-Scale IQ (PFSIQ). The NART-R has very good interrater and test-retest reliability, and good validity, although suffers from a ceiling effect limiting prediction of IQ scores beyond 125.

(4) Memory was assessed using the following:

(a) The Warrington Words and Faces Recognition Memory Tests (RMTs) [76] were used to assess recognition memory. The RMT correlates well with other measures of memory and has adequate reliability for patients with neurological disorders [77, 78].

(b) The People and Shapes subtests from the Doors and People Test were used to assess verbal and visual recall memory (D&P) [79]. These tests have sufficient validity and reliability [80] and are recommended for assessing recall in PD [81].

(5) The Graded Naming Test (GNT) [82] was used to assess language. The GNT has good test-retest reliability and is well suited for detecting any gradual changes in performance over time [83]. Moreover, it is sensitive to cognitive impairment in Parkinson's disease [84].

(6) The Silhouettes subtest from the Visual Object and Space Perception Battery (VOSP) [85] was used to assess visuoperceptual functioning. This test has been validated as a test of object perception [86] and is sensitive to visuospatial impairment seen in PD dementia [87] and atypical PD [88].

(7) Elevator Counting and Elevator Counting with Distraction subtests from the Test of Everyday Attention (TEA) [89] were used to assess sustained and selective attention. These tests have high test-retest reliability and correlate with other measures of attention. Furthermore, these tests have been shown to be sensitive to Parkinsonian disorders, including Lewy body dementia [90].

(8) Executive functioning was assessed using the following:

(a) FAS and Category subtests from the Delis–Kaplan Executive Function System (DKEFS) [91] were used to assess verbal fluency. The tests have been standardised and found to be sufficiently reliable [92].

(b) The Stroop [93] was used to assess verbal inhibition. It has high reliability [94] and is sensitive to cognitive deficits in PD [95].

(c) The Hayling and Brixton tests [96] were used to assess verbal suppression/strategy formation [97] and nonverbal set-shifting, respectively. They have moderate sensitivity and specificity for detecting executive dysfunction [98] and are sensitive to PD [99, 100].

(9) The Symbol Search and Digit Symbol Coding subtests from the WAIS-III [72] were used to assess processing speed. These tests have been shown to be sensitive to PD [101].

2.3. Mood Assessment. All patients were screened for mood disorder using the Hospital Anxiety and Depression Scale (HADS) [102] and the Apathy Evaluation Scale (AES) [103]. These tests have been validated for use in PD [104, 105].

2.4. Case Note Review. The case notes were reviewed by one clinical neuropsychologist (JAF) to identify any change in cognition, mood, or behaviour since DBS, as highlighted by the surgery team, neurologists, or nursing staff. Any mention of decline in memory, attention, perception, language, reasoning, mood, anxiety, depression, or motivation was recorded, along with number of months elapsed since surgery. As discussed before, any mention of a de novo impulse control disorder was recorded.

2.5. Statistical Analysis. Scores for each of the neuropsychological assessments were compared with published normative data. For each measure, patients were judged to be impaired if scores were ≤2 SD. When multiple measures were used, performance was classified as impaired when ≤2 SD on at least one of the measures used.

Normality of distribution was assessed using the Kolmogorov–Smirnov test and, if significant, by examining the z-scores for skewness and kurtosis. Homogeneity of variance was assessed using Levene's test. Unless otherwise stated, all data met the assumptions of normality and homogeneity of variance. Baseline scores of the STN and GPi DBS groups were compared using t-tests or Mann–Whitney tests, as appropriate. Pre- and after DBS scores were compared using t-tests for related samples or Wilcoxon signed-ranks, as appropriate. Pearson's correlations, chi-squared analyses, and logistic regression techniques were used to detect any significant associations. All analyses were conducted using IBM SPSS Statistics Data Editor, version 19.

The research was done in accordance with the Helsinki Declaration and the Institute of Neurology Joint Research Ethics Committee UCLH, NHS Trust Research and Development Directorate.

3. Results

3.1. Patient Demographics. As shown in Table 1, the STN and GPi DBS patient groups did not significantly differ in

TABLE 1: Patient demographic characteristics.

	STN ($n = 28$)	GPi ($n = 12$)	p
Gender (male)	17	8	0.72
Age (at first assessment, years)	57.50 ± 7.32	61.33 ± 6.30	0.12
NART Predicted Full-Scale IQ	111.57 ± 11.08	103.42 ± 15.43	0.07
Age at PD diagnosis (years)	45.55 ± 7.80	48.60 ± 6.35	0.29
PD disease duration (years)	18.77 ± 6.12	19.00 ± 4.55	0.92
History of impulse control disorder (n, %)	9, 28.1%	1, 3.1%	0.08

terms of age, gender split, or premorbid level of intellectual functioning, as estimated by the NART. They also did not significantly differ in age at diagnosis, duration of disease, or history of impulse control disorder.

3.2. Clinical Characteristics before and after DBS. At baseline, there were no significant differences between the STN and GPi DBS patient groups in UPDRS-III scores off or on medication, nor in baseline levodopa-equivalent dosage (as shown in Tables 2 and 3). STN DBS was successful in improving UPDRS-III scores off medication ($t(23) = 6.50$, $p < 0.001$), with a corresponding reduction in levodopa-equivalent dosage ($t(21) = 4.50$, $p < 0.001$). There was no significant difference in UPDRS-III scores on medication. In the GPi DBS group, there was no significant change in levodopa-equivalent dosage and change in motor performance was not examined because of insufficient collection of postsurgery motor performance data.

There were also no significant differences between the STN and GPi DBS patients groups in proportion of patients receiving dopamine agonist treatment before or after DBS.

3.3. Cognitive Performance before and after DBS. When baseline neuropsychological assessment scores were compared with published normative data, impairment was documented on at least one domain of cognitive function in 85% of all patients (STN: $n = 22$, 64.7%; GPi: $n = 12$, 100%). In both groups, impairments were frequently in intellectual functioning, memory, attention, and executive function (Table 4). The GPi DBS group also demonstrated frequent impairments in the additional domains of cognitive screen and speed. There was a significant association between DBS location and frequency of impairment, with the GPi group having more frequent impairments on the cognitive screen ($\chi^2(1) = 9.20$, $p < 0.05$), measures of memory ($\chi^2(1) = 5.80$, $p < 0.05$), executive function ($\chi^2(1) = 9.20$, $p < 0.05$), and speed ($\chi^2(1) = 9.20$, $p < 0.05$).

When investigated further, we found that the GPi DBS patients obtained lower baseline scores on tests of general intellectual functioning (VIQ: $t(38) = 4.24$, $p < 0.001$; PIQ: $t(38) = 2.33$, $p < 0.05$), recognition memory (RMT words: $U = 65.5$, $p < 0.05$; RMT faces: $t(37) = 3.74$, $p < 0.01$), attention (TEA EC with distraction: $t(37) = 2.76$, $p < 0.05$), and executive functioning (category fluency: $t(37) = 2.75$, $p < 0.05$; Stroop: $t(35) = 3.49$, $p < 0.01$; Brixton: $t(33) = 4.12$,

TABLE 2: Patient motor characteristics before and after DBS.

	STN			GPi		
	Before DBS ($n = 28$)	After DBS ($n = 24$)	p	Before DBS ($n = 11$)	After DBS ($n = 4$)	p
UPDRS-III off medication	48.68 ± 14.10	28.67 ± 9.99	0.00	50.73 ± 11.09	35.20 ± 15.32	—
UPDRS-III on medication	17.29 ± 7.967	15.83 ± 7.20	0.49	24.64 ± 10.97	20.75 ± 11.56	—

TABLE 3: Patient medication characteristics before and after DBS.

	STN ($n = 28$)			GPi ($n = 12$)		
	Before DBS	After DBS	p	Before DBS	After DBS	p
Levodopa-equivalent dosage (mg/d)	1321.82 ± 638.68	863.73 ± 583.92	0.00	1263.40 ± 971.08	1205.10 ± 626.68	0.81
Dopamine agonist treatment (n, %)	15, 46.9%	6, 18.8%	0.01	7, 21.9%	5, 15.6%	0.16

TABLE 4: Cognitive performance before DBS: proportion impaired in each domain.

Cognitive domain	STN ($n = 28$)	GPi ($n = 12$)	p
Screen	**1, 3.7%**	**5, 41.7%**	**0.01**
IQ	12, 42.9%	8, 66.7%	0.30
Memory	**9, 33.3%**	**9, 75.0%**	**0.04**
Language	1, 3.7%	3, 27.3%	0.07
Perception	2, 7.4%	1, 8.3%	1.00
Attention	5, 18.5%	4, 33.3%	0.42
Executive function	**4, 14.8%**	**8, 66.7%**	**0.01**
Speed	**2, 7.4%**	**4, 36.4%**	**0.05**

Results are given as number and percentage. Chi-squared significant group comparisons are indicated in bold.

$p < 0.01$). Thus, all subsequent analyses of cognitive performance were split according to site of DBS.

As shown in Table 5, there was a significant drop in phonemic and category fluency following both STN and GPi DBS. In the STN patients, there was also a significant decline in performance on Symbol Search, and in the GPi patients, there was also a decline in PIQ. There were also near-significant declines in Stroop performance and VIQ following STN DBS. There were no other significant or near-significant differences in cognitive performance following either STN or GPi DBS.

Case note review revealed mention of decline in cognitive function in 15% ($n = 6$) of patients after DBS (4 STN DBS, 14.3%; 2 GPi DBS, 16.7%). There was no significant association between DBS location and subsequent cognitive decline ($\chi^2(5) = 4.73$, $p = 48$). Number of months elapsed since surgery had a bimodal distribution, with two patients demonstrating marked decline immediately (STN and GPi DBS, resp.), but others demonstrating decline at least a year after surgery ($n = 4$, range = 13–72 months). When considering those who declined immediately, one demonstrated confusion and hallucinations immediately after GPi DBS surgery, thought to be associated with a urinary tract infection and which improved with appropriate treatment consistent with a diagnosis of delirium rather than dementia. However, the other deteriorated physically and cognitively after STN DBS (as confirmed by repeat cognitive assessment), without any subsequent improvement.

3.4. Predictors of Cognitive Decline following DBS.

Pearson correlational analysis revealed no significant baseline cognitive, mood, or motor correlates of decline in phonemic fluency after either STN or GPi DBS. Greater decline in category verbal fluency following STN DBS was associated with higher levels of apathy ($r = 0.47$, $p < 0.05$) and levodopa-equivalent dosages at baseline ($r = -0.43$, $p < 0.05$) and greater change in cognitive speed, as indexed by change in performance on both Digit Symbol Coding ($r = 0.49$, $p < 0.05$) and Symbol Search ($r = -0.53$, $p < 0.01$). However, only the correlation between decline in category fluency and Symbol Search survived the Bonferroni adjustment for multiple comparisons. Greater decline in category fluency following GPi DBS was associated with worse UPDRS-III scores off medication at baseline ($r = 0.70$, $p < 0.05$), but this did not survive the Bonferroni adjustment.

There were also no significant baseline correlates of decline in Symbol Search after STN DBS. However, greater decline in PIQ following GPi DBS was associated with slower baseline performance on the Digit Symbol Coding subtest. There were no other significant predictors of decline following DBS.

In order to identify baseline predictors of the subsequent global and irreversible cognitive decline following STN DBS noted in the one patient, Crawford and Howell [106] single-case methodology was used. This revealed that this patient was significantly older (68 years) than the mean age (59.15 years) of the STN DBS patients who remained stable ($t = 1.86$, $p < 0.05$). Indeed, although the baseline neurology assessment revealed no atypical symptoms, it did raise concerns about the older age. MMSE performance was flawless, but the patient demonstrated mild baseline impairments in all domains, including language and visuoperceptual functioning. Indeed, this patient was the only patient to demonstrate baseline impairment in language and subsequently undergo STN DBS. Another patient also demonstrated baseline impairment in visuoperceptual and subsequently underwent STN DBS, which proved successful, but it is noted that this patient was younger (55 years) than the mean age of the STN DBS group.

When considering the remaining patients who demonstrated cognitive decline at least a year after surgery (as identified

TABLE 5: Cognitive performance before and after DBS: mean scores on each test.

Assessment	STN (n = 28)			GPi (n = 12)		
	Before DBS	After DBS	p	Before DBS	After DBS	p
MMSE (30)	28.64 ± 1.41	28.64 ± 1.68	1.00[a]	26.75 ± 3.14	25.75 ± 2.87	0.31[a]
WAIS-VIQ	111.21 ± 12.40	107.54 ± 15.93	0.05[a]	92.75 ± 13.10	92.67 ± 10.71	0.97[a]
Vocabulary (66)	51.57 ± 9.61	49.96 ± 10.00	0.13[a]	40.64 ± 15.02	37.27 ± 14.14	0.16[a]
Similarities (33)	**24.71 ± 4.51**	**22.75 ± 5.64**	**0.02[a]**	19.36 ± 5.43	18.36 ± 5.12	0.43[a]
Arithmetic (22)	**15.61 ± 2.94**	**14.04 ± 4.64**	**0.01[a]**	10.36 ± 2.94	9.64 ± 3.04	0.90[a]
Digit span (30)	**17.57 ± 4.15**	**16.43 ± 4.26**	**0.04[a]**	14.08 ± 3.09	14.00 ± 3.16	0.41[a]
WAIS-PIQ	106.37 ± 15.17	104.04 ± 19.57	0.50[a]	**93.64 ± 15.11**	**84.45 ± 12.91**	**0.01[a]**
Picture Completion (25)	17.96 ± 4.25	17.19 ± 4.86	0.33[a]	12.92 ± 3.66	11.33 ± 3.53	0.07[a]
Matrix Reasoning (26)	16.35 ± 5.61	15.31 ± 5.90	0.24[a]	11.10 ± 4.33	9.20 ± 4.21	0.09[a]
RMT-W (50)	46.81 ± 3.50	45.12 ± 5.35	0.10[b]	39.20 ± 9.45	40.30 ± 8.68	0.16[a]
RMT-F (50)	41.88 ± 4.13	41.08 ± 5.68	0.54[a]	33.60 ± 6.85	34.00 ± 7.92	0.80[a]
D&P People delayed (12)	7.21 ± 3.68	7.50 ± 4.30	0.59[b]	6.40 ± 4.65	5.60 ± 3.95	0.57[a]
D&P Shapes delayed (12)	10.50 ± 3.28	10.25 ± 2.82	0.22[b]	8.86 ± 3.63	7.43 ± 3.78	0.30[a]
GNT (30)	23.69 ± 3.42	23.69 ± 3.28	1.00[a]	17.91 ± 8.11	19.45 ± 6.65	0.34[a]
VOSP Silhouettes (30)	22.81 ± 3.25	21.92 ± 3.91	0.13[a]	20.82 ± 3.52	19.00 ± 5.88	0.41[a]
DKEFS FAS (SS)	**13.42 ± 4.89**	**11.54 ± 4.61**	**0.01[a]**	**10.92 ± 5.18**	**8.00 ± 4.88**	**0.01[a]**
DKEFS Category (SS)	**12.31 ± 4.21**	**10.00 ± 4.99**	**0.01[a]**	**8.50 ± 3.00**	**5.00 ± 3.30**	**0.01[a]**
Stroop (112)	91.81 ± 21.36	83.77 ± 22.94	0.06[a]	63.00 ± 20.44	58.50 ± 23.45	0.12[a]
Hayling (SS)	5.68 ± 1.07	5.32 ± 1.52	0.28[b]	4.60 ± 1.84	4.70 ± 1.83	0.89[a]
Brixton (SS)	4.91 ± 1.53	5.00 ± 2.28	0.83[a]	2.33 ± 1.66	2.56 ± 2.07	0.72[a]
TEA EC (7)	6.67 ± 0.96	6.75 ± 0.44	0.85[b]	6.50 ± 1.41	5.88 ± 1.55	0.26[b]
TEA EC-Distraction (SS)	9.91 ± 2.66	8.96 ± 2.92	0.15[a]	7.13 ± 3.14	5.75 ± 1.91	0.17[a]
WAIS-SS (SS)	**9.62 ± 2.25**	**8.46 ± 2.82**	**0.02[a]**	7.89 ± 3.33	6.11 ± 2.42	0.86[a]
WAIS-DSC (SS)	8.20 ± 2.52	7.48 ± 2.65	0.22	4.89 ± 2.67	4.67 ± 1.87	0.86[a]

Results are given as mean ± SD ([a]paired t-test; [b]Wilcoxon signed-rank). Significant differences are indicated in bold. MMSE: Mini-Mental Status Examination; WAIS-VIQ, PIQ: Wechsler Adult Intelligence Scale-Third Edition-Verbal IQ, Performance IQ; RMT-W, F: Warrington Recognition Memory Test for Words, Faces; D&P: Doors and People Test; GNT: Graded Naming Test; VOSP: Visual Object and Space Perception Battery; DKEFS: Delis–Kaplan Executive Function System; SS: scaled score; TEA EC, ECD: Test of Everyday Attention Elevator Counting, Elevator Counting with Distraction; WAIS-III SC, DSC: Wechsler Adult Intelligence Scale-Third Edition Symbol Search, Digit Symbol Coding.

TABLE 6: Mood scores before and after DBS.

Assessment	STN (n = 28)			GPi (n = 12)		
	Before DBS	After DBS	p	Before DBS	After DBS	p
HADS anxiety (21)	7.50 ± 3.23	6.27 ± 4.85	0.19[b]	8.55 ± 3.30	9.00 ± 4.12	0.69[a]
HADS depression (21)	6.15 ± 4.42	6.00 ± 4.04	0.86[a]	7.00 ± 3.85	7.73 ± 4.63	0.67[a]
Apathy (54)	10.75 ± 6.02	13.96 ± 11.16	0.15[b]	14.57 ± 6.71	20.86 ± 11.11	0.67[a]

Results are given as mean ± SD ([a]paired t-test; [b]Wilcoxon signed-rank).

in the case note review), no significant difference in demographics or cognitive performance at baseline was identified.

3.5. Mood before and after DBS.
Baseline mood assessment revealed high rates of anxiety disorder (n = 22, 56.4%), depression (n = 14, 35.9%), and apathy (n = 14, 38.9%) but no significant association between frequency of mood disorder and subsequent DBS location. There were also no significant differences in anxiety, depression, or apathy mean scores between the two surgery groups after DBS (Table 6). Case note review indicated mention of mood and/or motivation disorder in a high proportion of patients following DBS (STN: n = 17, 60.7%; GPi: n = 8, 66.7%), documented a mean of 23.16 months (SD = 18.09) after surgery. There was no significant association between DBS location and likelihood of mood disorder and no significant difference in time since surgery between the two DBS patient groups.

Incidence of case note indication of cognitive impairment or mood disorder, as a function of time, is depicted in Figure 1.

One patient also developed de novo impulse control disorder, namely, hypersexuality, after GPi DBS.

3.6. Predictors of Mood Disorder following DBS.
Patients who had subsequent mood disorder were found to have significantly higher baseline levels of depression (t(36.65) = −0 3.56, p < 0.01) and underwent a greater reduction in levodopa medication than those who did not (t(30) = −3.43, p < 0.01; Figure 2). There were no other significant baseline predictors of subsequent mood disorder, including DBS target.

Logistic regression confirmed these as significant predictors of subsequent mood disorder ($\chi^2(2) = 24.13$, p < 0.001), explaining 72.2% of the variance (Nagelkerke R^2). Significant and independent associations were found

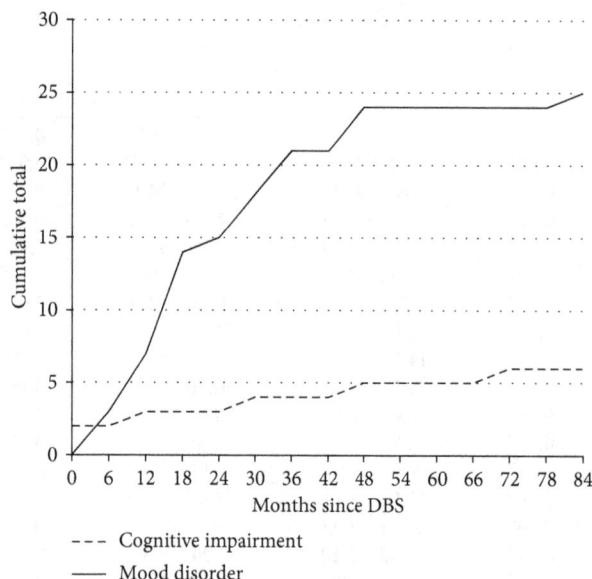

FIGURE 1: Cumulative cases of cognitive impairment and mood disorder as a function of time following DBS.

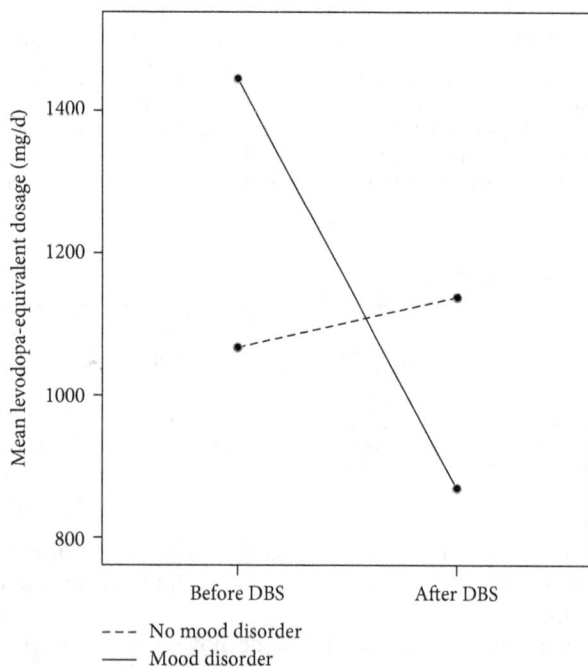

FIGURE 2: Mean levodopa-equivalent dosage of patients before and after DBS in patients split according to subsequent onset of mood disorder.

for both baseline depression ($p < 0.05$; odds ratio: 2.23; 95% confidence intervals: 1.17–4.25) and levodopa reduction ($p < 0.05$; odds ratio: 1.00; 95% confidence intervals: 1.00–1.00). Classification analysis revealed only one false negative.

The patient who developed impulse control disorder following GPi DBS did not experience a reduction in levodopa-equivalent dosage but rather an increase, with ongoing dopamine agonist treatment.

4. Discussion

Neuropsychological assessment is considered to be an important part of the screening for selection of candidates for DBS. However, to the best of our knowledge, no standardised assessment procedure currently exists, with many studies relying upon brief screening tools only. Neuropsychological screening should comprise tests with sufficient reliability and validity, which are sensitive to cognitive impairment and dementia in PD, able to disambiguate between PD and other disorders, including atypical Parkinsonian syndromes, and be sensitive to the changes in cognitive and mood functioning associated with DBS.

In this study, we examined the use of our standardised neuropsychological assessment in a sample of patients undergoing DBS for PD. Our assessment tested a wide range of neuropsychological domains, including general intellectual functioning, verbal and visual recognition and recall memory, language, visuoperceptual functioning, attention, verbal fluency, executive functioning, and speed of processing. The tests were all standardised, with adequate psychometric properties, easy to administer, and suitable for routine clinical services.

Our neuropsychological assessment was sensitive to the cognitive impairment found in PD. At baseline, we documented frequent impairments in intellectual functioning, memory, attention, and executive function, with more frequent impairments, as expected, in the GPi group. Indeed, only six of all DBS patients (15%) did not demonstrate impairment in at least one cognitive domain. Despite this only one patient demonstrated immediate and irreversible cognitive decline following DBS. This highlights the limitation of using the presence of any baseline cognitive impairment as an exclusionary criterion for DBS. As low test scores may reflect a number of cognitive and noncognitive variables, such as high levels of fatigue, low scores on any one test should not be used to preclude surgery.

Our neuropsychological assessment was also sensitive to the cognitive impairments that warrant caution before proceeding with DBS. In the patient who demonstrated immediate and irreversible global cognitive decline, single-case statistics revealed that this patient was significantly older than the mean age of those who remained stable and had greater deficits in language and visuoperceptual processing at baseline. Of course, this is a single case, and therefore, these results may not be generalizable, but this finding supports earlier reports that decline in cognitive functioning following DBS is more common in patients who are older [12, 28, 29, 34] and who have greater or more encompassing cognitive deficits at baseline [36, 68].

Although previous guidance on patient selection has tended to focus on memory impairment as a core contraindication for surgery [45, 124], PD patients often demonstrate patchy performance on tests of memory, likely reflecting the role of frontosubcortical-mediated cognition on memory functioning [107]. In our study, we observed common impairments in memory at baseline, but frank deficits in language and visuoperceptual processing were considerably less common and likely betrayed a greater level of general cognitive impairment. Previous guidance has warned that lower cognitive functioning at baseline is predictive of poorer cognitive outcome, but hitherto, there have been no recommendations on what level of impairment should constitute a contraindication to surgery. Our data suggest that, when using the present neuropsychological assessments, caution must be advised if any deficits are revealed in language and/or visuoperceptual processing (scores <5th percentiles), particularly in patients who are older and under consideration for STN DBS.

Previous studies describing negative cognitive outcomes following DBS may have failed to identify such risk factors because of insufficient scrutiny of baseline cognitive performance. Previous reports of immediate and global decline following DBS have often stated that such deterioration has occurred despite satisfactory performance on neuropsychological testing at baseline [11, 12]). Closer examination reveals that such testing has often been limited to a few screening measures of cognitive function (e.g., the MMSE) or focused on executive function, rather than explicitly assessing the presence of impairment in others, more atypical domains, such as language and visual processing. For example, York and colleagues [12] report the immediate and global cognitive decline in one gentleman aged 73 years but limit discussion of baseline cognitive performance to MMSE only, which was notably intact with a score of 28/30.

In keeping with this, our patient who demonstrated immediate and permanent cognitive decline performed flawlessly on the MMSE and performed poorly on only two out of four tests of executive function but demonstrated unexpected impairments, most clearly in language and visual perception. This underlines the importance of a broad neuropsychological assessment, interrogating a wide range of cognitive domains, to reveal the full cognitive profile.

Our neuropsychological assessment was also sensitive to the changes in cognitive functioning associated with DBS. Pre- and after DBS assessments revealed that alongside improvements in the motor status and medication load are noted in the STN group at least, and our assessment detected significant declines in verbal fluency in both groups following DBS. This confirms the mild changes frequently noted in this cognitive function following DBS [18, 35].

Although the exact cause of verbal fluency decline remains unclear, it has been linked with reductions in self-generation [18, 22]. Accordingly, the present study found that greater decline in verbal fluency was associated with higher levels of apathy at baseline. Although this did not persist after the Bonferroni adjustment for multiple comparisons, several studies have described increases in apathy following DBS [16, 18, 22, 60, 108–110]. Such behavioural adynamia, as witnessed by the reduced fluency and increased apathy, may in part relate to changes in cognitive speed [29]. We found that reduction in fluency was significantly associated with greater changes on at least one measure of speed of processing. These changes did not seem to simply reflect withdrawal of dopaminergic medication [111, 112], as although reductions in verbal fluency were related to higher levels of baseline levodopa dosage and there was no correlation with change in dosage following DBS. It has also

been suggested that the surgery itself may contribute to increases in apathy [60, 113], possibly caused by microlesions to the subthalamic area during implantation of the electrode [114].

Irrespective of the underlying mechanism, deterioration in verbal fluency can deleteriously affect activities of daily living and quality of life [115] and is correlated with reduced independence in everyday functional tasks [116]. Therefore, it is recommended that patients and their families are counselled about this significant risk before deciding to proceed with surgery, particularly those who present with higher levels of apathy at baseline.

In addition to this finding of reduced verbal fluency, our assessment detected declines in other aspects of cognitive functioning. Specifically, STN patients demonstrated significant slowing on the Symbol Search test and near-significant slowing on the Stroop and reduction in VIQ. GPi patients demonstrated significant reductions in PIQ. These findings confirm a slowing in the STN patients at least. In the absence of any other focal deficits, the heterogeneous reductions in performance on the WAIS (in both DBS groups) may also reflect the composite nature of this measure and the effortful, sustained, and speeded aspects of attentional functioning that it requires. Such reductions in speed of processing after DBS have rarely been discussed as most studies investigating cognitive changes have failed to include any measure of processing speed [115]. In previous studies, there have been conflicting reports of faster responding following STN DBS. However, further inspection suggests this may be due to a speed-accuracy trade-off [1, 117]. In our study, we have shown that deleterious changes in speed of processing are present, with likely important consequences for general intellectual functioning.

When considering the patients who went on to report cognitive decline at least a year after surgery (as identified by case note review), there were no significant predictors at baseline. This may suggest that the observed decline reflects the normal progression of the disease, rather than any preexisting vulnerability in the cognitive profile. It is important to recognise that the case note review was limited to qualitative and subjective comments only, precluding comment on the severity of any cognitive decline. However, the current findings do support previous studies which suggest that the risk of developing dementia following DBS is equivalent to that in medically treated patients [34, 118, 119]. This should be validated through future research that involves a medically treated control group.

Our study indicated no significant changes in mood or apathy, as measured by questionnaires, following DBS. However, case note review revealed a very high incidence of depression, anxiety, and/or apathy after surgery. These contrasting findings may be explained by the fact that assessment of mood relied upon self-reported symptoms of depression, anxiety, or depression, whereas case note review simply indicated clinicians' observations. Discrepancy between self- and proxy-ratings of mood in Parkinson's disease has been reported previously [45, 120, 125] and may be explained by patients' lack of insight and cognitive dysfunction [121].

Mood disorder emerging after DBS has been largely attributed to reduction in dopaminergic medications [111, 112]. Accordingly, we found that deterioration in mood was significantly correlated with reductions in levodopa medication, irrespective of DBS location. There was no association with discontinuation of dopamine agonists, suggesting that overall levodopa load was more important than the type of medication. These findings are in keeping with previous reports of mood disorder occurring as a nonmotor dopamine withdrawal syndrome after DBS [70, 112].

Furthermore, the chance of developing mood disorder, as identified in the case notes, was even higher in those who endorsed clinically significant levels of depression at baseline. This may suggest that those who have a preexisting vulnerability in mood are at high risk of developing profound mood disorder following DBS. Of course, the high incidence of mood disorder as noted in the case notes may simply reflect clinicians' recognition of (stable) low mood. However, its timing of onset and high incidence is consistent with several other studies [22, 59, 60, 122]. Therefore, we recommend careful and systematic longitudinal psychological follow-up for all PD DBS patients.

High levels of postoperative apathy or mood disorder can negate any improvement in quality of life [63, 126], but few studies have researched the presence of any baseline correlates of such decline. This study has found that a higher rating of depression at baseline is a predictor of poorer psychosocial outcome following DBS. We found high rates of depression, apathy, and anxiety in our patients at baseline, which may reflect elements of both reactive mood disorder and dysregulation of reward and motivation processing [123]. Indeed, previous research has suggested that mood disorder following DBS may reflect the effects of impaired extrastriatal dopaminergic pathways not sufficiently compensated for by STN stimulation [70]. Therefore, we would suggest that rather than excluding such patients from DBS, any dopamine withdrawal following surgery should be done cautiously.

One of our patients developed de novo impulse control disorder following GPi DBS. The onset of hypersexuality occurred in the context of increased levodopa dosages following surgery, with ongoing use of dopamine agonists. Our findings were of course limited to clinician ratings only and may have missed other cases. Future research should further investigate the incidence of impulse control disorder following DBS by using a semistructured interview, such as the QUIP [127]. Nevertheless, this case reflects the challenges of balancing treatment of motor and nonmotor symptoms in PD (cf. [128]).

4.1. Recommended Battery. Following our findings, we propose an abbreviated version of our neuropsychological protocol, suitable for routine clinical use. We recommend that this protocol includes our measures of current and premorbid intellectual functioning (prorated version of the WAIS-III, NART-R) to gauge overall level of intellectual decline; memory recognition and recall (RMT Words and Faces and D&P People and Shapes) to ensure cognitive profile is not amnestic and thus atypical for PD; language and visuoperceptual function (GNT and VOSP Silhouettes)

to detect the identified red flags for DBS; verbal fluency (DKEFS FAS and Category) and another measure of executive function (Stroop) to determine severity of executive dysfunction; speed of processing (Digit Symbol Coding and Symbol Search); and measures of mood and behavioural functioning, targeting depression, apathy (HADS and AES), and impulse control disorder (using a measure such as the QUIP). Of course, analysis of neuropsychological performance should consider any relevant cultural or linguistic factors, and it may be appropriate to replace some of the present neuropsychological assessments with suitable substitutions for specific populations.

5. Conclusion

This study has presented a standardised neuropsychological assessment procedure suitable for the selection of appropriate candidates with PD for DBS and identified clear baseline risk factors for subsequent decline in cognitive functioning and mood.

Acknowledgments

This work was undertaken at UCLH/UCL, which received a proportion of funding from the Department of Health's National Institute for Health Research Biomedical Research Centre's funding scheme. The Unit of Functional Neurosurgery, UCL Institute of Neurology, is supported by the Sainsbury Monument Trust and Parkinson's Appeal for Deep Brain Stimulation.

References

[1] M. Jahanshahi, C. M. A. Ardouin, R. G. Brown et al., "The impact of deep brain stimulation on executive function in Parkinson's disease," Brain, vol. 123, no. 6, pp. 1142–1154, 2000.

[2] M. S. Okun, R. L. Rodriguez, A. Mikos et al., "Deep brain stimulation and the role of the neuropsychologist," Clinical Neuropsychologist, vol. 21, no. 1, pp. 162–189, 2007.

[3] J. Massano and C. Garrett, "Deep brain stimulation and cognitive decline in Parkinson's disease: a clinical review," Frontiers in Neurology, vol. 3, pp. 1–13, 2002.

[4] M. S. Okun, M. Tagliati, M. Pourfar et al., "Management of referred deep brain stimulation failures: a retrospective analysis from two movement disorders centres," Archives of Neurology, vol. 65, no. 8, pp. 1250–1255, 2005.

[5] J. M. Bronstein, M. Tagliati, R. L. Alterman et al., "Deep brain stimulation for Parkinson's disease: an expert consensus and review of key issues," Archives of Neurology, vol. 68, no. 2, pp. 165–171, 2011.

[6] V. C. Anderson, K. J. Burchiel, P. Hogarth, J. Favre, and J. P. Hammerstad, "Pallidal vs subthalamic nucleus deep brain stimulation in Parkinson's disease," Archives of Neurology, vol. 62, no. 4, pp. 554–560, 2005.

[7] K. A. Follett, F. M. Weaver, M. Stern et al., "Pallidal versus subthalamic deep-brain stimulation for Parkinson's disease,"

New England Journal of Medicine, vol. 362, no. 22, pp. 2077–2091, 2010.

[8] L. L. Trépanier, R. Kumar, A. M. Lozano, A. E. Lang, and J. A. Saint-Cyr, "Neuropsychological outcome of GPi pallidotomy and GPi or STN deep brain stimulation in Parkinson's disease," *Brain and Cognition*, vol. 42, no. 3, pp. 324–347, 2000.

[9] V. J. J. Oderkerken, J. A. Boel, and B. A. Schmand, "GPi vs STN deep brain stimulation for Parkinson's disease: three-year follow-up," *Neurology*, vol. 86, no. 8, pp. 755–761, 2016.

[10] J. C. Rothlind, M. K. York, K. Carlson et al., "Neuropsychological changes following deep brain stimulation surgery for Parkinson's disease: comparisons of treatment at pallidal and subthalamic targets versus best medical therapy," *Journal of Neurology, Neurosurgery & Psychiatry*, vol. 86, no. 6, pp. 622–629, 2015.

[11] P. Krack, A. Batir, N. Van Blercom et al., "Five-year follow up of bilateral stimulation of the subthalamic nucleus in advanced Parkinson's disease," *New England Journal of Medicine*, vol. 349, no. 20, pp. 1925–1934, 2003.

[12] M. K. York, M. Dulay, A. Macias et al., "Cognitive declines following bilateral subthalamic nucleus deep brain stimulation for the treatment of Parkinson's disease," *Journal of Neurology, Neurosurgery and Psychiatry*, vol. 79, no. 7, pp. 789–795, 2008.

[13] M. Alegret, C. Junqué, F. Valldeoriola et al., "Effects of bilateral subthalamic stimulation on cognitive function in Parkinson's disease," *Archives of Neurology*, vol. 58, no. 8, pp. 1223–1227, 2001.

[14] A. Antonini, I. U. Isaias, G. Rodolfi, A. Landi, and F. Natuzzi, "A 5-year prospective assessment of advanced Parkinson's disease patients treated with subcutaneous apomorphine infusion or deep brain stimulation," *Journal of Neurology*, vol. 258, no. 4, pp. 579–585, 2011.

[15] C. Ardouin, B. Pillon, E. Peiffer et al., "Bilateral subthalamic or pallidal stimulation for Parkinson's disease affects neither memory nor executive functions: a consecutive series of 62 patients," *Annals of Neurology*, vol. 46, no. 2, pp. 217–223, 1999.

[16] L. Castelli, M. Lanotte, M. Zibetti et al., "Apathy and verbal fluency in STN-stimulated PD patients: an observational follow-up study," *Journal of Neurology*, vol. 254, no. 9, pp. 1238–1243, 2007.

[17] A. Daniele, A. Albanese, M. F. Contarino et al., "Cognitive and behavioural effects of chronic stimulation of the subthalamic nucleus in patients with Parkinson's disease," *Journal of Neurology, Neurosurgery and Psychiatry*, vol. 74, no. 2, pp. 175–182, 2003.

[18] D. De Gaspari, C. Siri, M. Di Dioia et al., "Clinical correlates and cognitive underpinnings of verbal fluency impairment after chronic subthalamic stimulation in Parkinson's disease," *Parkinsonism and Related Disorders*, vol. 12, no. 5, pp. 289–295, 2006.

[19] K. Dujardin, P. Krystokowiak, L. Defebvre, S. Blond, and A. Destée, "A case of severe dysexecutive syndrome consecutive to chronic bilateral pallidal stimulation," *Neuropsychologia*, vol. 38, no. 9, pp. 1305–1315, 2000.

[20] K. Dujardin, L. Defebvre, P. Krystkowiak, S. Blond, and A. Destée, "Influence of chronic bilateral stimulation of the subthalamic nucleus on cognitive function in Parkinson's disease," *Journal of Neurology*, vol. 248, no. 7, pp. 603–611, 2001.

[21] K. Dujardin, S. Blairy, L. Defebvre et al., "Subthalamic nucleus stimulation induces deficits in decoding emotional facial expressions in Parkinson's disease," *Journal of Neurology, Neurosurgery and Psychiatry*, vol. 75, no. 2, pp. 202–208, 2004.

[22] A. Funkiewiez, C. Ardouin, E. Caputo et al., "Long term effects of bilateral subthalamic nucleus stimulation on cognitive function, mood, and behaviour in Parkinson's disease," *Journal of Neurology, Neurosurgery and Psychiatry*, vol. 75, no. 6, pp. 834–839, 2004.

[23] J. Ghika, J.-G. Villemure, H. Fankhauser, J. Favre, G. Assal, and F. Ghika-Schmid, "Efficiency and safety of bilateral contemporaneous pallidal stimulation (deep brain stimulation) in levodopa-responsive patients with Parkinson's disease with severe motor fluctuations: a two-year follow-up review," *Journal of Neurosurgery*, vol. 89, no. 5, pp. 713–718, 1998.

[24] A. Gironell, J. Kulisevsky, L. Rami et al., "Effects of pallidotomy and bilateral subthalamic stimulation on cognitive function in Parkinson disease: a controlled comparative study," *Journal of Neurology*, vol. 250, no. 8, pp. 917–923, 2003.

[25] R. Moretti, P. Torre, R. M. Antonello et al., "Neuropsychological changes after subthalamic nucleus stimulation: a 12 month follow-up in nine patients with Parkinson's disease," *Parkinsonism and Related Disorders*, vol. 10, no. 2, pp. 73–79, 2003.

[26] C. E. Morrison, J. C. Borod, K. Perrine et al., "Neuropsychological functioning following bilateral subthalamic nucleus stimulation in Parkinson's disease," *Archives of Clinical Neuropsychology*, vol. 19, no. 2, pp. 165–181, 2004.

[27] B. Pillon, C. Ardouin, P. Danier et al., "Neuropsychological changes between "off" and "on" STN or GPi stimulation in Parkinson's disease," *Neurology*, vol. 55, no. 3, pp. 411–418, 2000.

[28] J. A. Saint-Cyr, L. L. Trépanier, R. Kumar, A. M. Lozano, and A. E. Lang, "Neuropsychological consequences of chronic bilateral stimulation of the subthalamic nucleus in Parkinson's disease," *Brain*, vol. 123, no. 10, pp. 2091–2108, 2000.

[29] H. M. M. Smeding, J. D. Speelman, H. M. Huizenga, P. R. Schuurman, and B. Schmand, "Predictors of cognitive and psychosocial outcome after STN DBS in Parkinson's disease," *Journal of Neurology, Neurosurgery and Psychiatry*, vol. 82, no. 7, pp. 754–760, 2011.

[30] A. I. Tröster, S. P. Woods, J. A. Fields, C. Hanisch, and W. W. Beatty, "Declines in switching underlie verbal fluency changes after unilateral pallidal surgery in Parkinson's disease," *Brain and Cognition*, vol. 50, no. 2, pp. 207–217, 2002.

[31] H. Russmann, J. Ghika, J. G. Villemure et al., "Subthalamic nucleus deep brain stimulation in Parkinson disease patients over age 70 years," *Neurology*, vol. 63, no. 10, pp. 1952–1954, 2004.

[32] M. Tagliati, J. Miravite, A. Koss, J. Shils, and R. L. Alterman, "Is advanced age a poor predictor of motor outcome for subthalamic DBS in Parkinson's disease?," *Neurology*, vol. 62, pp. A395–A396, 2004.

[33] M. Tagliati, M. H. Pourfar, and R. L. Alterman, "Subthalamic nucleus deep brain stimulation in Parkinson disease patient over age 70 years," *Neurology*, vol. 65, pp. 179–180, 2000.

[34] S. Aybek, A. Gronchi-Perrin, A. Berney et al., "Long-term cognitive profile and incidence of dementia after STN-DBS in Parkinson's disease," *Movement Disorders*, vol. 22, no. 7, pp. 974–981, 2007.

[35] S. P. Woods, J. A. Fields, and A. I. Troster, "Neuropsychological sequelae of subthalamic nucleus deep brain

stimulation in Parkinson's disease: a critical review," *Neuropsychological Review*, vol. 12, no. 2, pp. 111–126, 2002.

[36] A. E. Lang and H. Widner, "Deep brain stimulation for Parkinson's disease: patient selection and evaluation," *Movement Disorders*, vol. 17, no. 3, pp. S94–S101, 2002.

[37] R. L. Rodriguez, H. H. Fernandez, I. Haq, and M. S. Okun, "Pearls in patient selection for deep brain stimulation," *Neurologist*, vol. 13, no. 5, pp. 253–260, 2007.

[38] A. E. Lang, J.-L. Houeto, P. Krack et al., "Deep brain stimulation: preoperative issues," *Movement Disorders*, vol. 21, no. 14, pp. S171–S196, 2006.

[39] British Psychological Society, *Psychological Services for People with Parkinson's Disease*, British Psychological Society, Leicester, UK, 2009.

[40] P. Silberstein, R. G. Bittar, R. Boyle et al., "Deep brain stimulation for Parkinson's disease: Australian referral guidelines," *Journal of Clinical Neuroscience*, vol. 16, no. 8, pp. 1001–1008, 2009.

[41] M. Folstein, S. E. Folstein, and P. R. McHugh, ""Mini-mental state" a practical method for grading cognitive state of patients for the clinician," *Journal of Psychiatric Research*, vol. 12, no. 3, pp. 189–198, 1975.

[42] C. A. Bouquet, V. Bonnaud, and R. Gil, "Investigation of supervisory attentional system functions in patients with Parkinson's disease using the Hayling Task," *Journal of Clinical and Experimental Neuropsychology*, vol. 25, no. 6, pp. 751–760, 2003.

[43] R. Cools, R. Rogers, R. A. Barker, and T. W. Robbins, "Top-down attentional control in Parkinson's disease: salient considerations," *Journal of Cognitive Neuroscience*, vol. 22, no. 5, pp. 848–859, 2010.

[44] J. D. E. Gabrieli, J. Singh, G. T. Stebbins, and C. G. Goetz, "Reduced working memory span in Parkinson's disease: Evidence for the role of frontostriatal system in working and strategic memory," *Neuropsychology*, vol. 10, no. 3, pp. 322–332, 1996.

[45] A. McKinlay, R. C. Grace, J. C. Dalrymple-Alford, and D. Roger, "Characteristics of executive function impairment in Parkinson's disease patients without dementia," *Journal of the International Neuropsychological Society*, vol. 16, no. 2, pp. 268–277, 2010.

[46] A. M. Owen, A. C. Roberts, J. R. Hodges, B. A. Summers, C. E. Polkey, and T. W. Robbins, "Contrasting mechanisms of impaired attentional set-shifting in patients with frontal lobe damage or Parkinson's disease," *Brain*, vol. 116, no. 5, pp. 1159–1175, 1993.

[47] C. H. Williams-Gray, A. Hampshire, R. A. Barker, and A. M. Owen, "Attentional control in Parkinson's disease is dependent on COMT val158 met genotype," *Brain*, vol. 131, no. 2, pp. 397–408, 2008.

[48] J. Uekermann, I. Daum, M. Bielawski et al., "Differential executive control impairments in early Parkinson's disease," in *Focus on Extrapyramidal Dysfunction*, T. Müller and P. Riederer, Eds., pp. 39–51, Springer-Verlag GmbH, Berlin, Germany, 2004.

[49] M. Grossman, E. Surif, C. Lee et al., "Information processing speed and sentence comprehension in Parkinson's disease," *Neuropsychology*, vol. 16, no. 2, pp. 174–181, 2002.

[50] A. M. Johnson, Q. J. Almeida, C. Stough et al., "Visual inspection time in Parkinson's disease: deficits in early stages of cognitive processing," *Neuropsychologia*, vol. 42, no. 5, pp. 577–583, 2004.

[51] J. G. Phillips, T. Schiffter, M. E. Nicholls, J. L. Bradshaw, R. Iansek, and L. L. Saling, "Does old age or Parkinson's disease cause bradyphrenia?," *Journals of Gerontology Series A: Biomedical Sciences and Medical Sciences*, vol. 54, no. 8, pp. M404–M409, 1999.

[52] B. A. Shipley, I. J. Deary, J. Tan, G. Christie, and J. M. Starr, "Efficiency of temporal order discrimination as an indicator of bradyphrenia in Parkinson's disease: the inspection time loop task," *Neuropsychologia*, vol. 40, no. 8, pp. 1488–1493, 2002.

[53] E. Mamikonyan, P. J. Moberg, A. Siderowf et al., "Mild cognitive impairment is common in Parkinson's disease patients with normal Mini-Mental State Examination (MMSE) scores," *Parkinsonism & Related Disorders*, vol. 15, no. 3, pp. 226–231, 2009.

[54] C. Zadikoff, S. H. Fox, D. F. Tang-Wai et al., "A comparison of the mini mental state exam to the Montreal cognitive assessment in identifying cognitive deficits in Parkinson's disease," *Movement Disorders*, vol. 23, no. 2, pp. 297–299, 2008.

[55] S. Hoops, S. Nazem, A. D. Siderowf et al., "Validity of the MoCA and MMSE in the detection of MCI and dementia in Parkinson disease," *Neurology*, vol. 73, no. 21, pp. 1738–1745, 2009.

[56] L. J. Launer, M. A. Dinkgreve, C. Jonker, C. Hooijer, and J. Lindeboom, "Are age and education independent correlates of the Mini-Mental State Exam performance of community-dwelling elderly?," *Journal of Gerontology*, vol. 48, no. 6, pp. P271–P277, 1993.

[57] T. N. Tombaugh and N. J. McIntyre, "The mini-mental state examination: a comprehensive review," *Journal of the American Geriatrics Society*, vol. 40, no. 9, pp. 922–935, 1992.

[58] P. Limousin and I. Martinez-Torres, "Deep brain stimulation for Parkinson's disease," *Neurotherapeutics*, vol. 5, no. 2, pp. 309–319, 2008.

[59] D. Drapier, S. Drapier, P. Sauleau et al., "Does subthalamic nucleus stimulation induce apathy in Parkinson's disease?," *Journal of Neurology*, vol. 253, no. 8, pp. 1083–1091, 2006.

[60] F. Le Jeune, D. Drapier, A. Bourguignon et al., "Subthalamic nucleus stimulation in Parkinson's disease induces apathy: a PET study," *Neurology*, vol. 73, no. 21, pp. 1746–1751, 2009.

[61] S. E. Starkstein and S. Brockman, "Apathy and Parkinson's disease," *Current Treatment Options in Neurology*, vol. 13, no. 3, pp. 267–273, 2011.

[62] A. Berney, F. Vingerhoets, A. Perrin et al., "Effect on mood of subthalamic DBS for Parkinson's disease: a consecutive series of 24 patients," *Neurology*, vol. 59, no. 9, pp. 1427–1429, 2002.

[63] V. Voon, P. Krack, A. E. Lang et al., "A multicentre study on suicide outcomes following subthalamic stimulation for Parkinson's disease," *Brain*, vol. 131, no. 10, pp. 2720–2728, 2008.

[64] R. Martinez-Fernandez, P. Pelissier, J.-L. Quesada et al., "Postoperative apathy can neutralise benefits in quality of life after subthalamic stimulation for Parkinson's disease," *Journal of Neurology, Neurosurgery and Psychiatry*, vol. 87, no. 3, pp. 311–318, 2015.

[65] P. R. Burkhard, F. J. G. Vingerhoets, A. Berney et al., "Suicide after successful deep brain stimulation for movement disorders," *Neurology*, vol. 63, no. 11, pp. 2170–2172, 2004.

[66] V. Voon, J. A. Saint-Cyr, A. M. Lozano, E. Moro, K. Dujardin, and A. E. Lang, "Suicide risk in patients with Parkinson's disease undergoing subthalamic stimulation," *Movement Disorders*, vol. 19, p. S323, 2004.

[67] E. Bell, B. Maxwell, M. P. McAndrews, A. F. Sadikot, and E. Racine, "A review of social and relational aspects of deep brain stimulation in Parkinson's disease informed by

healthcare provider experiences," *Parkinson's Disease*, vol. 2011, Article ID 871874, 8 pages, 2011.

[68] M. S. Okun, S. S. Wu, K. D. Foote et al., "Do stable patients with a premorbid depression history have a worse outcome after deep brain stimulation for Parkinson's disease?," *Neurosurgery*, vol. 69, no. 2, pp. 357–361, 2011.

[69] T. Stefurak, D. Mikulis, H. Mayberg et al., "Deep brain stimulation for Parkinson's disease dissociates mood and motor circuits: a functional MRI case study," *Movement Disorders*, vol. 18, no. 12, pp. 1508–1516, 2003.

[70] J. L. Houeto, V. Mesnage, L. Mallet et al., "Behavioural disorders, Parkinson's disease and subthalamic stimulation," *Journal of Neurology, Neurosurgery and Psychiatry*, vol. 72, no. 6, pp. 701–707, 2002.

[71] J. Herzog, J. Volkmann, P. Krack et al., "Two-year follow-up of subthalamic deep brain stimulation in Parkinson's disease," *Movement Disorder*, vol. 18, no. 11, pp. 1332–1337, 2003.

[72] D. Wechsler, *WAIS-III*, Psychological Corporation, San Antonio, TX, USA, 1997.

[73] M. J. Taylor and R. K. Heaton, "Sensitivity and specificity of WAIS-III/WMS-III demographically corrected factor scores in neuropsychological assessment," *Journal of the International Neuropsychological Society*, vol. 7, no. 7, pp. 867–874, 2001.

[74] J. Zhu, D. S. Tulsky, L. Price, and H. Y. Chen, "WAIS-III reliability data for clinical groups," *Journal of the International Neuropsychological Society*, vol. 7, no. 7, pp. 862–866, 2001.

[75] H. E. Nelson, *National Adult Reading Test*, NFER-Nelson, Windsor, UK, 1982.

[76] E. K. Warrington, *Recognition Memory Test: RMT*, NFER-Nelson, Windsor, UK, 1984.

[77] C. M. Bird, K. Papadopoulou, P. Ricciardelli, M. N. Rossor, and L. Cipolotti, "Test-retest reliability, practice effects and reliable change indices for the recognition memory test," *British Journal of Clinical Psychology*, vol. 42, no. 4, pp. 407–425, 2003.

[78] V. M. Soukup, A. Bimbela, and M. C. Schiess, "Recognition memory for faces: reliability and validity of the Warrington Recognition Memory Test (RMT) in a neurological sample," *Journal of Clinical Psychology in Medical Settings*, vol. 6, no. 3, pp. 287–293, 1999.

[79] A. D. Baddeley, H. Emslie, and I. Nimmo-Smith, *Doors and People: A Test of Visual and Verbal Recall and Recognition*, Thames Valley Test Company, Bury St Edmunds, UK, 1994.

[80] C. Davis, C. M. Bradshaw, and E. Szabadi, "The doors and people memory test: validation of norms and some new correction formulae," *British Journal of Clinical Psychology*, vol. 38, no. 3, pp. 305–314, 1999.

[81] C. Metzler-Baddeley, "A review of cognitive impairments in dementia with Lewy bodies relative to Alzheimer's disease and Parkinson's disease with dementia," *Cortex*, vol. 43, no. 5, pp. 583–600, 2007.

[82] P. McKenna and E. K. Warrington, *The Graded Naming Test*, NFER-Nelson, Windsor, UK, 1983.

[83] C. M. Bird and L. Cipolotti, "The utility of the recognition memory test and the graded naming test for monitoring neurological patients," *British Journal of Clinical Psychology*, vol. 46, no. 2, pp. 223–234, 2007.

[84] T. A. Hughes, H. F. Ross, S. Musa et al., "A 10-year study of the incidence of and factors predicting dementia in Parkinson's disease," *Neurology*, vol. 54, no. 8, pp. 1596–1603, 2000.

[85] E. K. Warrington and M. James, *The Visual Object and Space Perception Battery*, Thames Valley Test Company, Bury St Edmunds, UK, 1991.

[86] L. J. Rapport, S. R. Millis, and P. J. Bonello, "Validation of the Warrington theory of visual processing and the visual object and space perception battery," *Journal of Clinical and Experimental Neuropsychology*, vol. 20, no. 2, pp. 211–220, 1998.

[87] J. Barnes, L. Boubert, J. Harris, A. Lee, and A. S. David, "Reality monitoring and visual hallucinations in Parkinson's disease," *Neuropsychologia*, vol. 41, no. 5, pp. 565–574, 2003.

[88] T. H. Bak, D. Caine, V. C. Hearn, and J. R. Hodges, "Visuospatial functions in atypical Parkinsonian syndromes," *Journal of Neurology, Neurosurgery & Psychiatry*, vol. 77, no. 4, pp. 454–456, 2006.

[89] I. H. Robertson, T. Ward, V. Ridgeway, and I. Nimmo-Smith, *The Test of Everyday Attention: TEA*, Thames Valley Test Company, Bury St Edmunds, UK, 1994.

[90] J. Calderon, R. J. Perry, S. W. Erzinclioglu et al., "Perception, attention, and working memory are disproportionately impaired in dementia with Lewy bodies compared with Alzheimer's disease," *Journal of Neurology, Neurosurgery & Psychiatry*, vol. 70, no. 2, pp. 157–164, 2001.

[91] D. C. Delis, E. Kaplan, and J. H. Kramer, *Delis–Kaplan Executive Function System*, Psychological Corporation, San Antonio, TX, USA, 2001.

[92] S. Homack, D. Lee, and C. A. Riccio, "Test review: Delis–Kaplan executive function system," *Journal of clinical and experimental neuropsychology*, vol. 27, no. 5, pp. 599–609, 2005.

[93] M. R. Trenerry, B. Crosson, J. DeBoe, and W. R. Lebere, *Stroop Neuropsychological Screening Test*, Psychological Assessment Resources, Odessa, FL, USA, 1989.

[94] G. P. Strauss, D. N. Allen, M. L. Jorgensen, and S. L. Cramer, "Test-retest reliability of standard and emotional Stroop tasks: an investigation of color-word and picture-word versions," *Assessment*, vol. 12, no. 3, pp. 330–337, 2005.

[95] A. Henik, J. Singh, D. J. Beckley, and R. D. Rafal, "Disinhibition of automatic word reading in Parkinson's disease," *Cortex*, vol. 29, no. 4, pp. 589–599, 1993.

[96] P. W. Burgess and T. Shallice, *The Hayling and Brixton Tests*, Thames Valley Test Company, Bury St Edmunds, UK, 1997.

[97] L. Cipolotti, B. Spanò, C. Healy et al., "Inhibition processes are dissociable and lateralized in human prefrontal cortex," *Neuropsychologia*, vol. 93, pp. 1–12, 2016.

[98] P. W. Halligan and D. T. Wade, *The Effectiveness of Rehabilitation for Cognitive Deficits*, Oxford University Press, New York, NY, USA, 2005.

[99] I. Obeso, L. Wilkinson, E. Casabona et al., "Deficits in inhibitory control and conflict resolution on cognitive and motor tasks in Parkinson's disease," *Experimental Brain Research*, vol. 212, no. 3, pp. 371–384, 2011.

[100] L. Yáguez, A. Costello, J. Moriarty et al., "Cognitive predictors of cognitive change following bilateral subthalamic nucleus deep brain stimulation in Parkinson's disease," *Journal of Clinical Neuroscience*, vol. 21, no. 3, pp. 445–450, 2014.

[101] D. Muslimović, B. Post, J. D. Speelman, R. J. De Haan, and B. Schmand, "Cognitive decline in Parkinson's disease: a prospective longitudinal study," *Journal of the International Neuropsychological Society*, vol. 15, no. 3, pp. 426–437, 2009.

[102] A. S. Zigmond and R. P. Snaith, "The hospital anxiety and depression scale," *Acta Psychiatrica Scandinavica*, vol. 67, no. 6, pp. 361–370, 1983.

[103] R. S. Marin, R. C. Biedrzycki, and S. Fririnciogullari, "Reliability and validity of the apathy evaluation scale," *Psychiatry Research*, vol. 38, no. 2, pp. 143–162, 1991.

[104] J. Marinus, C. Ramaker, J. J. van Hilten, and A. M. Stiggelbout, "Health related quality of life in Parkinson's disease: a systematic review of disease specific instruments," *Journal of Neurology, Neurosurgery & Psychiatry*, vol. 72, no. 2, pp. 241–248, 2002.

[105] G. C. Pluck and R. G. Brown, "Apathy in Parkinson's disease," *Journal of Neurology, Neurosurgery & Psychiatry*, vol. 73, no. 6, pp. 636–642, 2002.

[106] J. R. Crawford and D. C. Howell, "Comparing and individual's test score against norms derived from small samples," *Clinical Neuropsychologist*, vol. 12, no. 4, pp. 482–486, 1998.

[107] L. B. Zahodne, D. Bowers, C. C. Price et al., "The case for testing memory with both stories and word lists prior to DBS surgery for Parkinson's disease," *Clinical Neuropsychology*, vol. 25, no. 3, pp. 348–358, 2011.

[108] A. L. Benabid, S. Chabardes, J. Mitrofanis, and P. Pollak, "Deep brain stimulation of the subthalamic nucleus for the treatment of Parkinson's disease," *The Lancet Neurology*, vol. 8, no. 1, pp. 67–81, 2009.

[109] F. Ory-Magne, C. Brefel-Courbon, M. Simonetta-Moreau et al., "Does ageing influence deep brain stimulation outcomes in Parkinson's disease?," *Movement Disorders*, vol. 22, no. 10, pp. 1457–1463, 2007.

[110] O. Porat, O. S. Cohen, R. Schwartz, and S. Hassin-Baer, "Association of preoperative symptom profile with psychiatric symptoms following subthalamic nucleus stimulation in patients with Parkinson's disease," *Journal of Neuropsychiatry and Clinical Neurosciences*, vol. 21, no. 4, pp. 398–405, 2009.

[111] V. Czernecki, M. Schüpbach, S. Yaici et al., "Apathy following subthalamic stimulation in Parkinson disease: a dopamine responsive symptom," *Movement Disorders*, vol. 23, no. 7, pp. 964–969, 2008.

[112] S. Thobois, C. Ardouin, E. Lhommée et al., "Non-motor dopamine withdrawal syndrome after surgery for Parkinson's disease: predictors and underlying mesolimbic denervation," *Brain*, vol. 133, no. 4, pp. 1111–1127, 2010.

[113] P. K. Doshi, N. Chhaya, and M. H. Bhatt, "Depression leading to attempted suicide after bilateral subthalamic nucleus stimulation for Parkinson's disease," *Movement Disorders*, vol. 17, no. 5, pp. 1084-1085, 2002.

[114] P. P. Derost, L. Ouchchane, D. Morand et al., "Is DBS-STN appropriate to treat severe Parkinson's disease in an elderly population?," *Neurology*, vol. 68, no. 17, pp. 1345–1355, 2007.

[115] T. D. Parsons, S. A. Rogers, A. J. Braaten, S. P. Woods, and A. I. Tröster, "Cognitive sequelae of subthalamic nucleus deep brain stimulation in Parkinson's disease: a meta-analysis," *The Lancet Neurology*, vol. 5, no. 7, pp. 578–588, 2006.

[116] D. A. Cahn-Weiner, P. A. Boyle, and P. F. Malloy, "Tests of executive function predict instrumental activities of daily living in community-dwelling older individuals," *Applied Neuropsychology*, vol. 9, no. 3, pp. 187–191, 2002.

[117] M. Jahanshahi, I. Obeso, C. Baunez, M. Alegre, and P. Krack, "Parkinson's disease, the subthalamic nucleus, inhibition and impulsivity," *Movement Disorders*, vol. 30, no. 2, pp. 128–140, 2015.

[118] A. E. Williams, G. Marina Arzola, A. M. Strutt, R. Simpson, J. Jankovic, and M. K. York, "Cognitive outcome and reliable change indices two years following bilateral subthalamic nucleus deep brain stimulation," *Parkinsonism and Related Disorders*, vol. 17, no. 5, pp. 321–327, 2011.

[119] W. M. N. Schuepbach, J. Rau, K. Knudsen et al., "Neurostimulation for Parkinson's disease with early motor complications," *New England Journal of Medicine*, vol. 368, no. 7, pp. 610–622, 2013.

[120] M. S. Duenas and M. S. Serrano, "The incongruities of the NPI-Q score obtained by the caregiver versus that obtained directly from the non-demented patient with Parkinson's disease," *Revista Ecuatoriana De Neurologia*, vol. 16, p. 12, 2007.

[121] W. Fitts, D. Weintraub, L. Massimo et al., "Caregiver report of apathy predicts dementia in Parkinson's disease," *Parkinsonism and Related Disorders*, vol. 21, no. 8, pp. 992–995, 2015.

[122] M. S. Okun, H. H. Fernandez, S. Wu et al., "Cognition and mood in Parkinson's disease in STN versus GPi DBS: the COMPARE trial," *Annals of Neurology*, vol. 65, no. 5, pp. 586–595, 2009.

[123] C. Vriend, T. Pattij, Y. D. van der Werf et al., "Depression and impulse control disorders in Parkinson's disease: two sides of the same coin?," *Neuroscience & Biobehavioral Reviews*, vol. 38, pp. 60–71, 2014.

[124] M. S. Okun, H. H. Fernandez, R. L. Rodriguez, and K. D. Foote, "Identifying candidates for deep brain stimulation in Parkinson's disease: the role of the primary care physician," *Geriatrics*, vol. 62, no. 5, pp. 18–24, 2004.

[125] A. McKinlay, R. C. Grace, J. C. Dalrymple-Alford, T. J. Anderson, J. Fink, and D. Roger, "Neuropsychiatric problems in Parkinson's disease: comparisons between self and caregiver report," *Aging & Mental Health*, vol. 12, no. 5, pp. 647–653, 2008.

[126] L. Kirsch-Darrow, L. B. Zahodne, M. Marsiske, M. S. Okun, K. D. Foote, and D. Bowers, "The trajectory of apathy after deep brain stimulation: from pre-surgery to 6 months post-surgery in Parkinson's disease," *Parkinsonism and Related Disorders*, vol. 17, no. 3, pp. 182–188, 2011.

[127] D. Weintraub, E. Mamikonyan, K. Papay, J. A. Shea, S. X. Xie, and A. Siderowf, "Questionnaire for impulsive-compulsive disorders in Parkinson's disease-rating scale," *Movement Disorders*, vol. 27, no. 2, pp. 242–247, 2011.

[128] E. Lhommée, H. Klinger, S. Thobois et al., "Subthalamic stimulation in Parkinson's disease: restoring the balance of motivated behaviours," *Brain*, vol. 135, no. 5, pp. 1463–1477, 2012.

The Sources of Reactive Oxygen Species and Its Possible Role in the Pathogenesis of Parkinson's Disease

Minrui Weng,[1] Xiaoji Xie,[1] Chao Liu,[2] Kah-Leong Lim,[2] Cheng-wu Zhang ⓘ,[1] and Lin Li ⓘ[1]

[1]*Key Laboratory of Flexible Electronics (KLOFE) & Institute of Advanced Materials (IAM), Jiangsu National Synergetic Innovation Center for Advanced Materials (SICAM), Nanjing Tech University (Nanjing Tech), 30 South Puzhu Road, Nanjing 211816, China*
[2]*Department of Physiology, Yong Loo Lin School of Medicine, National University of Singapore, Singapore,117593*

Correspondence should be addressed to Cheng-wu Zhang; iamcwzhang@njtech.edu.cn and Lin Li; iamlli@njtech.edu.cn

Academic Editor: Giuseppina Martella

Parkinson's disease (PD) is the second most common neurodegenerative disorder characterized by progressive loss of dopaminergic neurons in the substantia nigra. The precise mechanism underlying pathogenesis of PD is not fully understood, but it has been widely accepted that excessive reactive oxygen species (ROS) are the key mediator of PD pathogenesis. The causative factors of PD such as gene mutation, neuroinflammation, and iron accumulation all could induce ROS generation, and the later would mediate the dopaminergic neuron death by causing oxidation protein, lipids, and other macromolecules in the cells. Obviously, it is of mechanistic and therapeutic significance to understand where ROS are derived and how ROS induce dopaminergic neuron damage. In the present review, we try to summarize and discuss the main source of ROS in PD and the key pathways through which ROS mediate DA neuron death.

1. Introduction

Parkinson's disease (PD) is an age-dependent, progressive neurodegenerative disease, characterized by selective loss of dopaminergic (DA) neurons residing in an area of the midbrain known as the substantia nigra [1, 2]. As the second most common neurodegenerative disease, PD remains incurable, which might be underlined by the fact that mechanism for PD pathogenesis is not fully illustrated.

With the intensive studies, it is now widely accepted that genetic background, environment factors, and aging are the key contributors of PD pathogenesis. In recent years, some PD-associated genes have been identified, including α-synuclein (SNCA), PTEN-induced putative kinase 1 (PINK1), parkin, DJ-1 (PARK7), and leucine rich repeat kinase 2 (LRRK2), mutations of which lead to the familial forms of PD (early-onset) [3]. Even in the rest of 90% of the sporadic cases of PD, mutations of those genes could also increase the PD susceptibility [4]. Environmental factors such as heavy metals, drugs, and exposure to neurotoxic compounds can induce PD via interfering dopamine transporter activity, dopamine metabolism, mitochondrial function, and proteasome activity [5–7]. Aging could result in misfolding of proteins as well as mitochondrial dysfunction, which are all closely related to the PD pathogenesis [8]. Although the underlying mechanisms of neuronal degeneration in PD remain to be better understood, it is well established that all of the PD-related factors mentioned above can cause excessive generation of ROS [9].

ROS, as the by-products of cellular metabolism, are defined as a group of reactive molecules derived from molecular oxygen, which include superoxide anion (O_2^-), hydroxyl radical ($\cdot OH$), and hydrogen peroxide (H_2O_2) [10]. ROS are essential for maintaining many physiological processes such as apoptosis, autophagy, and immunological defense [11]. But if the balance between production and elimination of ROS is disturbed, pathogenic consequences such as neurodegeneration would happen [12].

In this review, we will focus on discussing how the PD-associated factors induce ROS generation and how ROS lead to dopaminergic neuron death in PD (Figure 1).

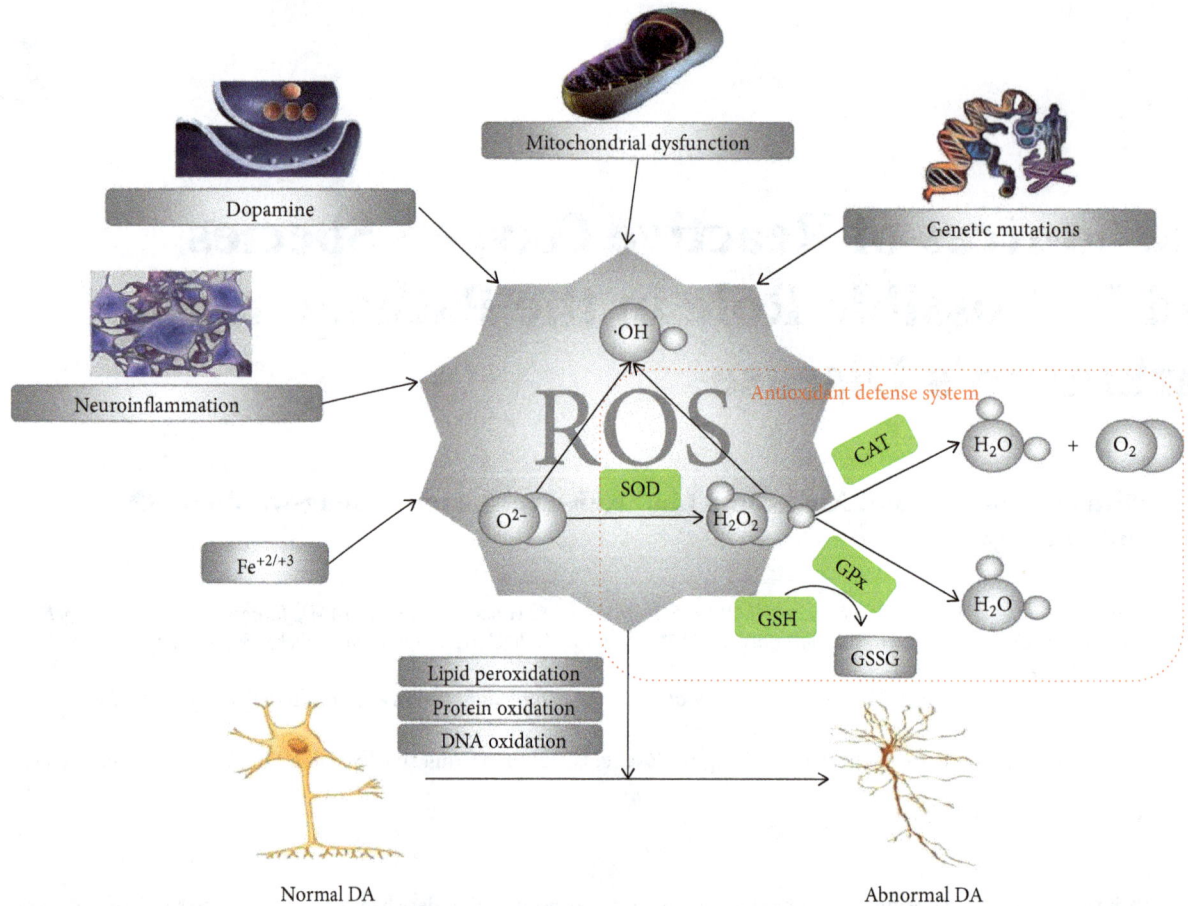

FIGURE 1: Schematic pathway of ROS generation and induction of DA neurons death. Mitochondria dysfunction, dopamine, neuro-inflammation, iron, and genetic mutations solely or synergistically induce ROS generation, which could induce dopaminergic neurons death via protein, lipid, and DNA oxidation.

2. ROS and PD-Associated Factors

Numerous evidences suggest that PD-associated factors such as genes mutation, mitochondrial dysfunction, dopamine auto-oxidation, neuroinflammation, iron accumulation, and external toxicants accumulation, all could induce ROS generation.

2.1. PD-Related Genetic Mutations and ROS. It has been recognized that the genetic mutations such as α-synuclein, PINK1, parkin, DJ-1, and LRRK2 are causative factors of the familial forms of PD [13, 14]. Mutation or multiplication of the α-synuclein gene facilitates the accumulation of α-synuclein, which is a major component of Lewy bodies, the pathological hallmark of PD [15]. It was indicated that accumulation of α-synuclein caused oxidative stress by two parallel pathways: directly stimulating the generation of excessive ROS or indirectly interfering scavenge of damaged mitochondria from which majority of ROS were derived [16, 17]. PINK1 is the kinase that could phosphorylate and activate parkin in the process of damaged mitochondria clearance by autophagy, which exerts neuroprotection against ROS overproduction [18]. It was reported that loss of

PINK1 or parkin induced mitochondrial dysfunction and consequent overproduction of ROS, while overexpression of PINK1 or parkin protected against ROS-induced cell death [19, 20]. Parkin is an E3 ubiquitin ligase, and loss of function leads to autosomal recessive PD [21]. Mutation of parkin impairs its function in the elimination of damaged mitochondria, the latter generated ROS [22]. DJ-1 is a small compact protein that localized on the outer mitochondrial membrane (OMM). The sulfhydryl group of DJ-1 could react with ROS to form the cysteine sulfinic acid, which functions as a ROS quencher [23]. Loss of DJ-1 renders increased ROS levels and ultimately caused dopaminergic neuron death [19]. LRRK2 is a large multidomain protein and its mutation leads to autosomal dominant PD. A proposed mechanism for the increased vulnerability of LRRK2 mutant cells to oxidative stress is via the kinase-dependent interaction between LRRK2 and dynamin-like protein (DLP1), which facilitates DLP1 translocation to mitochondria and subsequent mitochondrial fission [24, 25]. Another mechanism is through the interaction of LRRK2 with peroxiredoxin 3 (PRDX3), which is a mitochondrial member of the antioxidant family of thioredoxin peroxidases. Mutations in the LRRK2 kinase domain increase phosphorylation of PRDX3 leading to decreased peroxidase activity, increased ROS production, and increased cell death [26, 27]. Notably, postmortem analysis of brains from PD patients carrying the G2019S mutation in the kinase domain of LRRK2 has shown marked increase in phosphorylated PRDX3 compared to normal brains [28].

2.2. Mitochondrial Dysfunction and ROS.

Mitochondria are known as the "power houses" of cells, the place generating adenosine triphosphate (ATP) through oxidative phosphorylation (OXPHOS) [29]. During ATP production, ROS also generate from the electron transport chain [30]. The ROS from complex I are released to the mitochondrial matrix, while the ROS from complex III are released to both the mitochondrial matrix and the inner membrane space (IMS) [31]. Mitochondrial dysfunction leads to increased ROS generation; in return, ROS are also harmful to the electron transport chain itself, leading to even higher production of ROS [32, 33]. It was suggested that mitochondria-induced overproduction of ROS was a key factor responsible for cell death and the progression of late-onset neurodegenerative diseases, particularly in idiopathic PD [32, 34]. Mitochondrial dysfunction leads to the deficiency of ATP, which is indispensable especially to dopaminergic neurons to propagate electrical signals, maintain ionic gradients and secrete dopamine [35]. The fact that the activity of the mitochondrial electron transport chain in the substantia nigra of PD patients was decreased compared with age-matched controls, further supported the role of mitochondrial dysfunction in PD [36]. In summary, mitochondrial dysfunction can cause PD though the overproduction of ROS, which underlines the dopaminergic neuron death in PD.

2.3. Dopamine and ROS.

Dopamine (DA), the neurotransmitter produced from DA neurons, is responsible for the regulation of excitatory and inhibitory synaptic transmission for ensuring smooth coordinated movement [37]. The movement disorder displayed in PD patients is basically underlined by the deficiency of DA. Noteworthy, dopamine is an unstable molecule that may auto-oxidize to form quinones and H_2O_2 [38, 39]. H_2O_2 could react with iron or oxygen to form more active OH [40]. DA quinones could react with the sulfhydryl groups of the cysteine in proteins, particularly glutathione (GSH), a ROS scavenger, resulting in lower GSH levels, and higher ROS level [41]. In addition, ROS, especially H_2O_2, are generated as by product in the process of dopamine oxidative metabolism by monoamine oxidases B [42, 43]. Besides the synthesis and degradation, the transport and storage of dopamine also contribute to elevated ROS production. Dopamine is synthesized in the cytosol and rapidly stored into synaptic vesicles for providing a stable environment for DA before released out [15], which is dependent on vesicular monoamine transporter 2 (VMAT2). Dopamine reuptake, occurred with the help of dopamine active transporter (DAT), is essential for precisely tuning the dopamine level in synaptic cleft [44]. Obviously, any perturbation to the storage and reuptake of dopamine would elevate cytoplasmic dopamine, which enhances the susceptibility to be oxidation. Consist with that, mutant α-synuclein, which linked to inherited forms of PD, is associated with enhanced dopamine reuptake and down regulates VMAT2 [45]. In addition, DAT is involved in dopamine neurotoxicity by reuptake dopamine from extracellular space to cytosol leading to accumulation of dopamine [46]. Conclusively, dopamine is an unstable molecule and prone to auto-oxidize in cytoplasm. Any perturbation elevating cytoplasmic dopamine can increase dopamine auto-oxidization and subsequently ROS and eventually PD pathogenesis.

2.4. Neuroinflammation and ROS.

Neuroinflammation is a protective response of nervous system to various kinds of tissue insults and damage. It would induce release of trophic factors and ROS to protect against stimulus so as to facilitate the regeneration and the repair [47]. Once inflammation is overwhelmed, it would cause accumulation of ROS and consequently cell death [48]. A large body of research shows that chronic inflammation involves in chronic neurodegenerative diseases, particularly the pathogenesis of PD.

Microglial cells, resident immune cells in the central nervous system (CNS), are main participants of the inflammatory response. Activated microglia releases various cytokines and chemokines to initiate corresponding processes to recruit additional microglia and leukocytes to the site of injury [49]. Cytokines such as, TNF-α, IL-1β, and IFN-γ, are proinflammatory, which will activate NADPH oxidases (Nox). Nox2, one isoform of Nox, is mainly expressed in the nervous system involved in the production of ROS as a result of the catalyzing the electron transfer from NADPH to oxygen [50]. In addition, TNF-α could cause the depletion of endogenous antioxidants such as GSH of DA neurons, which renders DA neurons more susceptible to ROS [51]. IL-1β causes aberrant mitochondrial membrane potential and the depletion of ATP through facilitating the formation of peroxynitrite, ultimately leading to mitochondria dysfunction and consequent increased ROS [52, 53]. Beside cytokines and chemokines, microglia can also be activated by endogenous proteins such as α-synuclein [54]. α-Synuclein directly promotes activation of Nox$_2$ in microglia leading to a burst of ROS. Conclusively, cytokines and chemokines released by microglia can induce NAPDH oxidase activity, which are capable of markedly enhancing the level of ROS and therefore PD pathogenesis.

2.5. Iron and ROS.

Iron accumulation is another important hallmark of PD, which has been supported by multiple of evidences, especially increased iron level observed in the substantia nigra of PD patients compared to age-matched controls [55]. Iron is indispensable for many fundamental biological processes, but excessive iron is cytotoxic. Neurons therefore tightly regulate iron levels via controlling both iron uptake and iron storage. As established, the homeostasis of cellular iron is coordinated mainly by two iron regulatory proteins (IRP1 and IRP2) [56, 57], which could bind to DNA iron-response elements (IREs) and regulate their translations [58]. With aging, the regulation machinery of iron

TABLE 1: Antioxidant defense systems and proposed mechanisms against ROS.

Classifications	Antioxidants	Functions
Enzymatic antioxidant defenses	Superoxide dismutase (SOD)	SOD catalyzes two O^{2-} anions to convert into a molecule of H_2O_2 and oxygen $$2\,O^{2-} + 2H^+ \rightarrow H_2O_2 + O_2$$
	Glutathione peroxidase (GPx)	GPx, a family of multiple isoenzymes containing selenium, catalyzes the degradation of H_2O_2 and lipid peroxides. Moreover, GPx can utilize GSH as an electron donor for the reduction of peroxides [64].
	Catalase (GPx)	Catalase, mainly existing in peroxisomes, is responsible for converting H_2O_2 into water $$2\,H_2O_2 \rightarrow 2\,H_2O + O_2$$
Nonenzymatic antioxidants	Ascorbic acid (vitamin C)	Vitamin C, a water-soluble antioxidant, is capable of removing ROS by electron transfer. In addition, vitamin C can act as a cofactor for antioxidant enzymes [88]; [90]
	α-Tocopherol (vitamin E)	Vitamin E, a lipid-soluble antioxidant, can attenuate the effects of peroxide. In particular, it can protect against lipid peroxidation in cell membranes [88]
	Glutathione (GSH)	GSH, in its reduced form, is known to react with ROS for the removal of ROS. Moreover, GSH is the electron donor for the reduction of peroxides in the GPx reaction [64]

tends to be compromised and abnormal iron accumulation and increased free iron concentration subsequently occurred [59].

Excessive iron ions can cause an exacerbated ROS production via Fenton and Haber–Weiss reactions. Iron also catalyzes the conversion of excess dopamine to neuromelanin, during which ROS are generated [60]. Consistent with that, N-acetyl-l-cysteine (NAC), an antioxidant, which could decrease iron levels, showed neuroprotective effect in PD models [61]. Moreover, desferrioxamine (DFO) and VAR10303 (VAR), two kinds of iron chelator, reduced the ROS and rescued the MPTP induced PD mouse phenotypes [62, 63]. Collectively, iron can also contribute to pathogenesis of PD via aggravating ROS production.

3. Pathological Role of ROS in the PD Pathogenesis

In cells, ROS are strictly regulated by antioxidant defense systems, which mainly consist of superoxide dismutase (SOD), glutathione peroxidase (GPx), catalase (CAT), ascorbic acid (vitamin C), α-tocopherol (vitamin E), and GSH [64] (Table 1). Once the formation of ROS overwhelms the antioxidant defense system, oxidative stress will be induced. As motioned above, various PD causative factors can lead to excessive ROS generation, which further emphasizes the pivotal role of ROS in the PD pathogenesis. ROS participated in PD pathogenesis involving the peroxidation of lipid, protein, and nucleic acid [65].

3.1. ROS-Induced Lipid Peroxidation.
Lipid is the main component of the membrane for cell as well as the organelles, such as mitochondria and nuclear. Lipid, especially polyunsaturated fatty acids, is very vulnerable to the attack of ROS [66]. A hydrogen moiety of unsaturated carbon of

polyunsaturated fatty acids could easily be attacked and consequently captured by ROS to form water, leaving an unpaired electron on the polyunsaturated fatty acids, which was converted into a peroxyl radical [67]. Once formed, peroxyl radicals would eventually produce malondialdehyde (MDA), 4-hydroxynonenal (4-HNE), and other toxic products [68, 69]. It was suggested that MDA was the major mutagenic and carcinogenic product of lipid peroxidation, whereas 4-HNE was less mutagenic and carcinogenic but the most toxic [70]. 4-HNE could trigger caspase activation and ultimately cause neuronal apoptosis [71]. In addition, 4-HNE could also reduce the GSH levels via interplaying with sulfhydryl groups [72]. Peroxided lipid reacts with polyunsaturated fatty acids leading to further oxidation, ultimately disrupting plasma membranes [73]. Accordingly, ROS-induced lipid peroxidation can cause neuronal damage and contribute to PD progression.

3.2. ROS-Induced Protein Oxidation.
It has been demonstrated that ROS initiates protein oxidation by two parallel pathways: directly inducing protein chain and side chain oxidation and indirectly inducing protein oxidation in the process of lipid peroxidation and glycosylation [74, 75]. Protein oxidation includes the cross-linking and fragmentation of protein and carbonyl group formation [76–78]. It is noteworthy that surface-exposed methionine and cysteine residues of proteins are particularly sensitive to oxidation by almost all forms of ROS. ROS-induced protein oxidation potentially effects cell survival via disrupting the active site of enzymes and consequently protein-protein and protein-DNA interactions [79]. It was demonstrated that loss function mutation in DJ-1, one familial PD-related gene, leaded to protein oxidative damage [80]. Supplementation of antioxidant, vitamin C, could decrease the H_2O_2 and

oxidized protein level [81]. Therefore, protein oxidation by ROS involves in PD pathogenesis.

3.3. ROS-Induced DNA Oxidation. It is acknowledged that OH can bind with DNA molecule, leading to oxidation of bases and the deoxyribose backbone [82]. The key product of DNA oxidation is 8-hydroxy-deoxyguanosine (8-OHdG), which results in transcriptional mutagenesis and generation of mutated species of protein that contributed to PD pathogenesis [83, 84]. Notably, mitochondrial DNA (mtDNA) oxidation by ROS would lead to mtDNA abnormality and consequently trigger the expression of aberrant mitochondrial proteins and mitochondrial dysfunction, collectively exacerbating ROS production [85, 86]. It is therefore unsurprising to note that there is a vicious cycle between mtDNA oxidation and increased ROS production, which ultimately leads to neuronal death and PD pathogenesis.

4. Anti-ROS with Compounds for the Therapeutics of PD

In light of the above-mentioned evidence on the crucial role of ROS in the pathogenesis of PD, anti-ROS therapy has been an attractive strategy to counteract the oxidative stress-induced neuronal cell death in PD [87]. Classic antioxidants mainly include vitamin C, vitamin E, Coenzyme Q10 (CoQ10), GSH, NAC, and creatine. Vitamin C and vitamin E are members of antioxidant defense systems. Vitamin E could scavenge hydroxyl and peroxyl radicals, thus protecting against lipid peroxidation [88]. Vitamin C could not only directly remove O_2^- and OH, but also indirectly facilitate vitamin E to counteract overproduced ROS to show neuroprotection in PD [89, 90]. It was reported that a combination of vitamin C and vitamin E administered to patients with early PD may slow the progression of the disease [91, 92]. CoQ10, a constituent of the mitochondrial electron transport chain (ETC), prevented electrons leaking along the ETC which would generate ROS [93]. It was reported that oral administration of CoQ10 in PD animal models and PD patients attenuated mitochondrial dysfunction and deficit of dopamine [94]. Mechanically, CoQ10 acted as antioxidant to scavenge H_2O_2 or as a cofactor and activator of mitochondrial uncoupling proteins to decrease the generation of ROS [93, 95]. GSH, the major endogenous antioxidant molecule, was found to reduce in the substantia nigra of PD patients [96]. However, direct administration of GSH did not achieve expected effect of scavenging ROS due to its susceptibility to oxidation by various ROS [97]. NAC, a precursor of GSH, was alternatively utilized to restore GSH levels by providing the rate-limiting substrate for GSH synthesis [98]. Moreover, NAC could also directly act as a scavenger of ROS and ameliorate dopaminergic neuronal loss in PD models [99, 100]. Creatine is a nitrogenous guanidine molecule with antioxidant properties, which could retain mitochondrial dysfunction and protect DA neuron death in PD models [101, 102]. As known, most of the ROS are produced during ATP production though

OXPHOS. Resveratrol, a natural polyphenolic compound, is showed to protect against Parkin deficiency-induced mitochondria dysfunction and oxidative stress via activating AMPK/SIRT1/PGC-1α axis [103]. Pinocembrin (PB) could mitigate MPP (+) induced SH-SY5Y cells oxidative stress and apoptosis [104].

Nuclear factor erythroid 2-related factor 2 (Nrf2) controls the antioxidant and detoxifying response in mammalian [105]. Recently, it was reported that carnosic acid (CA) exerts antioxidant effects through activation of Nrf2, the latter upregulating expression of some of endogenous antioxidants such as GPx, glutathione reductase (GR) [106]. Moreover, isothiocyanate sulforaphane (SFN), another Nrf2 activator, also displays neuroprotective effects in PD models [107]. All those studies suggest that Nrf2 is a pivotal mediator of cellular antioxidative stress system.

Noteworthy, antioxidants show the promising effect for antagonizing oxidative stress in animal PD models, and they do not display the equivalent efficacy in clinical trials. More work need to do before antioxidant could be applied for PD treatment in clinic.

5. Conclusions

PD is the second most common neurodegenerative disorder, and the mechanisms of neuronal degeneration in PD are poorly known and remain to be fully illustrated. It is widely accepted that genetic mutations, mitochondrial dysfunction, dopamine auto-oxidation, neuroinflammation, and iron accumulation contribute significantly to the pathogenesis of PD. Interestingly, all of the PD-related factors can cause excessive generation of ROS. Once ROS overwhelm antioxidant defense systems, excess ROS can induce lipid peroxidation, protein oxidation, and DNA oxidation to trigger PD-related cell loss in the SN. In the future, the molecular signal pathway of ROS inducing PD pathogenesis needs be further explored. Antioxidants which could be utilized for PD treatment should be developed.

Acknowledgments

This study was supported by the National Science Foundation of China (Grant nos. 81672508 and 61505076), Jiangsu Provincial Foundation for Distinguished Young Scholars (BK20170041), Key University Science Research Project of Jiangsu Province (no. 16KJA180004), and Jiangsu key Research and Development program (BE2015699).

References

[1] K. Jellinger, "Neuropathological substrates of Alzheimers disease and Parkinsons disease," *Journal of Neural Transmission*, vol. 24, pp. 109–129, 1987.

[2] H. E. Moon and S. H. Paek, "Mitochondrial dysfunction in Parkinson's disease," *Experimental Neurobiology*, vol. 24, pp. 103–116, 2015.

[3] A. J. Whitworth and L. J. Pallanck, "Genetic models of Parkinson's disease: mechanisms and therapies," *SEB Experimental Biology Series*, vol. 60, pp. 93–113, 2008.

[4] M. I. Shadrina and P. A. Slominsky, "Molecular genetics of Parkinson's disease," *Russian Journal of Genetics*, vol. 42, no. 8, pp. 858–871, 2006.

[5] A. P. Chou, N. Maidment, R. Klintenberg et al., "Ziram causes dopaminergic cell damage by inhibiting e1 ligase of the proteasome," *Journal of Biological Chemistry*, vol. 283, no. 50, pp. 34696–34703, 2008.

[6] J. A. Doorn, V. R. Florang, J. H. Schamp, and B. C. Vanle, "Aldehyde dehydrogenase inhibition generates a reactive dopamine metabolite autotoxic to dopamine neurons," *Parkinsonism & Related Disorders*, vol. 20, pp. S73–S75, 2014.

[7] J. Zhang, V. A. Fitsanakis, G. Y. Gu et al., "Manganese ethylene-bis-dithiocarbamate and selective dopaminergic neurodegeneration in rat: a link through mitochondrial dysfunction," *Journal of Neurochemistry*, vol. 84, no. 2, pp. 336–346, 2003.

[8] J. M. Ross, L. Olson, and G. Coppotelli, "Mitochondrial and ubiquitin proteasome system dysfunction in ageing and disease: two sides of the same coin?," *International Journal of Molecular Sciences*, vol. 16, no. 8, pp. 19458–19476, 2015.

[9] K.-L. Lim and C.-W. Zhang, "Molecular events underlying Parkinson's disease—an interwoven tapestry," *Frontiers in Neurology*, vol. 4, 2013.

[10] B. Halliwell, "Oxidative stress and neurodegeneration: where are we now?," *Journal of Neurochemistry*, vol. 97, no. 6, pp. 1634–1658, 2006.

[11] L. Covarrubias, D. Hernandez-Garcia, D. Schnabel, E. Salas-Vidal, and S. Castro-Obregon, "Function of reactive oxygen species during animal development: passive or active?," *Developmental Biology*, vol. 320, no. 1, pp. 1–11, 2008.

[12] I. Casetta, V. Govoni, and E. Granieri, "Oxidative stress, antioxidants and neurodegenerative diseases," *Current Pharmaceutical Design*, vol. 11, no. 16, pp. 2033–2052, 2005.

[13] C. Chai and K.-L. Lim, "Genetic insights into sporadic Parkinson's disease pathogenesis," *Current Genomics*, vol. 14, no. 8, pp. 486–501, 2013.

[14] R. Youle, "Autophagy functions of genes mutated in ALS and Parkinson's disease," *Free Radical Biology and Medicine*, vol. 112, p. 15, 2017.

[15] S. Basu, G. Je, and Y.-S. Kim, "Transcriptional mutagenesis by 8-oxodG in α-synuclein aggregation and the pathogenesis of Parkinson's disease," *Experimental and Molecular Medicine*, vol. 47, no. 8, p. e179, 2015.

[16] R. Di Maio, P. J. Barrett, E. K. Hoffman et al., "Alpha-Synuclein binds to TOM20 and inhibits mitochondrial protein import in Parkinson's disease," *Science Translational Medicine*, vol. 8, no. 342, 2016.

[17] E. Junn and M. M. Mouradian, "Human alpha-synuclein over-expression increases intracellular reactive oxygen species levels and susceptibility to dopamine," *Neuroscience Letters*, vol. 320, no. 3, pp. 146–150, 2002.

[18] Q. Zheng, C. Huang, J. Guo et al., "Hsp70 participates in PINK1-mediated mitophagy by regulating the stability of PINK1," *Neuroscience Letters*, vol. 662, no. 1, pp. 264–270, 2018.

[19] H. Yang, J. Zuo, and W. Liu, "Parkin, PINK1, DJ-1 and mitochondria dysfunction with Parkinson's disease," *Chinese Bulletin of Life Sciences*, vol. 22, pp. 1009–1012, 2010.

[20] H.-T. Zhang, L. Mi, T. Wang et al., "PINK1/parkin-mediated mitophagy play a protective role in manganese induced apoptosis in SH-SY5Y cells," *Toxicology In Vitro*, vol. 34, pp. 212–219, 2016.

[21] C. W. Zhang, L. T. Hang, T. P. Yao, and K. L. Lim, "Parkin regulation and neurodegenerative disorders," *Frontiers in Aging Neuroscience*, vol. 7, 2016.

[22] D. Cartelli, A. Amadeo, A. M. Calogero et al., "Parkin absence accelerates microtubule aging in dopaminergic neurons," *Neurobiology of Aging*, vol. 61, pp. 66–74, 2017.

[23] E. Junn, W. H. Jang, X. Zhao, B. S. Jeong, and M. M. Mouradian, "Mitochondrial localization of DJ-1 leads to enhanced neuroprotection," *Journal of Neuroscience Research*, vol. 87, no. 1, pp. 123–129, 2009.

[24] J. Niu, M. Yu, C. Wang, and Z. Xu, "Leucine-rich repeat kinase 2 disturbs mitochondrial dynamics via dynamin-like protein," *Journal of Neurochemistry*, vol. 122, no. 3, pp. 650–658, 2012.

[25] X. Wang, M. H. Yan, H. Fujioka et al., "LRRK2 regulates mitochondrial dynamics and function through direct interaction with DLP1," *Human Molecular Genetics*, vol. 21, no. 9, pp. 1931–1944, 2012.

[26] D. C. Angeles, B.-H. Gan, L. Onstead et al., "Mutations in LRRK2 increase phosphorylation of peroxiredoxin 3 exacerbating oxidative stress-induced neuronal death," *Human Mutation*, vol. 32, no. 12, pp. 1390–1397, 2011.

[27] W. M. Johnson, C. Yao, S. Chen, A. L. Wilson-Delfosse, and J. J. Mieyal, "Loss of redoxin proteins exacerbates LRRK2-mediated Parkinson's disease phenotype in *C. elegans*," *FASEB Journal*, vol. 27, pp. 20–24, 2013.

[28] D. C. Angeles, P. Ho, L. L. Chua et al., "Thiol peroxidases ameliorate LRRK2 mutant-induced mitochondrial and dopaminergic neuronal degeneration in Drosophila," *Human Molecular Genetics*, vol. 23, no. 12, pp. 3157–3165, 2014.

[29] R. Banerjee, A. A. Starkov, M. F. Beal, and B. Thomas, "Mitochondrial dysfunction in the limelight of Parkinson's disease pathogenesis," *Biochimica et Biophysica Acta (BBA)-Molecular Basis of Disease*, vol. 1792, no. 7, pp. 651–663, 2009.

[30] E. Cadenas and K. J. A. Davies, "Mitochondrial free radical generation, oxidative stress, and aging," *Free Radical Biology and Medicine*, vol. 29, pp. 222–230, 2000.

[31] F. Muller, Y. H. Liu, and H. Van Remmen, "Complex III releases superoxide to both sides of the inner mitochondrial membrane," *Journal of Biological Chemistry*, vol. 279, no. 47, pp. 49064–49073, 2004.

[32] A. H. Bhat, K. B. Dar, S. Anees et al., "Oxidative stress, mitochondrial dysfunction and neurodegenerative diseases; a mechanistic insight," *Biomedicine & Pharmacotherapy*, vol. 74, pp. 101–110, 2015.

[33] L. Hang, J. Thundyil, K.-L. Lim, and N. Y. A. Sci, "Mitochondrial dysfunction and Parkinson disease: a Parkin-AMPK alliance in neuroprotection," *Mitochondrial Research in Translational Medicine*, vol. 1350, no. 1, pp. 37–47, 2015.

[34] P. H. Reddy and M. F. Beal, "Amyloid beta, mitochondrial dysfunction and synaptic damage: implications for cognitive decline in aging and Alzheimer's disease," *Trends in Molecular Medicine*, vol. 14, no. 2, pp. 45–53, 2008.

[35] Y.-H. Su, Y.-L. Lee, S.-F. Chen et al., "Essential role of ss-human 8-oxoguanine DNA glycosylase 1 in mitochondrial oxidative DNA repair," *Environmental and Molecular Mutagenesis*, vol. 54, no. 1, pp. 54–64, 2013.

[36] A. H. V. Schapira, "Mitochondria in the aetiology and pathogenesis of Parkinson's disease," *The Lancet Neurology*, vol. 7, no. 1, pp. 97–109, 2008.

[37] W. Hauber, "Involvement of basal ganglia transmitter systems in movement initiation," *Progress In Neurobiology*, vol. 56, pp. 507–540, 1998.

[38] A. Biosa, I. Arduini, M. E. Soriano, L. Bubacco, and M. Bisaglia, "Analysis of the functional effects mediated by dopamine oxidation products at the mitochondrial level," *Journal of Neurochemistry*, vol. 142, p. 106, 2017.

[39] T. G. Hastings, "The role of dopamine oxidation in mitochondrial dysfunction: implications for Parkinson's disease," *Journal of Bioenergetics and Biomembranes*, vol. 41, pp. 469–472, 2009.

[40] P. Dusek, S. A. Schneider, and J. Aaseth, "Iron chelation in the treatment of neurodegenerative diseases," *Journal of Trace Elements in Medicine and Biology*, vol. 38, pp. 81–92, 2016.

[41] S. U. Park, J. V. Ferrer, J. A. Javitch, and D. M. Kuhn, "Peroxynitrite inactivates the human dopamine transporter by modification of cysteine 342: potential mechanism of neurotoxicity in dopamine neurons," *Journal of Neuroscience*, vol. 22, no. 11, pp. 4399–4405, 2002.

[42] S. Saller, L. Kunz, D. Berg et al., "Dopamine in human follicular fluid is associated with cellular uptake and metabolism-dependent generation of reactive oxygen species in granulosa cells: implications for physiology and pathology," *Human Reproduction*, vol. 29, no. 3, pp. 555–567, 2014.

[43] M. B. H. Youdim, D. Edmondson, and K. F. Tipton, "The therapeutic potential of monoamine oxidase inhibitors," *Nature Reviews Neuroscience*, vol. 7, no. 4, pp. 295–309, 2006.

[44] R. R. Gainetdinov and M. G. Caron, "Monoamine transporters: from genes to behavior," *Annual Review of Pharmacology and Toxicology*, vol. 43, no. 1, pp. 261–284, 2003.

[45] F. J. S. Lee, F. Liu, Z. B. Pristupa, and H. B. Niznik, "Direct binding and functional coupling of alpha-synuclein to the dopamine transporters accelerate dopamine-induced apoptosis," *FASEB Journal*, vol. 15, no. 6, pp. 916–926, 2001.

[46] P. Su and F. Liu, "A peptide disrupting the D2R-DAT interaction protects against dopamine neurotoxicity," *Experimental Neurology*, vol. 295, pp. 176–183, 2017.

[47] A. A. Farooqui, L. A. Horrocks, and T. Farooqui, "Modulation of inflammation in brain: a matter of fat," *Journal of Neurochemistry*, vol. 101, no. 3, pp. 577–599, 2007.

[48] H.-L. Hsieh and C.-M. Yang, "Role of redox signaling in neuroinflammation and neurodegenerative diseases," *BioMed Research International*, vol. 2013, Article ID 484613, 18 pages, 2013.

[49] S. T. Dheen, C. Kaur, and E.-A. Ling, "Microglial activation and its implications in the brain diseases," *Current Medicinal Chemistry*, vol. 14, no. 11, pp. 1189–1197, 2007.

[50] T. Seredenina, S. Schiavone, G. Maghzal et al., "Inhibition of NOX NADPH oxidases as a potential treatment for neuroinflammation," *Free Radical Biology and Medicine*, vol. 65, p. S14, 2013.

[51] H. L. Hayter, B. J. Pettus, F. Ito, L. M. Obeid, and Y. A. Hannun, "TNF alpha-induced glutathione depletion lies downstream of cPLA(2) in L929 cells," *FEBS Letters*, vol. 507, no. 2, pp. 151–156, 2001.

[52] E. K. Kim, K. B. Kwon, M. J. Han et al., "Coptidis rhizoma extract protects against cytokine-induced death of pancreatic beta-cells through suppression of NF-kappa B activation," *Experimental and Molecular Medicine*, vol. 39, no. 2, pp. 149–159, 2007.

[53] K. Ramdial, M. C. Franco, and A. G. Estevez, "Cellular mechanisms of peroxynitrite-induced neuronal death," *Brain Research Bulletin*, vol. 133, no. 4, pp. 4–11, 2017.

[54] M. L. Block, L. Zecca, and J.-S Hong, "Microglia-mediated neurotoxicity: uncovering the molecular mechanisms," *Nature Reviews Neuroscience*, vol. 8, no. 1, pp. 57–69, 2007.

[55] R. D. Wang, "Iron metabolism in Parkinson's disease patients with olfactory disorder," *Journal of the American Geriatrics Society*, vol. 64, p. S374, 2016.

[56] D. W. Lee and J. K. Andersen, "Iron elevations in the aging parkinsonian brain: a consequence of impaired iron homeostasis.," *Journal of Neurochemistry*, vol. 112, no. 2, pp. 332–339, 2010.

[57] E. C. Theil and R. S. Eisenstein, "Combinatorial mRNA regulation: Iron regulatory proteins and iso-iron-responsive elements (Iso-IREs)," *Journal of Biological Chemistry*, vol. 275, no. 52, pp. 40659–40662, 2000.

[58] D. Kaur and J. Andersen, "Does cellular iron dysregulation play a causative role in Parkinson's disease?," *Ageing Research Reviews*, vol. 3, no. 3, pp. 327–343, 2004.

[59] J. Sian-Huelsmann, S. Mandel, M. B. H. Youdim, and P. Riederer, "The relevance of iron in the pathogenesis of Parkinson's disease," *Journal of Neurochemistry*, vol. 118, no. 6, pp. 939–957, 2011.

[60] F. A. Zucca, J. Segura-Aguilar, E. Ferrari et al., "Interactions of iron, dopamine and neuromelanin pathways in brain aging and Parkinson's disease," *Progress in Neurobiology*, vol. 155, pp. 96–119, 2017.

[61] C. Nunez-Millacura, V. Tapia, P. Munoz, R. B. Maccioni, and M. T. Nunez, "An oxidative stress-mediated positive-feedback iron uptake loop in neuronal cells," *Journal of Neurochemistry*, vol. 82, no. 2, pp. 240–248, 2002.

[62] O. Bar-Am, T. Amit, L. Kupershmidt et al., "Neuroprotective and neurorestorative activities of a novel iron chelator-brain selective monoamine oxidase-A/monoamine oxidase-B inhibitor in animal models of Parkinson's disease and aging," *Neurobiology of Aging*, vol. 36, no. 3, pp. 1529–1542, 2015.

[63] M. P. Gotsbacher, T. J. Telfer, P. K. Witting, K. L. Double, D. I. Finkelstein, and R. Codd, "Analogues of desferrioxamine B designed to attenuate iron-mediated neurodegeneration: synthesis, characterisation and activity in the MPTP-mouse model of Parkinson's disease," *Metallomics*, vol. 9, no. 7, pp. 852–864, 2017.

[64] R. Dringen, "Metabolism and functions of glutathione in brain," *Progress in Neurobiology*, vol. 62, no. 6, pp. 649–671, 2000.

[65] M. Valko, D. Leibfritz, J. Moncol, M. T. D. Cronin, M. Mazur, and J. Telser, "Free radicals and antioxidants in normal physiological functions and human disease," *International Journal of Biochemistry & Cell Biology*, vol. 39, no. 1, pp. 44–84, 2007.

[66] P. R. Angelova, M. H. Horrocks, D. Klenerman, S. Gandhi, A. Y. Abramov, and M. S. Shchepinov, "Lipid peroxidation is essential for alpha-synuclein-induced cell death," *Journal of Neurochemistry*, vol. 133, no. 4, pp. 582–589, 2015.

[67] D. A. Patten, M. Germain, M. A. Kelly, and R. S. Slack, "Reactive oxygen species: stuck in the middle of neurodegeneration," *Journal of Alzheimers Disease*, vol. 20, no. s2, pp. S357–S367, 2010.

[68] J. Miletic, T. Ilic, A. Stefanovic, M. Miljkovic, and M. Stojanov, "4-Hydroxynonenal in Parkinson's disease," *Amino Acids*, vol. 47, p. 1675, 2015.

[69] A. Sharma, P. Kaur, B. Kumar, S. Prabhakar, and K. D. Gill, "Plasma lipid peroxidation and antioxidant status of Parkinson's disease patients in the Indian population," *Parkinsonism & Related Disorders*, vol. 14, no. 1, pp. 52–57, 2008.

[70] L. T. McGrath, B. M. McGleenon, S. Brennan, D. McColl, S. McIlroy, and A. P. Passmore, "Increased oxidative stress in Alzheimer's disease as assessed with 4-hydroxynonenal but

not malondialdehyde," *QJM-Monthly Journal of the Association of Physicians*, vol. 94, pp. 485–490, 2001.

[71] M. A. Siddiqui, V. Kumar, M. P. Kashyap et al., "Short-term exposure of 4-hydroxynonenal induces mitochondria-mediated apoptosis in PC12 cells," *Human & Experimental Toxicology*, vol. 31, pp. 336–345, 2012.

[72] I. Ahmed, A. John, C. Vijayasarathy, M. A. Robin, and H. Raza, "Differential modulation of growth and glutathione metabolism in cultured rat astrocytes by 4-hydroxynonenal and green tea polyphenol, epigallocatechin-3-gallate," *Neurotoxicology*, vol. 23, no. 3, pp. 289–300, 2002.

[73] J. K. Andersen, "Oxidative stress in neurodegeneration: cause or consequence?," *Nature Reviews Neuroscience*, vol. 10, no. 7, pp. S18–S25, 2004.

[74] F. Sesti, S. Liu, and S. Q. Cai, "Oxidation of potassium channels by ROS: a general mechanism of aging and neurodegeneration?," *Trends in Cell Biology*, vol. 20, no. 1, pp. 45–51, 2010.

[75] L.-J. Yan, "Positive oxidative stress in aging and aging-related disease tolerance," *Redox Biology*, vol. 2, pp. 165–169, 2014.

[76] G. A. Czapski, W. Szypula, M. Kudlik et al., "Assessment of antioxidative activity of alkaloids from Huperzia selago and Diphasiastrum complanatum using in vitro systems," *Folia Neuropathologica*, vol. 52, no. 4, pp. 394–406, 2014.

[77] E. Floor and M. G. Wetzel, "Increased protein oxidation in human substantia nigra pars compacta in comparison with basal ganglia and prefrontal cortex measured with an improved dinitrophenylhydrazine assay," *Journal of Neurochemistry*, vol. 70, no. 1, pp. 268–275, 1998.

[78] S. Mukherjee, E. A. Kapp, A. Lothian et al., "Characterization and identification of dityrosine cross-linked peptides using tandem mass spectrometry," *Analytical Chemistry*, vol. 89, no. 11, pp. 6137–6146, 2017.

[79] Y. Jammes, J. G. Steinberg, F. Bregeon, and S. Delliaux, "The oxidative stress in response to routine incremental cycling exercise in healthy sedentary subjects," *Respiratory Physiology & Neurobiology*, vol. 144, no. 1, pp. 81–90, 2004.

[80] S. Xu, X. Yang, Y. Qian, and Q. Xiao, "Parkinson disease-related DJ-1 modulates the expression of uncoupling protein 4 against oxidative stress," *Journal of Neurochemistry*, vol. 145, no. 4, pp. 312–322, 2018.

[81] L. H. Sanders, J. McCoy, X. Hu et al., "Mitochondrial DNA damage: Molecular marker of vulnerable nigral neurons in Parkinson's disease," *Neurobiology of Disease*, vol. 70, pp. 214–223, 2014.

[82] Z. I. Alam, A. Jenner, S. E. Daniel et al., "Oxidative DNA damage in the parkinsonian brain: an apparent selective increase in 8-hydroxyguanine levels in substantia nigra," *Journal of Neurochemistry*, vol. 69, no. 3, pp. 1196–1203, 1997.

[83] D. Bregeon, P.-A. Peignon, and A. Sarasin, "Transcriptional Mutagenesis Induced by 8-Oxoguanine in Mammalian Cells," *PLoS Genetics*, vol. 5, no. 7, article e1000577, 2009.

[84] K. Gmitterova, J. Gawinecka, U. Heinemann, P. Valkovic, and I. Zerr, "DNA versus RNA oxidation in Parkinson's disease: which is more important?," *Neuroscience Letters*, vol. 662, pp. 22–28, 2018.

[85] A. Bender, K. J. Krishnan, C. M. Morris et al., "High levels of mitochondrial DNA deletions in substantia nigra neurons in aging and Parkinson disease," *Nature Genetics*, vol. 38, no. 5, pp. 515–517, 2006.

[86] D. J. Surmeier, J. N. Guzman, J. Sanchez-Padilla, and J. A. Goldberg, "The origins of oxidant stress in Parkinson's disease and therapeutic strategies," *Antioxidants & Redox Signaling*, vol. 14, no. 7, pp. 1289–1301, 2011.

[87] L. T. Hang, A. H. Basil, and K. L. Lim, "Nutraceuticals in Parkinson's disease," *NeuroMolecular Medicine*, vol. 18, no. 3, pp. 306–321, 2016.

[88] S. Gandhi and A. Y. Abramov, "Mechanism of oxidative stress in neurodegeneration," *Oxidative Medicine and Cellular Longevity*, vol. 2012, Article ID 428010, 11 pages, 2012.

[89] A. Y. Chen, J.-M. Lu, Q. Yao, and C. Chen, "Entacapone is an antioxidant more potent than vitamin C and vitamin E for scavenging of hypochlorous acid and peroxynitrite, and the inhibition of oxidative stress-induced cell death," *Medical Science Monitor*, vol. 22, pp. 687–696, 2016.

[90] K. Dasuri, L. Zhang, and J. N. Keller, "Oxidative stress, neurodegeneration, and the balance of protein degradation and protein synthesis," *Free Radical Biology and Medicine*, vol. 62, pp. 170–185, 2013.

[91] M. Baunthiyal, V. Singh, and S. Dwivedi, "Insights of antioxidants as molecules for drug discovery," *International Journal of Pharmacology*, vol. 13, no. 7, pp. 874–889, 2017.

[92] G. P. Paraskevas, E. Kapaki, O. Petropoulou, M. Anagnostouli, V. Vagenas, and C. Papageorgiou, "Plasma levels of antioxidant vitamins C and E are decreased in vascular parkinsonism," *Journal of the Neurological Sciences*, vol. 215, no. 1-2, pp. 51–55, 2003.

[93] C. W. Shults, D. Oakes, K. Kieburtz et al., "Effects of coenzyme Q(10) in early Parkinson disease-evidence of slowing of the functional decline," *Archives of Neurology*, vol. 59, no. 10, pp. 1541–1550, 2002.

[94] A. Storch, "Coenzyme Q(10) in Parkinson's disease," *Der Nervenarzt*, vol. 78, no. 12, pp. 1378–1382, 2007.

[95] K. Kieburtz, B. Ravina, W. R. Galpern et al., "A randomized clinical trial of coenzyme Q(10) and GPI-1485 in early Parkinson disease," *Neurology*, vol. 68, no. 1, pp. 20–28, 2007.

[96] J. Ehrhart and G. D. Zeevalk, "Cooperative interaction between ascorbate and glutathione during mitochondrial impairment in mesencephalic cultures," *Journal of Neurochemistry*, vol. 86, no. 6, pp. 1487–1497, 2003.

[97] H. J. Sun, Y. Wang, T. Hao, C.-Y. Wang, Q.-Y. Wang, and X.-X. Jiang, "Efficient GSH delivery using PAMAM-GSH into MPP-induced PC12 cellular model for Parkinson's disease," *Regenerative Biomaterials*, vol. 3, no. 5, pp. 299–307, 2016.

[98] L. D. Coles, P. J. Tuite, G. Oz et al., "Repeated-dose oral N-acetylcysteine in Parkinson's disease: pharmacokinetics and effect on brain glutathione and oxidative stress," *Journal of Clinical Pharmacology*, vol. 58, no. 2, pp. 158–167, 2018.

[99] S. Penugonda, S. Mare, G. Goldstein, W. A. Banks, and N. Ercal, "Effects of N-acetylcysteine amide (NACA), a novel thiol antioxidant against glutamate-induced cytotoxicity in neuronal cell line PC12," *Brain Research*, vol. 1056, no. 2, pp. 132–138, 2005.

[100] P. Sozio, A. Lannitelli, L. S. Cerasa et al., "New L-dopa codrugs as potential antiparkinson agents," *Archiv Der Pharmazie*, vol. 341, no. 7, pp. 412–417, 2008.

[101] A. Bender, W. Koch, M. Elstner et al., "Creatine supplementation in Parkinson disease: a placebo-controlled randomized pilot trial," *Neurology*, vol. 67, no. 7, pp. 1262–1264, 2006a.

[102] M. Loehe and H. Reichmann, "Clinical neuroprotection in Parkinson's disease-still waiting for the breakthrough," *Journal of the Neurological Sciences*, vol. 289, no. 1-2, pp. 104–114, 2010.

[103] A. Ferretta, A. Gaballo, P. Tanzarella et al., "Effect of resveratrol on mitochondrial function: implications in parkin-associated familiar Parkinson's disease," *Biochimica et Biophysica Acta (BBA)-Molecular Basis of Disease*, vol. 1842, no. 7, pp. 902–915, 2014.

[104] Y. Wang, J. Gao, Y. Miao et al., "Pinocembrin protects SH-SY5Y cells against MPP(+)-induced neurotoxicity through the mitochondrial apoptotic pathway," *Journal of Molecular Neuroscience*, vol. 53, no. 4, pp. 537–545, 2014.

[105] N. Esteras, A. T. Dinkova-Kostova, and A. Y. Abramov, "Nrf2 activation in the treatment of neurodegenerative diseases: a focus on its role in mitochondrial bioenergetics and function," *Biological Chemistry*, vol. 397, no. 5, pp. 382–400, 2016.

[106] M. R. de Oliveira, I. C. C. de Souza, and C. R. Fürstenau, "Carnosic acid induces anti-inflammatory effects in paraquat-treated SH-SY5Y cells through a mechanism involving a crosstalk between the Nrf2/HO-1 axis and NF-κB," *Molecular Neurobiology*, vol. 55, no. 1, pp. 890–897, 2018.

[107] F. Morroni, G. Sita, A. Djemil et al., "Comparison of adaptive neuroprotective mechanisms of sulforaphane and its interconversion product erucin in in vitro and in vivo models of Parkinson's disease," *Journal of Agricultural and Food Chemistry*, vol. 66, no. 4, pp. 856–865, 2018.

24

Rivastigmine as a Symptomatic Treatment for Apathy in Parkinson's Dementia Complex: New Aspects for This Riddle

Rita Moretti,[1] **Paola Caruso,**[1] **and Matteo Dal Ben**[2,3]

[1]*Clinica Neurologica, Dipartimento Universitario Clinico di Scienze Mediche, Chirurgiche e della Salute,*
 Università degli Studi di Trieste, Trieste, Italy
[2]*FIF Science Park, University of Trieste, Trieste, Italy*
[3]*Dipartimento Universitario Clinico di Scienze Mediche, Chirurgiche e della Salute, Università degli Studi di Trieste, Trieste, Italy*

Correspondence should be addressed to Rita Moretti; moretti@units.it

Academic Editor: Nir Qvit

Over 90% of PDD patients show at least one neuropsychiatric symptom (NPS); in the 60–70% two or more NPS are present. Their incidence is important in terms of prognosis and severity of pathology. However, among all NPS, apathy is often the most disturbing, associated with greater caregiver's burden. Similar to other NPS, apathy may be due to a dysfunction of the nigrostriatal pathway, even though, not all the PD patients become apathetic, indicating that apathy should not entirely be considered a dopamine-dependent syndrome, and in fact it might also be related to acetylcholine defects. Apathy has been treated in many ways, without sure benefits; among these, Rivastigmine may present benefic properties. We present a series of 48 patients, suffering from PDD, treated with Rivastigmine, and followed-up for one year; they have been devotedly studied for apathy, even though all the other NPS disorders have been registered. Rivastigmine did not have a prolonged benefic effect on apathy, in our work, on the contrary of what had been observed in the literature, probably due to the longer follow-up of our patients.

1. Introduction

Behavior and cognitive symptoms are common in Parkinson's Disease (PD) and in Parkinson's Disease Dementia (PDD) [1–6]. As well pointed out by a recent study [7], 90% of PDD patients showed at least one neuropsychiatric symptom (NPS) and a percentage up to 60–70% two or more NPS [8]; NPS are important predictive factors for prognosis, institutionalization, and overall mortality [9–13]. There is no clinical consensus on how to treat NPS; antipsychotics drugs are widely employed, but they should be used only for small amount of time, and they are recommended to treat hallucinations, delusions, and aggressiveness. Major warning has been given by FDA to atypical neuroleptics [8] and the American Geriatric Society (AGS) Beers consensus criteria for safe medication use in the elderly [14] recommend avoiding antipsychotics to treat NPS of dementia due to the increased mortality and CVAE risk [14, 15]. Cholinesterase and butirrylcholinesterase inhibitors and NMDA antagonists have been used to treat primary cognitive disturbance in PDD [16], but there are some data, which give reason for their benefits also in the management of NPS [17–21].

However, among all the NPS, one of the most intriguing (for the complicate pathophysiological mechanism underlying it) [22] and one of the most disturbing (for caregivers and for patients) is apathy. The presence of apathy has been associated with greater cognitive impairment [[23–27]; see data in [22]], and its prevalence in PDD varies between 16.5% and 51%, depending upon the instrument for assessment and on the samples examined [28–30]. It has been hypothesized that dysfunction of the nigrostriatal pathway might be involved in the pathophysiology of apathy in PD, [29], confirmed by functional connectivity study which documented a conspicuous impairment of striatal and ventrolateral prefrontal regions connections [31]. Data are not univocal, since two other studies [32, 33] did not find out any structural differences when comparing apathetic to nonapathetic PD patients, after applying appropriate correction for multiple comparisons [34].

To be precise, the extension of brain networks involved in apathy in PDD is enormous, and many other neuroimaging and functional studies indicate different brain areas involvement, not only nigrostriatal pathways [data and literature in [22]] documented it. Reijnders et al. [25] found an association between higher apathy and lower gray matter density in the bilateral inferior frontal gyrus and precentral gyrus, in the bilateral inferior parietal gyrus, and right precuneus, confirmed by Skidmore et al. [35], who showed that the severity of apathy was best predicted by a greater sufferance of the right middle orbitofrontal cortex and bilateral subgenual cingulate cortex, of the left supplementary motor cortex, and of the left inferior parietal lobule and left fusiform gyrus [35]. (FDG) PET-studies specifically found a positive correlation of apathy and cerebral metabolism during rest in the right middle frontal gyrus, right inferior frontal gyrus, left anterior insula [26], bilateral orbitofrontal lobes and bilateral anterior cingulate [32], and left posterior cingulate cortex [26]. Much more interesting is that not all the PD patients become apathetic, indicating that apathy should not entirely be considered a dopamine-dependent syndrome in PD, and is in fact present even in not-purely dopaminergic alterations [11, 36, 37]. As strongly pointed out by Kos et al., [34] an inverse correlation between catecholaminergic binding potential, indicative of a specific combined loss of dopamine and noradrenaline innervation, and apathy was found in the bilateral ventral striatum in an exploratory resting-state analysis in PD [38]. Some studies tried to involve acetylcholine in driving motivation and its lack related to apathy [39].

Apathy has been treated in many different ways [17, 40–42]. Some recently published studies [5, 6] suggested some benefic properties of Rivastigmine on this NPS symptom too, in complete accordance with the results obtained by Devos et al. [17].

We present a series of patients, suffering from PDD, treated with Rivastigmine, and devotedly studied for apathy, within a complex sequence of NPS disorders; we did not have the same successful results showed by the previous studies; we discuss the results, trying to give pathological explanation to a different possible mechanism outstanding apathy in PDD.

2. Materials and Methods

50 patients diagnosed with PDD, from 1 December 2010 up to 31 December 2013, referring to the Neurological Unit Research of Trieste, were enrolled.

The diagnosis was based on UK PD Society Brain Bank clinical diagnostic criteria and clinical diagnostic criteria for probable PDD [43–45]. Data from a physical and neurological examinations, laboratory tests, and brain magnetic resonance imaging (or CT for 6 patients, claustrophobic and therefore not possible for them to attend MRI) were obtained. Patients with a history of stroke or brain hemorrhage or other psychiatric disorders, atypical PD, or secondary Parkinsonism have not been enrolled for this study.

The patients must completely fulfill the criteria for probable PDD, as presented by Goetz et al. [45]: core features must be present, as well as a typical profile of impaired attention, fluctuation of executive functions, an impairment in visuospatial functions, or impaired free recall; it should be associated with at least one behavioral symptom (such as apathy, depression, and anxiety). Patients must fulfill the diagnostic rating sheet for probable PDD, with a history of PD, with a PD disease developed before dementia, with MMSE' scores less than 26, with an impairment in ADLs, with impaired cognition for the 4 items (sevens backwards; lexical fluency; MMSE pentagons; 3-word recall), with absence of major depression; absence of delirium; and absence of other neuropsychiatric diseases [46].

All patients were diagnosed for the first time as PDD, upon enrollment in this study.

All patients were on antiparkinsonian medications.

The equivalent daily dose of levodopa was calculated as the international standard converting measure [47] as follows: dose of levodopa plus dose of dopamine-agonists multiplied by equivalents (= 1 × levodopa dose + 0.75 × controlled release dose + 0.33 × entacapone + 20 × ropinirole dose + 100 × pramipexole + 10 × selegiline + 1 × amantadine) [47]. Each caregiver's patient gave informed consent for participation before entry. All procedures complied with ethical standards for human investigations and the principles of the Declaration of Helsinki.

2.1. Outcome Measures. This was a prospective, longitudinal, open-label, observational, single center, 12-month clinical trial on the effect of Rivastigmine for improving BPSD, with particular reference to apathy. Baseline second level testing data were obtained before starting Rivastigmine, which has been titrated to all patients for eight weeks. All subjects were administered a maintenance dose of Rivastigmine for 12 months. The main outcomes of the study were as follows:

(1) Global performance was assessed using the Montreal Cognitive Assessment (MoCA) [48–50]; the test comprises 6 parts, which have been administered in extenso (memory recall-5 scores; visuospatial construction 4 scores; executive functions 4 scores; attention and working memory 6 scores; language 5 scores; orientation: 6 scores). We considered the results as a whole, and not by subscores. The most significant parts, however, are attention, executive function, and visuospatial construction.

(2) Executive functions, attention, judgment, and analogical reasoning were assessed by Frontal Assessment Battery (FAB) [51].

(3) Apathy was assessed by the Clinician/Researcher Rated Version of the Apathy Evaluation Scale (AES-C) and the parallel Self-Report Version of the same instrument (AES-S) [52]; total score ranges from 18 to 72 points (higher score indicates more severe apathy). The cutoff score ≥ 37 was used to divide apathetic from nonapathetic patients. In the present study, we

considered to be apathetic a patient who showed a total AES-S score ≥37.

(4) Global behavioral symptoms were assessed by the Neuropsychiatric Inventory, NPI [53]; symptom frequency was rated on a scale of 1 to 4 (1 = less than once a week; 2 = once a week; 3 = several times a week; 4 = everyday), and severity was rated on a scale of 1 to 3 (1 = mild; 2 = moderate; 3 = severe). A composite score ranging from 1 to 12, defined as the product of frequency and severity, was calculated. The important aspect of caregiver distress was also recorded and scored for each neuropsychiatric symptom complex (as the study by Oh et al., 2015-A) [6]. The caregiver was asked to rate their own emotional or psychological distress caused by each symptom on a scale of 0 to 5 (0 = no distress; 1 = minimal; 2 = mild; 3 = moderate; 4 = moderately severe; 5 = very severe). A total caregiver distress score was obtained by summing the individual scores on the 12 items (as the study by Oh et al., 2015-A [6]).

2.2. Statistical Analyses. Statistical analyses were performed using the Statistical Package for the Social Sciences (SPSS, version 16.0). Within group changes from baseline to 12 months were tested using the Wilcoxon Signed Ranks test. This was done for the overall scores for each efficacy variable.

In addition, subanalyses of Spearman's Rho correlation and 2-tailed analyses were performed between behavioral data obtained using the NPI, the FAB scores, and apathy scores.

Results are presented as mean changes from baseline with standard deviations, and *p* values are presented where appropriate.

3. Results

Of the 50 patients enrolled, 2 abandoned the study, so 48 patients have been fully studied and followed for 12 months (28 males, 20 women). They have been diagnosed as PDD in accordance with the complete fulfillment of the eight items of the diagnostic rating sheet for probable PDD, as recommended by the Movement Disorder Task Force [46], and their mean scores have been reported in Table 1. Their mean age is 70.4 ± 2.34 years old; their mean educational level is 8.5 ± 2.5 years of school attendance. The mean L-dopa equivalent dosage was 660 ± 130.5 mg/day. 42 patients received dopamine-agonists, 17 entacapone during their cure. Patients have been followed for a mean period of three years (2.5 ± 0.6 years) for motor disturbances, and they have been diagnosed as PDD during the first visit in our Unit. They have never assumed anticholinesterase inhibitors before our diagnosis. Patients were titrated in three months to receive the mean patch dose of transdermal Rivastigmine of 9.5 mg/24 hrs. The most salient side effects at every titration are nausea and disequilibrium; nobody refused the therapy and abandoned the study for conspicuous side effects. Heart frequency and blood pressure are measured at each visit but

TABLE 1: Cognitive parameters. Values are mean (SD). NS = not significant. *MMSE corrected for the adjustments according to age and education.

	Recruitment
MMSE*	23.7 (0.6)
Pill Questionnaire	2.1 (0.2)
Attention, months reversed	3.1 (0.4)
Lexical fluency	8.2 (0.7)
MMSE pentagons	0.1 (0.1)
3-word recall	2.1 (0.3)
GDS-15	3.6 (0.5)

the caregivers have been instructed to measure by themselves at home three times a week.

Table 2 reproduced the summary of the most salient cognitive aspects, compared with a Wilcoxon Signed Rank test (12 months versus baseline).

Tables 3, 4, and 5 represent the behavior aspect resumed by NPI subscores, in order of their prevalence in the studied population, their relevance (the product of severity for frequency), and the derived caregiver stress parameters (as derived by the scores they gave).

Table 6 reflects a sum-up of the possible coexistence of more than 1 NPS for each patient, during the 12-month follow-up.

Table 7 reflects the qualitative results of apathy evaluation, as self-reported (AES-S) and clinically evaluated (AES-C). We have considered as apathetic a patient with a score of >37; all our patients satisfied the criteria, and we report the differences, according to a Wilcoxon rank signed test from the cutoff.

There is a slight, but significant decrease in global cognitive functions and in frontal executive functions, as reported in Table 2. From the very beginning, all the patients showed behavior symptoms, as reported in Table 3; the first evaluation indicates that 77% of patients manifested apathy, with a severe impact on daily living (8, as the product of frequency × severity, maximum score 12), and with a severe relevance for caregivers (4, in a scale from 0 to 5); the second more relevant symptom is anxiety (54% of patients), with an important impact in daily living (6, as the product of frequency × severity), and with a limited relevance for caregivers (2, in a scale from 0 to 5); the third symptom is depression (46% of patients), with a discrete impact in daily living (4, as the product of frequency × severity), and with a limited relevance for caregivers (2, in a scale from 0 to 5); the fourth symptom is hallucinations (42% of patients), with a limited impact on daily living (2, as the product of frequency × severity) and with a limited relevance for caregivers (1, in a scale from 0 to 5). It should be noted that all the other NPS symptoms have been reported, within a limited number of patients, and with limited consequences in daily living. Qualitative assessment of apathy (AES-S and AES-C) is online with this report, as shown in Table 7; as shown in Table 6, 25% of patients showed only one NPS symptom; 42% showed two or more NPS symptoms and 33% three or more. The mean total NPI

TABLE 2: Cognitive parameters at baseline and at 12 months. Values are mean (SD). NS = not significant. *MoCA are reported as raw scores, and in square brackets corrected for the adjustments according to age and education expressed as years of schooling-Conti et al., 2015; Santangelo et al., 2015.

	Baseline	12 months	Within groups (12 months versus baseline) p value
MoCA*	24.1 (0.9) [22.01 (0.8)]	21.3 (0.2) [18.1 (0.7)]	$p < 0.05$
FAB total score	8.2 (0.5)	7.1 (1.3)	$p < 0.05$
Analogies	1.1 (0.2)	1.1 (0.6)	$p < 0.05$
Phonemic fluency	1.2 (0.2)	0.9 (0.5)	NS
Motor series	2.1 (0.7)	1.6 (0.2)	$p < 0.05$
Contrast instructions	2.1 (0.8)	1.4 (0.5)	$p < 0.05$
Go/no-go	0.6 (0.5)	0.2 (0.4)	$p < 0.05$
Prehension behavior	1.1 (0.9)	0.9 (0.8)	NS

TABLE 3: Baseline NPI results.

Subitems NPI	Number of patients/48 (%)	Frequency × severity	Caregiver distress
hallucinations	20 (42%)	2	1
Delusions	10 (21%)	1	1
Agitation/aggression	5 (10%)	2	1
Dysphoria/depression	22 (46%)	4	2
Anxiety	26 (54%)	6	2
Irritability	7 (15%)	4	2
Disinhibition	2 (4%)	2	2
Euphoria	3 (6%)	2	2
Apathy	37 (77%)	8	4
Aberrant motor behavior	3 (6%)	2	2
Sleep behavior change	6 (12%)	4	3
Appetite change	2 (4%)	2	2

TABLE 4: 6-month NPI results; in the first and third rows it has been reported the within group comparison with baseline.

Subitems NPI	Number of patients/48 (%) within groups (6 months versus baseline)	Frequency × severity	Caregiver distress
hallucinations	16 (33%) ($p < 0.001$)	2	1 (NS)
Delusions	7 (15%) ($p < 0.05$)	1	1 (NS)
Agitation/aggression	4 (8%) (NS)	2	1 (NS)
Dysphoria/depression	17 (35%) ($p < 0.001$)	3	1 ($p < 0.05$)
Anxiety	20 (42%) ($p < 0.001$)	4	1 ($p < 0.05$)
Irritability	4 (8%) ($p < 0.001$)	3	1 ($p < 0.05$)
Disinhibition	1 (2%) ($p < 0.001$)	2	1 ($p < 0.05$)
Euphoria	2 (4%) (NS)	2	1 ($p < 0.05$)
Apathy	30 (62%) ($p < 0.001$)	8	4 (NS)
Aberrant motor behavior	2 (4%) (NS)	2	2 ($p < 0.05$)
Sleep behavior change	4 (8%) ($p < 0.001$)	2	3 ($p < 0.05$)
Appetite change	1 (2%) ($p < 0.001$)	2	2 ($p < 0.05$)

TABLE 5: 12-month NPI results. In the first and third rows it has been reported the within group comparison with baseline and with 6-month results.

Subitems NPI	Number of patients/48 (%) within groups (12 months versus baseline) (12 months versus 6 months)	Frequency × severity	Caregiver distress within groups (12 months versus baseline) (12 months versus 6 months)
Hallucinations	15 (31%) ($p < 0.001$) (NS)	2	1 (NS) (NS)
Delusions	8 (17%) ($p < 0.05$) (NS)	1	1 (NS) (NS)
Agitation/aggression	3 (8%) (NS) (NS)	2	1 (NS) (NS)
Dysphoria/depression	19 (40%) ($p < 0.05$) (NS)	3	1 ($p < 0.05$) (NS)
Anxiety	21 (44%) ($p < 0.001$) (NS)	4	1 ($p < 0.05$) (NS)
Irritability	1 (2%) ($p < 0.001$) ($p < 0.001$)	3	1 ($p < 0.05$) (NS)
Disinhibition	0 (0%) ($p < 0.001$) ($p < 0.001$)	0	1 ($p < 0.05$) (NS)
Euphoria	0 (0%) ($p < 0.001$) ($p < 0.001$)	0	1 ($p < 0.05$) (NS)
Apathy	33 (69%) ($p < 0.05$) (NS)	8	8 (NS) (NS)
Aberrant motor behavior	1 (4%) (NS) (NS)	1	1 ($p < 0.05$) (NS)
Sleep behavior change	5 (10%) ($p < 0.001$) (NS)	3	2 ($p < 0.05$) (NS)
Appetite change	1 (2%) ($p < 0.001$) (NS)	1	1 ($p < 0.05$) (NS)

TABLE 6: A synopsis of the presence of a single or more than one NPS for each patient, during follow-up.

	3 or more NPS num pts/48 (%)	2 or more NPS num pts/48 (%)	1 NPS num pts/48 (%)
NPI baseline	16 (33%)	20 (42%)	12 (25%)
NPI 6 months	12 (25%)	26 (54%)	10 (21%)
NPI 12 months	8 (17%)	28 (58%)	12 (25%)

composite score at baseline was 39.4±12.1 and total caregiver distress score was 24.6 ± 11.1.

At 6-month evaluation, all the patients presented behavior symptoms, as reported in Table 4; the evaluation indicates that 62% of patients manifested apathy (decrease within group, 6 month versus baseline, with a Wilcoxon rank signed

test, -7 ± 0.5, $p < 0.001$), with a severe impact on daily living (8, as the product of frequency × severity, maximum score 12), and with a severe relevance for caregivers (4, in a scale from 0 to 5, not significant from baseline); the second more relevant symptom remains anxiety (42% of patients; decrease within group, 6 months versus baseline, with a Wilcoxon rank

TABLE 7: Apathy scores, AES-C, clinician rated apathy evaluation scale; AES-S, self-report rated apathy evaluation scale. Values are mean (SD). NS = not significant. We report the differences from the cutoff score.

	Baseline cutoff > 37	12- month cutoff > 37	Within group baseline/12 months
AES-S	+16.3 (4.1)	+ 19.9 (2.1)	NS
AES-C	+15.5 (3.7)	+21.5 (2.7)	$p < 0.05$

signed test: -6 ± 0.8, $p < 0.001$), with a decreased impact on daily living (4, as the product of frequency × severity), and with a limited relevance for caregivers (1, in a scale from 0 to 5, $p < 0.05$ versus baseline); the third symptom is depression (35% of patients; decrease within group, 6 months versus baseline, with a Wilcoxon rank signed test: -4 ± 0.9, $p < 0.001$), with a modest impact on daily living (3, as the product of frequency × severity), and with a limited relevance for caregivers (1, in a scale from 0 to 5, $p < 0.05$); the fourth symptom is hallucinations (33% of patients; decrease within group, 6 months versus baseline, with a Wilcoxon rank signed test: -4 ± 0.9, $p < 0.001$), with a limited impact on daily living (2, as the product of frequency × severity), and with a limited relevance for caregivers (1, in a scale from 0 to 5, $p < 0.05$). It should be noted that all the other NPS symptoms have been reported, and caregivers reflect a relief of their distress; nonsignificant results have been found for agitation/aggression, euphoria, and aberrant motor behavior parameters, but they had very limited consequences in daily living and were minor cause of caregiver' distress. Moreover, as shown in Table 6, 21% of patients showed only one NPS symptom; 54% showed two or more NPS symptoms and 25% three or more. The mean total NPI composite score at baseline was 33.1 ± 17.1 (according to a Wilcoxon Signed rank test, within group, -6.3 ± 5.0, $p < 0.05$) and total caregiver distress score was 16.7 ± 7.1 (according to a Wilcoxon Signed rank test, within group, -5.9 ± 4.0, $p < 0.05$).

At 12-month evaluation, all the patients presented behavior symptoms, as reported in Table 5; results here have been compared within groups (12 months versus baseline and 6 months versus baseline); there is a general stability of the results; there is a slight decrease in the irritability scores, associated with a decrease in the disinhibition scores and in the euphoria scores ($p < 0.001$), in comparison with the results obtained at 6-month evaluation; apathy increased, up to 69% of patients (decrease within group, 12 month versus baseline, with a Wilcoxon rank signed test (-4 ± 0.7, $p < 0.05$)), with a severe impact on daily living (8, as the product of frequency × severity, maximum score 12) and with a severe relevance for caregivers (4, in a scale from 0 to 5, not significant from baseline and from 6 months); the second more relevant symptom remains anxiety, increasing up to 44% of patients up to 6 months (decrease within group, 12 months versus baseline, with a Wilcoxon rank signed test (-5 ± 0.8, $p < 0.05$)), with a stable impact on daily living (4, as the product of frequency × severity), but with a limited

relevance for caregivers (1, in a scale from 0 to 5, $p < 0.05$ versus baseline, stable versus 6 month); the third symptom is depression, rising up to 40% from 6-month evaluation (decrease within group, 12 months versus baseline, with a Wilcoxon rank signed test (-3 ± 0.3, $p < 0.05$)), with a modest, stable, impact on daily living (3, as the product of frequency × severity), and with a limited relevance for caregivers (1, in a scale from 0 to 5, $p < 0.05$ versus baseline, stable versus 6 months); the fourth stable symptom is hallucinations (31% of patients, decrease within group, 12 months versus baseline, with a Wilcoxon rank signed test (-5 ± 0.4, $p < 0.001$)), with a limited impact on daily living (2, as the product of frequency × severity), and with a limited relevance for caregivers (1, in a scale from 0 to 5, not significant versus baseline and versus 6-month evaluation). Moreover, as shown in Table 6, 25% of patients showed only one NPS symptom; 58% showed two or more NPS symptoms and 17% three or more. The mean total NPI composite score at baseline was 28.7 ± 11.3 (according to a Wilcoxon Signed rank test, within group, versus baseline -4.4 ± 5.8, $p < 0.05$) and an increased total caregiver distress score, which was 20.3 ± 6.2 (according to a Wilcoxon Signed rank test, within group, $+3.9 \pm 1.1$, $p < 0.05$). Qualitative assessment of apathy (AES-S and C) is online with this report, as shown in Table 7 with a significant increase of AES-C, above the cutoff scores (according to a Wilcoxon Signed rank test, within group, versus baseline $+6.2 \pm 2.1$, $p < 0.05$).

Spearman's rank correlation analyses (made at 12 months) indicated that there was a significant correlation, in both the groups, between

(1) NPI high scores and caregiver's distress ($r = 0.78$, $p < 0.01$);

(2) NPI apathy score and AES-S and AES-C ($r = 0.71$, $p < 0.01$ and $r = 0.78$, $p < 0.01$, respectively);

(3) FAB scores and apathy score (NPI and AES-C) ($r = 0.75$, $p < 0.01$ for NPI subscore and $r = 0.79$, $p < 0.01$, for AES-C).

4. Discussion

This work shares many points with the most recent published on the topic [5, 6, 42]; the principal and most significant of them is that NPS are the most salient aspects of PDD intellective disruption and the most relevant for their caregivers.

On the contrary of what merged from the other studies, where depression and anxiety are the most cited NPS, in this study we have found that apathy is the most constant NPS; its impact for frequency and severity is heavy and constant in the time and is onerous for the caregivers.

Rivastigmine works well and improves NPS symptoms, reducing caregivers' stress, in line with many other studies [5, 6, 54], in PD psychosis [55], in AD [56, 57], and in sVAD [20, 21] at the very beginning, and, in line with what has been previously described, we assist a first-step (6-month evaluation) global general amelioration of signs and symptoms in NPS, with a relief of caregiver's distress. That concerns practically all the NPS, a part from agitation and aberrant motor behavior; the results are so good to reflect on a significant decrease of NPI total score and an effective decrease on caregiver's burden. But even at this point, apathy, in our cases, maintains its hard impact, and for its frequency and severity it is related to caregiver's stress. Rivastigmine does not ameliorate that score. At 12-month evaluation, results in our study differ, even more, from the previous reported studies: there is a slight reduction of NPS signs, as demonstrated by the comparison with baseline results, but results are quite superimposable to what has been revealed at 6-month evaluation. On the contrary, caregivers burden increase significantly. That relates quite well with the qualitative perceive of apathy, as demonstrated by AES-S and AES-C, which remains stable from baseline throughout the entire follow-up. So, we can conclude that Rivastigmine might help for NPS symptoms in PDD, but its efficacy is limited in time, varies for symptoms, and does not have benefit for apathy in daily living.

Apathy increments in PDD the burden of the other motor and intellectual dysfunctions and worsens all the other behavioral symptoms. As reported in many dedicated studies, apathy is tightly related to PD or, better say, to a sufferance of the nigrostriatal pathway [13, 29, 58, 59]. Functional connectivity within the striatum and between striatal and ventrolateral prefrontal regions has been demonstrated in support of those studies, in patients with PD with high apathy compared to low [31], but results are not univocal, as they have been rejected by other studies [32, 33]. In general, many others are the brain networks related to apathy in PD, extending from the nigrostriatal up to frontal, cingulate, and limbic areas, precuneus, parietal inferior lobule, and so on (see data and literature in [22, 34]). If functional localization of networks underlying apathy is uncertain, even more complex is the neurochemical and pharmacological face. Hence, seeming quite conclusive that basal forebrain, striatum, parietal, and frontal cortex are strongly involved in apathy, three major neurotransmitters should be taken into account for its determination: acetylcholine, noradrenaline, and dopamine. An inverse correlation between catecholaminergic binding potential, indicative of a specific loss of dopamine and noradrenaline innervation, and apathy in PD was found in the bilateral ventral striatum [38]. But again, data are not so certain and are verified by studies in AD patients, although dopaminergic neurotransmission is thought to underline many goal-directed behaviors including addiction, and there is evidence for the efficacy of dopaminergic agents for apathy in AD [60]; there was no association between dopamine D2/D3 receptor density and apathy in AD [61]. We have no data, at the moment, for the studies of D2-D3 concentrations in PD or PDD with or without apathy.

Since many NPS respond to acetylcholinestease and butyrrylcholinesterase inhibitors, it can be documented a pivotal role of Ach in vivo. Rivastigmine works quite well, at least at the very beginning for NPS, but not for apathy. What seems highly probable is that in PDD there is a very precarious equilibrium between dopamine and Ach and that disequilibrium might potentiate the resistance of specific symptoms such as apathy, probably determined by the alteration of multineurotransmitters synaptic networks.

Our study has some strengths:

(1) We enrolled first-diagnosed PDD patients who began Rivastigmine in our study and have been studied for 12 months.

(2) All the patients can be fully examined and have a strenuous assistance of a caregiver, who is the other actor of the study.

(3) We employed some similar method as those described by Oh et al. (2015-A) [6] and implement some other measures, but as Oh et al., [6] we strictly surveyed the pharmacological intake of our patients in order to avoid any other interference bias.

(4) All the patients have been supplied by transdermal Rivastigmine patch.

However, our study has several weaknesses:

(1) It is a single center study, and the number of patients is very small to infer definite results.

(2) It is an open-label and not blinded study.

(3) It has no pathological confirmation.

Data deriving from our study suggest that

(1) apathy should be considered from the very initial phases of PD (and PDD) by devoted neuropsychological instrument;

(2) multireceptor approach should be employed to treat it, so many potential sites could be employed, such as SSRI, NARI, dopaminergic agonists, and probably modulating also Ach;

(3) apathy should be discussed with and explained to patients and to caregivers: it might help to confront it better;

(4) neurologists should think more overtly about apathy, in order to understand it and possibly treat it; apathy inside a specific disease, such as PD, or AD, or sVAD might become something different. It must be said, forwardly, that, as well as in AD, it seems difficult to find a neurodegenerative complex clinical condition, such as PDD, in which apathy is an isolated symptom. AS in our study, even if devotedly constructed to define it, apathy can coexist with other NPS, and therefore, its anatomical and biochemical core could be modified and worsened, by the interference of many other neurochemical substrates, which underline opposite symptoms, such as anxiety, aggression, and euphoria.

5. Conclusion

In conclusion, our study confirmed some results of many other precedent studies, on the positive results of Rivastigmine for the reduction of NPS symptoms, but we are more circumspect on its effect on apathy, suggesting that polyvalent and multireceptor treatment should be desirable and employed; larger, placebo-controlled studies should be required to define, adequately combat, and give long-lasting relief to such a difficult symptom, as apathy is.

Acknowledgments

The authors thank Mary Louise Spencer-Wallace, Ph.D., for her precious assistance.

References

[1] C. H. Williams-Gray, T. Foltynie, S. J. G. Lewis, and R. A. Barker, "Cognitive deficits and psychosis in Parkinson's disease: a review of pathophysiology and therapeutic options," *CNS Drugs*, vol. 20, no. 6, pp. 477–505, 2006.

[2] J. S. A. M. Reijnders, U. Ehrt, W. E. J. Weber, D. Aarsland, and A. F. G. Leentjens, "A systematic review of prevalence studies of depression in Parkinson's disease," *Movement Disorders*, vol. 23, no. 2, pp. 183–189, 2008.

[3] A. Schrag, M. Jahanshahi, and N. Quinn, "What contributes to quality of life in patients with Parkinson's disease?" *Journal of Neurology, Neurosurgery & Psychiatry*, vol. 69, no. 3, pp. 308–312, 2000.

[4] D. Weintraub, P. J. Moberg, J. E. Duda, I. R. Katz, and M. B. Stern, "Effect of psychiatric and other nonmotor symptoms on disability in Parkinson's disease," *Journal of the American Geriatrics Society*, vol. 52, no. 5, pp. 784–788, 2004.

[5] S. Y. Oh, J. S. Kim, and P. H. Lee, "Effect of rivastigmine on behavioral and psychiatric symptoms of Parkinson's disease dementia," *Journal of Movement Disorders*, vol. 8, no. 2, pp. 98–102, 2015.

[6] Y. S. Oh, J. E. Lee, P. H. Lee, and J. S. Kim, "Neuropsychiatric symptoms in Parkinson's disease dementia are associated with increased caregiver burden," *Journal of Movement Disorders*, vol. 8, no. 1, pp. 26–32, 2015.

[7] K. H. Karlsen, J. P. Larsen, E. Tandberg, and J. G. Mæland, "Influence of clinical and demographic variables on quality of life in patients with Parkinson's disease," *Journal of Neurology, Neurosurgery & Psychiatry*, vol. 66, no. 4, pp. 431–435, 1999.

[8] L. M. Shulman, R. L. Taback, A. A. Rabinstein, and W. J. Weiner, "Non-recognition of depression and other non-motor symptoms in Parkinson's disease," *Parkinsonism and Related Disorders*, vol. 8, no. 3, pp. 193–197, 2002.

[9] D. Aarsland, I. Litvan, and J. P. Larsen, "Neuropsychiatric symptoms of patients with progressive supranuclear palsy and Parkinson's disease," *Journal of Neuropsychiatry and Clinical Neurosciences*, vol. 13, no. 1, pp. 42–49, 2001.

[10] D. Aarsland, J. Zaccai, and C. Brayne, "A systematic review of prevalence studies of dementia in Parkinson's disease," *Movement Disorders*, vol. 20, no. 10, pp. 1255–1263, 2005.

[11] R. G. Brown and G. Pluck, "Negative symptoms: the 'pathology' of motivation and goal-directed behaviour," *Trends in Neurosciences*, vol. 23, no. 9, pp. 412–417, 2000.

[12] R. Erro, C. Vitale, M. Amboni et al., "The heterogeneity of early Parkinson's disease: a cluster analysis on newly diagnosed untreated patients," *PLoS ONE*, vol. 8, no. 8, Article ID e70244, 2013.

[13] G. Santangelo, C. Vitale, L. Trojano et al., "Relationship between apathy and cognitive dysfunctions in de novo untreated Parkinson's disease: a prospective longitudinal study," *European Journal of Neurology*, vol. 22, no. 2, pp. 253–260, 2015.

[14] The American Geriatrics Society 2012 Beers Criteria Update Expert Panel, "American Geriatrics Society updated Beers Criteria for potentially inappropriate medication use in older adults," *Journal of the American Geriatrics Society*, vol. 60, no. 4, pp. 616–631, 2012.

[15] M. Steinberg and C. G. Lyketsos, "Atypical antipsychotic use in patients with dementia. Managing safety concerns," *American Journal of Psychiatry*, vol. 169, no. 9, pp. 900–906, 2012.

[16] K. Seppi, D. Weintraub, M. Coelho et al., "The movement disorder society evidence-based medicine review update: treatments for the non-motor symptoms of Parkinson's disease," *Movement Disorders*, vol. 26, supplement 3, pp. S42–S80, 2011.

[17] D. Devos, C. Moreau, D. Maltête et al., "Rivastigmine in apathetic but dementia and depression-free patients with Parkinson's disease: a double-blind, placebo-controlled, randomised clinical trial," *Journal of Neurology, Neurosurgery & Psychiatry*, vol. 85, no. 6, pp. 668–674, 2014.

[18] C. G. Parsons, W. Danysz, A. Dekundy, and I. Pulte, "Memantine and cholinesterase inhibitors: complementary mechanisms in the treatment of Alzheimer's disease," *Neurotoxicity Research*, vol. 24, no. 3, pp. 358–369, 2013.

[19] J. Birks, "Cholinesterase inhibitors for Alzheimer's disease," *The Cochrane Database of Systematic Reviews*, no. 1, Article ID CD005593, 2006.

[20] R. Moretti, P. Torre, R. M. Antonello, G. Cazzato, S. Griggio, and A. Bava, "An open-label pilot study comparing rivastigmine and low-dose aspirin for the treatment of symptoms specific to patients with subcortical vascular dementia," *Current Therapeutic Research*, vol. 63, no. 7, pp. 443–458, 2002.

[21] R. Moretti, P. Torre, R. M. Antonello, G. Cazzato, and A. Bava, "Rivastigmine in subcortical vascular dementia: an open 22-month study," *Journal of the Neurological Sciences*, vol. 203-204, pp. 141–146, 2002.

[22] R. Moretti and R. Signori, "Neural correlates for apathy: frontal-prefrontal and parietal cortical-subcortical circuits," *Frontiers in Aging Neuroscience*, vol. 8, article 289, 2016.

[23] S. E. Starkstein, H. S. Mayberg, T. J. Preziosi, P. Andrezejewski, R. Leiguarda, and R. G. Robinson, "Reliability, validity, and clinical correlates of apathy in Parkinson's disease," *The Journal of Neuropsychiatry and Clinical Neurosciences*, vol. 4, no. 2, pp. 134–139, 1992.

[24] S. E. Starkstein and A. F. Leentjens, "The nosological position of apathy in clinical practice," *Journal of Neurology, Neurosurgery, and Psychiatry*, vol. 10, pp. 202–209, 2008.

[25] J. S. A. M. Reijnders, B. Scholtissen, W. E. J. Weber, P. Aalten, F. R. J. Verhey, and A. F. G. Leentjens, "Neuroanatomical correlates of apathy in Parkinson's disease: a magnetic resonance imaging study using voxel-based morphometry," *Movement Disorders*, vol. 25, no. 14, pp. 2318–2325, 2010.

[26] G. Robert, F. Le Jeune, C. Lozachmeur et al., "Apathy in patients with Parkinson disease without dementia or depression: a PET study," *Neurology*, vol. 79, no. 11, pp. 1155–1160, 2012.

[27] B. N. Cuthbert and T. R. Insel, "Toward the future of psychiatric diagnosis: the seven pillars of RDoC," *BMC Medicine*, vol. 11, article 126, 2013.

[28] D. T. Stuss, R. Van Reekum, and K. J. Murphy, "Differentiation of states and causes of apathy," in *The Neuropsychology of Emotion*, J. C. Borod, Ed., pp. 340–363, Oxford University Press, Oxford, UK, 2000.

[29] K. Dujardin, P. Sockeel, M. Delliaux, A. Destée, and L. Defebvre, "Apathy may herald cognitive decline and dementia in Parkinson's disease," *Movement Disorders*, vol. 24, no. 16, pp. 2391–2397, 2009.

[30] J. Cummings, J. H. Friedman, G. Garibaldi et al., "Apathy in neurodegenerative diseases: recommendations on the design of

clinical trials," *Journal of Geriatric Psychiatry and Neurology*, vol. 28, no. 3, pp. 159–173, 2015.

[31] H. C. Baggio, B. Segura, J. L. Garrido-Millan et al., "Resting-state frontostriatal functional connectivity in Parkinson's disease-related apathy," *Movement Disorders*, vol. 30, no. 5, pp. 671–679, 2015.

[32] C. Huang, L. D. Ravdin, M. J. Nirenberg et al., "Neuroimaging markers of motor and nonmotor features of Parkinson's disease: an [^{18}F]fluorodeoxyglucose positron emission computed tomography study," *Dementia and Geriatric Cognitive Disorders*, vol. 35, no. 3-4, pp. 183–196, 2013.

[33] V. Isella, P. Melzi, M. Grimaldi et al., "Clinical, neuropsychological, and morphometric correlates of apathy in Parkinson's disease," *Movement Disorders*, vol. 17, no. 2, pp. 366–371, 2002.

[34] C. Kos, M. J. van Tol, J. B. C. Marsman, H. Knegtering, and A. Aleman, "Neural correlates of apathy in patients with neurodegenerative disorders, acquired brain injury, and psychiatric disorders," *Neuroscience and Biobehavioral Reviews*, vol. 69, pp. 381–401, 2016.

[35] F. M. Skidmore, M. Yang, L. Baxter et al., "Apathy, depression, and motor symptoms have distinct and separable resting activity patterns in idiopathic Parkinson disease," *NeuroImage*, vol. 81, pp. 484–495, 2013.

[36] M. L. Levy, J. L. Cummings, L. A. Fairbanks et al., "Apathy is not depression," *Journal of Neuropsychiatry and Clinical Neurosciences*, vol. 10, no. 3, pp. 314–319, 1998.

[37] R. Moretti, P. Torre, R. M. Antonello et al., "Apathy: a complex symptom specific to the clinical pattern of presentation of Parkinson's disease?" *American Journal of Alzheimer's Disease and Other Dementias*, vol. 27, no. 3, pp. 196–201, 2012.

[38] P. Remy, M. Doder, A. Lees, N. Turjanski, and D. Brooks, "Depression in Parkinson's disease: loss of dopamine and noradrenaline innervation in the limbic system," *Brain*, vol. 128, no. 6, pp. 1314–1322, 2005.

[39] K. Martinowich, K. M. Cardinale, R. J. Schloesser, M. Hsu, N. H. Greig, and H. K. Manji, "Acetylcholinesterase inhibition ameliorates deficits in motivational drive," *Behavioral and Brain Functions*, vol. 8, article 15, 2012.

[40] S. Thobois, E. Lhommée, H. Klinger et al., "Parkinsonian apathy responds to dopaminergic stimulation of D2/D3 receptors with piribedil," *Brain*, vol. 136, no. 5, pp. 1568–1577, 2013.

[41] A. Chatterjee and S. Fahn, "Methylphenidate treats apathy in Parkinson's disease," *Journal of Neuropsychiatry and Clinical Neurosciences*, vol. 14, no. 4, pp. 461–462, 2002.

[42] A. Schrag, A. Sauerbier, and K. R. Chaudhuri, "New clinical trials for nonmotor manifestations of Parkinson's disease," *Movement Disorders*, vol. 30, no. 11, pp. 1490–1504, 2015.

[43] W. R. G. Gibb and A. J. Lees, "The relevance of the Lewy body to the pathogenesis of idiopathic Parkinson's disease," *Journal of Neurology, Neurosurgery and Psychiatry*, vol. 51, no. 6, pp. 745–752, 1988.

[44] M. Emre, D. Aarsland, R. Brown et al., "Clinical diagnostic criteria for dementia associated with Parkinson's disease," *Movement Disorders*, vol. 22, no. 12, pp. 1689–1707, 2007.

[45] C. G. Goetz, M. Emre, and B. Dubois, "Parkinson's disease dementia: definitions, guidelines, and research perspectives in diagnosis," *Annals of Neurology*, vol. 64, supplement 2, pp. S81–S92, 2008.

[46] B. Dubois, D. Burn, C. Goetz et al., "Diagnostic procedures for Parkinson's disease dementia: recommendations from the movement disorder society task force," *Movement Disorders* vol. 22, no. 16, pp. 2314–2324, 2007.

[47] C. L. Tomlinson, R. Stowe, S. Patel, C. Rick, R. Gray, and C. E. Clarke, "Systematic review of levodopa dose equivalency reporting in Parkinson's disease," *Movement Disorders*, vol. 25, no. 15, pp. 2649–2653, 2010.

[48] Z. S. Nasreddine, N. A. Phillips, V. Bédirian et al., "The Montreal Cognitive Assessment, MoCA: a brief screening tool for mild cognitive impairment," *Journal of the American Geriatrics Society*, vol. 53, no. 4, pp. 695–699, 2005.

[49] G. Santangelo, M. Siciliano, R. Pedone et al., "Normative data for the montreal cognitive assessment in an Italian population sample," *Neurological Sciences*, vol. 36, no. 4, pp. 585–591, 2015.

[50] S. Conti, S. Bonazzi, M. LAiacona, M. Masina, and M. Vanelli Coralli, "Montreal Cognitive Assessment (MoCA)-Italian version: regression based norms and equivalent scores," *Neurological Sciences*, vol. 36, no. 2, pp. 209–214, 2015.

[51] B. Dubois, A. Slachevsky, I. Litvan, and B. Pillon, "The FAB: a frontal assessment battery at bedside," *Neurology*, vol. 55, no. 11, pp. 1621–1626, 2000.

[52] R. S. Marin, R. C. Biedrzycki, and S. Firinciogullari, "Reliability and validity of the apathy evaluation scale," *Psychiatry Research*, vol. 38, no. 2, pp. 143–162, 1991.

[53] J. L. Cummings, M. Mega, K. Gray, S. Rosenberg-Thompson, D. A. Carusi, and J. Gornbein, "The neuropsychiatric inventory: comprehensive assessment of psychopathology in dementia," *Neurology*, vol. 44, no. 12, pp. 2308–2314, 1994.

[54] M. Emre, D. Aarsland, A. Albanese et al., "Rivastigmine for dementia associated with Parkinson's disease," *The New England Journal of Medicine*, vol. 351, no. 24, pp. 2509–2518, 2004.

[55] P. J. Reading, A. K. Luce, and I. G. McKeith, "Rivastigmine in the treatment of parkinsonian psychosis and cognitive impairment: preliminary findings from an open trial," *Movement Disorders*, vol. 16, no. 6, pp. 1171–1174, 2001.

[56] E. Cumbo and L. D. Ligori, "Differential effects of current specific treatments on behavioral and psychological symptoms in patients with Alzheimer's disease: a 12-month, randomized, open-label trial," *Journal of Alzheimer's Disease*, vol. 39, no. 3, pp. 477–485, 2014.

[57] B. Winblad, G. Grossberg, L. Frölich et al., "IDEAL: a 6-month, double-blind, placebo-controlled study of the first skin patch for Alzheimer disease," *Neurology*, vol. 69, no. 4, supplement 1, pp. S14–S22, 2007.

[58] G. Santangelo, C. Vitale, M. Picillo et al., "Apathy and striatal dopamine transporter levels in de-novo, untreated Parkinson's disease patients," *Parkinsonism and Related Disorders*, vol. 21, no. 5, pp. 489–493, 2015.

[59] R. David, M. Koulibaly, M. Benoit et al., "Striatal dopamine transporter levels correlate with apathy in neurodegenerative diseases. A SPECT study with partial volume effect correction," *Clinical Neurology and Neurosurgery*, vol. 110, no. 1, pp. 19–24, 2008.

[60] P. B. Rosenberg, K. L. Lanctôt, L. T. Drye et al., "Safety and efficacy of methylphenidate for apathy in Alzheimer's disease: a randomized, placebo-controlled trial," *Journal of Clinical Psychiatry*, vol. 74, no. 8, pp. 810–816, 2013.

[61] S. Reeves, R. Brown, R. Howard, and P. Grasby, "Increased striatal dopamine (D2/D3) receptor availability and delusions in Alzheimer disease," *Neurology*, vol. 72, no. 6, pp. 528–534, 2009.

25

Neuroprotective Effects of Salidroside in the MPTP Mouse Model of Parkinson's Disease: Involvement of the PI3K/Akt/GSK3β Pathway

Wei Zhang,[1] Hong He,[1] Hujie Song,[2] Junjie Zhao,[1] Tao Li,[1] Leitao Wu,[1]
Xiaojun Zhang,[3] and Jianzong Chen[1]

[1]Research Center of Traditional Chinese Medicine, Xijing Hospital, Fourth Military Medical University, Xi'an 710032, China
[2]Department of Encephalopathy, Xi'an Encephalopathy Hospital of Traditional Chinese Medicine, Xi'an 710032, China
[3]Department of Physics, Fourth Military Medical University, Xi'an 710032, China

Correspondence should be addressed to Xiaojun Zhang; zy04310@fmmu.edu.cn and Jianzong Chen; jzchen57@fmmu.edu.cn

Academic Editor: Palanisamy Arulselvan

The degenerative loss through apoptosis of dopaminergic neurons in the substantia nigra pars compacta plays a primary role in the progression of Parkinson's disease (PD). Our in vitro experiments suggested that salidroside (Sal) could protect against 1-methyl-4-phenylpyridine-induced cell apoptosis in part by regulating the PI3K/Akt/GSK3β pathway. The current study aims to increase our understanding of the protective mechanisms of Sal in the 1-methyl-4-phenyl-1,2,3,6-tetrahydropyridine- (MPTP-) induced PD mouse model. We found that pretreatment with Sal could protect against MPTP-induced increase of the time of turning downwards and climbing down to the floor. Sal also prevented MPTP-induced decrease of locomotion frequency and the increase of the immobile time. Sal provided a protection of in MPTP-induced loss of tyrosine hydroxylase-positive neurons in SNpc and the level of DA, DOPAC, and HVA in the striatum. Furthermore, Sal could increase the phosphorylation level of Akt and GSK3β, upregulate the ratio of Bcl-2/Bax, and inhibit the activation of caspase-3, caspase-6, and caspase-9. These results show that Sal prevents the loss of dopaminergic neurons and the PI3K/Akt/GSK3β pathway signaling pathway may have mediated the protection of Sal against MPTP, suggesting that Sal may be a potential candidate in neuroprotective treatment for PD.

1. Introduction

Parkinson's disease (PD), as one of the most common neurodegenerative disorders, displays characteristic motor and behavioral disturbances, including static tremor, rigidity, bradykinesia, and posture gait disorders. It is primarily caused by the degenerative deletion through apoptosis of dopaminergic (DA) neurons in the substantia nigra pars compacta (SNpc) [1]. Therapeutic approaches including numerous drugs have been greatly identified, but most of drugs which were explored for clinical approval cannot suspend or stop the progression of PD with inevitable obvious adverse effects [2–5]. Although its pathogenesis remains unclear, current evident indicates that Akt, also known as protein kinase B, plays a potential mechanistic role of defective signaling in PD [6–8]. It hypothesizes that pharmacological compounds which recover the defective Akt activity might be an operative method for striking neurotrophic and antiapoptotic effects.

The phosphoinositide 3-kinase (PI3K)/Akt pathway is a critical pathway related to survival, proliferation, and growth in response to extracellular signals in neurons [9–11]. PI3K phosphorylates the 3-position hydroxyl group in the inositol ring of phosphoinositides and then recruits Akt contained pleckstrin homology domain to translocate to the plasma membrane. As a serine/threonine-specific protein kinase, it has been found that Akt and phosphorylated Akt have a marked decrease in the SNpc of PD patients [6]. In addition, the active PI3K/Akt pathway increases the survival and growth of DA neuronal cells by inhibiting apoptosis [12–14]. Glycogen synthase kinase-3 (GSK-3), as one of the substrates of Akt, is a pleiotropic serine/threonine protein kinase [15,16].

It contains two isoforms of GSK-3α and GSK-3β. Some evidences discovered that Akt could inhibit the activity of GSK3 by phosphorylating at Ser21 in GSK-3α or Ser9 in GSK-3β [15, 17]. GSK-3β dysregulation results in Parkinson's-like pathophysiology; meanwhile, activation of GSK-3β has been shown to facilitate numerous apoptotic conditions in PD [18, 19].

Salidroside (Sal, 2-(4-hydroxyphenyl)ethyl β-D-glucopyranoside, $C_{14}H_{20}O_7$) is mainly extracted from *Rhodiola rosea* L., which grows at high altitude localities and usually is used as one of the herbal drugs in worldwide [20]. Sal has been shown to have numerous pharmacological effects, such as antioxidant effects [21, 22], antiapoptosis effects [23], and maintenance of mitochondrial function [24]. Our paper recently found that Sal protected DA neurons against 1-methyl-4-phenyl-1,2,3,6-tetrahydropyridine- (MPTP-)/1-methyl-4-phenyl-pyridinium- (MPP+-) induced toxicity in a dose-dependent manner through modulation of the ROS-NO related mitochondrial pathway both in vivo and in vitro [25]. Moreover, we also have shown that Sal could protect against MPP+-induced apoptosis through modulation of the PI3K/Akt pathway in vitro [26]. Based on the result, this study aimed to further evaluate the neuroprotective effects of Sal in the MPTP-induced PD mouse model and determine whether its protective mechanisms relate to the PI3K/Akt/GSK3β pathway, so that it can provide evidence for Sal as a potential target for effective neuroprotective treatment for PD.

2. Materials and Methods

2.1. Animals and Treatment. C57BL/6 mice (male, eight weeks old, weighing 23–28 g) were supplied by the Experimental Animal Center of the Fourth Military Medical University and fed in a 12 h on/off light cycle in a temperature-controlled room (23 ± 1°C). All mice were reared in a single cage with food and water provided ad libitum for 7 days before the start of experiments. All procedures were approved by the Animal Care and Use Committee of the Fourth Military Medical University.

The subacute MPTP mice model was carried out depending on the previously published methods [27]. All the mice were divided by the random number method into 5 groups (n = 10 per group): control group, in which mice were intraperitoneally injected with saline (30 mg/kg/day) for 12 days, Sal (HPLC ≥ 98%, National Institute for the Control of Pharmaceutical and Biological Products, Xi'an, China) group, in which mice were intraperitoneally injected with Sal (45 mg/kg/day) for 12 days, MPTP (Sigma-Aldrich, MO, USA) group, in which mice were intraperitoneally injected with saline (30 mg/kg/day) for 7 days and then MPTP (30 mg/kg/day) for 5 consecutive days, Sal + MPTP group I, in which mice were intraperitoneally injected with Sal (15 mg/kg/day) for 7 days and then MPTP (30 mg/kg/day) for 5 consecutive days, and Sal + MPTP group II, in which mice were intraperitoneally injected with Sal (45 mg/kg/day) for 7 days and then MPTP (30 mg/kg/day) for 5 consecutive days. After the last treatment at 24 h, the mice were managed to subsequent tests.

2.2. Pole Test. Pole tests were performed following a previously published protocol starting on the 1st day after treatment began [28]. Mice were permitted to adapt to the experimental environment for 2 days before the first test. Each mouse was placed on the top of a pole with a rough surface (1 cm in diameter and 55 cm in height) with its head facing upwards. The time in which the mouse completely turned downwards (T-turn) and climbed down to the floor (T-LA) was recorded.

2.3. Open Field Test. The open field test evaluated the change of locomotory capacity according to the previously published protocol [29]. A wooden box ($40 \times 40 \times 40$ cm³) was horizontally divided into 16 squares of equal size (10×10 cm²). The central 4 squares (20×20 cm²) were considered the center, and the surrounding 4 sides (10×10 cm²) and 4 corners (10×10 cm²) were considered the periphery. After a mouse was put in the center of the box, a 30 min test session was initiated. The dynamic activity of mice was recorded by an automatic video tracking system (Shanghai Jiliang Software Technology Co., Ltd., Shanghai, China). The percentage of speed and time spent in the center of the arena was used to assess the motor and behavioral changes.

2.4. Immunofluorescence Staining. Immunofluorescence histochemistry of mouse brain tissue was performed according to previously published protocols [30]. The tissue was cut into 30 μm slices with a sliding microtome. In the staining experiments, it was fixed in 4% paraformaldehyde for 15 min followed by incubation in 0.2% Triton X-100 permeabilization solution for 1 h and 1% bovine serum albumin for 2 h. Sections were then incubated in a chicken anti-mouse tyrosine hydroxylase (TH) antibody (Abcam, CA, USA) diluted at 1 : 200 in primary antibody dilution buffer at 4°C overnight. After rinsing three times in PBS for 5 minutes, slides were incubated with Alexa Fluor® 594 Goat Anti-Chicken IgG secondary antibody (Life Technologies, NY, USA) for 2 h at room temperature in the dark. Cover slips were mounted onto slides with 0.5% glycerin. The section was analyzed on an immunofluorescence microscopy (IX51, Olympus, Japan). The TH-positive neuron cells in 5 position-matched sections of each mouse were manually counted by ImageJ software (version 1.48) by a technician who was blinded to this study [31]. The average number of immunoreactive neurons per section represents the livability.

2.5. High Performance Liquid Chromatography (HPLC) Analysis of Striatal Dopamine and Its Metabolite Level. High performance liquid chromatography (HPLC) was used to analyze the dopamine (DA) and its metabolites, including dihydroxyphenyl acetic acid (DOPAC) and homovanillic acid (HVA), in the striatum, as previously described [32]. The striatum was rapidly isolated and was homogenized by 100 μL ice-cold 0.2 N perchloric acid. After the homogenization, it was centrifuged at 13,000 ×g for 15 min at 4°C. The supernatant was filtered by the 0.45 mm of filter and then tested by electrochemical detection (Eicom, Kyoto, Japan) for HPLC. The concentration was expressed as ng/mg tissue.

2.6. Western Blots. The tissue was collected and ground and combined with a cell lysate solution. Protein quantification was performed with a bicinchoninic acid protein assay kit (Life Technologies, NY, USA). In Western blot tests, after electrophoresis, the transferred PVDF membranes were incubated overnight with antibodies against Akt, phospho-Akt (Ser473), GSK-3β, and phospho-GSK-3β (Ser9) (Cell Signaling Technology, MA, USA), B-cell lymphoma-2 (Bcl-2), Bax, or cleaved cysteine-dependent aspartate-directed proteases (caspase-3, caspase-6, or caspase-9) (Abcam, CA, USA). All antibodies were diluted to 1:500–1:3000 and were incubated at 4°C. Membranes were subjected to 3 times × 5 min washes in PBS and were then incubated for 2 h with HRP-conjugated anti-rabbit IgG antibody. Protein levels were measured with Quantity One analysis software (Bio-Rad, CA, USA). All experiments were conducted in triplicate.

2.7. Statistical Analyses. Data were expressed as the mean ± SEM from at least three independent experiments. Statistical significance was analyzed by one-way analysis of variance (ANOVA) or Student's *t*-test in SPSS version 20.0. A value of $P < 0.05$ was considered statistically significant.

3. Results

3.1. Sal Prevents Behavioral Disorders. The protective effect of Sal against PD-related behavioral disorders was evaluated by pole test and open field test in the MPTP-induced PD mouse model. In the pole test, MPTP treatment significantly extended the time of T-turn to 3.9 ± 0.5 s ($P < 0.01$) and that of T-LA to 18.0 ± 1.4 s ($P < 0.01$) compared with the control group (Figures 1(a) and 1(b)). Pretreatment with Sal significantly blocked the increase of T-turn and T-LA time in the Sal + MPTP group I ($P < 0.05$; $P < 0.01$) and Sal + MPTP group II ($P < 0.01$; $P < 0.01$) compared with the MPTP group; however, it merely had no significant difference in Sal + MPTP group II when compared with control group ($P > 0.05$). In the open field test, the locomotion frequency significantly reduced to 35.1 ± 7.2 times ($P < 0.05$) and immobility time increased to 19.3 ± 4.2 s ($P < 0.01$) in the MPTP group when compared with the control group (Figures 1(c) and 1(d)). Pretreatment with Sal had no significant changes in either locomotion frequency or immobile time in the Sal + MPTP group I ($P > 0.05$). However, pretreatment with Sal significantly prevented the locomotion frequency ($P < 0.01$) and decreased the immobile time ($P < 0.01$) in the Sal + MPTP group II (Figures 1(c) and 1(d)), and it had no significant difference when compared with control group ($P > 0.05$).

3.2. Sal Prevents the Loss of TH-Positive Neurons. There was no significant difference in the number of TH-positive neurons (100.0 ± 5.2%) in the control group and in the Sal group (95.3 ± 3.6%) (Figures 2(a), 2(b), and 2(f)). However, a significant reduction was observed in the number of TH-positive neurons in the MPTP group compared with the control group ($P < 0.01$) (Figures 2(a), 2(c), and 2(f)). Compared with MPTP group, although pretreatment with Sal significantly restored the number of TH-positive neurons in

the Sal + MPTP group I (50.2 ± 6.4% versus 30.4 ± 4.2%) ($P < 0.05$), it was still lower than that in control group ($P < 0.05$). However, pretreatment with Sal could significantly restore that number to 70.2 ± 5.7% in the Sal + MPTP group II ($P < 0.01$) (Figures 2(c), 2(e), and 2(f)), and it had no significant difference when compared with control group ($P > 0.05$).

3.3. Sal Prevents the Loss of Striatal DA, DOPAC, and HVA Level. DA, DOPAC, and HVA can directly express the content of dopamine in the striatum of mice. It was found that the level of DA, DOPAC, and HVA had no statistical obvious change in the Sal group, when compared with control group (Figure 3). It significantly reduced these levels in the MPTP group ($P < 0.01$); however, it statistically significantly increased all of them in a dose-dependent way in the Sal + MPTP group I ($P < 0.05$) and in the Sal + MPTP group II ($P < 0.01$). And they merely had no significant difference in the Sal + MPTP group II when compared with control group ($P > 0.05$).

3.4. Sal Prevents the Level of pSer473-Akt and pSer9-GSK-3β. Next the role of Akt and GSK-3β in Sal protection against MPTP-induced toxicity is explored. There was no difference in the total level of Akt and GSK-3β among all groups (Figures 4(a) and 4(c)). MPTP treatment induced a decrease in pSer473-Akt/Akt ratio compared with the control group (45.0 ± 5.1% versus 100.0 ± 4.5%) ($P < 0.01$) (Figures 4(a) and 4(b)). Pretreatment with Sal could prevent the pSer473-Akt level to 70.0 ± 3.2% in the Sal + MPTP group I ($P < 0.05$) and 95.1 ± 5.1% in the Sal + MPTP group II ($P < 0.01$); however, it merely had no significant difference in Sal + MPTP group II when compared with control group ($P > 0.05$). In addition, MPTP treatment induced a decrease in pSer9-GSK-3β/GSK-3β ratio compared with the control group (40.5 ± 13.2% versus 100.0 ± 4.0%) ($P < 0.01$) (Figures 4(c) and 4(d)). It significantly prevented the pSer9-GSK-3β/GSK-3β level to 65.2 ± 4.1% in the Sal + MPTP group I ($P < 0.05$) and 101.1 ± 7.0% in the Sal + MPTP group II ($P < 0.01$); however, it also had no significant difference in Sal + MPTP group II when compared with control group ($P > 0.05$).

3.5. Sal Prevents the Ratio of Bcl-2 and Bax. The balance of the Bcl-2/Bax ratio is an indicator of the activation of proapoptotic signaling and is related to cell survival or death. It investigated whether treatment with Sal protected against MPTP-induced toxicity involving Bcl-2 and Bax in vivo. It significantly reduced the Bcl-2/Bax ratio of 31.2 ± 8.0% in the MPTP Group ($P < 0.01$) (Figures 5(a) and 5(b)). Pretreatment with Sal significantly restored the Bcl-2/Bax ratio to 55.5 ± 8.3% in the Sal + MPTP group I ($P < 0.05$) and 90.4 ± 9.1% in the Sal + MPTP group II ($P < 0.01$); however, it merely had no significant difference in the Sal + MPTP group II when compared with control group ($P > 0.05$).

3.6. Sal Inhibits the Cleavage of Caspase-3, Caspase-6, and Caspase-9. Caspase family members are key mediators that activate apoptotic pathways. Western blot showed that MPTP significantly increased the cleaved level of caspase-3 to 4.2 ± 0.3-fold, caspase-6 to 3.8 ± 0.3-fold, and caspase-9 to 4.0 ±

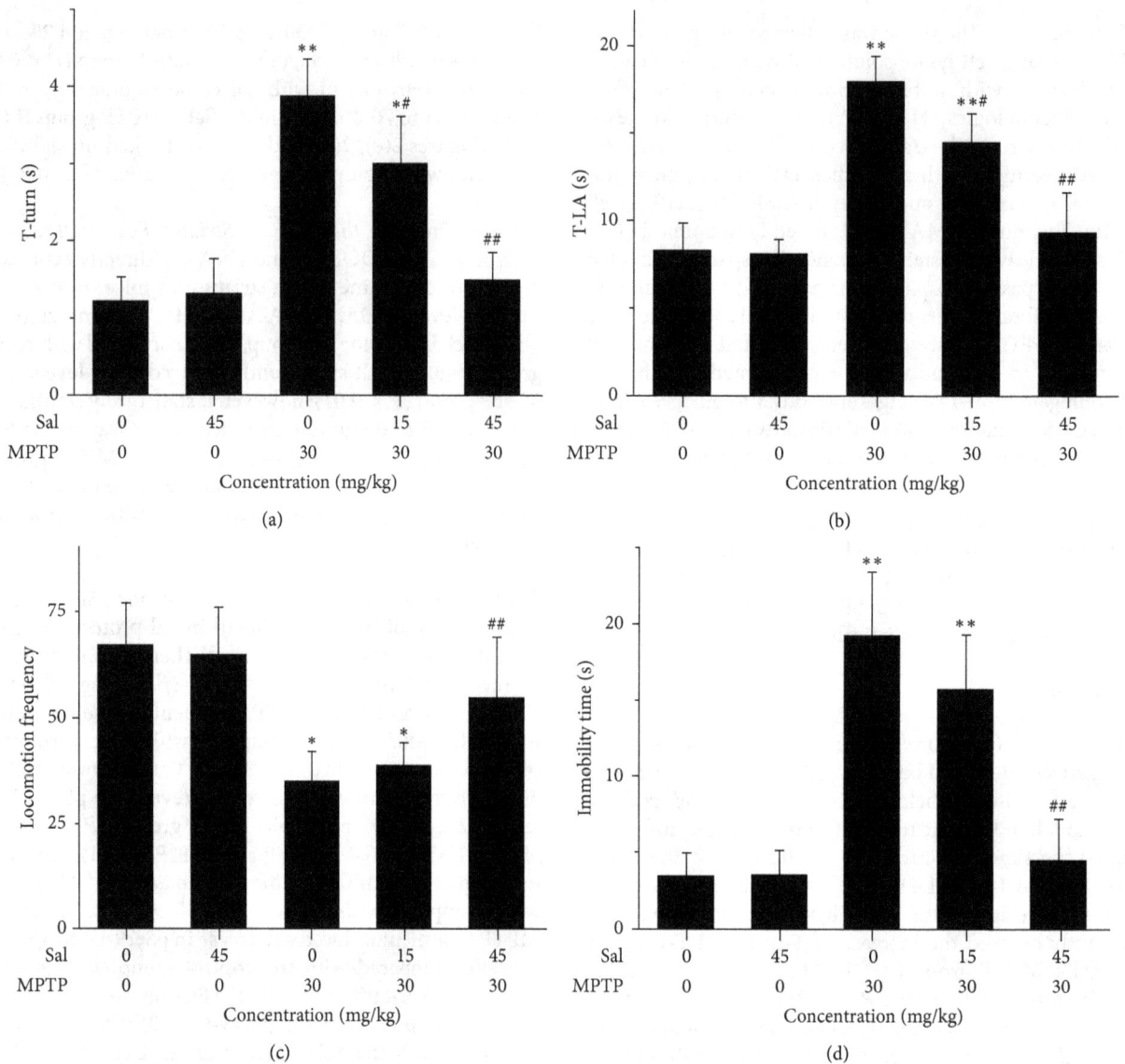

FIGURE 1: Sal improved behavior disorders in the MPTP-induced PD mouse model in pole tests and open field tests. Mice were pretreated with a sham solution or Sal (15 or 45 mg/kg). (a) Time spent to completely turn downward (T-turn). (b) Time spent getting from the top of the pole to the floor (T-LA). (c) Locomotion frequency. (d) Time spent immobile. Each column represents the mean ± SEM ($n = 10$). $^*P < 0.05$ and $^{**}P < 0.01$ compared with the control group; $^{\#}P < 0.05$ and $^{\#\#}P < 0.01$ compared with the MPTP group.

0.5-fold in the MPTP group compared with the control group ($P < 0.01$) (Figures 6(a) and 6(b)). Compared with the MPTP group, although pretreatment with Sal significantly decreased the cleavage of these caspases to 2.0±0.2-, 1.9±0.4-, and 2.5± 0.2-fold, respectively, in the Sal + MPTP group I ($P < 0.05$), the cleavages were still higher than those in control group ($P < 0.05$). Pretreatment with Sal significantly reduced caspases cleavage in the Sal + MPTP group II compared with the MPTP group ($P < 0.01$); and the cleavages had no significant difference when compared with control group ($P > 0.05$).

4. Discussion

The present study shows that pretreatment with Sal prevents the behavioral disorders and the reduced numbers of TH-positive neurons in the SNpc and the level of DA, DOPAC,

and HVA in the striatum in the MPTP-induced PD mouse model. Sal protects against MPTP-induced toxicity in part through the regulation of the PI3K/Akt/GSK3β signaling pathway, the upregulation of Bcl-2/Bax ratio, and the inhibition of the cleavage of caspase-3, caspase-6, and caspase-9.

MPTP, as a selective toxin for DA neurons, can cause Parkinsonism which has been generally used for PD models in vivo [33, 34]. Postmortem brain biochemistry has revealed that the movement disorders associated with PD are caused by the degeneration of DA neurons in SNpc [35]. By appearance of PD symptoms, it was found that at least 50% of all nigral neurons have degenerated in SNpc, and 80% of DA levels were depleted in striatum [36–38]. In this study, pretreatment with the higher concentration of Sal (45 mg/kg) significantly blocked the increase of the time of T-turn and

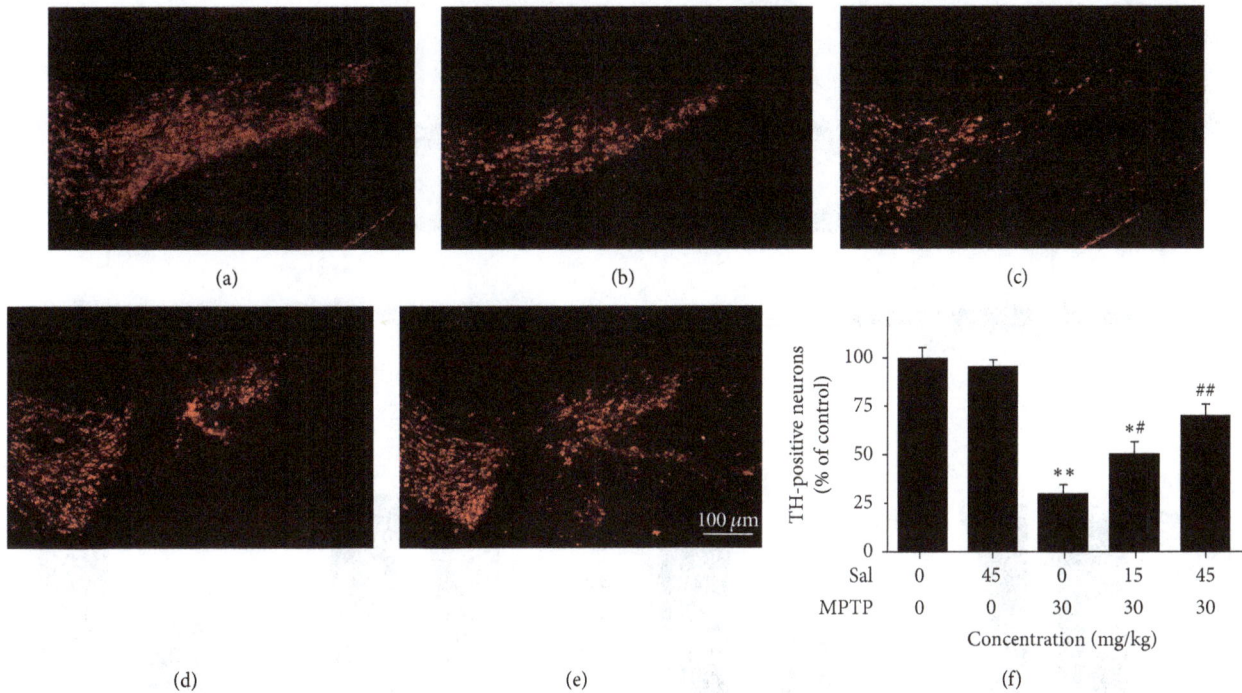

FIGURE 2: Sal protects the loss of TH-positive neurons in the SNpc in the MPTP-induced PD mouse model; (a) control group; (b) Sal group; (c) MPTP group; (d) Sal + MPTP group I; (e) Sal + MPTP group II. Bar = 100 μm. (f) Histogram shows the number of TH-positive neurons in the control group as standard. Each column represents mean ± SEM ($n = 10$). $^*P < 0.05$ and $^{**}P < 0.01$ compared with the control group; $^#P < 0.05$ and $^{##}P < 0.01$ compared with the MPTP group.

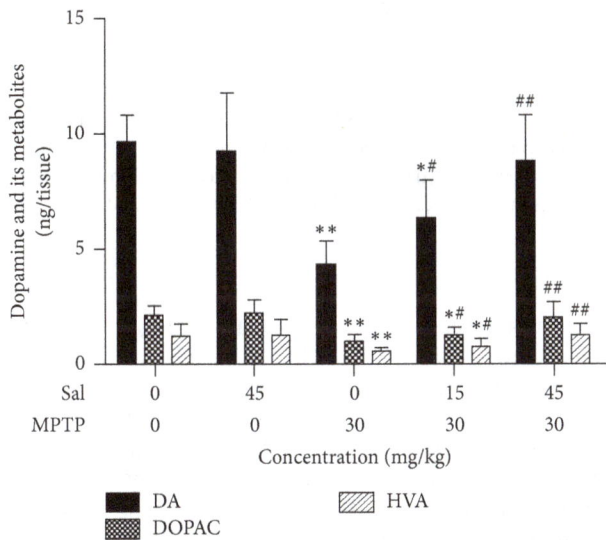

FIGURE 3: Sal increases the level of striatal DA and its metabolites in the MPTP-induced PD mouse model. DA and its metabolites (DOPAC and HVA) were measured by HPLC. Data represent three independent experiments. Each column represents the mean ± SEM ($n = 10$). $^*P < 0.05$ and $^{**}P < 0.01$ compared with the control group; $^#P < 0.05$ and $^{##}P < 0.01$ compared with the MPTP group.

T-LA compared with the MPTP group. It also prevented the locomotion frequency and decreased the immobile time.

The obvious loss of dopamine neurons in the SN is one of the typical pathological characteristics of PD. The nigrostriatal pathway as one of the four major DA pathways in the brain is particularly involved in the production of DA. TH plays a key regulatory role in cellular responses to changes in the rates of biosynthesis and release of catecholamines (DA, norepinephrine, and epinephrine) [2, 39]. Studies have shown that the presence of missense mutations in TH on both alleles could cause severe Parkinsonian-related phenotypes [40]. It was further found that kind of TH-deficient mice would die at an early age [3, 41]. In this study, MPTP-treated mice showed a 30.4% of remaining in TH-positive neurons, which is consistent with previous reports [37, 38]. However, 45 mg/kg of Sal provided the protection of TH-positive neurons in the higher concentration which compared with 15 mg/kg of Sal. In addition, it was also found that Sal (45 mg/kg) prevented the loss of striatal DA, DOPAC, and HVA level in the MPTP-induced mice without influencing the normal level of them in the Sal Group. These illustrate that Sal plays the important protective effect in order to prevent the reduced number of DA neurons and the level of DA and its metabolites in the nigrostriatal pathway in MPTP-induced mice.

PI3K/Akt pathway is one of critical components of cell survival, proliferation, and growth pathways in many different cell types including neurons [8, 42]. Akt, as the substrate of PI3K, plays a primary role in the antiapoptotic pathway [8, 42]. Active PI3K/Akt signaling pathway can prevent DA neurons loss in MPTP or MPTP-like neurotoxins [43, 44]. Many pharmacological compounds have been illustrated to

(a)

(c)

(b)

(d)

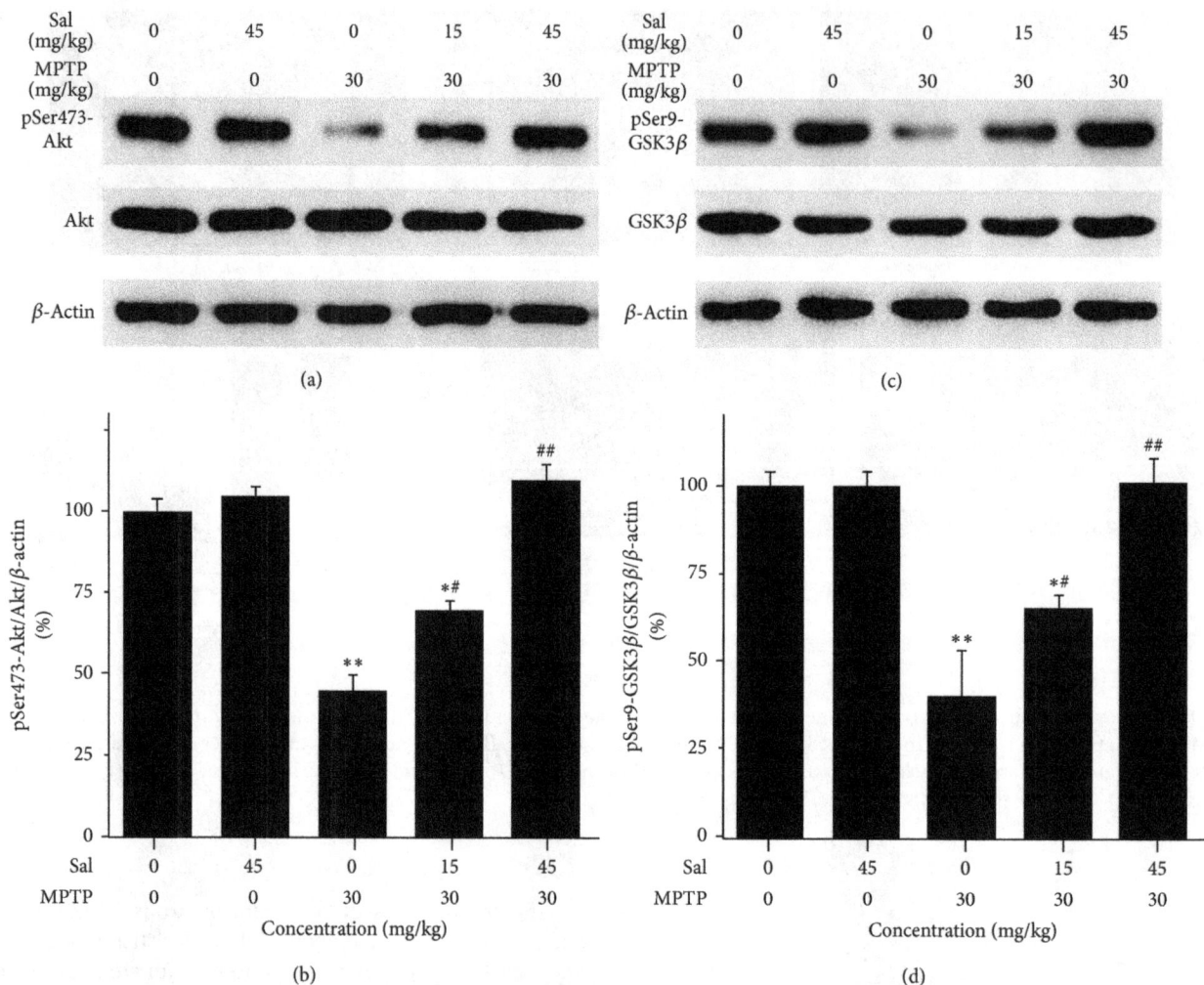

FIGURE 4: Sal increases the level of pSer473-Akt and pSer9-GSK-3β in the MPTP-induced PD mouse model. (a) Protein expression of pSer473-Akt and Akt. (b) Quantification is normalized to the control group of (a). Data represents three independent experiments. Each column represents the mean $\pm$ SEM ($n = 10$). (c) Protein expression of pSer9-GSK-3β and GSK-3β. (d) Quantification is normalized to the control group of (c). Data represents three independent experiments. Each column represents the mean $\pm$ SEM ($n = 10$). $^{#}P < 0.05$ and $^{##}P < 0.01$ compared with the MPTP group.

exert their neuroprotective effects against oxidative stress through activating the Akt pathway [45–48]. Moreover, stress stimulation could induce the translocation of Akt to mitochondria for phosphorylation, followed by the rapid inhibition of mitochondrial GSK-3β by phosphorylation at Ser9 [49]. The phosphorylation of GSK-3β, a determining factor for apoptosis, has been shown to result in neuronal cell death [13, 50, 51]. In this study, it was shown that MPTP treatment induced a decrease in pSer473-Akt/Akt level and pSer9-GSK-3β/GSK-3β level. Only the higher level of Sal (45 mg/kg) could prevent their level. Hence, combining our present study and previous studies [26], it is demonstrated that pretreatment with Sal could increase the level of pSer473-Akt and pSer9-GSK-3β both in vitro and in vivo.

Bcl-2 family members, as antiapoptotic or proapoptotic regulators, play a wide role in cellular activities [52]. The ratio of Bcl-2/Bax, as an indicator of the activation of proapoptotic signaling, is related to cell survival or death [19]. Akt upregulates the expression of Bcl-2 and thus leads to

cell survival by phosphorylating and inhibiting proapoptotic proteins such as Bax [14, 53, 54]. In this study, treatment with Sal (45 mg/kg) significantly inhibited the MPTP-induced decrease of Bcl-2 level and increase of Bax level. Caspases are essential in apoptosis [55]. Akt phosphorylates caspase-9 promoting the cell survival [14]. It also phosphorylates caspase-3 and caspase-6, thus inhibiting their proapoptotic functions in a variety of cell lines [42, 50, 51]. In this study, pretreatment with Sal (45 mg/kg) significantly decreased the cleavage of caspase-3, caspase-6, and caspase-9 compared with the MPTP group. It was indicated that pretreatment with Sal by an appropriate concentration could increase the antiapoptosis protein and decrease the proapoptosis protein for promoting the cell survival.

5. Conclusion

In conclusion, Sal not only prevents the behavioral disorders but also inhibits the reduced numbers of TH-positive neurons

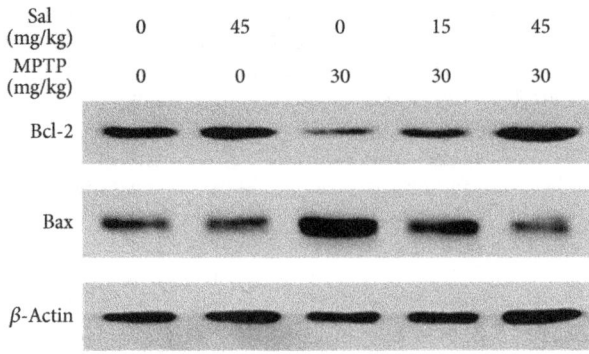

(a)

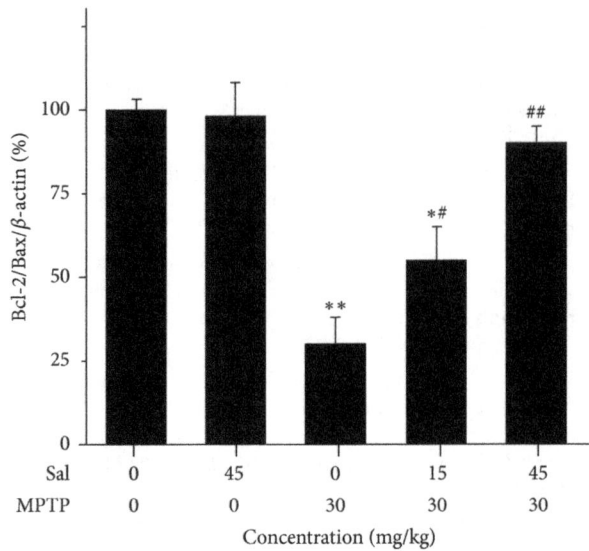

(b)

FIGURE 5: Sal upregulates the protein level of Bcl-2 and downregulates the protein level of Bax in the MPTP-induced PD mouse model. (a) Protein expression of Bcl-2 and Bax. (b) Quantification is normalized to the control group. Data represent three independent experiments. Each column represents the mean ± SEM ($n = 10$). $^{*}P < 0.05$ and $^{**}P < 0.01$ compared with control group; $^{#}P < 0.05$ and $^{##}P < 0.01$ compared with MPTP group.

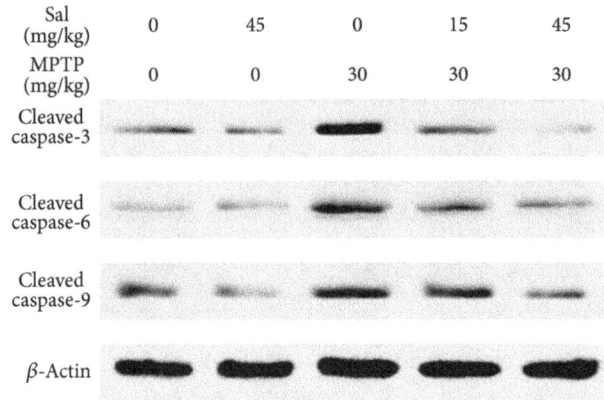

(a)

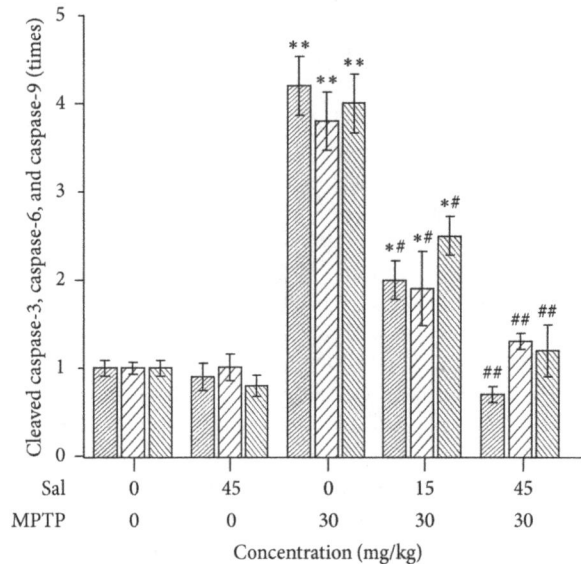

(b)

FIGURE 6: Sal inhibits the cleavage of caspase-3, caspase-6, and caspase-9 in the MPTP-induced PD mouse model. (a) Protein expression of cleaved caspase-3, caspase-6, and caspase-9. (b) Quantification is normalized to the control group. Data represent three independent experiments. Each column represents the mean ± SEM ($n = 10$). $^{*}P < 0.05$ and $^{**}P < 0.01$ compared with the control group; $^{#}P < 0.05$ and $^{##}P < 0.01$ compared with the MPTP group.

and the level of DA, DOPAC, and HVA in the MPTP-induced PD mouse model. This closely related with the regulation of the PI3K/Akt/GSK3β signaling pathway, the upregulation of a normal Bcl-2/Bax ratio, and the inhibition of the cleaved caspase-3, caspase-6, and caspase-9. In accordance with recently reported results in vitro, these results indicate that activation of the PI3K/Akt/GSK3β signaling pathway by Sal protects against the neurotoxic conditions associated with the MPTP-induced PD mouse model.

Abbreviations

PD: Parkinson's disease
DA: Dopaminergic
SNpc: Substantia nigra pars compacta
PI3K: Phosphoinositide 3-kinase
GSK-3:   Glycogen synthase kinase-3
Sal: Salidroside

TH: Tyrosine hydroxylase
MPTP: 1-Methyl-4-phenyl-1,2,3,6-tetrahydropyridine
MPP^{+}:   1-Methyl-4-phenyl-pyridinium
Bcl-2:   B-cell lymphoma-2
Caspase: Cysteine-dependent aspartate-directed proteases.

Authors' Contributions

Wei Zhang and Hong He contributed equally to this study.

References

[1] F. Javoy-Agid, A. Ploska, and Y. Agid, "Microtopography of tyrosine hydroxylase, glutamic acid decarboxylase, and choline acetyltransferase in the substantia nigra and ventral tegmental area of control and Parkinsonian brains," *Journal of Neurochemistry*, vol. 37, no. 5, pp. 1218–1227, 1981.

[2] H.-C. Fan, S.-J. Chen, H.-J. Harn, and S.-Z. Lin, "Parkinson's disease: from genetics to treatments," *Cell Transplantation*, vol. 22, no. 4, pp. 639–652, 2013.

[3] D. Athauda and T. Foltynie, "The ongoing pursuit of neuroprotective therapies in Parkinson disease," *Nature Reviews Neurology*, vol. 11, no. 1, pp. 25–40, 2015.

[4] G. Zhang, N. Xiong, Z. Zhang et al., "Effectiveness of traditional chinese medicine as an adjunct therapy for Parkinson's disease: a systematic review and meta-analysis," *PLoS ONE*, vol. 10, no. 3, Article ID e0118498, 2015.

[5] S. T. Masoud, L. M. Vecchio, Y. Bergeron et al., "Increased expression of the dopamine transporter leads to loss of dopamine neurons, oxidative stress and l-DOPA reversible motor deficits," *Neurobiology of Disease*, vol. 74, pp. 66–75, 2015.

[6] S. Timmons, M. F. Coakley, A. M. Moloney, and C. O' Neill, "Akt signal transduction dysfunction in Parkinson's disease," *Neuroscience Letters*, vol. 467, no. 1, pp. 30–35, 2009.

[7] S. K. Jha, N. K. Jha, R. Kar, R. K. Ambasta, and P. Kumar, "p38 MAPK and PI3K/AKT signalling cascades in Parkinson's disease," *International Journal of Molecular and Cellular Medicine*, vol. 4, no. 2, pp. 67–86, 2015.

[8] B. D. Manning and L. C. Cantley, "AKT/PKB signaling: navigating downstream," *Cell*, vol. 129, no. 7, pp. 1261–1274, 2007.

[9] C. M. Coelho and S. J. Leevers, "Do growth and cell division rates determine cell size in multicellular organisms?" *Journal of Cell Science*, vol. 113, part 17, pp. 2927–2934, 2000.

[10] M. J. Fry, "Phosphoinositide 3-kinase signalling in breast cancer: how big a role might it play?" *Breast Cancer Research*, vol. 3, no. 5, pp. 304–312, 2001.

[11] R. Katso, K. Okkenhaug, K. Ahmadi, S. White, J. Timms, and M. D. Waterfield, "Cellular function of phosphoinositide 3-Kinases: implications for development, immunity, homeostasis, and cancer," *Annual Review of Cell and Developmental Biology*, vol. 17, pp. 615–675, 2001.

[12] K.-X. Sun, H.-W. Xia, and R.-L. Xia, "Anticancer effect of salidroside on colon cancer through inhibiting JAK2/STAT3 signaling pathway," *International Journal of Clinical and Experimental Pathology*, vol. 8, no. 1, pp. 615–621, 2015.

[13] Y. Wu, Y. Shang, S. Sun, H. Liang, and R. Liu, "Erythropoietin prevents PC12 cells from 1-methyl-4-phenylpyridinium ion-induced apoptosis via the Akt/GSK-3β/caspase-3 mediated signaling pathway," *Apoptosis*, vol. 12, no. 8, pp. 1365–1375, 2007.

[14] M. H. Cardone, N. Roy, H. R. Stennicke et al., "Regulation of cell death protease caspase-9 by phosphorylation," *Science*, vol. 282, no. 5392, pp. 1318–1321, 1998.

[15] D. A. E. Cross, D. R. Alessi, P. Cohen, M. Andjelkovich, and B. A. Hemmings, "Inhibition of glycogen synthase kinase-3 by insulin mediated by protein kinase B," *Nature*, vol. 378, no. 6559, pp. 785–789, 1995.

[16] A. K. Srivastava and S. K. Pandey, "Potential mechanism(s) involved in the regulation of glycogen synthesis by insulin," *Molecular and Cellular Biochemistry*, vol. 182, no. 1-2, pp. 135–141, 1998.

[17] L. Yao, W. Li, H. She et al., "Activation of transcription factor MEF2D by bis(3)-cognitin protects dopaminergic neurons and ameliorates Parkinsonian motor defects," *Journal of Biological Chemistry*, vol. 287, no. 41, pp. 34246–34255, 2012.

[18] D. Hernandez-Baltazar, M. E. Mendoza-Garrido, and D. Martinez-Fong, "Activation of GSK-3β and caspase-3 occurs in nigral dopamine neurons during the development of apoptosis activated by a striatal injection of 6-hydroxydopamine," *PLoS ONE*, vol. 8, no. 8, Article ID e70951, 2013.

[19] D. W. Li, Z. Q. Liu, W. Chen et al., "Association of glycogen synthase kinase-3beta with Parkinson's disease (review)," *Molecular Medicine Reports*, vol. 9, no. 6, pp. 2043–2050, 2014.

[20] A. Booker, B. Jalil, D. Frommenwiler et al., "The authenticity and quality of Rhodiola rosea products," *Phytomedicine*, vol. 23, no. 7, Article ID 00318, pp. 754–762, 2016.

[21] L. Xiao, H. Li, J. Zhang et al., "Salidroside protects caenorhabditis elegans neurons from polyglutamine-mediated toxicity by reducing oxidative stress," *Molecules*, vol. 19, no. 6, pp. 7757–7769, 2014.

[22] X. Li, J. Sipple, Q. Pang, and W. Du, "Salidroside stimulates DNArepair enzyme Parp-1 activity in mouse HSC maintenance," *Blood*, vol. 119, no. 18, pp. 4162–4173, 2012.

[23] L. Zhu, T. Wei, J. Gao et al., "The cardioprotective effect of salidroside against myocardial ischemia reperfusion injury in rats by inhibiting apoptosis and inflammation," *Apoptosis*, vol. 20, no. 11, pp. 1433–1443, 2015.

[24] W. Zhang, M. Peng, Y. Yang, Z. Xiao, B. Song, and Z. Lin, "Protective effects of salidroside on mitochondrial functions against exertional heat stroke-induced organ damage in the rat," *Evidence-Based Complementary and Alternative Medicine*, vol. 2015, Article ID 504567, 11 pages, 2015.

[25] S. Wang, S. He, L. Chen, W. Zhang, X. Zhang, and J. Chen, "Protective effects of salidroside in the MPTP/MPP+-induced model of Parkinson's disease through ROS-NO-related mitochondrion pathway," *Molecular Neurobiology*, vol. 51, no. 2, pp. 718–728, 2015.

[26] L. Zhang, W. Ding, H. Sun et al., "Salidroside protects PC12 cells from MPP+-induced apoptosis via activation of the PI3K/Akt pathway," *Food and Chemical Toxicology*, vol. 50, no. 8, pp. 2591–2597, 2012.

[27] N. A. Tatton and S. J. Kish, "In situ detection of apoptotic nuclei in the substantia nigra compacta of 1-methyl-4-phenyl-1,2,3,6-tetrahydropyridine-treated mice using terminal deoxynucleotidyl transferase labelling and acridine orange staining," *Neuroscience*, vol. 77, no. 4, pp. 1037–1048, 1997.

[28] K. Matsuura, H. Kabuto, H. Makino, and N. Ogawa, "Pole test is a useful method for evaluating the mouse movement disorder caused by striatal dopamine depletion," *Journal of Neuroscience Methods*, vol. 73, no. 1, pp. 45–48, 1997.

[29] P. Simon, R. Dupuis, and J. Costentin, "Thigmotaxis as an index of anxiety in mice. Influence of dopaminergic transmissions," *Behavioural Brain Research*, vol. 61, no. 1, pp. 59–64, 1994.

[30] W. Wang, Y. Yang, C. Ying et al., "Inhibition of glycogen synthase kinase-3β protects dopaminergic neurons from MPTP toxicity," *Neuropharmacology*, vol. 52, no. 8, pp. 1678–1684, 2007.

[31] V. Jackson-Lewis, M. Jakowec, R. E. Burke, and S. Przedborski, "Time course and morphology of dopaminergic neuronal death caused by the neurotoxin 1-methyl-4-phenyl-1,2,3,6-tetrahydropyridine," *Neurodegeneration*, vol. 4, no. 3, pp. 257–269, 1995.

[32] Z. Lin, C. A. Dodd, and N. M. Filipov, "Short-term atrazine

exposure causes behavioral deficits and disrupts monoaminergic systems in male C57BL/6 mice," *Neurotoxicology and Teratology*, vol. 39, pp. 26–35, 2013.

[33] E. Grünblatt, S. Mandel, and M. B. H. Youdim, "MPTP and 6-hydroxydopamine-induced neurodegeneration as models for Parkinson's disease: neuroprotective strategies," *Journal of Neurology*, vol. 247, supplement 2, pp. Ii95–Ii102, 2000.

[34] S. Przedborski and M. Vila, "The 1-methyl-4-phenyl-1,2,3,6-tetrahydropyridine mouse model: a tool to explore the pathogenesis of Parkinson's disease," *Annals of the New York Academy of Sciences*, vol. 991, pp. 189–198, 2003.

[35] J. Segura-Aguilar, I. Paris, P. Muñoz, E. Ferrari, L. Zecca, and F. A. Zucca, "Protective and toxic roles of dopamine in Parkinson's disease," *Journal of Neurochemistry*, vol. 129, no. 6, pp. 898–915, 2014.

[36] C. D. Marsden, "Parkinson's disease," *The Lancet*, vol. 335, no. 8695, pp. 948–952, 1990.

[37] H. Bernheimer, W. Birkmayer, O. Hornykiewicz, K. Jellinger, and F. Seitelberger, "Brain dopamine and the syndromes of Parkinson and Huntington Clinical, morphological and neurochemical correlations," *Journal of the Neurological Sciences*, vol. 20, no. 4, pp. 415–455, 1973.

[38] P. Riederer and S. Wuketich, "Time course of nigrostriatal degeneration in Parkinson's disease. A detailed study of influential factors in human brain amine analysis," *Journal of Neural Transmission*, vol. 38, no. 3-4, pp. 277–301, 1976.

[39] L. Brichta and P. Greengard, "Molecular determinants of selective dopaminergic vulnerability in Parkinson's disease: an update," *Frontiers in Neuroanatomy*, vol. 8, article 152, 2014.

[40] D. B. Miller and J. P. O'Callaghan, "Biomarkers of Parkinson's disease: present and future," *Metabolism: Clinical and Experimental*, vol. 64, no. 3, supplement 1, pp. S40–S46, 2015.

[41] Z. Arraf, T. Amit, M. B. H. Youdim, and R. Farah, "Lithium and oxidative stress lessons from the MPTP model of Parkinson's disease," *Neuroscience Letters*, vol. 516, no. 1, pp. 57–61, 2012.

[42] M. Pap and G. M. Cooper, "Role of glycogen synthase kinase-3 in the phosphatidylinositol 3- kinase/Akt cell survival pathway," *Journal of Biological Chemistry*, vol. 273, no. 32, pp. 19929–19932, 1998.

[43] H. Ruan, Y. Yang, X. Zhu, X. Wang, and R. Chen, "Neuroprotective effects of (±)-catechin against 1-methyl-4-phenyl-1,2,3,6-tetrahydropyridine (MPTP)-induced dopaminergic neurotoxicity in mice," *Neuroscience Letters*, vol. 450, no. 2, pp. 152–157, 2009.

[44] Y. Tasaki, T. Omura, T. Yamada et al., "Meloxicam protects cell damage from 1-methyl-4-phenyl pyridinium toxicity via the phosphatidylinositol 3-kinase/Akt pathway in human dopaminergic neuroblastoma SH-SY5Y cells," *Brain Research*, vol. 1344, pp. 25–33, 2010.

[45] M. Fukui, H. J. Choi, and B. T. Zhu, "Mechanism for the protective effect of resveratrol against oxidative stress-induced neuronal death," *Free Radical Biology and Medicine*, vol. 49, no. 5, pp. 800–813, 2010.

[46] R. Qin, X. Li, G. Li et al., "Protection by tetrahydroxystilbene glucoside against neurotoxicity induced by MPP$^+$: the involvement of PI3K/Akt pathway activation," *Toxicology Letters*, vol. 202, no. 1, pp. 1–7, 2011.

[47] C. Malagelada, Z. H. Jin, and L. A. Greene, "RTP801 is induced in Parkinson's disease and mediates neuron death by inhibiting Akt phosphorylation/activation," *The Journal of Neuroscience*, vol. 28, no. 53, pp. 14363–14371, 2008.

[48] J.-H. Liu, F. Yin, L.-X. Guo, X.-H. Deng, and Y.-H. Hu, "Neuroprotection of geniposide against hydrogen peroxide induced PC12 cells injury: involvement of PI3 kinase signal pathway," *Acta Pharmacologica Sinica*, vol. 30, no. 2, pp. 159–165, 2009.

[49] G. N. Bijur and R. S. Jope, "Glycogen synthase kinase-3 beta is highly activated in nuclei and mitochondria," *Neuroreport*, vol. 14, no. 18, pp. 2415–2419, 2003.

[50] V. V. Senatorov, M. Ren, H. Kanai, H. Wei, and D.-M. Chuang, "Short-term lithium treatment promotes neuronal survival and proliferation in rat striatum infused with quinolinic acid, an excitotoxic model of Huntington's disease," *Molecular Psychiatry*, vol. 9, no. 4, pp. 371–385, 2004.

[51] A. R. Alvarez, P. C. Sandoval, N. R. Leal, P. U. Castro, and K. S. Kosik, "Activation of the neuronal c-Abl tyrosine kinase by amyloid-β-peptide and reactive oxygen species," *Neurobiology of Disease*, vol. 17, no. 2, pp. 326–336, 2004.

[52] D. T. Chao and S. J. Korsmeyer, "BCL-2 family: regulators of cell death," *Annual Review of Immunology*, vol. 16, pp. 395–419, 1998.

[53] S. Pugazhenthit, A. Nesterova, C. Sable et al., "Akt/protein kinase B up-regulates Bcl-2 expression through cAMP-response element-binding protein," *The Journal of Biological Chemistry*, vol. 275, no. 15, pp. 10761–10766, 2000.

[54] L. C. Cantley, "The phosphoinositide 3-kinase pathway," *Science*, vol. 296, no. 5573, pp. 1655–1657, 2002.

[55] E. S. Alnemri, D. J. Livingston, D. W. Nicholson et al., "Human ICE/CED-3 protease nomenclature," *Cell*, vol. 87, no. 2, p. 171, 1996.

26

Antidyskinetic Treatment with MTEP Affects Multiple Molecular Pathways in the Parkinsonian Striatum

Jing-ya Lin, Zhen-guo Liu, Cheng-long Xie, Lu Song, and Ai-juan Yan

Department of Neurology, Xin Hua Hospital Affiliated to Shanghai Jiao Tong University School of Medicine,
1665 Kongjiang Road, Shanghai 200092, China

Correspondence should be addressed to Zhen-guo Liu; zhenguoliu2004@aliyun.com

Academic Editor: Francisco Grandas

Parkinson's disease is characterized by dopaminergic neuron loss and dopamine (DA) depletion in the striatum. Standard treatment is still focused on the restoration of dopamine with exogenous L-Dopa, which however causes L-Dopa-induced dyskinesia (LID). Several studies have shown that antagonism of the metabotropic glutamate receptor 5 alleviates LID, but the underlying mechanisms have remained unclear. We set out to determine where this alleviation may depend on restoring the equilibrium between the two main striatofugal pathways. For this purpose, we examined molecular markers of direct and indirect pathway involvement (prodynorphin and proenkephalin, resp.) in a rat model of LID treated with the mGluR5 antagonist MTEP. Our results show that MTEP cotreatment significantly attenuates the upregulation of prodynorphin mRNA induced by L-Dopa while also decreasing the expression levels of proenkephalin mRNA. We also examined markers of the mGluR5-related PKC/MEK/ERK1/2 signaling pathway, finding that both the expression of PKC epsilon and the phosphorylation of MEK and ERK1/2 had decreased significantly in the MTEP-treated group. Taken together, our results show that pharmacological antagonism of mGluR5 normalizes several abnormal molecular responses in the striatum in this experimental model of LID.

1. Introduction

The loss of dopaminergic neurons in the substantia nigra and the depletion of dopamine are main neuropathological features of Parkinson's disease (PD) [1, 2]. Current standard treatment for PD still focuses on the dopamine replacement therapy with L-Dopa [2]. However, long-term use of this drug causes a decrease in the efficacy and disabling abnormal involuntary movement (AIM), which was known as L-Dopa-induced dyskinesia (LID) [3].

The striatum is deeply involved in handling the motor information that comes from the cortex. In the classic model of striatal connectivity, there are direct and indirect pathways in the striatum [4]. Both direct and indirect pathways originate from medium spiny efferent neurons (MSNs). In the indirect pathway, the MSNs express enkephalin, while in the direct pathway the MSNs express dynorphin [5]. The first report of a direct correlation between prodynorphin level and LID was provided by Cenci et al. [6]; furthermore, they also proposed that an imbalance between the direct and indirect pathways leads to the appearance of the motor signs

of parkinsonism [7]. In a recent research, it was also reported that both the dynorphin and enkephalin expression levels were involved in the development of motor complications while being treated with L-Dopa. Sgroi et al. pointed out that, on the one hand, the preproenkephalin level was increased before the use of L-Dopa after 6-OHDA lesion, and it remained high after L-Dopa washout; on the other hand, there is a correlation between the rotational AIM and preproenkephalin level in the on state [8]. All these phenomenons suggested that the increased proenkephalin mRNA level may be a prerequisite to the locomotor sensitization before L-Dopa treatment [8]. On the other hand, the association of prodynorphin with LID is clearer than that with proenkephalin, because it has been consistently proven in several studies [5, 8–10].

We also know that overactivation of glutamatergic signaling and the hypersensitivity of the glutamatergic system in the basal ganglia play an important role in the pathophysiology of LID. Several groups of researchers reported that the blockade of the metabotropic glutamate receptor 5 (mGluR5) could attenuate the LID [11–16]; emerging evidence has come to

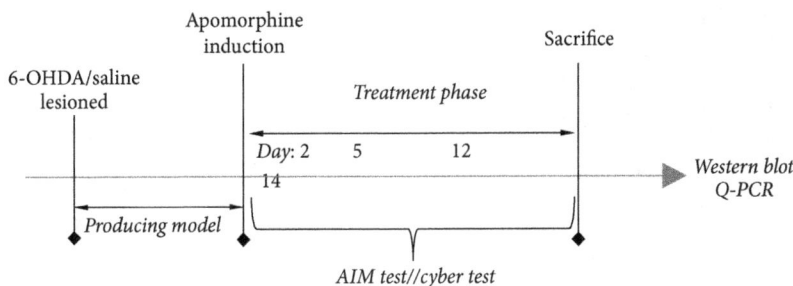

FIGURE 1: The protocol of the experiment. Dopamine depletion was induced by 6-OHDA injections in the medial forebrain bundle (MFB) while the sham group was injected with saline in the MFB. Three weeks later, the rats that exhibited apomorphine-induced rotations exceeding 7 turns/min in the apomorphine induction test were put to the subsequent experiment. The sham and PD groups were injected with saline once daily; the LID group received L-Dopa (25 mg/kg) and benserazide (6.25 mg/kg) cocktail once daily, while the MTEP group received MTEP (5 mg/kg) 30 min before the injection of L-Dopa and benserazide. All treatments were performed for 14 days; behavior tests like AIM test, open field test, and cylinder test were performed on days 2, 5, 12, and 14. Two hours after the last injection on the 14th day, all groups were sacrificed for western blot and Q-PCR.

support the important role of mGluR5 in the development of LID [17]. But the mechanism behind the alleviation effect is unclear [18]. It is of great importance to investigate the extent to which the blockade of the metabotropic receptor 5 affects the imbalance between direct and indirect pathways and to investigate what the molecular alterations in the mGluR5-related signaling pathway are, in order to interpret the antidyskinesia effect of the antagonists of mGluR5. In order to address these questions, we tested the protein level of protein kinase C (PKC), MEK, and extracellular signal-regulated kinase 1/2 (ERK1/2) in the mGluR5 mediated PKC/MEK/ERK1/2 signaling pathway; we also tested the mRNA expression level of prodynorphin (PDyn) and proenkephalin (PEnk) in order to verify the effect of the blockade of mGluR5 on the direct and indirect pathways.

2. Materials and Methods

2.1. Experimental Design. As shown in Figure 1, Sprague-Dawley rats were given 6-OHDA injections in the medial forebrain bundle (MFB) in the right side of the brain, while five SD rats were given saline injections instead as sham group. Contralateral turning behavior was tested on the 6-OHDA rats after the apomorphine injection. The rats whose apomorphine-induced rotations are more than 7 turns/min were enrolled in the follow-up experiments as the Parkinson disease model animals. The selected rats were distributed into 3 groups randomly. The first group was given L-Dopa (25 mg/kg, i.p.) plus benserazide (6.25 mg/kg, i.p.) once daily for 14 days, labeled as LID group; the second group was given saline once daily for 14 days, labeled as PD group; and the third group was given MTEP (5 mg/kg, i.p.) 20 mins before the injection of L-Dopa plus benserazide for 14 days, labeled as MTEP group. During this period, AIM and open field tests were conducted in all the groups on days 2, 5, 8, 12, and 14 by a new assigned observer who did not know the details of each group. The animals were sacrificed 2 h after the last injection for western blot and Q-PCR.

2.2. Animals. The study was conducted on adult female Sprague-Dawley rats (Sprague-Dawley, 180–220 g, Sippr-BK

Ltd., Shanghai, China). The maintenance of the animals followed the guidelines of the National Institutes of Health for the care and use of laboratory animals. All experimental protocols involving animals were approved by the Ethical Committee of the Medical School of Shanghai Jiaotong University.

2.3. Drugs. L-Dopa and benserazide were purchased from Sigma-Aldrich (Spain), and MTEP was purchased from Abcam (UK). All drugs were freshly prepared in 0.9% saline before use. L-Dopa (Sigma-Aldrich) plus benserazide (Sigma-Aldrich) was administrated once daily. MTEP (3-[(2-methyl-1,3-thiazol-4-yl)ethynyl]-pyridine, Abcam, UK) preceded the L-Dopa cocktail 20 minutes earlier once daily for 2 weeks.

2.4. 6-OHDA Lesions and Treatment. For the stereotaxic procedure, the rats (weighing 180~220 g) were anesthetized with 10% chloral hydrate (0.5 ml/100 g) deeply. As previously described [19, 20], the surgery was performed on the right side medial forebrain bundle (MFB) by unilateral injection of 6-OHDA (20 mmol/L, containing 0.02% ascorbic acid; Sigma-Aldrich, Spain) at the coordination of MFB. Sham-operated rats received the vehicle at the same spot. A volume of 4 μl was injected in each spot. 21 days later, all the rats were tested with 0.05 mg/kg subcutaneous injection of apomorphine (i.p. WOKO, Japan). Contralateral rotation test was performed and the animals exhibiting full body turns of over 7 turns/min towards the unlesioned side were enrolled and started on a 2-week course of daily i.p. injections of MTEP (5 mg/kg) followed by L-Dopa (25 mg/kg) plus benserazide (6.25 mg/kg) 20 min later.

2.5. Behavior Assessment. To evaluate LID, we used the combined "time * amplitude" scale which was first applied by Rylander et al. [21]; mice were observed in a clear-glass cylinder and were observed and evaluated by a trained experimenter. Rat abnormal involuntary movements (AIMs) were classified into three subtypes: axial, limb, and orolingual dyskinesia. Each individual dyskinesia subtype scores from 0 to 4. During a period of 120 min following levodopa injection, the severity of AIM was assessed at a 20 min interval (20, 40, 60, 80, 100, and 120 min). The ALO AIM scores were rated at 2, 5, 12, and 14 days during levodopa treatment. Motor coordination was evaluated with the cylinder test at 2, 5, 12, and 14 days and the locomotor activities were tested by the open field test on the 2nd and 14th days during levodopa treatment. The open field test and cylinder test were the index of Parkinsonian disability. In the cylinder test, the rats were placed in a glass cylinder with a diameter of 22 cm and a height of 35 cm to record forelimb use during vertical exploration for 60 min. During a period of 60 min before levodopa treatment, the forelimb functional test was assessed every 15 min (3 min monitoring period for each). The final value was expressed in terms of the percentage use of the impaired forelimb compared with the total number of limb use movements. All the behavioral experiments were carried out with the observer blinded to the groups and treatment.

2.6. Western Blot. Striatum tissue of rats was harvested 2 hours after the last injection of L-Dopa and homogenized in RIPA lysis buffer (Beyotime Institute of Biotechnology) and fresh-added protease inhibitor cocktail and phosphatase inhibitor (Roche Diagnostics, Switzerland). And then the cytosol was prepared by centrifugation at 12000g for 10 min at 4°C. An equal amount of protein (40 ug) from each sample was added to 10% SDS-PAGE and separated by electrophoresis and transferred to polyvinylidene difluoride membranes in a Tris-glycine transfer buffer. Each sample was heated at 95°C previously for 5 min. The membrane was blocked for half an hour at room temperature (26°C) in 5% instant nonfat milk and then incubated with primary antibodies corresponding to epsilon PKC (1:1000, Abcam, UK), p-MEK and MEK (1:1000, Abcam, UK), p-ERK1/2 and ERK1/2 (1:1000, Cell Signaling Technology (CST), USA), and β-actin IgG (diluted 1:1000; Beyotime Institute of Biotechnology), respectively, at 4°C overnight (14–16 hours). The membranes were subsequently washed with TBST (50 mM Tris-HCl (pH 7.5), 150 mM NaCl, and 0.05% Tween 20) and then incubated with horseradish peroxidase conjugated secondary anti-rabbit and anti-mouse IgG (diluted 1:1000; Beyotime Institute of Biotechnology) for one hour at room temperature. The signal was visualized by ECL (A:B = 1:1; Millipore) and quantified using Quantity One software (Image Lab). All individual protein bands were compared with their internal control actin values in order to provide relative protein abundance. All the procedures were repeated 3 times.

2.7. Real-Time PCR. Striatal tissues of rats were homogenized and total ribonucleic acid (RNA) was extracted by TRIzol reagent (Invitrogen, USA). cDNA was generated from total RNA samples using the Revert Aid First Strand cDNA Synthesis Kit (Takara, Japan). Q-PCR was performed using the ABI 7500 Real-Time PCR System (Life Technologies, USA) according to the supplier's instructions. The primer sequences used in this study were as follows:

5-CTTGTGTTCCCTGTGTGCAGTG-3 (forward)

3-AGCAACCTCATTCTCCAAGTCA-5 (reverse) for PDyn mRNA

5-GAAGATGGATGAGCTTTACCCC-3 (forward)

3-CAAGGTGTCTCCCTCATCTGC-5 (reverse) for proenkephalin mRNA

Amplification was performed with 40 cycles of denaturation at 95°C for 15 s, annealing at 60°C for 60 s, and extension at 75°C for 20 s using the ABI 7300 Real-Time PCR System (Applied Biosystems, CA, USA). Results were expressed as relative expression corrected to the GAPDH gene. The detector used in real-time PCR reaction is SYBR Green.

2.8. Statistical Analysis. Data were expressed as the mean ± standard deviation (SD) unless stated otherwise. Behavioral data were analyzed using Kruskal-Wallis test followed by Dunn's test for multiple comparisons in the case of comparing data over multiple days, or a Mann–Whitney U test. The western blot and Q-PCR conformed to normal distribution, and analyses of their data were performed using one-way analysis of variance (ANOVA) followed by LSD post hoc comparisons when appropriate as indicated in the figure legends. p values < 0.05 were considered statistically significant. Analysis was performed with GraphPad Prism 5.

3. Result

3.1. MTEP Prevented the Development of L-Dopa-Induced Dyskinesia. The PD group received saline injection over 14 days, while the LID group was injected with L-Dopa (25 mg/kg) plus benserazide (6.25 mg/kg). The MTEP group was given MTEP (5 mg/kg, i.p.) 20 min before the L-Dopa cocktail injection. The evaluation of the AIM scores included 3 subtypes: axial, limb, and orolingual AIMs. The scores demonstrated a rat dyskinesia scale. We found that 2 weeks of L-Dopa treatment induced full development of LID features, as demonstrated by the increased ALO AIM scores in the LID rats ($p < 0.05$ for treatment effect, $p < 0.05$ for time effect, and $p < 0.01$ for treatment and time interaction, Figure 2). This result is in line with our previous study. AIM scores decreased in the MTEP group. MTEP treatment for 14 days significantly reduced the total dyskinesia scores while the rats of PD group that received saline for 14 days did not develop dyskinesia. Furthermore, the MTEP group demonstrated a reduction in all testing sessions. These data indicate that treatment with MTEP significantly inhibited the development of LID.

3.2. MTEP Did Not Compromise the Anti-Parkinsonian Effect of L-Dopa. We then sought to determine whether the administration of antagonists of mGluR5 ameliorated LID compromised the therapeutic response to L-Dopa in PD rats. The cylinder test was used to assess spontaneous forelimb use. We conducted the cylinder test on the 2nd, 5th, 12th, and 14th days. We observed that 6-OHDA-lesioned rats treated with L-Dopa prefer to use the contralateral forelimb to touch the inner wall of the cylinder compared with the 6-OHDA-lesioned rats treated with saline, but the preferential use of the contralateral forelimb was lower compared with the sham group rats (Figure 3, *$p < 0.01$). Data showed that

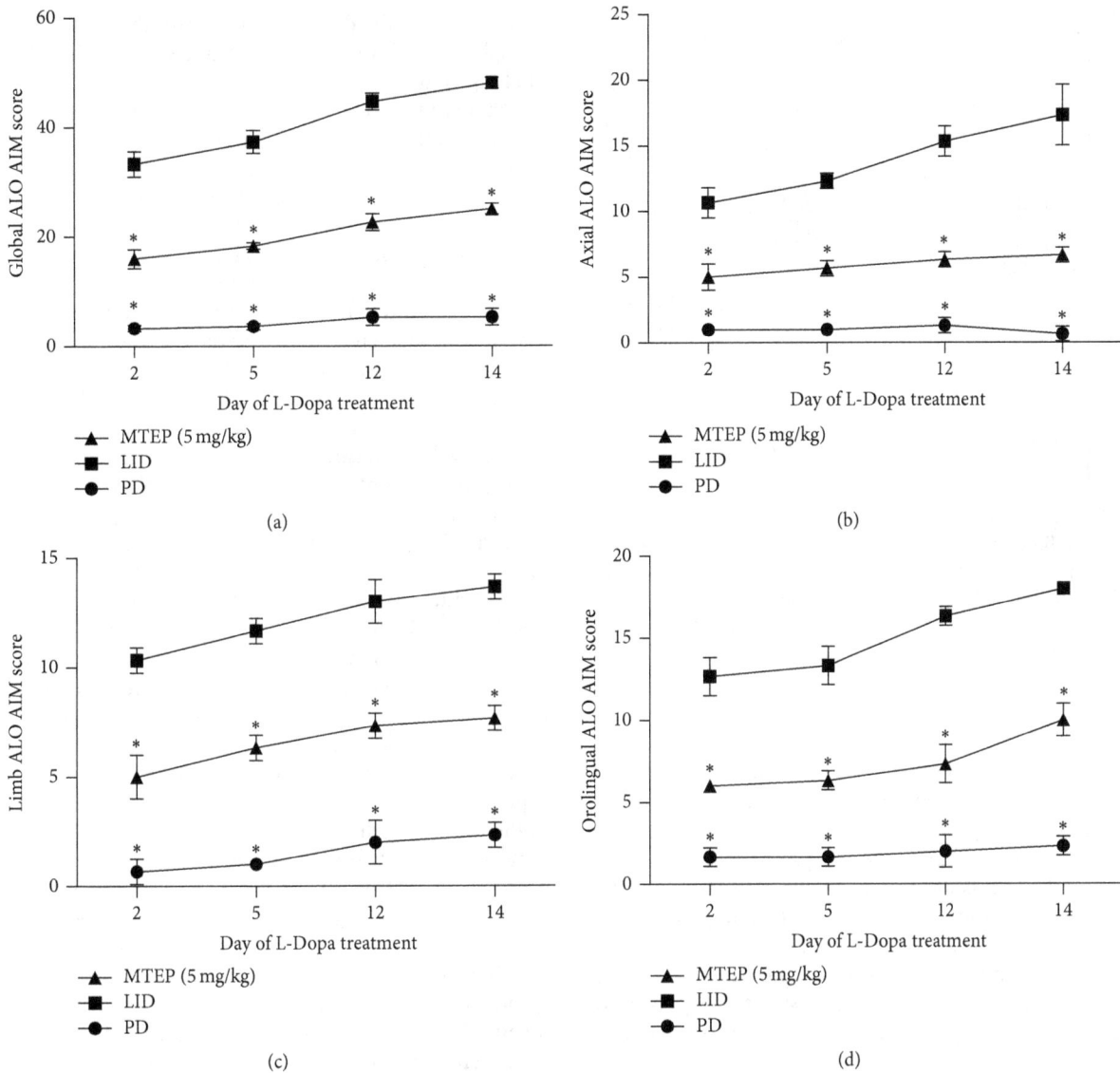

FIGURE 2: Effect of MTEP on the AIM scores. 14 days' use of MTEP significantly reduced AIM scores. At the 2nd, 5th, 12th, and 14th days, a total AIM score was calculated as the sum of the basic scores multiplied by the amplitude of the score for each AIM subtype: limb, orolingual, and axial, excluding the rotation subtype. (a) Time course of the total scores; sum of the axial, limb, and orolingual subtype scores; (b) time course of changes in the axial scores; (c) time course of changes in the limb score; and (d) time course of changes in the orolingual score. In each testing session, the AIM scores were rated following the administration of the drugs. Data are presented as the mean ± SD. $^*p < 0.01$ versus the LID group (Kruskal-Wallis test followed by Dunn's test for multiple comparisons or Mann–Whitney U test).

the coinjection of MTEP with L-Dopa did not impact the preferential use of the contralateral forelimb (Figure 3, $^#p < 0.05$). There is no significant difference between the LID group and the MTEP group.

3.3. Blockade of mGluR5 Prevents the Expression of PKC and Phosphorylation of MEK and ERK1/2 Protein Level. Protein kinase C was reported to contribute to the development of LID; in particular, the expression level of the novel PKC isoform, PKC epsilon, ipsilateral to the lesion side of the striatum, was increased after chronic L-Dopa treatment [22]. Here, we confirmed that intermittent administration of L-Dopa in hemi-Parkinsonian animals greatly increased the expression level of epsilon PKC, but this enhancement was

reversed by the injection of MTEP ($^#p < 0.05$, Figure 4(a)) compared with the LID group. It was documented that L-Dopa produces pronounced activation of ERK1/2 signaling in the dopamine-denervated striatum through a D1-receptor-dependent mechanism. This effect is associated with the development of dyskinesia [23]. In this study, we found that this elevation in p-MEK and p-ERK1/2 level was reduced in the MTEP group ($^#p < 0.05$, Figures 4(b) and 4(c)) compared with the LID group. The MTEP group also showed a minor but significant reduction compared with PD in the PKC expression level and phosphorylation of MEK ($^*p < 0.05$, Figures 4(b) and 4(c)), but there is no significant difference in the phosphorylation level of ERK1/2 between the PD and the MTEP groups ($p > 0.05$).

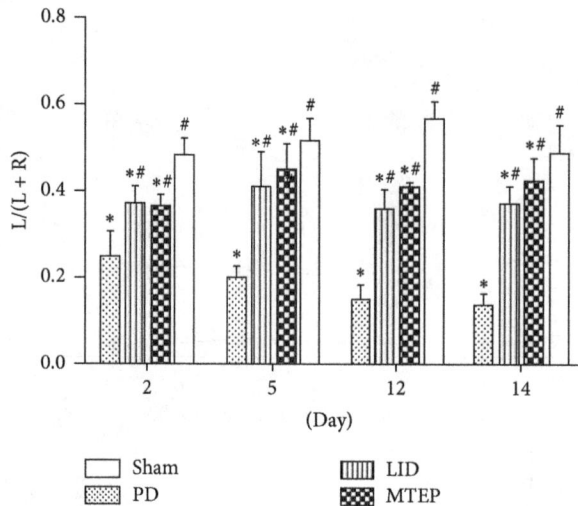

FIGURE 3: Spontaneous forelimb use of the rat in various experimental groups. Cylinder test. * indicates a significant decrease relative to the sham group (*$p < 0.01$), and # indicates a significant increase from PD group (#$p < 0.05$). Columns indicate the mean, and bars indicate the SD; the cylinder test was performed on the 2nd, 5th, 12th, and 14th days, using one-way ANOVA followed by Bonferroni post hoc tests.

3.4. MTEP Reduces the Expression of Prodynorphin and Proenkephalin in Parkinsonian Rats with LID. The mRNA expression levels of prodynorphin and proenkephalin were measured by real-time PCR. We found that prodynorphin (Figure 5(a)) expression has a minor reduction in the PD group, but it increased in the LID group; however, MTEP treatment significantly reversed the tendency. The proenkephalin (Figure 5(b)) levels were increased in PD rats primed with L-Dopa. However, MTEP significantly reduced the expression level of proenkephalin in PD rats primed with L-Dopa.

4. Discussion

Hypersensitivity and overactivation of glutamatergic signaling in the basal ganglia play a key role in the development of LID [24]. We used a hemi-Parkinsonian rat model of dyskinesia based on unilateral 6-OHDA striatal injection in the MFB, followed with the intraperitoneal administration of chronic L-Dopa daily at a dose of 25 mg/kg in the LID group and saline in the PD group and the injection of MTEP 20 min before the L-Dopa cocktail in the MTEP group. In accord with our previous work [20, 25, 26], these 6-OHDA-lesioned Parkinsonian rats developed progressive dyskinesia following the chronic use of L-Dopa (Figures 2(a)–2(d)). We also confirmed that antagonizing mGluR5 reduced the AIM scores in the rat model animals without ablating the anti-Parkinsonian effect of L-Dopa (Figure 3). In this present study, we explored the possible mechanism of the alleviation effect mediated by the antagonist of mGluR5. We found that PKC level increased in the LID group, which was consistent with the findings of Smith et al.; they also found that the antagonization of PKC could reduce the motor symptoms

of LID [22]. We also come up with the result that the phosphorylation of ERK1/2 and MEK was reduced in the MTEP group (Figures 4(a)–4(c)).

Numerous researches had already shown that the PKA signaling pathway in the striatum is closely related to the activation of D1R, which was deeply involved in the expression of LID [19, 20, 27]. After the enhancement of PKA signaling, many downstream molecules like ERK1/2 were upregulated. The phosphorylation of ERK1/2 was also closely correlated with the appearance of L-Dopa-induced dyskinesia [27–29].

It was well documented that there is a close functional interaction between the D1R and the mGluR5; with the long-term use of L-Dopa, the PKC/MEK/ERK1/2 pathway was activated [30], while blockade of the mGluR5 might call back the overactivated signal pathways.

It is well established that the opioidergic neuropeptides dynorphin and enkephalin are also involved in the striatal control of motor and behavioral function [8]. Changes in the striatal expression of proenkephalin and prodynorphin mRNA level have been reported in Parkinsonian rats with L-Dopa-induced dyskinesia. It is known that increased PDyn mRNA is attributed to increased activity in the direct pathway; the expression level of PDyn mRNA has also been reported to be closely related to the genesis of LID [31]. Enkephalin is an important striatal marker in the indirect pathway. In the classic model of the basal ganglia circuit, the enhancement of activities in the direct pathway increases the expression level of prodynorphin mRNA, and the inhibition of the indirect pathway was also reinforced [8, 32]. All these molecular changes lead to further asymmetrical pathological changes and further asymmetrical dysfunction of the neural circuit in the basal ganglia. To our knowledge, it is now established that 6-OHDA-lesioned Parkinsonian rats have an abnormal increase in the mRNA level of the direct (prodynorphin) and indirect (proenkephalin) markers [5, 7, 8]; in this present study, we found that striatal mRNA of proenkephalin was increased in PD rats and continued to increase after intermittent use of L-Dopa; as for the mRNA level of prodynorphin, it exhibited a minor drop in 6-OHDA-lesioned PD rats and this tendency reversed (increased) significantly after priming with L-Dopa in the following days (Figures 5(a) and 5(b)); these were consistent with the findings of Sgroi et al. [8]. After the use of the antagonist of mGluR5, as is shown in Figure 2, coadministration of MTEP (5 mg/kg, i.p.) with L-Dopa (25 mg/kg, i.p.) did not develop severe dyskinesia over the 14-day treatment; the antagonization of the mGluR5 downregulated the overactivated phosphorylation of the ERK1/2 via PKC/MEK/ERK1/2 pathways. On the other hand, the overactivation of the PKA pathway induced the enhancement in both prodynorphin and proenkephalin mRNA expression level after L-Dopa priming. In this study, we demonstrated that, with the antagonizing of the mGluR5, the L-Dopa induced an increase of the expression level of the phosphorylation of ERK1/2, and the mRNA expression levels of prodynorphin and proenkephalin were reduced in the 6-OHDA lesioned rats. On the one hand, the downregulation of both prodynorphin and proenkephalin helps to restore the imbalance of the basal ganglia circuit in the direct and indirect pathways. On the

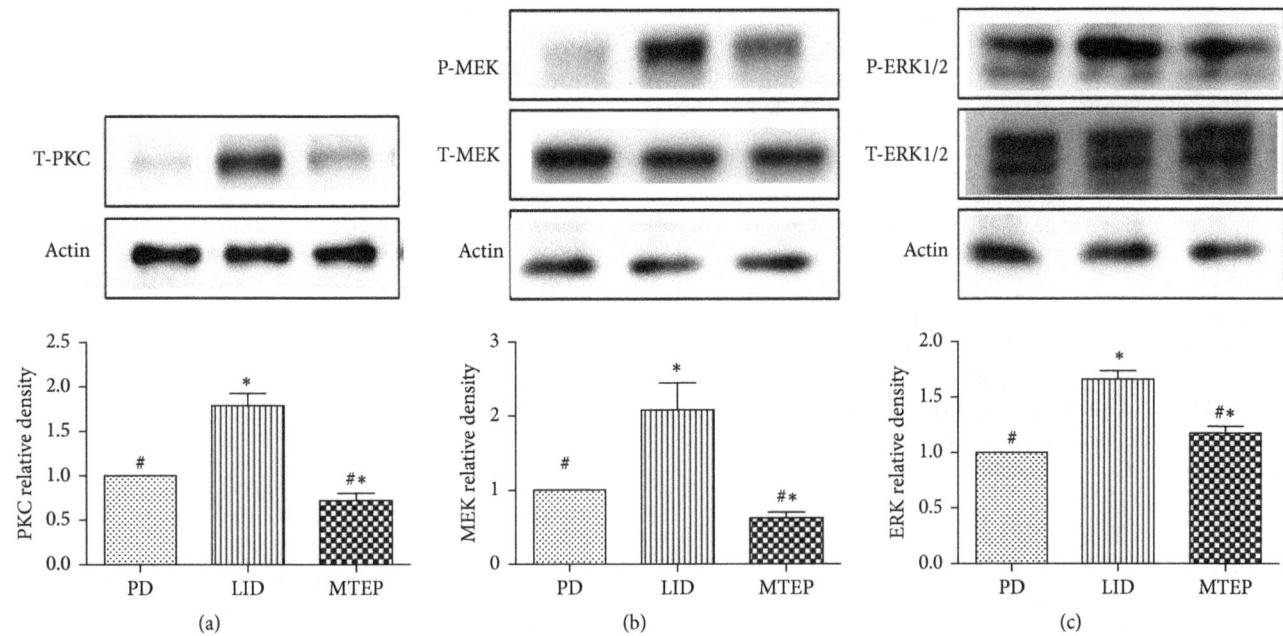

FIGURE 4: (a–c) Protein levels were evaluated by western blotting of samples from the lesioned side of the striatum (% of PD). (a) Protein level of PKC expressed relative to the level of β-actin in the 6-OHDA-lesioned rats treated with saline, L-Dopa (25 mg/kg) plus benserazide (6.25/kg), and MTEP. (b) Protein level of p-MEK level expressed relative to the total MEK level in the 6-OHDA-lesioned rats treated with saline, L-Dopa (25 mg/kg) plus benserazide (6.25/kg), and MTEP expressed relative to the level of β-actin in the sample. (c) p-ERK1/2 level expressed relative to the total ERK1/2 level in the 6-OHDA-lesioned rats treated with vehicle, L-Dopa (25 mg/kg) plus benserazide (6.25/kg), and MTEP expressed relative to the level of β-actin in the sample. Comparisons with the LID group revealed that MTEP prevented the increase of PKC, p-MEK, and p-ERK1/2 after chronic L-Dopa treatment ($^{#}p < 0.05$). Comparisons with the PD group revealed that PKC, p-MEK, and p-ERK levels were increased in the LID group, but there is a minor decrease in the PKC and MEK expression level ($^{*}p < 0.05$); there is no significant difference in the p-ERK1/2 expression level. The data represent the mean relative optical density ± SD (one-way ANOVA, $n = 4$ per group).

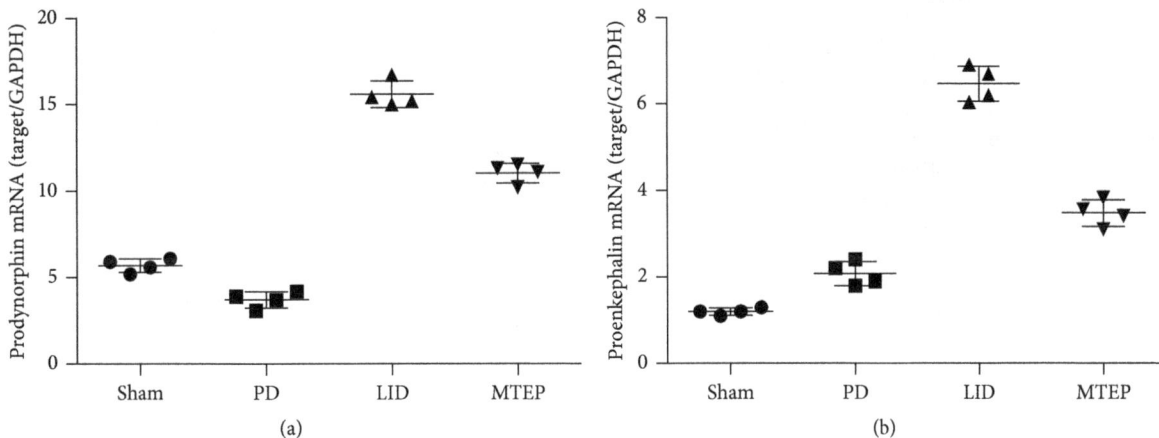

FIGURE 5: mRNA level of prodynorphin (a) and proenkephalin (b). MTEP reduced prodynorphin and proenkephalin mRNA levels in the striatum of dyskinetic rats. Striatal prodynorphin and proenkephalin mRNA expression levels were determined by real-time PCR. Increased levels of the two genes were found in LID rats. There is a minor but significant ($p < 0.05$) drop in the prodynorphin in the PD group. The antagonist of mGluR5 decreased the mRNA expression level in both prodynorphin and proenkephalin (one-way ANOVA, $n = 4$ per group).

other hand, according to the findings of Sgroi et al., the positive correlation between proenkephalin mRNA in off phase and the rotation AIMs in the on phase indicated that the improved enkephalin level probably represents a prerequisite for locomotor sensitization to subsequent L-Dopa

treatment [8]. The alleviation effect on proenkephalin mRNA level mediated by MTEP might reduce this hypersensitivity and contribute to the simultaneous reduction in AIM scores. The result we presented here seemed to have a contradiction with part of the figures provided by Mela et al. [15]; in their paper, they found that the acute injection of L-Dopa together with MTEP did not modify the upregulation of the proenkephalin mRNA induced by DA degeneration, but Mela et al. also confirmed in that very paper that, during the chronic L-Dopa treatment, the mGluR5 antagonism partially blocked the additional upregulation of both prodynorphin and proenkephalin, which was consistent with our presented data. Furthermore, on the one hand, it was reported that the DA can exert its effect on the D2 receptor through a non-cAMP-dependent way [33]; it upregulated the phosphorylation of Akt/GSK3$\beta\beta$ pathway to affect the DA-dependent behavior; on the other hand, recent research shows that the antagonism of mGluR5 could inhibit the phosphorylation of Akt/GSK3$\beta\beta$ [34]; this might contribute to the restoration of the activity of the indirect pathway and might be followed by a decrease of PPE.

5. Conclusion

Hypersensitivity and overactivation of glutamatergic signaling in the basal ganglia play a key role in the development of LID. Antagonizing mGluR5 could reduce the AIM scores in the rodent and primate PD model animals. While the antagonist downregulates the signaling on the PKC/MEK/ERK1/2 pathways, it also reduced the expression level of prodynorphin and proenkephalin mRNA significantly. Antidyskinetic treatment with MTEP affects multiple molecular pathways in the Parkinsonian striatum.

Authors' Contributions

Jing-ya Lin conceived the study and participated in the design of the manuscript and extracted data and helped draft the manuscript. Cheng-long Xie and Lu Song prepared figures and offered technical support during the whole process. Ai-juan Yan carried out the statistical analysis and interpretation of data. Zhen-guo Liu participated in the conceptualization and design of the experiment and data extraction and analysis and drafted the manuscript. All authors read and approved the final manuscript.

Acknowledgments

This study was supported by projects of the National Natural Science Foundation of China (81400925, 81471148, 81671273, 81771211, and 81703852), projects of the Shanghai Committee of Science and Technology (17401901000), National Key R&D Program of China (2017YFC1310300), and SHSMU-ION Research Center for Brain Disorders (2015NKX007).

References

[1] M. Feyder, A. Bonito-Oliva, and G. Fisone, "L-DOPA-induced dyskinesia and abnormal signaling in striatal medium spiny neurons: Focus on dopamine D1 receptor-mediated transmission," *Frontiers in Behavioral Neuroscience*, no. OCTOBER, 2011.

[2] P. Calabresi, M. D. Filippo, V. Ghiglieri, N. Tambasco, and B. Picconi, "Levodopa-induced dyskinesias in patients with Parkinson's disease: filling the bench-to-bedside gap," *The Lancet Neurology*, vol. 9, no. 11, pp. 1106–1117, 2010.

[3] F. Niccolini, L. Rocchi, and M. Politis, "Molecular imaging of levodopa-induced dyskinesias," *Cellular and Molecular Life Sciences*, vol. 72, no. 11, pp. 2107–2117, 2015.

[4] C. Winkler, D. Kirik, A. Björklund, and M. A. Cenci, "L-DOPA-induced dyskinesia in the intrastriatal 6-hydroxydopamine model of Parkinson's disease: Relation to motor and cellular parameters of nigrostriatal function," *Neurobiology of Disease*, vol. 10, no. 2, pp. 165–186, 2002.

[5] C. Marin, M. Bonastre, G. Mengod, R. Cortés, and M. C. Rodríguez-Oroz, "From unilateral to bilateral parkinsonism: Effects of lateralization on dyskinesias and associated molecular mechanisms," *Neuropharmacology*, vol. 97, pp. 365–375, 2015.

[6] M. A. Cenci, C. S. Lee, and A. Björklund, "L-DOPA-induced dyskinesia in the rat is associated with striatal overexpression of prodynorphin- and glutamic acid decarboxylase mRNA," *European Journal of Neuroscience*, vol. 10, no. 8, pp. 2694–2706, 1998.

[7] M. A. Cenci, "Dopamine dysregulation of movement control in l-DOPA-induced dyskinesia," *Trends in Neurosciences*, vol. 30, no. 5, pp. 236–243, 2007.

[8] S. Sgroi, C. Capper-Loup, P. Paganetti, and A. Kaelin-Lang, "Enkephalin and dynorphin neuropeptides are differently correlated with locomotor hypersensitivity and levodopa-induced dyskinesia in parkinsonian rats," *Experimental Neurology*, vol. 280, pp. 80–88, 2016.

[9] D. Rylander, A. Recchia, F. Mela, A. Dekundy, W. Danysz, and M. A. Cenci Nilsson, "Pharmacological modulation of glutamate transmission in a rat model of L-DOPA-induced dyskinesia: Effects on motor behavior and striatal nuclear signaling," *The Journal of Pharmacology and Experimental Therapeutics*, vol. 330, no. 1, pp. 227–235, 2009.

[10] X.-B. Cao, Q. Guan, Y. Xu, L. Wang, and S.-G. Sun, "Mechanism of over-activation in direct pathway mediated by dopamine D1 receptor in rats with levodopa-induced dyskinesias," *Neuroscience Bulletin*, vol. 22, no. 3, pp. 159–164, 2006.

[11] K. A. Johnson, P. J. Conn, and C. M. Niswender, "Glutamate receptors as therapeutic targets for Parkinson's disease," *CNS & Neurological Disorders—Drug Targets*, vol. 8, no. 6, pp. 475–491, 2009.

[12] F. Tison, C. Keywood, M. Wakefield et al., "A Phase 2A Trial of the Novel mGluR5-Negative Allosteric Modulator Dipraglurant for Levodopa-Induced Dyskinesia in Parkinson's Disease," *Movement Disorders*, vol. 31, no. 9, pp. 1373–1380, 2016.

[13] A. R. Salomons, N. E. Pinzon, H. Boleij et al., "Differential effects of diazepam and MPEP on habituation and neuro-behavioural processes in inbred mice," *Behavioral and Brain Functions*, vol. 8, article 30, 2012.

[14] O. Rascol, S. Perez-Lloret, and J. J. Ferreira, "New treatments for levodopa-induced motor complications," *Movement Disorders*, vol. 30, no. 11, pp. 1451–1460, 2015.

[15] F. Mela, M. Marti, A. Dekundy, W. Danysz, M. Morari, and M. A. Cenci, "Antagonism of metabotropic glutamate receptor type 5 attenuates L-DOPA-induced dyskinesia and its molecular and neurochemical correlates in a rat model of Parkinson's disease," *Journal of Neurochemistry*, vol. 101, no. 2, pp. 483–497, 2007.

[16] A. Dekundy, M. Pietraszek, D. Schaefer, M. A. Cenci, and W. Danysz, "Effects of group I metabotropic glutamate receptors blockade in experimental models of Parkinson's disease," *Brain Research Bulletin*, vol. 69, no. 3, pp. 318–326, 2006.

[17] V. Sgambato-Faure and M. A. Cenci, "Glutamatergic mechanisms in the dyskinesias induced by pharmacological dopamine replacement and deep brain stimulation for the treatment of Parkinson's disease," *Progress in Neurobiology*, vol. 96, no. 1, pp. 69–86, 2012.

[18] F. Nicoletti, J. Bockaert, G. L. Collingridge et al., "Metabotropic glutamate receptors: from the workbench to the bedside," *Neuropharmacology*, vol. 60, no. 7-8, pp. 1017–1041, 2011.

[19] L. Song, Z. Zhang, R. Hu et al., "Targeting the D1-N-methyl-D-aspartate receptor complex reduces L-dopa-induced dyskinesia in 6-hydroxydopamine-lesioned Parkinson's rats," *Drug Design, Development and Therapy*, vol. 10, pp. 547–555, 2016.

[20] C.-L. Xie, J.-Y. Lin, M.-H. Wang et al., "Inhibition of Glycogen Synthase Kinase-3β (GSK-3β) as potent therapeutic strategy to ameliorates L-dopa-induced dyskinesia in 6-OHDA parkinsonian rats," *Scientific Reports*, vol. 6, Article ID 23527, 2016.

[21] D. Rylander, H. Iderberg, Q. Li et al., "A mGluR5 antagonist under clinical development improves L-DOPA-induced dyskinesia in parkinsonian rats and monkeys," *Neurobiology of Disease*, vol. 39, no. 3, pp. 352–361, 2010.

[22] C. P. S. Smith, J. D. Oh, F. Bibbiani, M. A. Collins, I. Avila, and T. N. Chase, "Tamoxifen effect on L-DOPA induced response complications in parkinsonian rats and primates," *Neuropharmacology*, vol. 52, no. 2, pp. 515–526, 2007.

[23] J. E. Westin, L. Vercammen, E. M. Strome, C. Konradi, and M. A. Cenci, "Spatiotemporal pattern of striatal ERK1/2 phosphorylation in a rat model of L-DOPA-induced dyskinesia and the role of dopamine D1 receptors," *Biological Psychiatry*, vol. 62, no. 7, pp. 800–810, 2007.

[24] H. Awad, G. W. Hubert, Y. Smith, A. I. Levey, and P. J. Conn, "Activation of metabotropic glutamate receptor 5 has direct excitatory effects and potentiates NMDA receptor currents in neurons of the subthalamic nucleus," *The Journal of Neuroscience*, vol. 20, no. 21, pp. 7871–7879, 2000.

[25] S. Zhang, C. Xie, Q. Wang, and Z. Liu, "Interactions of CaMKII with dopamine D2 receptors: roles in levodopa-induced dyskinesia in 6-hydroxydopamine lesioned Parkinson's rats," *Scientific Reports*, vol. 4, article 6811, 2014.

[26] H. S. Lindgren, D. R. Andersson, S. Lagerkvist, H. Nissbrandt, and M. A. Cenci, "L-DOPA-induced dopamine efflux in the striatum and the substantia nigra in a rat model of Parkinson's disease: Temporal and quantitative relationship to the expression of dyskinesia," *Journal of Neurochemistry*, vol. 112, no. 6, pp. 1465–1476, 2010.

[27] X. Yang, H. Zhao, H. Shi et al., "Intranigral administration of substance P receptor antagonist attenuated levodopa-induced dyskinesia in a rat model of Parkinson's disease," *Experimental Neurology*, vol. 271, pp. 168–174, 2015.

[28] E. Santini, E. Valjent, and G. Fisone, "Parkinson's disease: levodopa-induced dyskinesia and signal transduction," *FEBS Journal*, vol. 275, no. 7, pp. 1392–1399, 2008.

[29] N. Pavón, A. B. Martín, A. Mendialdua, and R. Moratalla, "ERK phosphorylation and FosB expression are associated with L-DOPA-induced dyskinesia in hemiparkinsonian mice," *Biological Psychiatry*, vol. 59, no. 1, pp. 64–74, 2006.

[30] T. Fieblinger, I. Sebastianutto, C. Alcacer et al., "Mechanisms of dopamine D1 receptor-mediated ERK1/2 activation in the parkinsonian striatum and their modulation by metabotropic glutamate receptor type 5," *The Journal of Neuroscience*, vol. 34, no. 13, pp. 4728–4740, 2014.

[31] N. Yamamoto and J.-J. Soghomonian, "Metabotropic glutamate mGluR5 receptor blockade opposes abnormal involuntary movements and the increases in glutamic acid decarboxylase mRNA levels induced by L-DOPA in striatal neurons of 6-hydroxydopamine-lesioned rats," *Neuroscience*, vol. 163, no. 4, pp. 1171–1180, 2009.

[32] B. Henry, S. Duty, S. H. Fox, A. R. Crossman, and J. M. Brotchie, "Increased striatal pre-proenkephalin B expression is associated with dyskinesia in Parkinson's disease," *Experimental Neurology*, vol. 183, no. 2, pp. 458–468, 2003.

[33] J. M. Beaulieu, T. D. Sotnikova, S. Marion, R. J. Lefkowitz, R. R. Gainetdinov, and M. G. Caron, "An Akt/β-arrestin 2/PP2A signaling complex mediates dopaminergic neurotransmission and behavior," *Cell*, vol. 122, no. 2, pp. 261–273, 2005.

[34] M. Morissette, P. Samadi, A. H. Tahar, N. Bélanger, and T. Di Paolo, "Striatal Akt/GSK3 signaling pathway in the development of L-Dopa-induced dyskinesias in MPTP monkeys," *Progress in Neuro-Psychopharmacology & Biological Psychiatry*, vol. 34, no. 3, pp. 446–454, 2010.

27

Tremor Types in Parkinson Disease: A Descriptive Study Using a New Classification

Alexandre Gironell ⓘ, Berta Pascual-Sedano, Ignacio Aracil, Juan Marín-Lahoz, Javier Pagonabarraga, and Jaime Kulisevsky

Movement Disorders Unit, Department of Neurology, Hospital de la Santa Creu i Sant Pau, Autonomous University of Barcelona, Catalonia, Spain

Correspondence should be addressed to Alexandre Gironell; agironell@santpau.cat

Academic Editor: Seyed-Mohammad Fereshtehnejad

Background. The current classification of tremor types in Parkinson disease (PD) is potentially confusing, particularly for mixed tremor, and there is no label for pure resting tremor. With a view to better defining the clinical phenomenological classification of these tremors, our group relabeled the different types as follows: pure resting tremor (type I); mixed resting and action tremor with similar frequencies (type II) divided, according to action tremor presentation, into II-R when there is a time lag and II-C otherwise; pure action tremor (type III); and mixed resting and action tremor with differing frequencies (type IV). We performed a descriptive study to determine prevalence and clinical correlates for this new tremor classification. *Patient/Methods.* A total of 315 consecutively recruited patients with PD and tremor were clinically evaluated. X^2 tests were used to assess tremor type associations with categorical variables, namely, sex, family history of PD, motor fluctuations, and anticholinergic and beta-blocker use. With tremor type as the independent variable, ANOVA was performed to study the relationship between dependent quantitative variables, namely, age, age at PD diagnosis, disease duration, and UPDRS scores for rigidity. *Results.* The studied patients had tremor types as follows: type I, 30%; type II, 50% (II-R, 25% and II-C, 25%); type III, 19%; and type IV, 1%. No significant association was found between the studied clinical variables and tremor types. *Conclusions.* Mixed tremor was the most common tremor type in our series of patients with PD according to our proposed classification, which we hope will enhance understanding of the broad clinical phenomenology of PD.

1. Introduction

Tremor, one of the most characteristic manifestations of Parkinson disease (PD) and often the presenting sign, occurs in approximately 75% of patients with PD, who rank it as their second most troublesome symptom [1, 2].

PD tremor, whether resting or action tremor, is a highly variable symptom [3]. The classical tremor is reported as a resting tremor of 4–7 Hz, often asymmetric, which ceases with volitional movement [4]. Only resting tremor is a positive diagnostic criterion for PD [4, 5]. However, action tremor, whether pure or mixed with resting tremor, is often observed in PD and has a reported prevalence of as high as 92% [5].

In 1998, the Consensus Statement on Tremor issued by the Movement Disorder Society (MDS) classified the different tremor types observed in PD in 3 categories: type I, resting and action tremor with similar frequencies; type II, resting and action tremor with differing frequencies; and type III, pure action tremor. Finally, the term monosymptomatic rest tremor refers to patients with rest tremor and no other parkinsonian signs [6]. A more recent revised Consensus Statement does not modify the tremor type classification for PD [7]. In our opinion, this classification has led to some confusion regarding mixed tremor. In particular, differing tremor frequencies in type II tremor suggest that different tremor pacemakers are used and also possibly indicate the coexistence of different diseases. Furthermore, pure resting tremor does not appear as a separate tremor type.

With a view to better defining the clinical phenomenological classification of PD, our group relabeled the different PD tremor types in what appeared to us to be a more intuitive and logical way, as follows: type I, pure resting tremor; type II, mixed action and resting tremor with similar frequencies (subdivided into re-emergent and continuous tremors); type III, pure action tremor; and type IV, mixed action and resting tremor with different frequencies.

Below we describe a descriptive study of prevalence and clinical correlates for this new tremor classification, based purely on clinical phenomenology, for a consecutive series of patients with PD.

2. Patients and Methods

Included consecutively in the study were patients with PD and visibly detected tremor who attended the Movement Disorders Unit at Sant Pau Hospital Neurology Department between December 2015 and April 2017 (16 months). PD was diagnosed using the London Brain Bank criteria [8]. The study protocol was approved by the hospital ethics committee, and the study was performed in accordance with international ethical regulations. All subjects granted their signed informed consent to participate. The patients were clinically evaluated by neurologists specializing in movement disorders [9, 10].

Resting tremor was defined as a tremor present when arms were resting in the lap or by the side. Since it was not always easy to ensure that a patient was completely relaxed, when in doubt and in order to rule out gravitational force and muscle co-contraction, the patient was tested lying down on a bed or walking with their arms hanging at the sides. We also asked patients to complete tasks that increased tremor amplitude, either mental tasks (e.g., saying the months of the year backwards) or motor tasks (e.g., opening and closing the contralateral hand).

Action tremor can be either kinetic or postural. Kinetic tremor was defined as tremor present during hand movement (e.g., during a finger-to-nose movement or when writing). Postural tremor was assessed for stretched-out arms, the bat-wing position, and wrist extension.

For mixed tremor, accelerometric recordings were made using a previously described methodology [11]. Resting and action tremor were considered to have similar frequencies when the difference in frequency peaks was below 1.5 Hz. This is the described cutoff value for the coexistence of different tremor pacemakers and syndromes [12]. The clinical evaluation was performed in OFF time (12 hours after the last levodopa dose).

The tremor types are summarized in Table 1 and graphically explained in Figure 1. Type I is pure resting tremor, including the classical pill-rolling tremor. Type II is mixed resting and action tremor with similar frequencies, divided, according to action tremor presentation, into type II-R (re-emergent) when there is a time lag (usually 5–20 seconds) and type II-C (continuous) when there is no time lag. Type III is pure action tremor (essential tremor-like). Finally, type IV represents mixed resting and action tremor with differing frequencies, possibly indicating the coexistence of two tremor conditions (e.g., essential tremor and PD).

TABLE 1: Tremor types in Parkinson disease.

Type I. Pure resting tremor
Type II. Mixed resting and action tremor with similar frequencies*
II-R. Action tremor with a time lag
II-C. Action tremor without a time lag
Type III. Pure action tremor
Type IV. Mixed resting and action tremor with different frequencies**

*Difference <1.5 Hz; **difference >1.5 Hz.

In the neurological examination, for the most affected arm in each patient, the rigidity item from the motor evaluation section of the Unified Parkinson Disease Rating Scale (UPDRS) was used as a measure of parkinsonism severity. The Hoehn and Yahr scale for describing progression of PD symptoms was also scored. Also assessed based on a chart review and on patient reports were several clinical factors correlating with PD tremor types: age, sex, family history of tremor, disease duration, motor fluctuations, and treatment with anticholinergics or beta-blockers.

For the descriptive analysis, categorical variables were reported as percentages and number of cases, and quantitative variables were reported as mean ± standard deviation. X^2 tests were used to assess tremor type associations with the categorical variables of sex, family history of PD, presence of motor fluctuations, anticholinergic use, and beta-blocker use. Analysis of variance (ANOVA) was performed to study the relationship between dependent quantitative variables—age, age at PD diagnosis, disease duration, and UPDRS scores for rigidity—with tremor type as the independent variable. For all analyses, the statistical level of significance was established at 5% (alpha = 0.05, two-sided). The statistical package used was IBM-SPSS (ver. 22.0).

3. Results

A total of 315 patients (166 men and 149 women) with a mean age of 76.4 years (range 60–85 years) were included in the study. Table 2 shows the demographic and clinical characteristics of the patients in our series. Table 3 shows the accelerometric data for mixed tremor.

Around 30% of patients had tremor type I, 50% had type II (25% II-R and 25% II-C), 19% had type III, and 1% had type IV.

No significant association was found between the clinical variables studied and tremor types: age ($p = 0.232$), sex ($p = 0.092$), disease duration ($p = 0.238$), Hoehn and Yahr score ($p = 0.358$), family history of PD ($p = 0.766$), percentage of motor fluctuations ($p = 0.788$), and rigidity score ($p = 0.990$). There were no statistically significant differences in the percentage of patients with each tremor type in terms of anticholinergic use. No patient with type I tremor in our series was taking beta-blockers.

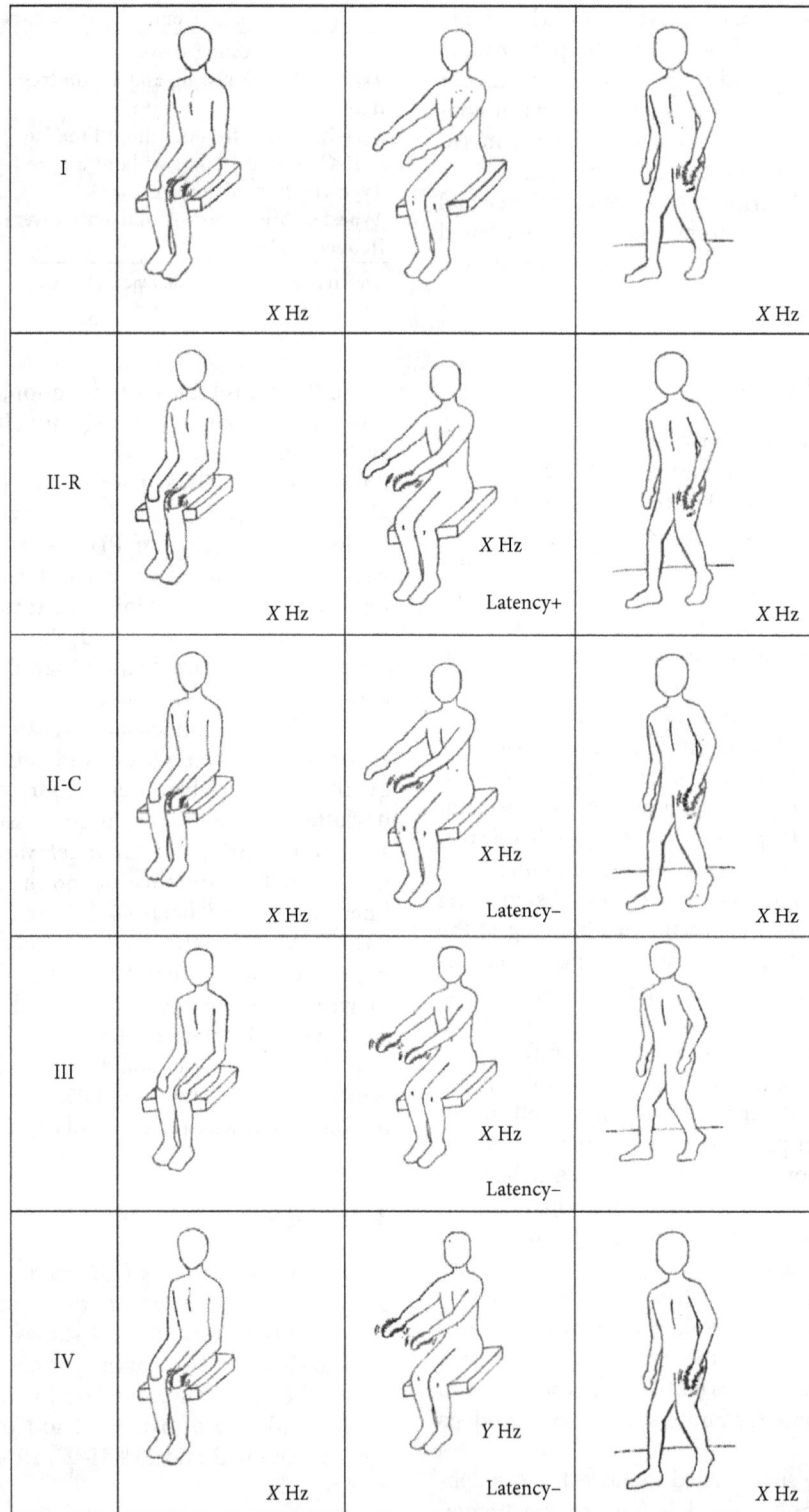

FIGURE 1: Tremor types in Parkinson disease graphically explained. Difference in X and Y frequency is above 1.5 Hz.

4. Discussion

We propose new labels for tremor types observed in PD based purely on clinical phenomenology. In our series, we found the most common tremor presentation in PD to be mixed resting and action tremor (51% of the patients). In our

opinion, this new classification improves on the MDS classification as it is more intuitive and logical. Our classification based on a descriptive cross-sectional study does not have a pathological, prognostic, or therapeutic value, but represents a first step for future pathological and prospective studies to determine its usefulness.

TABLE 2: Characteristics of patients with Parkinson disease by tremor type.

Characteristics	Tremor type					Association
	I	II-R	II-C	III	IV	
Number	96	78	78	60	3	—
Age	76.2 ± 9.2	76.2 ± 9.6	72.7 ± 9.1	74.0 ± 9.5	83.1 ± 1.4	$p = 0.232$
Female (%)	57	53	53	41	60	$p = 0.092$
Family history of PD (%)	5	10	17	16	20	$p = 0.766$
Disease duration (years)	5.2 ± 3.1	5.1 ± 3.2	7.3 ± 6.0	6.4 ± 4.7	5.5 ± 3.5	$p = 0.238$
Hoehn and Yahr I-II (%)	92	95	90	90	85	$p = 0.358$
Motor fluctuations (%)	12	10	12	9	10	$p = 0.788$
UPDRS rigidity	2.1 ± 0.3	2.0 ± 0.23	2.0 ± 0.3	2.2 ± 0.1	2.0 ± 0.3	$p = 0.990$
Anticholinergics (%)	15	25	24	10	10	$p = 0.110$
Beta-blockers (%)	0	10	30	50	60	$p = 0.090$

UPDRS, Unified Parkinson's Disease Rating Scale. Association: statistical association between clinical variable and tremor type.

TABLE 3: Accelerometric data for patients with mixed tremor.

Tremor type	Resting tremor (Hz)	Action tremor (Hz)	Time lag (seconds)
II-R	5.0 ± 0.8	4.9 ± 1.1	6.8 ± 2.2
II-C	5.2 ± 0.9	5.1 ± 0.7	0
IV	4.8 ± 1.1	7.5 ± 0.9	0

There are two main differences between our classification and the MDS classification [6, 7]. We include pure resting tremor (type I), and we emphasize mixed tremor with its respective categories, i.e., the same frequency (type II-R or II-C) or a different frequency (type IV).

Our study found that action tremor is prevalent in PD. In fact, pure or mixed action tremor was experienced by 70% of the patients in our series, a finding that corroborates previous studies reporting action tremor prevalence of as high as 92% in patients with PD [4, 5, 13, 14]. Nonetheless, only resting tremor is a diagnostic criterion for PD [15]. Yet pure resting tremor was experienced by only 30% of the patients in our study, whereas resting tremor including mixed tremor was experienced by 81% of our patients.

Interestingly, we found that 19% of our patients had pure action tremor, that is, essential tremor-like tremor. Our group has previously reported that this may be the first symptom of PD in about 6% of cases [16]. While some consider this tremor to be of minor importance, in clinical practice, moderate action tremor is regarded as more disabling than severe resting tremor [4, 5, 13, 14, 17].

The basis for action tremor in PD is not clear [5]. Several studies suggest that action tremor, like resting tremor, may be a manifestation of underlying basal ganglia disease [18]. Tremor has been reported to be more pronounced on the side of the body that is most affected by PD [19]. Single-dose challenges of dopaminergic and anticholinergic agents have been reported to significantly reduce action tremor amplitude [20]. Furthermore, a significant correlation between action tremor and resting tremor has been reported, suggesting that action tremor is a variant of resting tremor in patients with PD [21]. In a recent study, Dirkx et al. suggest that there are two distinct postural tremor phenotypes in PD: re-emergent tremor as a continuation of resting tremor during stable posturing, with a dopaminergic basis, and pure postural tremor as a less common type of tremor in PD, but with a largely nondopaminergic basis [22].

It has been hypothesized that re-emergent tremor (type II-R in our classification) is a form of resting tremor in PD [23]. Few studies have distinguished between re-emergent tremor and tremor that does not occur after a time lag [24]. In our study, we found similar prevalence for both re-emergent and continuous mixed tremor. Interestingly, a recent study reported a significantly shorter illness duration for patients with re-emergent tremor [25]. In our study, however, we found no difference in disease duration for the different tremor types. Furthermore, we found no relationship between tremor type and other clinical manifestations of PD, including rigidity, Hoehn and Yahr score, or PD family history.

The main limitation of our study is the small number of patients included, although we suggest that the sample is quite representative. Furthermore, we did not control for the effects of antiparkinsonian medication that might modify the tremor phenomenology. However, the patients in our study were evaluated in OFF time.

Furthermore, as a weighted limb test was not performed, some degree of misdiagnosis cannot be ruled out in cases of physiological action tremor. The classification of pure action tremor is difficult because rest tremor may be very mild and intermittent, especially when patients are treated with dopaminergic drugs.

Finally, another limitation of this cross-sectional study is that we did not study shifts between tremor subtypes; i.e., we did not assess how many patients switched from one type of tremor to another, although the absence of any significant correlation between disease duration and tremor type would suggest that shifting is not relevant. This issue, however, would need to be analyzed in future studies.

5. Conclusion

We propose new labels for tremor types observed in PD based purely on clinical phenomenology. Mixed tremor was the most common tremor type in our series of patients with PD according to our proposed classification, which we hope will enhance understanding of the broad clinical phenomenology of PD.

Acknowledgments

We thank Dr. Ignasi Gich for help with the statistical analysis and Ms. Mar Gironell for the drawings in Figure 1.

References

[1] A. Barbeau, "Parkinson's disease: clinical features and etiopathology," in *Handbook of Clinical Neurology. Vol. 5. Extrapyramidal Disorders*, P. J. Vinken, G. W. Bruyn, and H. L. Klawans, Eds., pp. 87–152, Elsevier Science Publishers B, New York, NY, USA, 1986.

[2] M. Politis, K. Wu, S. P. G. B. Molloy, K. E. Chaudhuri, and P. Piccini, "Parkinson's disease symptoms: the patient's perspective," *Movement Disorders*, vol. 25, no. 11, pp. 1646–1651, 2010.

[3] W. J. Zetusky, J. Jankovic, and F. J. Pirozzolo, "The heterogeneity of Parkinson's disease: clinical and prognostic implications," *Neurology*, vol. 35, no. 4, pp. 522–526, 1985.

[4] H. Teravainen and D. B. Calne, "Action tremor in Parkinson's disease," *Journal of Neurology, Neurosurgery and Psychiatry*, vol. 43, no. 3, pp. 257–263, 1980.

[5] W. E. Koller, B. Veter-Overfield, and R. Barter, "Tremors in early Parkinson's disease," *Clinical Neuropharmacology*, vol. 12, no. 4, pp. 293–297, 1989.

[6] G. Deuschl, P. Bain, and M. Brin, "Consensus statement of the movement disorder society on tremor," *Movement Disorders*, vol. 13, no. S3, pp. 2–23, 1998.

[7] K. P. Bhatia, P. Bain, N. Bajaj et al., "Consensus statement on the classification of tremors. Task force on tremor of the International Parkinson and Movement Disorder Society," *Movement Disorders*, vol. 33, no. 1, pp. 75–87, 2018.

[8] A. J. Hughes, S. E. Daniel, L. Kilford, and A. J. Lees, "Accuracy of clinical diagnosis of idiopathic Parkinson's disease. A clinicopathological study of 100 cases," *Journal of Neurology, Neurosurgery and Psychiatry*, vol. 55, no. 3, pp. 181–184, 1992.

[9] H. Zach, M. Dirk, B. R. Bloem, and R. C. Helmich, "The clinical evaluation of Parkinson's tremor," *Journal of Parkinson's Disease*, vol. 5, no. 3, pp. 471–474, 2015.

[10] C. W. Hess and S. L. Pullman, "Tremor: clinical phenomenology and assessment techniques," *Tremor and Other Hyperkinetic Movements*, pii:tre-02-65-365-1 2012.

[11] A. Gironell, J. Kulisevsky, B. Pascual, and M. Barbanoj, "Routine neurophysiological tremor analysis as a diagnostic

[12] G. Deuschl, P. Krack, M. Lauk, and J. Timmer, "Clinical neurophysiology of tremor," *Journal of Clinical Neurophysiology*, vol. 13, no. 2, pp. 110–121, 1996.

[13] H. Forssberg, P. E. Ingvarsson, N. Iwasaki, R. S. Johansson, and A. M. Gordon, "Action tremor during object manipulation in Parkinson's disease," *Movement Disorders*, vol. 15, no. 2, pp. 244–254, 2000.

[14] R. Zimmermann, G. Deuschl, A. Horning, J. Schulte-Monting, G. Fuchs, and C. H. Lucking, "Tremors in Parkinson's disease: symptom analysis and rating," *Clinical Neuropharmacology*, vol. 17, no. 4, pp. 303–314, 1994.

[15] A. H. Rajput, B. Rozdilsky, and L. Ang, "Occurrence of resting tremor in Parkinson's disease," *Neurology*, vol. 41, pp. 1298-1299, 1991.

[16] R Ribosa-Nogué and A Gironell, "Essential tremor and Parkinson's disease. Are they associated?," *Revista de Neurologia*, vol. 56, p. 351, 2013.

[17] J. W. Lance, R. S. Schwab, and E. A. Peterson, "Action tremor and the cogwheel phenomenon in Parkinson's disease," *Brain*, vol. 86, no. 1, pp. 95–110, 1963.

[18] M. Hallet, "Parkinson's disease tremor: pathophysiology," *Parkinsonism & Related Disorders*, vol. 18, no. S1, pp. S85-S86, 2012.

[19] M. Rivlin-Etzion, O. Marmor, G. Heimer, A. Raz, A. Nini, and H. Bergman, "Basal ganglia oscillations and pathophysiology of movement disorders," *Current Opinion in Neurobiology*, vol. 16, no. 6, pp. 629–637, 2006.

[20] A. Q. Rana, I. Siddiqui, A. A. Mosabbir, A. R. Qureshi, A. Fattah, and N. Awan, "Is action tremor in Parkinson's disease related to resting tremor?," *Neurological Research*, vol. 36, no. 2, pp. 107–111, 2014.

[21] A. Schrag, L. Schelosky, U. Scholz, and W. Poewe, "Reduction of Parkinsonian signs in patients with Parkinson's disease by dopaminergic versus anticholinergic single dose challenges," *Movement Disorders*, vol. 14, no. 2, pp. 252–255, 1999.

[22] M. F. Dirkx, H. Zach, B. R. Bloem, M. Hallet, and R. C. Helmich, "The nature of postural tremor in Parkinson disease," *Neurology*, vol. 90, no. 13, pp. e1095–e11103, 2018.

[23] E. D. Louis, G. Levy, L. J. Cote, H. Mejia, S. Fahn, and K. Marder, "Clinical correlates of action tremor in Parkinson disease," *Archives of Neurology*, vol. 58, no. 10, pp. 1630–1634, 2001.

[24] J. Jankovic, K. S. Schwartz, and W. Ondo, "Re-emergent tremor of Parkinson's disease," *Journal of Neurology, Neurosurgery and Psychiatry*, vol. 67, no. 5, pp. 646–650, 1999.

[25] P. Mailankody, K. Thennarasu, B. C. Nagaraju, R. Yadav, and P. K. Pal, "Re-emergent tremor in Parkinson's disease: a clinical and electromyographic study," *Journal of the Neurological Sciences*, vol. 366, pp. 33–36, 2016.

28

Aerobic Exercise Preserves Olfaction Function in Individuals with Parkinson's Disease

Anson B. Rosenfeldt,[1] Tanujit Dey,[2] and Jay L. Alberts[1,3,4]

[1]Department of Biomedical Engineering, Cleveland Clinic, 9500 Euclid Ave., Cleveland, OH 44119, USA
[2]Quantitative Health Sciences, Cleveland Clinic, 9500 Euclid Ave., Cleveland, OH 44119, USA
[3]Center for Neurological Restoration, Cleveland Clinic, 9500 Euclid Ave., Cleveland, OH 44119, USA
[4]Cleveland FES Center, L. Stokes Cleveland VA Medical Center, 10701 East Blvd, Cleveland, OH 44106, USA

Correspondence should be addressed to Jay L. Alberts; albertj@ccf.org

Academic Editor: Yuan-Han Yang

Introduction. Based on anecdotal reports of improved olfaction following aerobic exercise, the aim of this study was to evaluate the effects of an 8-week aerobic exercise program on olfaction function in individuals with Parkinson's disease (PD). *Methods.* Thirty-eight participants with idiopathic PD were randomized to either an aerobic exercise group ($n = 23$) or a nonexercise control group ($n = 15$). The aerobic exercise group completed a 60-minute cycling session three times per week for eight weeks while the nonexercise control group received no intervention. All participants completed the University of Pennsylvania Smell Identification Test (UPSIT) at baseline, end of treatment, and a four-week follow up. *Results.* Change in UPSIT scores between the exercise and nonexercise groups from baseline to EOT ($p = 0.01$) and from baseline to EOT+4 ($p = 0.02$) favored the aerobic exercise group. Individuals in the nonexercise group had worsening olfaction function over time, while the exercise group was spared from decline. *Discussion.* The difference in UPSIT scores suggested that aerobic exercise may be altering central nervous system pathways that regulate the physiologic or cognitive processes controlling olfaction in individuals with PD. While these results provide promising preliminary evidence that exercise may modify the disease process, further systematic evaluation is necessary.

1. Introduction

The majority of individuals with Parkinson's disease (PD) experience olfaction dysfunction [1, 2]. Hyposmia and anosmia are associated with loss of enjoyment of food, difficulty managing body weight, safety concerns (i.e., detecting gas and smoke), insecurities with body odor, and social isolation [3]. These factors lead to a decreased quality of life and increased rates of depression when compared to individuals with normal sense of smell [4].

Although the exact mechanism for olfaction loss in Parkinson's disease is unknown, it is likely that olfaction dysfunction is due to changes in the central nervous system (CNS) and is not a result of damage to the peripheral olfactory system [5]. It has been proposed that olfaction dysfunction in Parkinson's disease evolves from Lewy bodies formed in the olfactory bulb and progresses to brain stem nuclei such as the locus coeruleus and substantia nigra and eventually to the cerebral cortex [6]. In addition, neurotransmitters such as acetylcholine, norepinephrine, serotonin, and, to a lesser extent, dopamine, all of which are typically altered in Parkinson's disease, impact olfaction through various direct and indirect pathways [7].

The clinical importance of hyposmia continues to evolve, and in individuals with PD olfaction testing can be used at a diagnostic tool [8] and is predictive of long-term cognitive decline and postoperative delirium [9–11]. In a large cohort of de novo patients, it was reported that PD patients with hyposmia exhibit more severe motor symptoms and required greater levodopa-equivalent at a 2.5-year followup compared to those patients with normal olfactory function [12]. The growing importance of olfaction as a diagnostic and predictive tool in individual with PD highlights the need for further examination.

While hyposmia is not a target of PD treatment per se, antiparkinsonian medications have no effect on olfaction dysfunction [13, 14]. It has been proposed that deep brain stimulation (DBS) may indirectly affect olfaction; however, most large randomized DBS studies have not utilized an olfaction outcome measure, and the few DBS studies that have reported an olfaction outcome have been conducted on relatively small sample sizes and have yielded conflicting results [15–18]. There is preliminary evidence that exercise may have a positive impact on olfaction. In an 8-week swimming intervention in adult rats, synapsin and neurotrophic factors in the olfactory bulb were greater in the exercise group than the nonexercise control group [19]. In a longitudinal study of over 1800 older adults, those who exercised three times per week were at a lower risk of developing olfaction dysfunction over a 10-year follow-up period [20]. These studies provide rationale to investigate the idea that exercise may facilitate neuroplasticity of the olfaction system.

Aerobic exercise, in animal models of Parkinsonism, has been shown to have neuroprotective and neurorestorative effects, likely through modulation of neurotrophic factors that support angiogenesis and synaptogenesis, suppress oxidative stress, and enhance mitochondrial function [21]. Recently, we have demonstrated that a specific mode of aerobic exercise, forced exercise (FE), reduces motor symptoms as measured by blinded clinical assessments, improves upper extremity motor functioning and control, and produces changes in cortical and subcortical functional connectivity [22–25]. In our preliminary study examining forced and voluntary rate cycling, some participants with PD self-reported improvements in olfaction following aerobic exercise, thus leading to the hypothesis that aerobic exercise may be facilitating neuroplasticity within the olfactory system. The aim of this project was to formally evaluate the effects of an 8-week forced and voluntary aerobic exercise program on olfaction function in individuals with Parkinson's disease.

2. Methods

2.1. Participants.
Thirty-eight individuals with a diagnosis of idiopathic PD completed the informed consent process approved by the Cleveland Clinic Institutional Review Board. Primary inclusion criteria were clinical diagnosis of idiopathic PD by a neurologist, age between 30–75 years, and Hoehn and Yahr stages II-III when off antiparkinsonian medication. Primary exclusion criteria were existing cardiopulmonary disease or stroke, presence of dementia, and any medical or musculoskeletal contraindications to exercise. Participants completed a cardiopulmonary exercise (CPX) test on a stationary bicycle equipped with MedGraphics CardiO2/CP system with Breeze software and a twelve-lead electrocardiograph to screen for cardiac abnormalities that may warrant exclusion from the study.

2.2. Outcome Measure.
The University of Pennsylvania Smell Identification Test (UPSIT), a 40-item "scratch and sniff" test, has been established as a valid and reliable tool for individuals with olfaction dysfunction and healthy controls [26]. After scratching the scent area, the participant selects a smell from 4 options in a forced-choice paradigm. A higher score (out of 40 points) indicates better odor identification. The UPSIT is a self-administered test that is objectively scored with an answer key. Testing was completed at baseline, end of treatment (EOT), and 4-week followup after end of treatment (EOT+4). In order to test participants in the off-medication state, subjects were asked to refrain from taking their PD medications after 8 pm the night before.

A blinded rater completed the Unified Parkinson's disease Rating Scale (UPDRS) motor examination, a standardized test that assesses motor function in individuals with PD.

2.3. Experimental Design.
Following baseline testing, individuals were randomized into one of the following groups: (1) FE Cycling (FE), (2) Voluntary Exercise Cycling (VE), and (3) Nonexercise control group. Randomization was performed by having participants draw an envelope from a nonreplenished box. Of note, olfaction testing was added to the study testing protocol of an ongoing aerobic exercise study due to subjects' self-report of improved smell; thus the sample sizes were not evenly distributed.

2.4. Exercise Intervention.
Participants in the VE and FE groups attended exercise sessions in the Neural Control Laboratory of the Cleveland Clinic, three times per week for a total of eight weeks. Participants were asked to take their PD medication as prescribed by their neurologist on the day of each exercise session. During exercise session, participants in the VE groups performed a 10-minute warm-up, 40- minute exercise set, and a 10-minute cool-down on a semirecumbent bike at a self-selected pace. Participants were encouraged to maintain a target heart rate zone of 60–80% based on heart rate reserve (HRR) method using results from individual maximal CPX test.

The FE group exercised for an identical period of time and target heart rate zone on a semirecumbent stationary exercise cycle custom engineered with a motor and accompanying control algorithm designed to augment the individual's torque production during pedaling, thus resulting in a steady, high-rate cadence. It is important to note that the FE approach required active participation from the participant and that cycling was not passive. The motor assisted the individual in achieving a pedaling rate 30% greater than their preferred voluntary rate as determined during CPX testing, a percentage increase that resulted in global motor improvements in our previous work with PD [22, 27]. For both exercise groups, cadence in revolutions per minute (rpm) and heart rate were recorded for each session.

The control group received no exercise intervention and was asked to continue their current level of physical activity.

2.5. Statistical Analysis.
The primary outcome was the change in UPSIT scores from (1) baseline to EOT and (2) baseline to EOT+4. Shapiro-Wilk test was used to determine normality of the variables considered in the study. A 3×3 analysis of variance (ANOVA) model was used to examine UPSIT score changes at three time points (baseline, EOT, and EOT+4) for

TABLE 1: Participant baseline demographics.

	Nonexercise	Exercise (VE + FE)	p value
Sample size	15	FE = 9 VE = 14	
Age, years (SD)	60.9 (7.2)	60.5 (7.4)	0.85
Gender, male	8	16	0.33
Disease duration, years (SD)	3.3 (3.1)	3.3 (2.1)	0.93
Baseline UPSIT, points (SD)	24.0 (7.3)	21.6 (8.2)	0.35
Baseline UPDRS motor examination, points (SD)	21.9 (5.5)	23.5 (9.9)	0.52

FE: forced exercise; SD: standard deviation; UPDRS: Unified Parkinson's Disease Rating Scale; UPSIT: University of Pennsylvania Smell Identification Test; VE: voluntary exercise.

TABLE 2: Summary statistics for change in UPSIT scores from baseline to EOT and EOT+4.

	Mean of change in UPSIT (points)	Standard deviation (points)	Range (points)	p value
Baseline to EOT				
Nonexercise	(2.9)	2.3	(8.0)–0.0	
Exercise	(0.5)	3.3	(10.0)–5.0	0.01
Baseline to EOT+4				
Nonexercise	(2.7)	3.4	(10.0)–4.0	
Exercise	0.2	3.5	(7.0)–8.0	0.02

( ) indicates a score indicating a worsening in UPSIT score compared to baseline. A positive number indicates an improvement in UPSIT score.
EOT: end of treatment; EOT+4: end of treatment + 4 weeks; UPSIT: University of Pennsylvania Smell Identification Test.

three groups (FE, VE, and nonexercise) and the interaction between the time and group variables. A two-sample t-test was performed to determine the influence of exercise performance variables, cadence and HRR, between the two exercise groups. An analysis of covariance (ANCOVA) model was used to determine the association between the UPSIT and the exercise performance variables, HRR and cadence. All hypothesis testing was completed at 5% level of significance.

3. Results

Using UPSIT score as the dependent variable in the ANOVA model, neither group ($F_{2,105} = 0.09$, $p = 0.91$), time ($F_{2,105} = 0.30$, $p = 0.74$), nor the interaction between group and time ($F_{4,105} = 0.24$, $p = 0.92$) was significant. While a trend was present for the VE group to be exercising at a greater intensity as measured by HRR, there was no significant difference between exercise intensity for the VE and FE groups with means of 57.9 and 48.9 percent of HRR, respectively ($p = 0.06$). Results from the ANCOVA, using HRR as the dependent variable, revealed a nonsignificant interaction effect between HRR and changes in UPSIT scores between VE and FE ($p = 0.48$ at EOT; $p = 0.51$ at EOT+4). There was a significant difference in cadence between the VE and FE groups, with means of 69.7 and 82.9 rpms, respectively ($p < 0.01$); however, an ANCOVA model, using cadence as the dependent variable, revealed a nonsignificant interaction between cadence and change in UPSIT score between groups ($p = 0.13$ at EOT; $p = 0.59$ at EOT+4). Due to the similarities in exercise performance variables, data were collapsed across exercise groups for comparison to the nonexercise control group. Baseline demographics, provided in Table 1, were similar between the exercise and the nonexercise groups.

Table 2 and Figure 1 provide summary statistics for the exercise and control groups. A t-test indicated a significant difference in UPSIT scores between exercise and nonexercise groups from baseline to EOT ($p = 0.01$) and from baseline

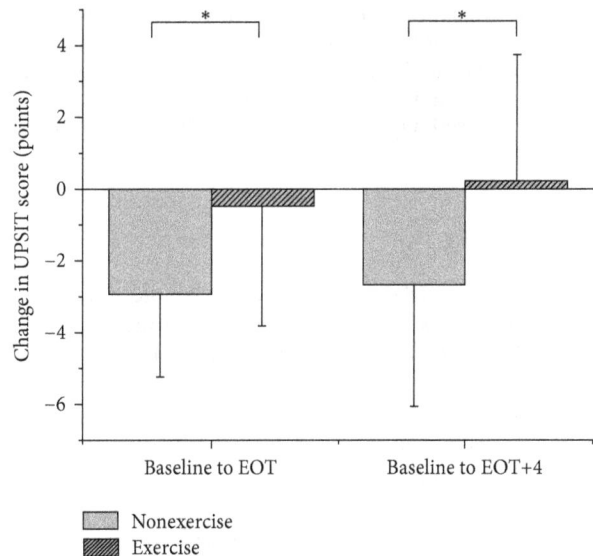

FIGURE 1: Mean change in UPSIT scores from baseline to EOT. There was a significant difference (indicated with *) between the exercise and nonexercise groups in change in UPSIT scores from baseline to EOT and EOT+4, respectively. A positive change in UPSIT score indicates improved odor identification.

to EOT+4 ($p = 0.02$). Figure 2 is a graphical depiction of the individual responses from each the groups from baseline to EOT. At EOT, no participants in the nonexercise group demonstrated an improvement on the UPSIT with a mean decrease of 2.9 (2.3) points. In contrast, 12 out of 23 individuals in the exercise group demonstrated an improvement in UPSIT scores; overall there was a mean decrease of 0.5 (3.3) points. From baseline to EOT+4, the nonexercise group had a decrease of 2.7 (3.4) points in UPSIT score while the exercise group exhibited a slight improvement of 0.2 (3.5) points.

There was no relationship between responders (those who improved their UPSIT score) and nonresponders (those who stayed the same or got worse in their UPSIT score) and the demographic variables listed in Table 1.

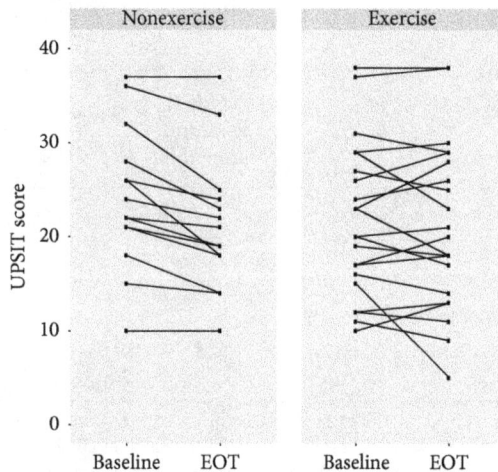

FIGURE 2: UPSIT scores at baseline and EOT for individuals in the exercise and nonexercise groups. At EOT, no participants in the nonexercise group demonstrated an improvement in UPSIT score; in contrast, 12 out of 23 individuals in the exercise group displayed an improvement in UPSIT score. Of note, 2 sets of individuals in the exercise group and 1 set of individuals in the nonexercise group scored identically from baseline to EOT; thus the lines are overlapping.

4. Discussion

Based on the UPSIT data, PD patients who did not exercise demonstrated a worsening of olfaction throughout the 8-week study and 4-week follow-up period, while those participating in aerobic exercise were spared from further worsening of olfaction function. The significant difference in UPSIT scores between the exercise and nonexercise groups suggests that aerobic exercise may be altering neurophysiological pathways or neurotransmitter function that regulate the physiologic or cognitive processes controlling olfaction [19, 20]. While we are not able to determine the exact mechanism underlying a sparring of olfaction, it is plausible, based on results from animal exercise studies, that the physiological changes (i.e., increased neurotrophins, neurotransmitters, and improved functional connectivity) and increases in cerebral blood flow associated with intensive aerobic exercise may have facilitated function of the olfaction system centrally or improved the higher level cognitive processes associated with odor detection [21, 28, 29]. While our previous imaging data supports altered CNS patterns of activation in the primary motor cortex, supplementary motor area, thalamus, globus pallidus, and putamen [24, 25], there is still much unknown about the role that aerobic exercise plays in modifying the structural and functional role of the CNS.

Although debated, olfaction function may worsen with disease duration [30], which is consistent with the nonexercise group demonstrating a decline in UPSIT scores over time. The wide range of change in UPSIT scores from the exercise group gives rise to the possibility that there is an individualized neurophysiological response to exercise ([28, 31, 32]). Individualized responses are reported with pharmacological interventions to PD, where some individuals exhibit a strong favorable response to levodopa therapy and

others experience modest benefits [33]. Since our previous research revealed acute bouts of FE that resulted in CNS changes similar to those seen with Parkinson's disease medications [24, 25], it is possible that, similar to medication, individuals experience varying responses to aerobic exercise. The genetic response to exercise continues to be evaluated; Bath and colleagues reported impaired odor discrimination associated with brain derived neurotrophic factor (BDNF) val66met polymorphism in mice and propose a mechanism of decreased neurogenesis in the olfactory bulb as a result of the polymorphism [34]. While we are unable to speculate if genetics played a role in our results, the role of genetics in response to exercise in individuals with PD is an area for future study.

There are limitations to the current study. First, the sample was a relatively small group of individuals with mild to moderate Parkinson's disease; thus the data should be interpreted within this context. A larger scale ($N = 100$) clinical trial is currently testing a similar cycling protocol that includes a variety of motor and nonmotor outcomes, including the UPSIT. Second, we did not screen for individuals who may have had preexisting nasal disease or olfactory dysfunction. Third, although the UPSIT is a well-studied test, the minimal clinical important difference is unknown; thus we are not able to determine if a change in the score is meaningful to the participant. Additionally, although the UPSIT is an odor identification test that is easily administered in a clinical setting, odor detection and threshold are not measured by this test. Notably, there was no difference in UPSIT scores between the FE and VE groups; thus it appears that the mode of cycling was less important than the aerobic nature of the exercise. In the future it will be important to determine the relationship between mode, frequency, duration, and intensity of aerobic exercise and olfaction dysfunction in PD.

These findings, although preliminary, have potential to impact quality of life in individuals with PD. Hyposmia is one of the top five symptoms in individuals diagnosed with PD ≤6 years in duration [35], and individuals with olfactory dysfunction are more likely to report difficulties with activities of daily living and to rely on community resources [36]. A meaningful implication of halting the progression of anosmia with aerobic exercise is the potential that exercise may modify the disease progression. The difference in UPSIT scores exhibited by the exercise group supports previous findings that intensive aerobic exercise is linked to global changes in PD function [22, 23]. This work may have significant implications regarding the relationship between exercise and brain function and the potential to modify the course of this progressive neurological disorder through exercise.

5. Conclusion

In this study, individuals with PD who participated in 24 sessions of aerobic exercise maintained their olfaction function as measured by the UPSIT, while individuals who did not exercise demonstrated a worsening in UPSIT scores. While these results provide promising preliminary evidence that exercise may modify the disease process, further systematic testing is needed.

Disclosure

The content is solely the responsibility of the authors and does not necessarily represent the views of the funding sources.

Acknowledgments

The authors would like to thank Amanda M. Penko and A. Elizabeth Jansen for their assistance with subject recruitment, protocol implementation, and data collection. This study was made possible by support from the National Institute of Health under Award no. R21HD056316 and B6678R VA Merit Review and the Davis Phinney Foundation.

References

[1] A. Haehner, S. Boesveldt, H. W. Berendse et al., "Prevalence of smell loss in Parkinson's disease—A Multicenter Study," *Parkinsonism and Related Disorders*, vol. 15, no. 7, pp. 490–494, 2009.

[2] C. H. Hawkes, B. C. Shephard, and S. E. Daniel, "Olfactory dysfunction in Parkinson's disease," *Journal of Neurology Neurosurgery and Psychiatry*, vol. 62, no. 5, pp. 436–446, 1997.

[3] A. Keller and D. Malaspina, "Hidden consequences of olfactory dysfunction: a patient report series," *BMC Ear, Nose and Throat Disorders*, vol. 13, article 8, 2013.

[4] B. Gopinath, K. J. Anstey, C. M. Sue, A. Kifley, and P. Mitchell, "Olfactory impairment in older adults is associated with depressive symptoms and poorer quality of life scores," *American Journal of Geriatric Psychiatry*, vol. 19, no. 9, pp. 830–834, 2011.

[5] A. Haehner, T. Hummel, and H. Reichmann, "Olfactory dysfunction as a diagnostic marker for Parkinson's disease," *Expert Review of Neurotherapeutics*, vol. 9, no. 12, pp. 1773–1779, 2009.

[6] D. R. Thal, K. Del Tredici, and H. Braak, "Neurodegeneration in normal brain aging and disease," *Science of Aging Knowledge Environment*, vol. 2004, no. 23, article pe26, 2004.

[7] R. L. Doty, "Olfaction in Parkinson's disease and related disorders," *Neurobiology of Disease*, vol. 46, no. 3, pp. 527–552, 2012.

[8] R. L. Doty, S. M. Bromley, and M. B. Stern, "Olfactory testing as an aid in the diagnosis of Parkinson's disease: development of optimal discrimination criteria," *Neurodegeneration*, vol. 4, no. 1, pp. 93–97, 1995.

[9] M. Vikdahl, M. E. Domellöf, L. Forsgren, and L. Håglin, "Olfactory function, eating ability, and visceral obesity associated with MMSE three years after Parkinson's disease diagnosis," *Journal of Nutrition, Health and Aging*, vol. 19, no. 9, pp. 894–900, 2015.

[10] M. E. Fullard, B. Tran, S. X. Xie et al., "Olfactory impairment predicts cognitive decline in early Parkinson's disease," *Parkinsonism & Related Disorders*, vol. 25, pp. 45–51, 2016.

[11] M. S. Kim, J. H. Yoon, H. J. Kim, S. W. Yong, and J. M. Hong, "Olfactory dysfunction is related to postoperative delirium in Parkinson's disease," *Journal of Neural Transmission*, vol. 123, no. 6, pp. 589–594, 2016.

[12] D. H. Lee, J. S. Oh, J. H. Ham et al., "Is normosmic Parkinson disease a unique clinical phenotype?" *Neurology*, vol. 85, no. 15, pp. 1270–1275, 2015.

[13] R. L. Doty, M. B. Stern, C. Pfeiffer, S. M. Gollomp, and H. I. Hurtig, "Bilateral olfactory dysfunction in early stage treated and untreated idiopathic Parkinson's disease," *Journal of Neurology Neurosurgery and Psychiatry*, vol. 55, no. 2, pp. 138–142, 1992.

[14] A. Haehner, T. Hummel, M. Wolz et al., "Effects of rasagiline on olfactory function in patients with Parkinson's disease," *Movement Disorders*, vol. 28, no. 14, pp. 2023–2027, 2013.

[15] M. Fabbri, L. C. Guedes, M. Coelho et al., "Subthalamic deep brain stimulation effects on odor identification in Parkinson's disease," *European Journal of Neurology*, vol. 22, no. 1, pp. 207–210, 2015.

[16] X. Guo, G. Gao, X. Wang et al., "Effects of bilateral deep brain stimulation of the subthalamic nucleus on olfactory function in Parkinson's disease patients," *Stereotactic and Functional Neurosurgery*, vol. 86, no. 4, pp. 237–244, 2008.

[17] T. Hummel, U. Jahnke, U. Sommer, H. Reichmann, and A. Müller, "Olfactory function in patients with idiopathic Parkinson's disease: effects of deep brain stimulation in the subthalamic nucleus," *Journal of Neural Transmission*, vol. 112, no. 5, pp. 669–676, 2005.

[18] D. P. Breen, H. L. Low, and A. Misbahuddin, "The impact of deep brain stimulation on sleep and olfactory function in Parkinson's disease," *Open Ophthalmology Journal*, vol. 9, pp. 70–72, 2015.

[19] C.-H. Chae, S.-L. Jung, S.-H. An et al., "Swimming exercise stimulates neuro-genesis in the subventricular zone via increase in synapsin I and nerve growth factor levels," *Biology of Sport*, vol. 31, no. 4, pp. 309–314, 2014.

[20] C. R. Schubert, K. J. Cruickshanks, D. M. Nondahl, B. E. K. Klein, R. Klein, and M. E. Fischer, "Association of exercise with lower long-term risk of olfactory impairment in older adults," *JAMA Otolaryngology—Head and Neck Surgery*, vol. 139, no. 10, pp. 1061–1066, 2013.

[21] M. J. Zigmond, J. L. Cameron, R. K. Leak et al., "Triggering endogenous neuroprotective processes through exercise in models of dopamine deficiency," *Parkinsonism and Related Disorders*, vol. 15, no. 3, pp. S42–S45, 2009.

[22] A. L. Ridgel, J. L. Vitek, and J. L. Alberts, "Forced, not voluntary, exercise improves motor function in Parkinson's disease patients," *Neurorehabilitation and Neural Repair*, vol. 23, no. 6, pp. 600–608, 2009.

[23] J. L. Alberts, S. M. Linder, A. L. Penko, M. J. Lowe, and M. Phillips, "It is not about the bike, it is about the pedaling: forced exercise and Parkinson's disease," *Exercise and Sport Sciences Reviews*, vol. 39, no. 4, pp. 177–186, 2011.

[24] E. B. Beall, M. J. Lowe, J. L. Alberts et al., "The effect of forced-exercise therapy for Parkinson's disease on motor cortex functional connectivity," *Brain Connectivity*, vol. 3, no. 2, pp. 190–198, 2013.

[25] J. L. Alberts, M. Phillips, M. J. Lowe et al., "Cortical and motor responses to acute forced exercise in Parkinson's disease," *Parkinsonism and Related Disorders*, vol. 24, pp. 56–62, 2016.

[26] R. L. Doty, P. Shaman, and M. Dann, "Development of the university of Pennsylvania smell identification test: a standardized microencapsulated test of olfactory function," *Physiology and Behavior*, vol. 32, no. 3, pp. 489–502, 1984.

[27] C. Shah, E. B. Beall, A. M. Frankemolle et al., "Exercise therapy for Parkinson's disease: pedaling rate is related to changes in motor connectivity," *Brain Connectivity*, vol. 6, no. 1, pp. 25–36, 2016.

[28] K. Knaepen, M. Goekint, E. Heyman, and R. Meeusen, "Neuro-

plasticity—exercise-induced response of peripheral brain-derived neurotrophic factor," *Sports Medicine*, vol. 40, pp. 765–801, 2010.

[29] M. W. Voss, C. Vivar, A. F. Kramer, and H. van Praag, "Bridging animal and human models of exercise-induced brain plasticity," *Trends in Cognitive Sciences*, vol. 17, no. 10, pp. 525–544, 2013.

[30] S. Boesveldt, D. Verbaan, D. L. Knol et al., "A comparative study of odor identification and odor discrimination deficits in Parkinson's disease," *Movement Disorders*, vol. 23, no. 14, pp. 1984–1990, 2008.

[31] E. Shimizu, K. Hashimoto, and M. Iyo, "Ethnic difference of the BDNF 196G/A (val66met) polymorphism frequencies: the possibility to explain ethnic mental traits," *American Journal of Medical Genetics Part B: Neuropsychiatric Genetics*, vol. 126, no. 1, pp. 122–123, 2004.

[32] P. G. da Silva, D. D. Domingues, L. A. de Carvalho, S. Allodi, and C. L. Correa, "Neurotrophic factors in Parkinson's disease are regulated by exercise: evidence-based practice," *Journal of the Neurological Sciences*, vol. 363, pp. 5–15, 2016.

[33] P. A. Kempster, D. R. Williams, M. Selikhova, J. Holton, T. Revesz, and A. J. Lees, "Patterns of levodopa response in Parkinson's disease: A Clinico-Pathological Study," *Brain*, vol. 130, no. 8, pp. 2123–2128, 2007.

[34] K. G. Bath, N. Mandairon, D. Jing et al., "Variant brain-derived neurotrophic factor (Val66Met) alters adult olfactory bulb neurogenesis and spontaneous olfactory discrimination," *The Journal of Neuroscience*, vol. 28, no. 10, pp. 2383–2393, 2008.

[35] M. Politis, K. Wu, S. Molloy, P. G. Bain, K. R. Chaudhuri, and P. Piccini, "Parkinson's disease symptoms: the patient's perspective," *Movement Disorders*, vol. 25, no. 11, pp. 1646–1651, 2010.

[36] B. Gopinath, K. J. Anstey, A. Kifley, and P. Mitchell, "Olfactory impairment is associated with functional disability and reduced independence among older adults," *Maturitas*, vol. 72, no. 1, pp. 50–55, 2012.

29

Identification of NURR1 (Exon 4) and FOXA1 (Exon 3) Haplotypes Associated with mRNA Expression Levels in Peripheral Blood Lymphocytes of Parkinson's Patients in Small Indian Population

Jayakrishna Tippabathani, Jayshree Nellore, Vaishnavie Radhakrishnan, Somashree Banik, and Sonia Kapoor

Department of Biotechnology, Sathyabama University, Chennai 600119, India

Correspondence should be addressed to Jayshree Nellore; sree_nellore@yahoo.com

Academic Editor: Cristine Alves da Costa

Here, we study the expression of NURR1 and FOXA1 mRNA in peripheral blood lymphocytes and its haplotypes in coding region in a small Chennai population of India. Thirty cases of Parkinson's patients (PD) with anti-PD medications (20 males aged 65.85 ± 1.19 and 10 females aged 65.7 ± 1.202) and 30 age matched healthy people (20 males aged 68.45 ± 1.282 and 10 females aged 65.8 ± 1.133) were included. The expression of NURR1 and FOXA1 in PBL was detected by Q-PCR and haplotypes were identified by PCR-SSCP. In the 30 PD cases examined, NURR1 and FOXA1 expression was significantly reduced in both male and female PD patients. However, NURR1 (57.631% reduced in males; 28.93% in females) and FOXA1 (64.42% in males; 55.76% in females) mRNA expression did differ greatly between male and female PD patients. Polymorphisms were identified at exon 4 of the NURR1 and at exon 3 of the FOXA1, respectively, in both male and female patients. A near significant difference in SSCP patterns between genders of control and PD population was analyzed suggesting that further investigations of more patients, more molecular markers, and coding regions should be performed. Such studies could potentially reveal peripheral molecular marker of early PD and different significance to the respective genders.

1. Introduction

Parkinson's disease (PD) is the second most common neurodegenerative disorder. PD is characterized by the loss of dopaminergic neurons in the substantia nigra pars compacta which leads to rigidity, bradykinesia, tremor, and postural instability. These symptoms do not develop until about 50–60% of the nigral neurons are lost and about 80–85% of the dopamine content of the striatum is depleted. The exact pathogenic mechanisms underlying the selective dopaminergic cell loss in PD are still not understood, although research points that the disease is caused by a combination of genetic and environmental factors. The prevalence and incidence of PD increase exponentially with age (~1-2% of the population above age 65 and 4–5% above age 85) and are slightly higher in men than in women. Recently in Deccan Chronicle, it has been published that in India the incidence is bound to double in ten years [1]. Magnetic resonance imaging (MRI) and computed tomography (CT) scan are usually unremarkable or may show age specific changes in Parkinson's disease. There is no lab test for PD, so it can be difficult to diagnose. Doctors use medical history and a neurological examination to diagnose it, but 70% of nigral neurons are lost when symptoms appear [2]. Late diagnosis hampers clinical development of new disease-modifying therapies; only alleviating symptoms is possible at present. For this reason, great interest in developing peripheral biomarker for PD has increased.

Molecular biomarkers in body fluids are likely to meet the expectation of unprecedented specificity together with costs that are lower than those of imaging/functional biomarkers.

Quantitative assays of cerebrospinal fluid proteomics, serum or plasma metabolomics, and gene expression profile in peripheral blood lymphocytes (PBL) are done in an attempt to identify potential peripheral biomarkers of the disease. Several studies have used PBL to quantity specific changes in dopamine (DA) content, tyrosine hydroxylase activity, DA receptors, and DA transporters in patients with PD [3, 4]. In addition, a significant decrease in mitochondrial complex I activity and a significant increase in caspase-3 activity have been reported in PBL of PD patients [5]. Likewise, genome-wide expression in PBL of PD patients and healthy controls identified co-chaperone protein ST13 as a potential molecular marker of early PD [6]. Based on these data, it has been proposed that PBL can be used for detecting the possible indicators of pathological mechanisms occurring in the brains of patients with PD.

Several studies demonstrated that transcription factors (TFs) like FOXA1/FOXA2, NURR1, PITX3, OTX2, LMX1a/b, and EN1/2 play a key role in mediating mesodiencephalic dopaminergic (mDA) neuron development and remain expressed in adulthood though dopaminergic neuronal maturation is completed [7]. Mutations or variations in genes coding for transcription factors involved in regulation of neuronal development and maintenance of nigrostriatal system function may be risk factors for PD [8, 9]. The human Nurr1 gene has been mapped on chromosome 2q22-23 and is composed of eight exons [10]. It is the key regulator for development of DA neurons and is also considered as a crucial regulator for the expression of several genes involved in PD pathology including DA transporter (DAT), tyrosine hydroxylase (TH), and vesicular monoamine transporter (VMAT2). In addition, variants in NURR1 gene have been found in association with sporadic and familial PD [11–14]. Also, deletion of FOXA1 and FOXA2 in embryonic DA neurons affects the binding of NURR1 to the promoter region of TH and aromatic L-amino acid decarboxylase (AADC) genes leading to a significant loss of TH and AADC expression in the SNpc of embryos and adult mice [15]. The deregulation of FOXA1/2 may also contribute to demise of DA neurons during PD progression in humans [16]. These observations suggest that Nurr1 and FOXA1 are potential candidate genes for PD susceptibility. However, there is no evidence on the genetic variations in FOXA1 gene in PD patients. Although we are diagnosing more patients with PD today, much needs to be done in the Indian context. Hence, the current study has been proposed to explore the peripheral NURR1 and FOXA1 gene expression in PD and to initially look for variation in exon 4 of NURR1 and exon 3 of FOXA1, respectively.

2. Subjects and Methods

2.1. Subjects. In the present study a total of 60 PBL samples, 20 male PD patients aged 65.85 ± 1.19, 10 female PD patients aged 65.7 ± 1.202, and 30 healthy controls (HC) matched by gender, age, and origin, were collected from Malar hospital, Chennai. The inclusion criteria for PD patients are as follows: being diagnosis with idiopathic PD, patients who are "on" medication (both male and female $N = 10$) and who are medically stable, Minimal Mini Mental State Examination 3

score of 24 or higher, and being able to walk independently indoors without an aid and outdoors with an aid. Control subjects were patient's spouses and volunteers who are free of neurological and psychiatric illnesses. All the female subjects were considered postmenopausal who self-reported the completion of menopause. All subjects or their legally authorized caregivers signed a written consent, approved by the Institutional Human Ethics Committee, Sathyabama University.

2.2. RNA Extraction and cDNA Synthesis. Whole blood (1 mL) was anticoagulated with ethylene diamine tetra acetic acid (EDTA), mixed with phosphate-buffered saline (PBS) 1:1, layered over HiSep LSM medium (HiMedia), and centrifuged at 400 ×g for 30 min according to the manufacturer's instructions. Peripheral blood mononuclear cells (PBMCs) were isolated and washed in ice-cold PBS for RNA extraction. Total RNA was isolated from PBMCs using the TRIzol Reagent method (Invitrogen) and then cDNA synthesis was performed according to the manufacturer's protocol (Applied Biosystem).

2.3. Q-PCR Assay of NURR1 and FOXA1 Gene Expression against Internal Control β-Actin. The detailed information on the NURR1, FOXA1, and β-actin primers is shown in Table 1. The experiment of QPCR was performed in duplicate with Applied Biosystem power SYBR green following protocol as described: initial denaturation for 5 min at 95°C, followed by 40 cycles of denaturation for 30 sec at 95°C, annealing for 45 sec at 61.5°C, and extension for 45 min at 72°C. β-Actin was used as a house keeping gene to standardize the results. The relative quantification of gene expression among the different groups was determined by the formation of $2^{-\Delta\Delta Ct}$ [17].

2.4. Detection of Haplotypes by Polymerase Chain Reaction and Single Stranded Conformation Polymorphism (PCR SSCP) Analysis

2.4.1. DNA Isolation and Amplification of DNA. Genomic DNA (200–300 ng) was isolated from each blood sample following the standard protocol [18]. 50 ng of this DNA was added to each 50 μL of polymerase chain reaction (PCR) mix which contained Amplicon master mix and 10 pmol of each primer. The detailed information of the primers used to explore haplotype variation in the exon 4 of NURR1 and exon 3 of FOXA1 are shown in Table 2. As the respective exons are too long for PCR-SSCP analysis it is divided into two reactions 1 and 2, respectively. PCR consisted of initial denaturation at 94°C for 5 minutes, 35 cycles of denaturation at 94°C for 45 seconds, annealing at 60.4°C for 45 seconds, and extension at 72°C for 45 seconds with final extension at 72°C for 10 minutes.

2.4.2. Single Strand Conformation Polymorphism Analysis (SSCP). Single strand conformation polymorphism (SSCP) is a reproducible, rapid, and quite simple method for the detection of deletions/insertions/rearrangements in the gene, which has been performed as described by Orita et al. [19]. Samples of purified double–stranded PCR product were added to formamide dye (95% formamide, 0.025%

TABLE 1: Genes with corresponding primers which are used for gene expression study.

Gene	Primers sequence	Size (bp)	Accession no.
NURR1	Forward primer 5′ CGGGTCGGTTTACTACAAG 3′ Reverse primer 5′ TGGTGGAAGTTGTGGAGAG 3′	111	AB017586.1
FOXA1	Forward primer 5′ GTTACAGGGAGGACTACCA 3′ Reverse primer 5′ TCCAAGGCAGTTCCAATAC 3′	111	NM_004496.3
ACTB	Forward primer 5′ TCGTGCGTACATTAAGG 3′ Reverse primer 5′ AAGGAAGGCTGGAAGAGT 3′	175	X00351.1

TABLE 2: Genes with corresponding primers which are used for SSCP analysis.

Gene		Primers sequence	Size (bp)
NURR1	Exon 4 (1)	Forward 5′ AGACACGGGCTCAAGGAACC 3′ Reverse 5′ ACTGCTCACACGGCTATCTCTG 3′	349
	Exon 4 (2)	Forward 5′ CCATTTCTGTAACCCTCCTAGC 3′ Reverse 5′ CCACCCACGCAACATTTAGT 3′	416
FOXA1	Exon 3 (1)	Forward 5′ TCGGAGCAGCAGCATAAG 3′ Reverse 5′ GGCAAGGAAGGAGGAGAAT 3′	488
	Exon 3 (2)	Forward 5′ GAGAACGGCTGCTACTTG 3′ Reverse 5′ GGAGGCTGGAGTCTTCAA 3′	300

xylenecyanol, 0.025% bromophenol blue, and 0.5 M EDTA), denatured at 95°C for 10 minutes, and immediately snap cooled on ice for 15 minutes. Aliquots were loaded on 12% polyacrylamide gel and subjected to electrophoresis for 10 hours at 200 V, 4°C. The gel was stained with 0.1% silver nitrate to visualize the reannealed single stranded PCR products.

2.5. Statistical Analysis. Quantitative data were expressed as SEM (standard error mean). The chi-square test or Student's t-test was used to test for differences between the PD patients and control subjects in the distribution of gender and age. Multivariate analysis was used to evaluate the differences in the mean value of the NURR1 and FOXA1 mRNA gene expression in PD Patients compared with controls.

3. Results and Discussion

This study aimed to detect differences in the expression of genes possibly related to the differentiation, survival, connectivity, and migration of dopamine neurons in peripheral blood of both male and female PD and respective control subjects.

3.1. Research Participants. We enrolled 30 consecutive PD patients who were ethnic Indians, diagnosed by the clinical assessments and stringent diagnosis criteria for PD [20] and 30 age matched healthy and neurodegenerative disease control individuals (Table 3) from Fortis Malar Hospital, Adyar. Amongst the PD patients, 20 were men and 10 were women. Further age matched, 30 healthy control individuals were enrolled where 20 were men and 10 were women. The age ranged from 58 to 76 with a mean of 65.85 ± 1.19 years for male PD patients and male controls 68.45 ± 1.282, while in the case of females the age ranged from 59 to 74 years with a mean

of 65.7 ± 1.202 for PD patients and female controls 65.8 ± 1.133. From Table 3, there is good evidence that the incidence of PD is more in male population when compared to women. Our finding is in concurrence with the previous reports where men in general are about 1.5 times more likely to develop PD than women, that is, in the ratio of 3 : 1 (male : female) [21].

3.2. NURR1 and FOXA1 Expression on PBL of All Study Groups. NURR1 is highly expressed in midbrain DAergic neurons [22] as well as other tissues, including PBL [23]. Emerging evidence indicates that impaired NURR1 function might contribute to the pathogenesis of PD: NURR1 and its transcriptional targets are downregulated in midbrain DA neurons that express high levels of the disease-causing protein α-synuclein. Recent studies indicated decreased expression in PBL in PD patients independent of medication, disease duration, or severity; NURR1 could be a useful biomarker for PD and related disorders [24, 25]. In our study, we observed reduction in mean mRNA expression of NURR1 in male patients with PD by 57.91% than healthy male controls ($p < 0.05$). To further determine the association of gender with the changes of NURR1 expression, we performed analyses in female PD and found that the NURR1 gene expression was reduced by 28.93% than healthy female controls ($p < 0.05$; Figure 1; Table 3). This data indicates that the decreased expression in NURR1 gene in PD was more robust in male patients and the difference between male PD and female PD was statistically significant ($p < 0.05$; Table 3). Moreover, NURR1 gene expression was more significantly decreased in older and female patients [25]. Focusing on the NURR1 levels in control samples, females showed lesser levels of NURR1 mRNA expression compared to men ($p < 0.05$; Table 3). Pérez-Sieira et al. demonstrated that estrogens are implicated in the upregulation of NURR1 in female rats [26]. Matsuki et al. confirmed that the levels of NURR1 in

TABLE 3: NURR1 gene expression versus β-actin as internal control in all groups.

Group	Gender	Age	Number of samples used	NURR1 mRNA mean ± SME	p value
HC	Male	68.45 ± 1.282	20	1.208 ± 0.36	<0.05
PD	Male	68.85 ± 1.19	20	0.5084 ± 0.35	
HC	Female	65.8 ± 1.133	10	1.13 ± 0.076	<0.05
PD	Female	65.7 ± 1.202	10	0.803 ± 0.028	

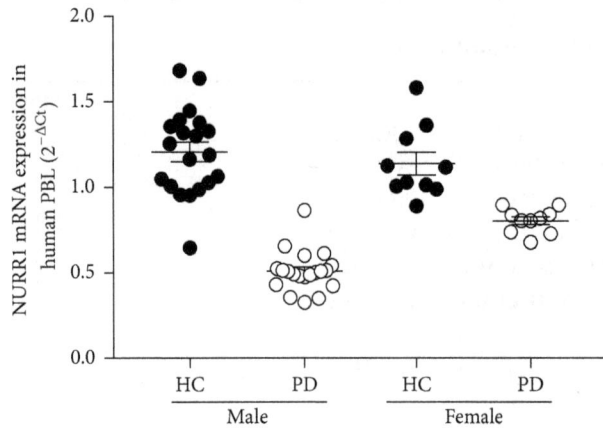

FIGURE 1: Scatter plot showing NURR1 mRNA expression on PBL in different study groups. Fluorescent reading from Q-PCR was quantitatively analyzed by determining the difference of Ct between Ct of NURR1 and β-actin. mRNA expression was determined by using the formation of $2^{-\Delta Ct}$. Bars represent mean ± SME measured from duplication assay in blind fashion. $p < 0.05$.

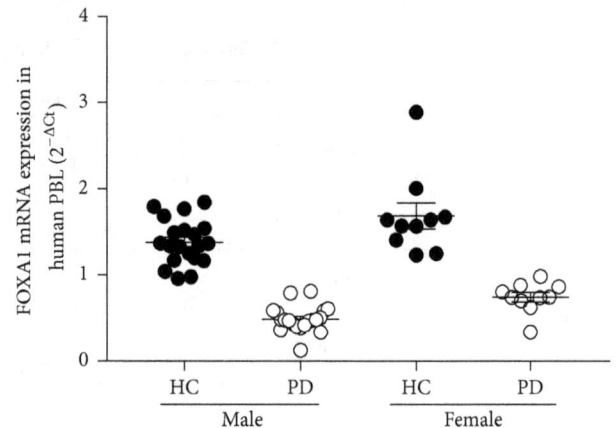

FIGURE 2: Scatter plot showing FOXA1 mRNA expression on PBL in different study groups. Fluorescent reading from Q-PCR was quantitatively analyzed by determining the difference of Ct between Ct of FOXA 1 and β-actin. mRNA expression was determined by using the formation of $2^{-\Delta Ct}$. Bars represent mean ± SME measured from duplication assay in blind fashion. $p < 0.05$.

blood samples from healthy women are associated with the levels of sex hormones, estradiol [E2], and progesterone [27]. As shown in Table 3, the control females in our current study might have lower sex hormones as they are in their postmenopausal phase which might have downregulated the NURR1 expression, a risk factor for PD.

Several datasets from PD patients and PD models showed the downregulation of FOXA1 and FOXA2 expression in the SNpc of PD patients [28–32]. In the current study, the mean mRNA expression of FOXA1 in patients' peripheral blood lymphocytes was analysed and results demonstrated diminished levels in male patients with PD by 64.46% than healthy male controls ($p < 0.05$). Moreover, in female patients it was reduced by 55.74% than healthy female controls ($p < 0.05$; Figure 2; Table 4). This finding suggests that the decreased expression in FOXA1 gene in PD was more robust in male patients and the difference between male PD and female PD was statistically significant ($p < 0.05$; Table 4).

Altogether, these data establishes that lower levels of NURR1 and FOXA1 gene expression were significantly associated with the increased risk for PD in male and female subjects, respectively. Furthermore, our results provide useful information that FOXA1 gene is reduced in PBL of Indian PD patients, indicating its possible systemic involvement in PD.

3.3. SSCP Polymorphisms. It is postulated that variants in NURR1 gene cause decrease in NURR1 mRNA and affect

the transcription of gene that encodes TH [9] that could cause dysfunction of dopaminergic neurons and lead to PD [33]. Various studies have reported coding missense mutation in exon 3 of NURR1 (709C>G and 711 C/A), −291Tdel and −245T→G sequence variation in the noncoding exon-1 within the $5'$ untranslated region, and mutations in exon 2 at 388 G/A, 35 A/G, and 21 C/G respectively, including some intron regions which markedly attenuates NURR1-induced transcriptional activation, leading to decreased expression being identified in a patient with PD [14, 34]. However, there is no evidence of the genetic variations in FOXA1 gene in PD patients. Hence in the current study, the amplified NURR1 and FOXA1 PCR products in both males and females (Figures 3(a) and 3(b)) were subjected to single-strand conformation polymorphism (SSCP) analysis to clarify whether the variants are disease causing mutations. The exon 4 of the NURR1 gene and the exon 3 of the FOXA1 gene were chosen for the SSCP analysis in two separate reactions, respectively, and the results are described below.

3.4. Exon 4 of NURR1. Two band patterns were identified for exon 4 of NURR1 gene in male PD controls: patterns A and B (Figure 4). Seventeen out of twenty (85%) male PD patients exhibited migration pattern D (pattern suggesting alterations) with respect to the two reactions of exon 4 of NURR1 gene. Three out of twenty (15%) male PD patients exhibited migration pattern D (pattern suggesting

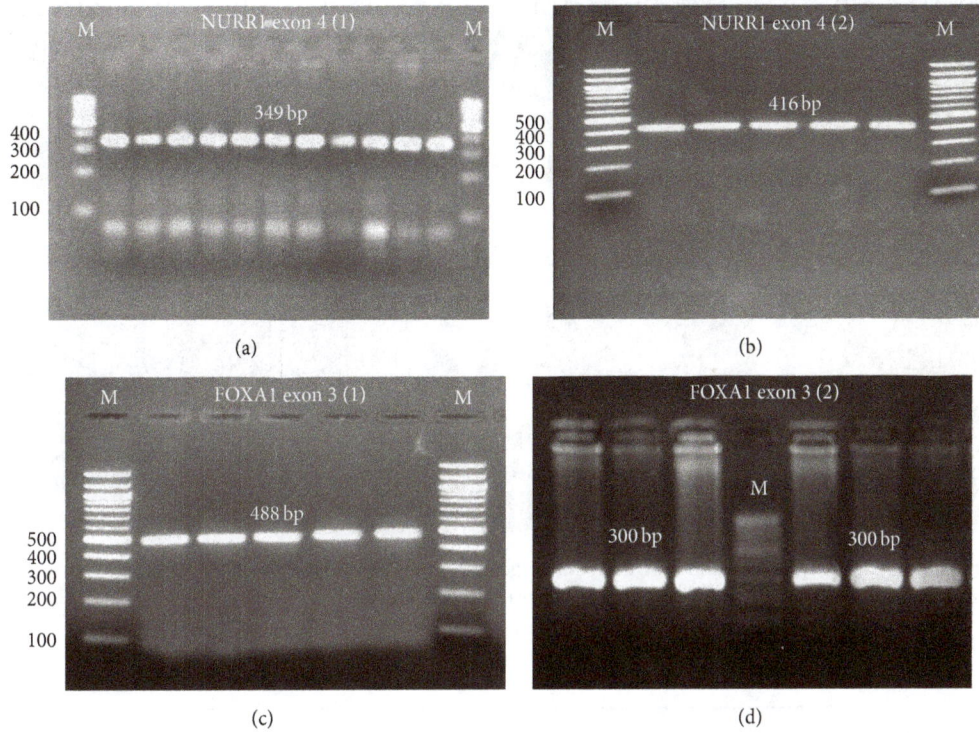

FIGURE 3: PCR amplification for exon 4 of the NURR1 gene (a-b) and exon 3 of the FOXA1 gene (c-d). The exons were divided into two reactions: 1 and 2, respectively.

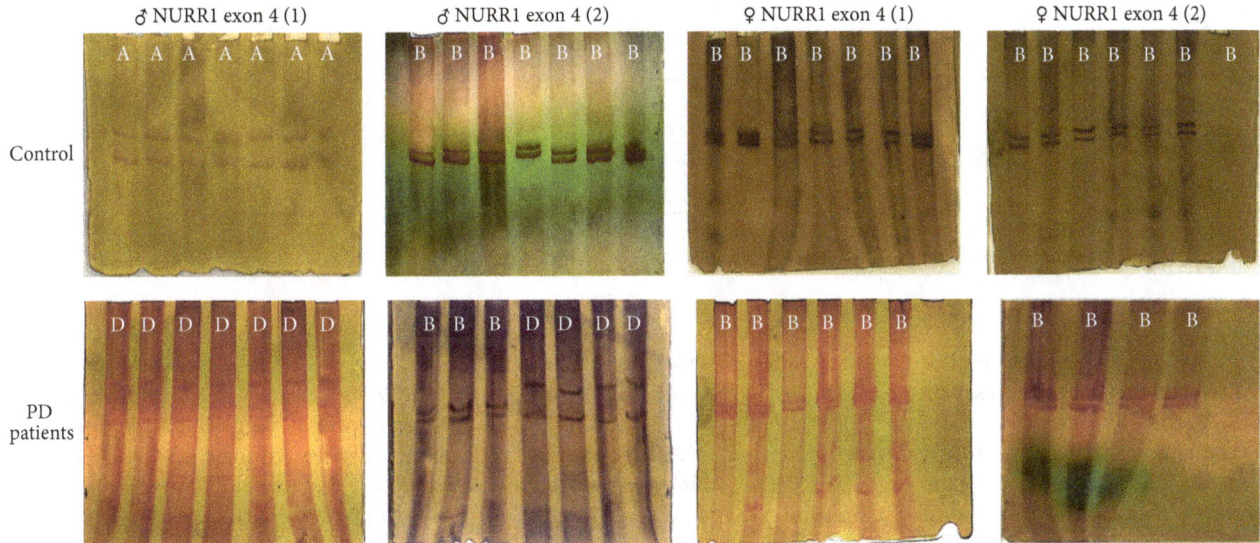

FIGURE 4: Representative SSCP analyses for exon 4 of the NURR1 gene in male and female PD patients. The exon was divided into two reactions: 1 and 2. A, B, and D represent conformational patterns of the bands found.

TABLE 4: FOXA 1 gene expression versus β-actin as internal control in all groups.

Group	Gender	Age	Number of samples used	FOXA1 mRNA mean ± SME	p value
HC	Male	68.45 ± 1.282	20	1.373 ± 0.77	<0.05
PD	Male	65.85 ± 1.19	20	0.4884 ± 0.045	
HC	Female	65.8 ± 1.133	10	1.681 ± 0.201	<0.05
PD	Female	65.7 ± 1.202	10	0.7436 ± 0.07	

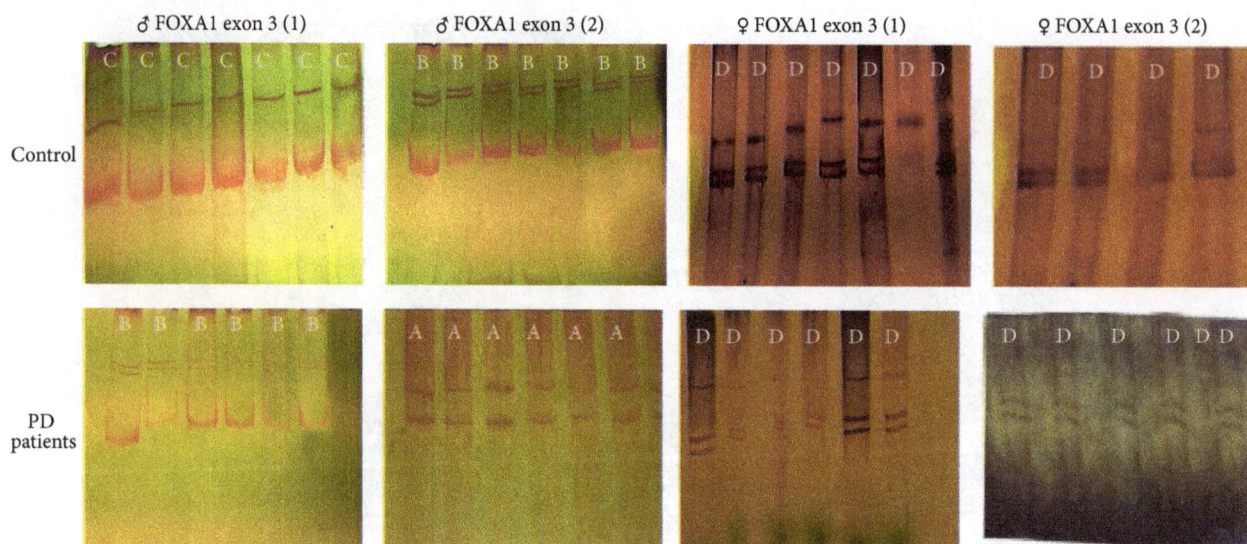

FIGURE 5: Representative SSCP analyses for exon 3 of the FOXA1 gene in male and female PD patients. The exon was divided into two reactions: 1 and 2. A, B, C, and D represents conformational patterns of the bands found.

TABLE 5: Mean values (±SEM) of mRNA expression ($2^{-\Delta ct}$) with PCR-SSCP patterns of NURR1 and FOXA1 gene.

Gene	Gender	Condition	$2^{-\Delta CT}$	SSCP patterns		Significance
				PCR1	PCR2	
NURR1	Male	HC	1.208	A	B	<0.05
		PD	0.508	D	B (0.2)	
					D (0.8)	
	Female	HC	1.13	B	B	NS
		PD	0.80	B	B	
FOXA1	Male	HC	1.327	C	B	<0.05
		PD	0.4884	B	A	
	Female	HC	1.681	D	D	NS
		PD	0.7436	D	D	

Note. NS represents "not significant" and B (0.2) and D (0.8) show frequency of the patterns B and D
PCR1: PCR amplification of exons in reaction 1; PCR2: PCR amplification of exons in reaction 2.

alterations) with respect to reaction 1 and migration pattern B (similar to control) with respect to reaction 2 of exon 4 of NURR1 gene.

The entire female PD controls revealed pattern B with respect to the two reactions of exon 4 of NURR1 gene, which suggested alteration in the pattern of migration, compared to male controls (Figure 4). Interestingly, all the twenty female PD patients exhibited migration pattern B (similar to controls) with respect to the two reactions of the exon 4 of NURR1 gene.

3.5. Exon 3 of FOXA1. Two band patterns were identified for exon 3 of FOXA1 gene in male PD controls: pattern C with respect to reaction 1 and B with respect to reaction 2 (Figure 5). The entire (100%) male PD patients exhibited migration pattern B (pattern suggesting alterations) with respect to reaction 1 and pattern A (pattern suggesting alterations) with respect to reaction 2 of the exon 3 of FOXA1 gene.

A single band pattern was revealed for the entire female PD controls: pattern D with respect to the two reactions of exon 3 of FOXA1 gene, which suggested alteration in the pattern of migration, compared to male controls (Figure 5). Interestingly, all the twenty female PD patients exhibited migration pattern B (similar to controls) with respect to the two reactions of exon 3 of FOXA1 gene.

3.6. Association Analysis. Table 5 shows the mean values showing the effect of SSCP patterns on NURR1 and FOXA1; SSCP analysis of the amplicon including exon 4 revealed that on average patterns B and D significantly ($p < 0.005$) influenced the NURR1 gene expression in male PD. SSCP band patterns B and A at FOXA1 exon 3 significantly ($p < 0.005$) influenced the FOXA1 gene expression in male PD. To our knowledge, this is the first report of male PD patients with gene variation in exon 4 of NURR1 and exon 3 of FOXA1. However, no genetic variation was found in exon 4 of NURR1 and exon 3 of FOXA1 in female PD patients. Furthermore, sex dependent genetic variation was demonstrated in exon 4 of NURR1 and exon 3 of FOXA1 of healthy controls, respectively.

4. Conclusions

In conclusion, these findings endorse the fact that common haplotype variation in transcription factors might have important and clinically relevant associations with PD. We anticipate that these findings will have implications for our understanding of gender differences in PD and also more broadly with potential applications in risk stratification, prognostication, and the development of appropriately targeted-treatment strategies. However, because only a small number of samples and only exon 4/3 region were investigated, a much larger association study is warranted in further studies.

Acknowledgments

The authors would like to thank patients, doctors, and other staff of Brain and Spine Care Unit, Fortis Malar Hospital, for their assistance. The authors would also like to thank the Genetics and Molecular Biology Laboratory, Directorate of Poultry Research, Hyderabad, for giving them access to their Q-PCR facility. The authors would like to extend great thanks to Sathyabama University for providing the opportunity to carry out this research work.

References

[1] A. S. John, "Multi-disciplinary care for Parkinson's must, say docs. Lifestyle Health and Wellbeing," Deccan Chronicle, http://www.deccanchronicle.com.

[2] C. W. Olanow, M. B. Stern, and K. Sethi, "The scientific and clinical basis for the treatment of Parkinson disease (2009)," Neurology, vol. 72, no. 21, S4, pp. S1–S136, 2009.

[3] M. Shi, B. R. Huber, and J. Zhang, "Biomarkers for cognitive impairment in parkinson disease," Brain Pathology, vol. 20, no. 3, pp. 660–671, 2010.

[4] R. Buttarelli, Francesca, A. Fanciulli, C. Pellicano, and F. E. Pontieri, "The dopaminergic system in peripheral blood lymphocytes: from physiology to pharmacology and potential applications to neuropsychiatric disorders," Current Neuropharmacology, vol. 9, no. 2, pp. 278–288, 2011.

[5] F. Blandini, A. Mangiagalli, M. Cosentino et al., "Peripheral markers of apoptosis in parkinson's disease: the effect of dopaminergic drugs," Annals of the New York Academy of Sciences, vol. 1010, no. 1, pp. 675–678, 2003.

[6] C. R. Scherzer, A. C. Eklund, L. J. Morse et al., "Molecular markers of early Parkinson's disease based on gene expression in blood," Proceedings of the National Academy of Sciences of the United States of America, vol. 104, no. 3, pp. 955–960, 2007.

[7] H. Doucet-Beaupré and M. Lévesque, "The role of developmental transcription factors in adult midbrain dopaminergic neurons," OA Neurosciences, vol. 1, no. 1, article no. 3, 2013.

[8] K. N. Alavian, C. Scholz, and H. H. Simon, "Transcriptional regulation of mesencephalic dopaminergic neurons: the full circle of life and death," Movement Disorders, vol. 23, no. 3, pp. 319–328, 2008.

[9] J. Jankovic, S. Chen, and W. D. Le, "The role of Nurr1 in the development of dopaminergic neurons and Parkinson's disease," Progress in Neurobiology, vol. 77, no. 1-2, pp. 128–138, 2005.

[10] T. Torii, T. Kawarai, S. Nakamura, and H. Kawakami, "Organization of the human orphan nuclear receptor Nurr1 gene," Gene, vol. 230, no. 2, pp. 225–232, 1999.

[11] K.-S. Kim, C.-H. Kim, D.-Y. Hwang et al., "Orphan nuclear receptor Nurr1 directly transactivates the promoter activity of the tyrosine hydroxylase gene in a cell-specific manner," Journal of Neurochemistry, vol. 85, no. 3, pp. 622–634, 2003.

[12] E. Hermanson, B. Joseph, D. Castro et al., "Nurr1 regulates dopamine synthesis and storage in MN9D dopamine cells," Experimental Cell Research, vol. 288, no. 2, pp. 324–334, 2003.

[13] S. M. Smits, T. Ponnio, O. M. Conneely, J. P. H. Burbach, and M. P. Smidt, "Involvement of Nurr1 in specifying the neurotransmitter identity of ventral midbrain dopaminergic neurons," European Journal of Neuroscience, vol. 18, no. 7, pp. 1731–1738, 2003.

[14] W.-D. Le, P. Xu, J. Jankovic et al., "Mutations in NR4A2 associated with familial Parkinson disease," Nature Genetics, vol. 33, no. 1, pp. 85–89, 2003.

[15] S. R. W. Stott, E. Metzakopian, W. Lin, K. H. Kaestner, R. Hen, and S.-L. Ang, "Foxa1 and Foxa2 are required for the maintenance of dopaminergic properties in ventral midbrain neurons at late embryonic stages," The Journal of Neuroscience, vol. 33, no. 18, pp. 8022–8034, 2013.

[16] G. T. Sutherland, N. A. Matigian, A. M. Chalk et al., "A cross-study transcriptional analysis of Parkinson's disease," PLoS ONE, vol. 4, no. 3, Article ID e4955, 2009.

[17] T. D. Schmittgen and K. J. Livak, "Analyzing real-time PCR data by the comparative CT method," Nature Protocols, vol. 3, no. 6, pp. 1101–1108, 2008.

[18] J. Sambrook and D. W. Russell, Molecular Cloning: A Laboratory Manual, Coldspring-Harbour Laboratory Press, London, UK, 3rd edition, 2001.

[19] M. Orita, H. Iwahana, H. Kanazawa, K. Hayashi, and T. Sekiya, "Detection of polymorphisms of human DNA by gel electrophoresis as single-strand conformation polymorphisms," Proceedings of the National Academy of Sciences of the United States of America, vol. 86, no. 8, pp. 2766–2770, 1989.

[20] N. Pankratz, W. C. Nichols, S. K. Uniacke et al., "Significant linkage of Parkinson disease to chromosome 2q36-37," American Journal of Human Genetics, vol. 72, no. 4, pp. 1053–1057, 2003.

[21] G. F. Wooten, L. J. Currie, V. E. Bovbjerg, J. K. Lee, and J. Patrie, "Are men at greater risk for Parkinson's disease than women?" Journal of Neurology, Neurosurgery & Psychiatry, vol. 75, no. 4, pp. 637–639, 2004.

[22] M. J. Bannon, B. Pruetz, A. B. Manning-Bog et al., "Decreased expression of the transcription factor NURR1 in dopamine neurons of cocaine abusers," Proceedings of the National Academy of Sciences of the United States of America, vol. 99, no. 9, pp. 6382–6385, 2002.

[23] T. Pan, W. Xie, J. Jankovic, and W. Le, "Decreased Nurr1 mRNA in peripheral blood lymphocytes in Parkinson's disease," Neurology, vol. 62, no. 7, article A108, 2004.

[24] W. Le, T. Pan, M. Huang et al., "Decreased NURR1 gene expression in patients with Parkinson's disease," Journal of the Neurological Sciences, vol. 273, no. 1-2, pp. 29–33, 2008.

[25] H. Liu, L. Wei, Q. Tao et al., "Decreased NURR1 and PITX3 gene expression in Chinese patients with Parkinson's disease," *European Journal of Neurology*, vol. 19, no. 6, pp. 870–875, 2012.

[26] S. Pérez-Sieira, M. López, R. Nogueiras, and S. Tovar, "Regulation of NR4A by nutritional status, gender, postnatal development and hormonal deficiency," *Scientific Reports*, vol. 4, article no. 4264, 2014.

[27] C. Matsuki, M. To, Y. Kondo et al., "Associations between brain-derived neurotrophic factor and estradiol in women's saliva," *Neuroendocrinology Letters*, vol. 35, no. 3, pp. 236–241, 2014.

[28] M. A. Hauser, Y.-J. Li, H. Xu et al., "Expression profiling of substantia nigra in Parkinson disease, progressive supranuclear palsy, and frontotemporal dementia with parkinsonism," *Archives of Neurology*, vol. 62, no. 6, pp. 917–921, 2005.

[29] Y. Zhang, M. James, F. A. Middleton, and R. L. Davis, "Transcriptional analysis of multiple brain regions in Parkinson's disease supports the involvement of specific protein processing, energy metabolism, and signaling pathways, and suggests novel disease mechanisms," *American Journal of Medical Genetics—Neuropsychiatric Genetics*, vol. 137, no. 1, pp. 5–16, 2005.

[30] L. B. Moran, D. C. Duke, M. Deprez, D. T. Dexter, R. K. B. Pearce, and M. B. Graeber, "Whole genome expression profiling of the medial and lateral substantia nigra in Parkinson's disease," *Neurogenetics*, vol. 7, no. 1, pp. 1–11, 2006.

[31] T. G. Lesnick, S. Papapetropoulos, D. C. Mash et al., "A genomic pathway approach to a complex disease: axon guidance and Parkinson disease," *PLoS Genetics*, vol. 3, no. 6, article e98, 2007.

[32] A. Domanskyi, H. Alter, M. A. Vogt, P. Gass, and I. A. Vinnikov, "Transcription factors Foxa1 and Foxa2 are required for adult dopamine neurons maintenance," *Frontiers in Cellular Neuroscience*, vol. 8, article no. 275, 2014.

[33] E.-K. Tan, H. Chung, Y. Zhao et al., "Genetic analysis of Nurr1 haplotypes in Parkinson's disease," *Neuroscience Letters*, vol. 347, no. 3, pp. 139–142, 2003.

[34] D. A. Grimes, F. Han, M. Panisset et al., "Translated mutation in the Nurr1 gene as a cause for Parkinson's disease," *Movement Disorders*, vol. 21, no. 7, pp. 906–909, 2006.

The Importance of Connection to Others in QoL in MSA and PSP

Louise Wiblin,[1] Rory Durcan,[1] Mark Lee,[2] and Katie Brittain[3]

[1]Clinical Ageing Research Unit, Newcastle University, Newcastle upon Tyne NE4 5PL, UK
[2]St Benedict's Hospice for Specialist Palliative Care, St. Benedict's Way, Sunderland SR2 0NY, UK
[3]Department of Nursing, Midwifery & Health, Northumbria University, Coach Lane Campus West, Room B128, Newcastle upon Tyne NE7 7XA, UK

Correspondence should be addressed to Louise Wiblin; louise.wiblin@gmail.com

Academic Editor: Pedro Chaná

Multiple System Atrophy (MSA) and Progressive Supranuclear Palsy (PSP) are atypical Parkinsonian disorders with extended morbidity and reduced lifespan, known to have marked and early impact upon quality of life (QoL). This study aimed to address the lack of studies in the literature regarding personal perspectives on QoL in MSA and PSP in both patients and carers. Participants took part in qualitative, in-depth interviews in the North East of England, exploring what impacts their QoL and their experiences of living with these complex conditions. Connection to others was found to be a prevailing theme, encompassing difficulty communicating, social isolation, impact on personal relationships, and stigma. This work is helpful in that it emphasises the personal experiences of these patients and carers, which can provide insights into important areas for clinical service planning and best clinical management of individual patients as well as considerations for future research into QoL in these rare disorders.

1. Introduction

Multiple System Atrophy (MSA) and Progressive Supranuclear Palsy (PSP) are sporadic atypical Parkinsonian disorders (AP) which have poor response to symptomatic treatment, rapid and relentless progression, and reduced life expectancy compared with Parkinson's disease (PD) [1–3]. As these diseases have an especially aggressive course, in recent years, particular attention has been given to maximise quality of life (QoL) in these conditions, including the introduction of a palliative approach. Research looking at QoL specifically in MSA and PSP is lacking compared with the current body of work on QoL in PD [4–6]. QoL is frequently described as one of the key domains to improve for patients and caregivers in the context of Parkinson's disease and related disorders and the importance ascribed to QoL is growing [7]. However, a definitive measure which succinctly captures the essence of QoL has not been described; though many tools exist to try and capture QoL using quantitative scales, particularly in Parkinson's disease and conditions such as MSA and PSP [4, 8, 9]. Qualitative work to explore the "how" and the "why"

of QoL and to gain an understanding from the patient and carer perspective has an important place in clinical research, particularly in QoL, as QoL is very much based upon an individual's perspective and reflection on the self. Qualitative methods are complementary to quantitative work, permitting access to the experiences of patients and carers that "other methods cannot reach" [10]. Qualitative work can act as a basis for developing clinical services or concepts for development of validated scales as well as reinforcing the important principles that lie at the heart of holistic medicine, understanding the patient's point of view and the diversity of experiences that patients and carers have [11, 12]. This study was carried out as part of a mixed methods project exploring QoL in MSA and PSP and a key finding in the qualitative portion of the investigation was the impact of connection to QoL in patients and in carers. Connection in this analysis refers to the way in which individuals are able to relate to others. This is via different means of communication, relating to people such as partners, family, or friends and how they felt others related to and perceived them. This has clinical implications, as good medical practice is built upon the development of patient and carer-relationships. Any barriers which patients and carers perceive should be identified wherever possible, to allow the best possible communication and rapport, as well as insight into their experience, and hence improve our management.

2. Methods and Ethics

This was an exploratory, qualitative project using semistructured interviews.

The study was approved by the Leeds-Bradford Research Ethics Committee. Participants were recruited from specialist atypical Parkinsonism clinics across three sites in the North East of England. All participants provided written informed consent. Participants were approached in clinic and provided with detailed information sheets informing them of the study aims, that participation was voluntary, that they could withdraw at any time, and that data would be treated confidentially. This qualitative study was part of a larger project exploring QoL in MSA and PSP using both quantitative and qualitative methods. Recruits to the project gave written consent if they wished to be approached to provide an interview. Any identifiable information was removed from transcripts, such as first names or surnames mentioned during interviews, to ensure the anonymity of interviewee and confidentiality was protected by the use of pseudonyms.

Patients had a diagnosis of MSA or PSP and carers were unpaid and voluntary. Purposive, pragmatic sampling was used to achieve a range and richness of experience with a balance of male, female, MSA, and PSP patients and a range of severities to give a more complete picture of living with AP. Particular effort was made to facilitate interviewing of participants with poor or negligible speech who used communication aids, as theirs is a poorly heard voice in clinical and research terms. In many articles in which interviews are performed with patients with Parkinsonian conditions, inability to communicate clearly is an exclusion criteria for participation, even in work on advanced disease. Indeed, few publications could be found by the authors (one included one patient with MSA and a mixture of neurodegenerative conditions and the other PD and stroke) describing the significant communication problems encountered in advanced neurological disease and allowing their participation [13, 14]. There was purposeful inclusion of these individuals into this qualitative study, permitting communication devices.

The interview schedule was produced with reference to the literature on MSA and PSP and QoL as well as qualitative work in PD (due to the lack of work looking at QoL and experience of living with MSA and PSP) [15–18]. It was developed by the interviewer (LW) with input from an experienced researcher in qualitative interviewing (KB). The schedule permitted broad coverage of key areas felt to be important after the literature review, encouraging a personalised response from each participant. The open questions of the interview guide could then be followed up by probes from the interviewer to explore elicited responses thoroughly. See Table 1.

Interviews were carried out by LW as a one-to-one meeting either in a clinical research setting or in participant's homes, depending on which environment they were most comfortable in. Interviews were recorded on a digital device

and transcribed verbatim. The interview transcripts were analysed using thematic analysis based upon the system described by Braun and Clarke [19]. See Figure 1.

In qualitative work, it is important in terms of transparency and rigour to describe the background of the researchers due to the influence this can have on their analysis. LW, the interviewer and primary researcher, is a training doctor in Neurology specialising in movement disorder with a particular interest in MSA and PSP and is an MD student looking at QoL and Palliative Care need in MSA and PSP. She undertook the main study design, participant recruitment, interviewing, analysis, and production of the manuscript. RD is a Geriatrics training doctor and movement disorder specialist who critiqued the analysis and contributed to the writing of the manuscript. ML is an advisor to the project and is a Consultant Physician and researcher in Palliative Care with an interest in movement disorder and was an advisor in the design of the project, the analysis process, and writing/review of the article. KB is an Associate Professor of Ageing & Health and is a Social Gerontologist. She advised on project design, reviewed and provided feedback on the coding process, and advised on project analysis and writing/review of the article.

QSR International NVIVO version 11 was used as an aid to analysis and data retrieval in thematic analysis. Coding was carried out as interviews were completed and were integrated into overarching themes; both data collection and analysis were an iterative process, whereby interviewing ceased when saturation took place, that is, when both LW and KB agreed that no more new, meaningful codes were being generated [20, 21].

Rigour was ensured by referring to qualitative guidelines such as COREQ and Yardley's criteria [22, 23]. See Table 2.

3. Results

Nineteen interviews were carried out in total, ten with patient participants and nine with carers. Four patients had MSA and there were four carers of individuals with MSA. There were six patients with PSP and five PSP-carers. Sixteen of the participants were patient-carer spouses and their relationships are described in Table 3.

A prevailing theme which was found in analysis was that of "connection to others." Other themes which emerged from the interviews using the topics covered in Table 1 were "transitions as a result of disease" and "accessing services." This paper will explore the "connection to others" theme, as it is beyond the scope of the article to cover all three aspects. "Connection to others" was made up of several subthemes which will be described below and illustrated with extracts from interview transcripts; see Figure 2. Connection in this study refers to the ways in which the participants relate to others and ultimately how their ability to connect impacts their relationships with others. Relationships are intrinsically about connection, the definition being *"The way in which two or more people or things are connected, or the state of being connected,"* Oxford English Dictionary [24].

3.1. Communication Difficulty. In order to relate to others and have meaningful interactions, communication is vital.

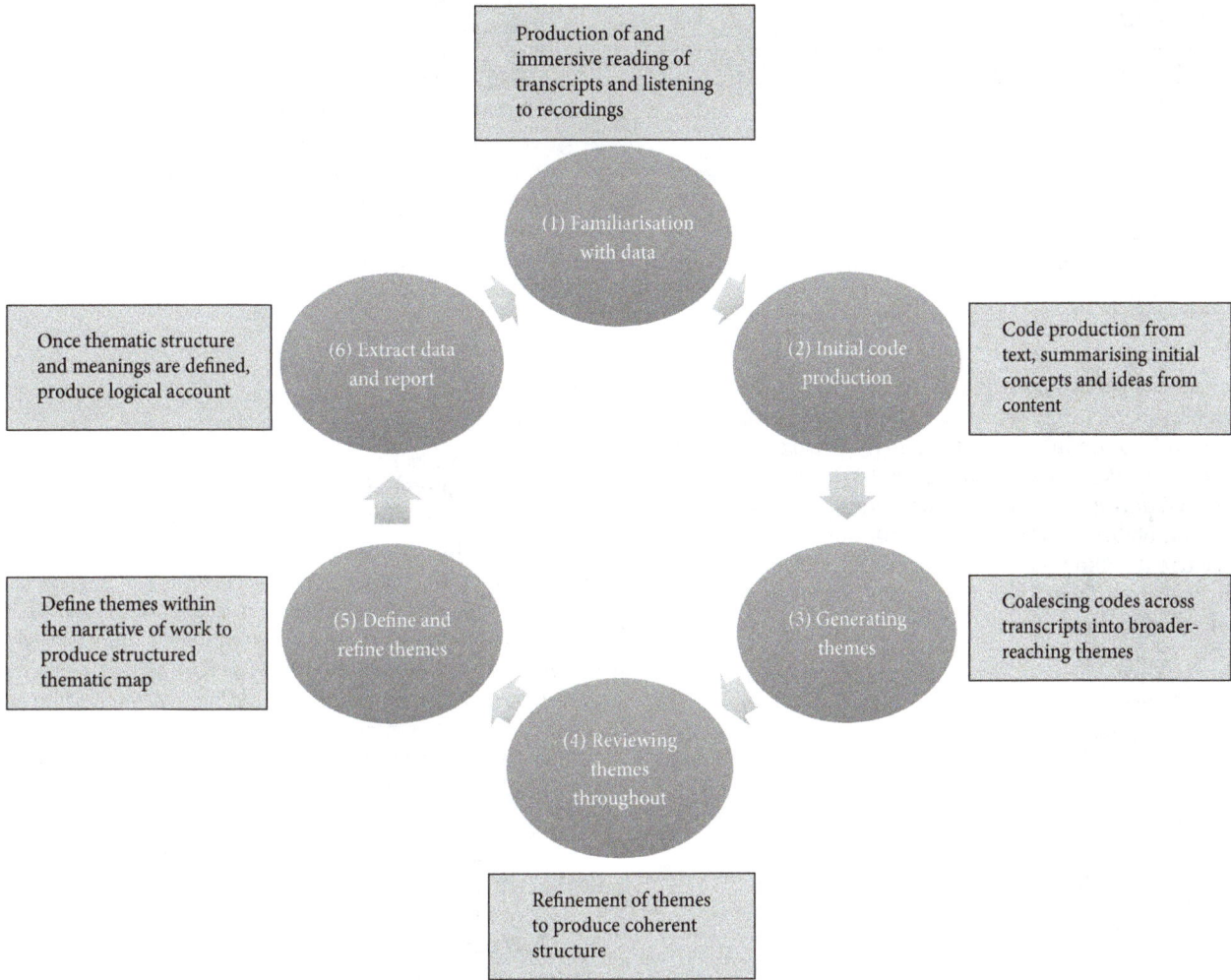

FIGURE 1: Stages of thematic analysis from Braun and Clarke 2006.

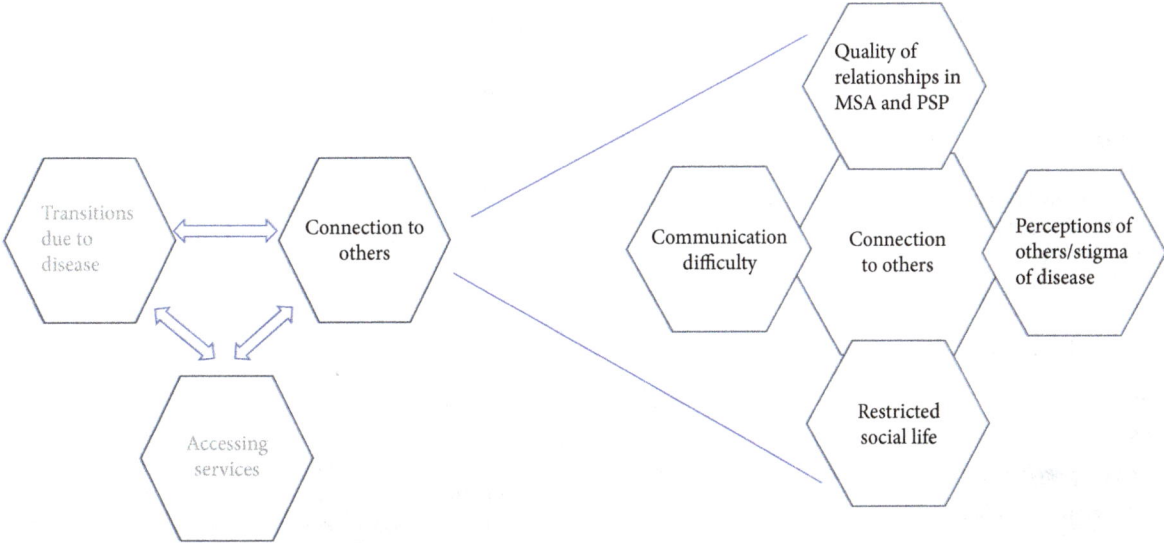

FIGURE 2: All prevailing themes from this project and their relationships to one another shown on the left. The theme "connection to others" and its associated subthemes are discussed in this article and are expanded on the right.

TABLE 1: Basic semistructured interview schedule. Structure derived from Patton [29].

Semistructured interview topics
Background of life before diagnosis
Process of diagnosis
How have things changed
Discussion of relationships
How is MSA/PSP challenging
Experiences with medical teams
What is your understanding of Palliative Care

The patient participants in this study had variable speech difficulty. Some were profound, necessitating the use of electronic communication devices (one participant used an adapted iPad and another a light-writer), whilst some remained intelligible. However, the majority of patients found that their ability to communicate with others was impaired. A recurrent subtheme was patients finding reassurance that their speech or fluency was not severe, frustrating, as they felt their struggles to communicate were being dismissed.

> Other people. . . I'll ask them, "Do I come across. . . ?" They always say, "Oh, you're fine." I don't believe them, but they always say I come across fine.

(Doris, age 59, participant with MSA)

> The social life has deteriorated because I'm scared I might be a bit caught short or not being able to speak properly. You said earlier that my voice seemed okay. To me, it doesn't seem okay, I'm not as confident as I used to be. I couldn't sit down at a meeting anymore, a complete meeting, because I feel embarrassed losing my voice.

(Gary, age 58, participant with PSP)

Gary, a participant with PSP, referred to a comment from LW prior to interview where the intent had been to encourage him that his voice would be clear when recording. This feedback is valuable in that it informs us that a social nicety of trying to give confidence to patients that their voice "isn't bad" may dismiss real concerns and distress which impact upon quality of life.

When the range of speech difficulty is considered, other participants were scarcely able to communicate verbally and needed to use electronic typing devices to "speak" for them.

> Interviewer: *do you think your main problem is. . . speech?*
>
> Sarah: **speech. . . yes. . .**
>
> Interviewer: *probably the speech*
>
> Sarah: *typing sounds for 5 min*
>
> Interviewer: *I think I can read what. . .*
>
> Sarah: *mmmm. . ..*

(Sarah, age 67, participant with PSP (bold text indicates "spoken" via light-writer device))

> First, I tried to put it down to the fact that she was doing this, but I don't think that is the case. I think she is starting to misspell words. . .and when it gets to, to, to press "Do", sometimes she presses it, and it repeats and repeats and repeats. And I'd say, "No, the wrong- thing that's wrong is, you've pressed it too many times with your finger," and I don't think she realizes. . ..

(Bob, 69, carer of Mary who has PSP)

Although these devices can enable people otherwise rendered unable to speak to make meaningful contact with others producing improvement in relationships and well-being as a consequence, the reality is that motor slowness, stiffness, and possible cognitive problems make communication devices increasingly difficult to use as the disease progresses. This can be frightening for patients and carers as they consider that their new "voice" may not be useable forever. This can be seen from Bob's statement above, as his wife Mary finds her light-writer more and more difficult to use and in Sarah who had profound slowness and rigidity, needing several minutes at a time to type short sentences or single words. This led to frustration where she tried to communicate with monosyllabic sounds when she was unable to type her thoughts.

3.2. Restricted Social Life. All participants in the study, across disease types, both patients and carers, described the negative impact of MSA or PSP on their ability to maintain a social life. This seemed to manifest in different ways. One frequent concern of patients with Parkinsonism is maintaining the volume of their voice. Work has suggested that patients with PD may have impaired ability to detect low volumes in their own voice, feeling that they are shouting when they are in fact difficult to hear. This likely adds to social awkwardness and feelings of effort or struggle in conversation [25, 26]. This can be seen by two patients with MSA, Doris and Rose, who particularly struggled to raise their voices and found themselves withdrawing socially as a consequence. This may lead to a profound change in perception of self and confidence.

> I know my speech. . . nine times out of ten, I've got to repeat myself, and then I'll think, "Oh, I can't be bothered." It's not worth it usually.

(Doris, age 59, participant with MSA)

> If I went to things, like the royalty dinners and things, there came to a certain point where really I couldn't take part in the conversation. Course you'd have a big round table. People were talking of course backwards and forwards, and they didn't, couldn't hear me. So I tended to just sort of sit back and just let things go on in front of me, and that was it, so I changed quite a bit.

(Rose, age 71, participant with MSA)

TABLE 2: Two criteria used to demonstrate quality and validity in qualitative work and how they apply to this study. From Tong et al. [22] and Yardley [23].

COREQ domain checklist summary	Yardley's qualitative validity criteria
Sampling method: purposive, pragmatic sampling	Sensitivity: study designed with respect to known literature with respect to patient input (patient/carer group consulted in design)
Setting: participant's homes or clinical research facility (choice given). One-to-one interviewing	Commitment and rigour: LW experienced in movement disorder and specialising in AP. Extensive review of literature, training in interviewing methods, and analysis overseen by KB, an academic with many years of experience in qualitative research
Method: thematic analysis. NVivo v. 11.0 used as analysis aid	Transparency: methods described in methods section, process used shown in Figure 1. Disclosure of researcher background and assumptions given
How was data recorded: recorded on digital device and transcribed verbatim	Impact and importance: having implications for planning of future services for AP and for improving best practice. Potential to impact QoL in a rare, underresearched group of conditions. Demonstrating the need for more work in the future
Description of themes: themes derived from data, not preselected then imposed	
Supporting extracts: quotations used throughout report	

TABLE 3: Participant demographics and relationships. * indicates these participants communicated with an electronic device.

Pseudonym	Sex	Condition	Role	Age	Profession	Marital status
Matthew (MP1)	Male	MSA	Patient	64	Retired lawyer	Married to Sally
Emma (CM1)	Female	MSA	Carer	61	Retired charity worker	Married to Matthew
Sally (CP1)	Female	PSP	Carer	70	Retired dental nurse	Married
Bryce (PP3)	Male	PSP	Patient	76	Retired technician	Single
Doris (MP2)	Female	MSA	Patient	59	Retired librarian	Married to Bill
Bill (CM2)	Male	MSA	Carer	57	Director	Married to Doris
Rose (MP3)	Female	MSA	Patient	71	Retired teacher	Married to Jackie
Jackie (CM3)	Male	MSA	Carer	73	Retired head teacher	Married to Rose
Julia (MP7)	Female	MSA	Patient	62	Retired hotelier	Married to Tiberius
Tiberius (CM7)	Male	MSA	Carer	66	Retired hotelier	Married to Julia
Sarah* (PP4)	Female	PSP	Patient	67	Retired teacher	Married to Tom
Tom (CP3)	Male	PSP	Carer	70	Retired oil chemist	Married to Sarah
Helen (PP18)	Female	PSP	Patient	68	Retired newsagent	Married to Earl
Earl (Cp17)	Male	PSP	Carer	70	Retired chartered accountant	Married to Helen
Mary* (PP24)	Female	PSP	Patient	69	Retired newsagent	Married to Bob
Bob (CP23)	Male	PSP	Carer	69	Retired newsagent	Married to Mary
Gary (PP20)	Male	PSP	Patient	58	Retired project manager	Married to Pat
Pat (CP19)	Female	PSP	Carer	62	Analyst	Married to Gary
Jack (PP19)	Male	PSP	Patient	71	Retired HGV manager	Married

Therefore, patients may be experiencing distress due to being less able to connect to others by speech, even if families and medical staff are not aware of any problem. The change may be innocuous, such as Rose's gradual shift during dinners to sitting back and letting the conversation flow around her as she realized her voice was becoming less able to cut through many voices in a loud social setting. This comparison with former selves and reducing abilities can produce a bereavement reaction for what has been lost.

From the carer's perspective, the burden of care and responsibility, especially the 24-hour nature of it, had an effect on social networks. Emma discussed the rare times she was able to meet with friends but found that she was unable to confide in them and she was afraid she would be unable to "click back" into a mindset which she uses to cope. This suggests that some barriers between carers and their old relationships and social lives grow because of their new responsibilities and experiences: perhaps not feeling that they share enough in common to confide in them. This produces a disconnect from society for the carer.

> Unless they're very close to you... it's hard to click back into the "hi, yes how you today?" when the day before you broken down in tears over coffee, but I find that even, with my good friends which I think I mentioned to you, that you think twice about opening up to them. I hardly see any friends.

(Emma, age 61, carer of Matthew who has MSA)

> What happens if I am not here, if she falls over?

(Earl, age 70, carer of Helen who has PSP)

> Because he has some horrendous falls...when he was at home before I went off for some respite he'd had- oh, he'd fallen and he was bruised. He looked like a car crash. He was always bumping into walls and stuff and falling back over and cracking his head. But I managed to keep him reasonably safe and intact as best I could.

(Sally, age 70, carer of partner with PSP)

Earl and Sally discussed a very common subtheme in carers of both groups but most prominently in carers for people with PSP, the constant vigilance due to fear of their partner falling and injuring themselves. This seemed to encompass the full-time nature of caring and the emotional as well as physical pressures it exerts. This need to protect their spouse leads to an ever-shrinking social circle as their partner becomes less able to leave the home, resulting in social networks reduced to care-giver, patient, and occasional visitors to the home.

3.3. Perceptions of Others/Stigma of Disease.
The ability to connect with others is influenced not only by the willingness and ability to communicate but also in how others perceive you (or possibly more importantly, how you believe others perceive you). Patients with MSA and PSP perceived stigma from others on the basis of their ability to interact. This was largely based on fear of perception from other from conversation, such as Gary feeling that his impaired fluency caused others to dismiss him or Rose's concern that her motor slowing would be seen as cognitive decline.

> Gary: Yes. I feel as it's difficult. The others will take what I say and they'll understand it, but then they'll question it.
>
> LW: What do you mean, Gary?
>
> Gary: It's the way you say things to people. Words get jumbled up. They'll then say they understood me, but they didn't.

(Gary, age 58, participant with PSP)

> ...you have people sort of waiting whilst I slowly spoke to them. I didn't want them to think that I'd sort of- I think everybody thinks when you've got that and you slow down it might be a mental thing, which obviously it isn't because inside your head, it's all, it's really going on.

(Rose, age 71, participant with MSA)

Mary, who used a light-writer to communicate, felt her inability to speak and the time she needed (due to a combination of bradykinesia and bradyphrenia) to type her responses caused her to believe herself judged by those around her. She felt that her combination of disabilities led to others believing that she was stupid and ignoring her, a powerful and profound insight into how these patients' symptoms impact upon their identity and well-being.

> Mary: *typing sounds* **I sometimes think** *typing sounds* ...**people don't understand**
>
> LW: what do people not understand that you want them to, can you pin that down?...
>
> Mary: **that I'm not stupid**
>
> Mary: *typing sounds* **it's very frustrating**
>
> LW: how do people react to your speech as it is?
>
> Mary: *typing sounds* **most people just ignore me**
>
> LW: ignore you?
>
> Mary: **yes.**

(Mary, age 69, participant with PSP (bold text indicates "spoken" via light-writer device))

3.4. Quality of Relationships in MSA and PSP.
Relationships and how they succeed or fail beyond a diagnosis of AP were a frequent theme. Relationships with others were frequently discussed within interviews. These relationships did not only include that between patient and carer (in this study, spouses) but also with other family members and friends.

As communication is so fundamental to relationships, the ability to have meaningful interactions with a partner is very important in maintaining that relationship through a diagnosis of a Parkinsonian disorder [27, 28]. This can be seen with Jackie, a carer who feels he can still communicate meaningfully with his wife Rose and with Sally, whose spouse is less able to speak (and was not able to give an interview) but she feels they are still able to communicate with each other.

> Well deep down, no, it doesn't matter at all. We can have a nice night in together and we can communicate with one another. [Rose] loves talking although she has difficulty talking now and I have difficulty hearing her. She is a little bit deaf, you might have noticed that but I think quality of life, it is defining quality of life. When you get to real hardcore values, they're probably undiminished in my view but you have to be single minded to be able to identify that and I count myself fortunate.

(Jackie, age 73, carer of Rose who has MSA)

Came back on the Sunday, I went straight to see [my husband]; tell him all about it and blah, blah, blah. He's happy to hear…we have quality time. We have meals together. I take him out; we go for a beer. I'm falling in love with him again.

(Sally, age 70, carer of husband with PSP)

Julia, a participant with MSA, spoke positively of the impact her marriage and the relationships with her family had on maintaining home life with a degenerative disease. The use of the term "rock" is an interesting one, suggesting her husband keeps her tethered or connected despite her illness.

Exactly. Which is why I always refer to him as my rock. Because he is a stable influence in my life. He is just so down-to-earth, his feet are just so firmly cranked on the ground. He keeps saying, "That's no bother. That's no bother."

(Julia, age 62, participant with MSA)

The relationship [changing]? No, not really. Still love each other.

(Tiberius, age 66, carer of Julia who has MSA)

Similarly, Julia's husband Tiberius, as he simply put it, did not feel that the quality of his relationship with his wife had changed, despite the change in her health and abilities and that they still loved each other. This support for people with chronic conditions is very valuable and may trigger medical and social teams to consider patients and carers more as a pair, supporting both, as the well-being of one is so fundamental to the other.

Interviewed participants discussed the difficulties in maintaining friendships which seemed to be multifactorial. The nature of friendship and even the friends themselves seemed to shift or change with diagnosis and increasing symptoms. Bryce, a participant with PSP, felt that certain friends were only interested in socializing when he was well enough to do so and lost interest in him when he became less physically able. From the statement below he feels discarded by his former peers.

Bryce: *No, because- well, your friends yes, used to be. When you were all right your friends used to come around and see you. Since I've took bad I never see them.*

LW: *Do you know why?*

Bryce: *Yes, because they don't care. That's my opinion like.*

(Bryce, age 76, participant with PSP)

Bryce was the only participant within the cohort who did not have a partner or spouse. Therefore, the impact of this loss of interaction with friends was especially profound for him. Friendship is often built upon mutual interests, and being less able to participate may mean less contact with friends as those activities become less accessible.

4. Discussion

This qualitative study suggests that maintaining connection and appreciating the possible barriers that MSA and PSP patients and carers face in this challenge are vital in enhancing QoL. There is evidence in the literature that connection to others is key to QoL in other chronic, life-limiting illnesses [15]. This study has shown that, in a cohort of individuals with MSA and PSP and their carers, connection was a prevailing concern, with subthemes of affected social life, communication impairment, perception of stigma, and impact on relationships. In neurological disorders, it has been shown that individuals who have wider social networks and better support tend to have better outcomes [30]. Social isolation has been found to be a predictor for further ischaemic events after stroke [31]. Although many studies apprise QoL using HR-QoL (Health-Related QoL) tools which focus on well-being within the scope of illness and disability, qualitative work in PD and stroke has shown that participants' concerns regarding QoL are frequently related to maintaining connection to others such as spouses or family and shrinking social lives [15, 32]. Northcott and Hilari [33] described how stroke affected friendships with particular impact if there was pronounced speech disturbance; this led to isolation from friends due to embarrassment on the patient's part or desertion from the friends as they found the stroke survivor more difficult to communicate with. Friendships were particularly imperiled if they were based upon activities which patients become too disabled to take part in anymore, such as sport. These factors are particularly applicable to AP and were described by participants with the added implication of progressing, worsening symptoms, unlike stroke in which the deficit is fixed and will stay stable or even improve.

Being able to communicate, verbally or otherwise, is integral to being able to connect to others, individuals, and communities. It has been shown that people with PD feel excluded from conversations as speech becomes more effortful, impacting upon their relationships, personal identity, and dignity; they, like some participants in this study, felt that their voices were impaired even if others said they were not. These perceived communication problems were correlated with depression [34, 35]. Efforts to reconnect individuals with speech problems due to neurodegenerative disease can be life-changing and increase QoL, such as providing electronic communication devices in MND [36]. However, progressing motor and cognitive problems in MSA and PSP (and indeed, in MND) can make these aids more challenging to use as the disease progresses, as the two participants who used lightwriters demonstrated in this work. Other practical measures we can take as medical practitioners include education, so clinicians, nurses, and therapists are aware of how these and similar conditions impede conversation, giving time and being creative in their approach in how to make connections to these patients. Simple signing, picture boards, and one-to-one sessions with trained specialists or volunteers may enable patients to relate their concerns, have these acknowledged, and improve QoL.

Stigma has been described in PD patients not just from physical changes in appearance but from decline in the ability to speak clearly and fluently [37]. It must also be recalled that stigma can be felt or enacted by others, but often the effect upon the person feeling this stigma is the same. PD patients in a review of a number of studies experienced impact on the quality of their interactions with others, producing a retreat from the social sphere [38]. Stigma has been found to predict negatively for QoL in PD [39]. When it is considered that speech problems in MSA and PSP are more severe and have an earlier onset and the conditions are overall less responsive to medication, these factors are especially important to consider in AP [40].

Finally, AP affects the care-giver's ability to connect to others. This is borne of the increasing support their relative needs, both physical and emotional, and the constant burden of vigilance and worry in keeping the patient safe. This can cut carers off from outside social life from the demands on their time and limited freedom [41]. This is seen in PD, though the rapidity and extended morbidity in AP would be likely to put more pressure on this carer group. Falls produce especial distress in carers, leading to fears of leaving the patient alone for any length of time, which has also been seen in PD, but again issues like motor recklessness in PSP may lead to these problems being more acute in AP [42].

5. Conclusions and Future Directions

This study is qualitative and based upon a group of participants in the North East of England; it is therefore not possible to conclude that its findings are generalisable. However, the strengths of this work include the subjective and personal insight into this group which is lacking in the literature; this is particularly meaningful when it is considered that QoL has a very personal and self-reflective element to it which may not be fully captured by quantitative survey data collection. Future work should consider QoL of patients and carers with AP, taking into account communication and relationships. The aim of this paper was to explore personal perspectives on QoL and how disease impacting connection to others can give clinicians insight into how AP affects patients and carers beyond a simple description of symptoms. The implications for practice are to emphasise the patient's need to communicate and feel connected to others, their carer, families, and friends and to feel they are involved in clinical decision-making. This is of paramount importance in maintaining QoL and allowing holistic assessment in these conditions for which we, as yet, have no curative treatment. Acknowledging the impact of speech issues on the QoL of patients and carers is key, giving time for patients to try and convey their concerns (even when very slow or needing many attempts to do so) and good, early speech and language input to maximise their ability to communicate by whatever means they have available. These findings also have wider societal implications. It is difficult for medical services to address these far-ranging issues of a disconnect from others in patients and carers alone. In the future, incorporating social care, the volunteer sector and even technological advancements to enhance communication and independence should complement medical services. QoL is often assessed using quantitative measures and whilst this is valuable, work with patient groups using qualitative methods has the potential to shine a light on concerns that we may never have known existed.

References

[1] J. Bükki, G. Nübling, and S. Lorenzl, "Managing Advanced Progressive Supranuclear Palsy and Corticobasal Degeneration in a Palliative Care Unit: Admission Triggers and Outcomes," *American Journal of Hospice and Palliative Medicine*, vol. 33, no. 5, pp. 477–482, 2014.

[2] Y. Ben-Shlomo, G. K. Wenning, F. Tison, and N. P. Quinn, "Survival of patients with pathologically proven multiple system atrophy: A meta-analysis," *Neurology*, vol. 48, no. 2, pp. 384–393, 1997.

[3] S. S. O'Sullivan, L. A. Massey, D. R. Williams et al., "Clinical outcomes of progressive supranuclear palsy and multiple system atrophy," *Brain*, vol. 131, no. 5, pp. 1362–1372, 2008.

[4] P. Martinez-Martin, M. Jeukens-Visser, K. E. Lyons et al., "Health-related quality-of-life scales in Parkinson's disease: critique and recommendations," *Movement Disorders*, vol. 26, no. 13, pp. 2371–2380, 2011.

[5] A. M. Kuopio, R. J. Marttila, H. Helenius, M. Toivonen, and U. K. Rinne, "The quality of life in Parkinson's disease," *Movement Disorder*, vol. 15, no. 2, pp. 216–223, 2000.

[6] I. J. Higginson, W. Gao, T. Z. Saleem et al., "Symptoms and Quality of Life in Late Stage Parkinson Syndromes: A Longitudinal Community Study of Predictive Factors," *PLoS ONE*, vol. 7, no. 11, Article ID e46327, 2012.

[7] J. Rees, C. O'Boyle, and R. MacDonagh, "Quality of life: Impact of chronic illness on the partner," *Journal of the Royal Society of Medicine*, vol. 94, no. 11, pp. 563–566, 2001.

[8] A. Schrag, F. Geser, M. Stampfer-Kountchev et al., "Health-related quality of life in multiple system atrophy," *Movement Disorders*, vol. 21, no. 6, pp. 809–815, 2006.

[9] A. Schrag, C. Selai, N. Quinn et al., "Measuring quality of life in PSP: The PSP-QoL," *Neurology*, vol. 67, no. 1, pp. 39–44, 2006.

[10] C. Pope and N. Mays, "Reaching the parts other methods cannot reach: an introduction to qualitative methods in health and health services research," *British Medical Journal*, vol. 311, no. 6996, pp. 42–45, 1995.

[11] A. Schrag, C. Selai, J. Davis, A. J. Lees, M. Jahanshahi, and N. Quinn, "Health-related quality of life in patients with progressive supranuclear palsy," *Movement Disorders*, vol. 18, no. 12, pp. 1464–1469, 2003.

[12] A. C. Klassen, J. Creswell, V. L. Plano Clark, K. C. Smith, and H. I. Meissner, "Best practices in mixed methods for quality of life research," *Quality of Life Research*, vol. 21, no. 3, pp. 377–380, 2012.

[13] S. Veronese, G. Gallo, A. Valle et al., "The palliative care needs of people severely affected by neurodegenerative disorders: A qualitative study," *Progress in Palliative Care*, vol. 23, no. 6, pp. 331–342, 2015.

[14] M. Walshe and N. Miller, "Living with acquired dysarthria: the speaker's perspective," *Disability and Rehabilitation*, vol. 33, no. 3, pp. 195–203, 2011.

[15] P. L. Hudson, C. Toye, and L. J. Kristjanson, "Would people with Parkinson's disease benefit form palliative care?" *Palliative Medicine*, vol. 20, no. 2, pp. 87–94, 2006.

[16] F. Hasson, W. G. Kernohan, M. McLaughlin et al., "An exploration into the palliative and end-of-life experiences of carers of people with Parkinson's disease," *Palliative Medicine*, vol. 24, no. 7, pp. 731–736, 2010.

[17] S. Fox, A. Cashell, W. G. Kernohan et al., "Palliative care for Parkinson's disease: Patient and carer's perspectives explored through qualitative interview," *Palliative Medicine*, vol. 31, no. 7, 2017.

[18] T. Moore and M. Guttman, "Challenges Faced by Patients With Progressive Supranuclear Palsy and their Families," *Movement Disorders Clinical Practice*, vol. 1, no. 3, pp. 188–193, 2014.

[19] V. Braun and V. Clarke, "Using thematic analysis in psychology," *Qualitative Research in Psychology*, vol. 3, no. 2, pp. 77–101, 2006.

[20] R. E. Boyatzis, *Transforming Qualitative Information: Theamtic Analysis and Code Development*, Sage Publications Ltd., London, UK, 1st edition, 1998.

[21] V. Clarke and V. Braun, "Teaching thematic analysis," *The Psychologist*, vol. 26, no. 2, pp. 120–123, 2013.

[22] A. Tong, P. Sainsbury, and J. Craig, "Consolidated criteria for reporting qualitative research (COREQ): a 32-item checklist for interviews and focus groups," *International Journal for Quality in Health Care*, vol. 19, no. 6, pp. 349–357, 2007.

[23] L. Yardley, "Dilemmas in qualitative health research," *Psychology and Health*, vol. 15, no. 2, pp. 215–228, 2000.

[24] Oxford English Dictionary, "Oxford English Dictionary: 'Relationship', in Oxford English Dictionary," 2017, https://en.oxford-dictionaries.com/definition/relationship.

[25] N. Miller, "Speech, voice and language in Parkinson's disease: changes and interventions," *Neurodegenerative Disease Management*, vol. 2, no. 3, pp. 279–289, 2012.

[26] L. C. Kwan and T. L. Whitehill, "Perception of speech by individuals with Parkinson's disease: a review," *Parkinson's Disease*, vol. 2011, Article ID 389767, 11 pages, 2011.

[27] B. Goldsworthy and S. Knowles, "Caregiving for Parkinson's disease patients: an exploration of a stress-appraisal model for quality of life and burden," *Journals of Gerontology—Series B Psychological Sciences and Social Sciences*, vol. 63, no. 6, pp. P372–P376, 2008.

[28] K. Greenwell, W. K. Gray, A. van Wersch, P. van Schaik, and R. Walker, "Predictors of the psychosocial impact of being a carer of people living with Parkinson's disease: a systematic review," *Parkinsonism and Related Disorders*, vol. 21, no. 1, pp. 1–11, 2015.

[29] M. Q. Patton, "Qualitative interviewing," in *Qualitative Interviewing, in Qualitiative Research & Evaluation Methods*, pp. 423–444, Sage Publications Inc., Thousand Oaks, Calif, USA, 2015.

[30] A. Dhand, D. A. Luke, C. E. Lang, and J.-M. Lee, "Social networks and neurological illness," *Nature Reviews Neurology*, vol. 12, no. 10, pp. 605–612, 2016.

[31] B. Boden-Albala, E. Litwak, M. S. V. Elkind, T. Rundek, and R. L. Sacco, "Social isolation and outcomes post stroke," *Neurology*, vol. 64, no. 11, pp. 1888–1892, 2005.

[32] E. B. Lynch, Z. Butt, A. Heinemann et al., "A qualitative study of quality of life after stroke: The importance of social relationships," *Journal of Rehabilitation Medicine*, vol. 40, no. 7, pp. 518–523, 2008.

[33] S. Northcott and K. Hilari, "Why do people lose their friends after a stroke?" *International Journal of Language and Communication Disorders*, vol. 46, no. 5, pp. 524–534, 2011.

[34] N. Miller, E. Noble, D. Jones, and D. Burn, "Life with communication changes in Parkinson's disease," *Age and Ageing*, vol. 35, no. 3, pp. 235–239, 2006.

[35] N. Miller, E. Noble, D. Jones, L. Allcock, and D. J. Burn, "How do I sound to me? Perceived changes in communication in Parkinson's disease," *Clinical Rehabilitation*, vol. 22, no. 1, pp. 14–22, 2008.

[36] S. Körner, M. Siniawski, K. Kollewe et al., "Speech therapy and communication device: Impact on quality of life and mood in patients with amyotrophic lateral sclerosis," *Amyotrophic Lateral Sclerosis and Frontotemporal Degeneration*, vol. 14, no. 1, pp. 20–25, 2013.

[37] F. Corallo, M. C. De Cola, V. Lo Buono, G. Di Lorenzo, P. Bramanti, and S. Marino, "Observational study of quality of life of Parkinson's patients and their caregivers," *Psychogeriatrics*, vol. 17, no. 2, pp. 97–102, 2017.

[38] M. Maffoni, A. Giardini, A. Pierobon, D. Ferrazzoli, and G. Frazzitta, "Stigma Experienced by Parkinson's Disease Patients: A Descriptive Review of Qualitative Studies," *Parkinson's Disease*, vol. 2017, Article ID 7203259, 2017.

[39] H.-I. Ma, M. Saint-Hilaire, C. A. Thomas, and L. Tickle-Degnen, "Stigma as a key determinant of health-related quality of life in Parkinson's disease," *Quality of Life Research*, vol. 25, no. 12, pp. 3037–3045, 2016.

[40] J. Rusz, C. Bonnet, J. Klempíř et al., "Speech disorders reflect differing pathophysiology in Parkinson's disease, progressive supranuclear palsy and multiple system atrophy," *Journal of Neurology*, vol. 262, no. 4, pp. 992–1001, 2015.

[41] D. McLaughlin, F. Hasson, W. G. Kernohan et al., "Living and coping with Parkinson's disease: perceptions of informal carers," *Palliative Medicine*, vol. 25, no. 2, pp. 177–182, 2011.

[42] A. Schrag, A. Hovris, D. Morley, N. Quinn, and M. Jahanshahi, "Caregiver-burden in parkinson's disease is closely associated with psychiatric symptoms, falls, and disability," *Parkinsonism & Related Disorders*, vol. 12, no. 1, pp. 35–41, 2006.

Permissions

All chapters in this book were first published in PD, by Hindawi Publishing Corporation; hereby published with permission under the Creative Commons Attribution License or equivalent. Every chapter published in this book has been scrutinized by our experts. Their significance has been extensively debated. The topics covered herein carry significant findings which will fuel the growth of the discipline. They may even be implemented as practical applications or may be referred to as a beginning point for another development.

The contributors of this book come from diverse backgrounds, making this book a truly international effort. This book will bring forth new frontiers with its revolutionizing research information and detailed analysis of the nascent developments around the world.

We would like to thank all the contributing authors for lending their expertise to make the book truly unique. They have played a crucial role in the development of this book. Without their invaluable contributions this book wouldn't have been possible. They have made vital efforts to compile up to date information on the varied aspects of this subject to make this book a valuable addition to the collection of many professionals and students.

This book was conceptualized with the vision of imparting up-to-date information and advanced data in this field. To ensure the same, a matchless editorial board was set up. Every individual on the board went through rigorous rounds of assessment to prove their worth. After which they invested a large part of their time researching and compiling the most relevant data for our readers.

The editorial board has been involved in producing this book since its inception. They have spent rigorous hours researching and exploring the diverse topics which have resulted in the successful publishing of this book. They have passed on their knowledge of decades through this book. To expedite this challenging task, the publisher supported the team at every step. A small team of assistant editors was also appointed to further simplify the editing procedure and attain best results for the readers.

Apart from the editorial board, the designing team has also invested a significant amount of their time in understanding the subject and creating the most relevant covers. They scrutinized every image to scout for the most suitable representation of the subject and create an appropriate cover for the book.

The publishing team has been an ardent support to the editorial, designing and production team. Their endless efforts to recruit the best for this project, has resulted in the accomplishment of this book. They are a veteran in the field of academics and their pool of knowledge is as vast as their experience in printing. Their expertise and guidance has proved useful at every step. Their uncompromising quality standards have made this book an exceptional effort. Their encouragement from time to time has been an inspiration for everyone.

The publisher and the editorial board hope that this book will prove to be a valuable piece of knowledge for researchers, students, practitioners and scholars across the globe.

List of Contributors

Mariana Babayeva, Haregewein Assefa, Paramita Basu, Sanjeda Chumki and Zvi Loewy
Touro College of Pharmacy, 230 West 125th Street, Room 530, New York, NY 10027, USA

Susanne Iwarsson
Department of Health Sciences, Faculty of Medicine, Lund University, Lund, Sweden
Department of Neurology and Rehabilitation, Skåne University Hospital, Lund, Sweden

Stina B. Jonasson
Department of Health Sciences, Faculty of Medicine, Lund University, Lund, Sweden
Department of Neurology and Rehabilitation, Skåne University Hospital, Lund, Sweden

Maria H. Nilsson
Department of Health Sciences, Faculty of Medicine, Lund University, Lund, Sweden
Memory Clinic, Skåne University Hospital, Malmö, Sweden

Peter Hagell
The PRO-CARE Group, School of Health and Society, Kristianstad University, Kristianstad, Sweden

Gun-Marie Hariz
Department of Community Medicine and Rehabilitation, Occupational Therapy, Umeå University, Umeå, Sweden

Yuan Zhang, Li Shu, Xun Zhou, Hongxu Pan
Department of Neurology, Xiangya Hospital, Central South University, Changsha, Hunan 410008, China
National Clinical Research Center for Geriatric Disorders, Changsha, Hunan 410078, China
Key Laboratory of Hunan Province in Neurodegenerative Disorders, Central South University, Changsha, Hunan 410008, China
Parkinson's Disease Center of Beijing Institute for Brain Disorders, Beijing 100069, China
Collaborative Innovation Center for Brain Science, Shanghai 200032, China
Collaborative Innovation Center for Genetics and Development, Shanghai 200438, China
Department of Geriatrics, Xiangya Hospital, Central South University, Changsha, Hunan 410008, China
Center for Medical Genetics, School of Life Sciences, Central South University, Changsha, Hunan 410008, China

Qian Xu
Department of Neurology, Xiangya Hospital, Central South University, Changsha, Hunan 410008, China
National Clinical Research Center for Geriatric Disorders, Changsha, Hunan 410078, China
Key Laboratory of Hunan Province in Neurodegenerative Disorders, Central South University, Changsha, Hunan 410008, China

Jifeng Guo
Department of Neurology, Xiangya Hospital, Central South University, Changsha, Hunan 410008, China
National Clinical Research Center for Geriatric Disorders, Changsha, Hunan 410078, China
Key Laboratory of Hunan Province in Neurodegenerative Disorders, Central South University, Changsha, Hunan 410008, China
Parkinson's Disease Center of Beijing Institute for Brain Disorders, Beijing 100069, China
Collaborative Innovation Center for Brain Science, Shanghai 200032, China
Collaborative Innovation Center for Genetics and Development, Shanghai 200438, China

Beisha Tang
Department of Neurology, Xiangya Hospital, Central South University, Changsha, Hunan 410008, China
National Clinical Research Center for Geriatric Disorders, Changsha, Hunan 410078, China
Key Laboratory of Hunan Province in Neurodegenerative Disorders, Central South University, Changsha, Hunan 410008, China
Parkinson's Disease Center of Beijing Institute for Brain Disorders, Beijing 100069, China
Collaborative Innovation Center for Brain Science, Shanghai 200032, China
Collaborative Innovation Center for Genetics and Development, Shanghai 200438, China
Department of Geriatrics, Xiangya Hospital, Central South University, Changsha, Hunan 410008, China
Center for Medical Genetics, School of Life Sciences, Central South University, Changsha, Hunan 410008, China

Qiying Sun
National Clinical Research Center for Geriatric Disorders, Changsha, Hunan 410078, China
Key Laboratory of Hunan Province in Neuro-degenerative Disorders, Central South University, Changsha, Hunan 410008, China

Department of Geriatrics, Xiangya Hospital, Central South University, Changsha, Hunan 410008, China

Wei Di
Department of Neurology, Xiangya Hospital, Central South University, Changsha, Hunan 410008, China
Department of Neurology, Shaanxi Provincial People's Hospital, Third Affiliated Hospital of Medical College, Xi'an Jiaotong University, Xi'an, Shaanxi 710068, China

Jingyan Li Xiaoling Liu and Hua Lv
Department of Neurology, Shaanxi Provincial People's Hospital, Third Affiliated Hospital of Medical College, Xi'an Jiaotong University, Xi'an, Shaanxi 710068, China

Zhiyong Zeng
Pediatric Department, The Second People's Hospital of Longgang District, Shenzhen, Guangdong 518112, China

Minzhi Bo
Xi'an Medical College, Xi'an, Shaanxi 710068, China

Jennifer Pate and Steven P. Millard
Veterans Affairs Puget Sound Health Care System, Seattle, WA, USA

Hojoong M. Kim, Shu-Ching Hu, Marie Y. Davis, Ali Samii and Cyrus P. Zabetian
Veterans Affairs Puget Sound Health Care System, Seattle, WA, USA
Department of Neurology, University of Washington School of Medicine, Seattle, WA, USA

James B. Leverenz
Lou Ruvo Center for Brain Health, Cleveland Clinic, Cleveland, OH, USA

Daniel J. Burdick
Booth Gardner Parkinson's Care Center, EvergreenHealth Medical Center, Kirkland, WA, USA

Sindhu Srivatsal
Virginia Mason Medical Center, Seattle, WA, USA

Andrew Paget
National Hospital for Neurology and Neurosurgery, Queen Square, London, UK

Jennifer A. Foley, Kailash P. Bhatia, Simon F. Farmer, Paul R. Jarman and Patricia Limousin
National Hospital for Neurology and Neurosurgery, Queen Square, London, UK
UCL Institute of Neurology, Queen Square, London, UK

Lisa Cipolotti
National Hospital for Neurology and Neurosurgery, Queen Square, London, UK

UCL Institute of Neurology, Queen Square, London, UK
Dipartimento di Scienze Psicologiche, Pedagogiche e della Formazione, Università degli Studi di Palermo, Palermo, Italy

Thomas T. Warner
National Hospital for Neurology and Neurosurgery, Queen Square, London, UK
Reta Lila Weston Institute of Neurological Studies, UCL Institute of Neurology, Queen Square, London, UK

Huw R. Morris
National Hospital for Neurology and Neurosurgery, Queen Square, London, UK
Department of Clinical Neuroscience, UCL Institute of Neurology, Queen Square, London, UK

Elaine H. Niven
School of Social Sciences (Psychology), University of Dundee, Dundee, UK

Thomas H. Bak and Sharon Abrahams
Human Cognitive Neuroscience–PPLS, University of Edinburgh, Edinburgh, UK
Centre for Cognitive Ageing and Cognitive Epidemiology, University of Edinburgh, Edinburgh, UK
Anne Rowling Regenerative Neurology Clinic, University of Edinburgh, Edinburgh, UK

Scott J. Sherman
Department of Neurology, College of Medicine, University of Arizona, Tucson, AZ 85724, USA

Beatrice Caballero
Department of Neurology, College of Medicine, University of Arizona, Tucson, AZ 85724, USA
Department of Cellular and Molecular Medicine, College of Medicine, University of Arizona, Tucson, AZ 85724, USA

Torsten Falk
Department of Neurology, College of Medicine, University of Arizona, Tucson, AZ 85724, USA
Department of Pharmacology, College of Medicine, University of Arizona, Tucson, AZ 85724, USA

Dominique Eichelberger and Pasquale Calabrese
Division of Molecular and Cognitive Neuroscience, Neuropsychology and Behavioural Neurology Unit, University of Basel, Basel, Switzerland

Antonia Meyer Menorca Chaturvedi Florian Hatz Peter Fuhr and Ute Gschwandtner
Department of Neurology, Hospital of the University of Basel, Petersgraben 4, 4031 Basel, Switzerland

Jing Huang, Wenyan Zhuo, Hongchun Sun, Huan Chen, Peipei Zhu, Xiaobo Pan and Jianhao Yang
Department of Neurology, Zhuhai People's Hospital, Zhuhai 519000, China

Yuhu Zhang and Lijuan Wang
Department of Neurology, Guangdong Neuroscience Institute, Guangdong General Hospital and Guangdong Academy of Medical Sciences, Guangzhou 510080, China

Raquel N. Taddei, Seyda Cankaya, Sandeep Dhaliwal and K. Ray Chaudhuri
MauriceWohl Clinical Neuroscience Institute and NIHR Biomedical Research Centre, Institute of Psychiatry, Psychology and Neuroscience, King's College Hospital, London, UK

Yang-Pei Chang
Department of Neurology, Kaohsiung Municipal Ta-Tung Hospital, Kaohsiung Medical University, Kaohsiung, Taiwan

Yuan-Han Yang
Department of Neurology, Kaohsiung Municipal Ta-Tung Hospital, Kaohsiung Medical University, Kaohsiung, Taiwan
Department of Neurology, Faculty of Medicine, College of Medicine, Kaohsiung Medical University, Kaohsiung, Taiwan

Chiou-Lian Lai and Li-Min Liou
Department of Neurology, Faculty of Medicine, College of Medicine, Kaohsiung Medical University, Kaohsiung, Taiwan
Department of Neurology, Kaohsiung Medical University Hospital, Kaohsiung, Taiwan

Clarissa Loureiro das Chagas Campêlo
Memory Studies Laboratory, Department of Physiology, Universidade Federal do Rio Grande do Norte, Natal, RN, Brazil

Regina Helena Silva
Behavioral Neuroscience Laboratory, Department of Pharmacology, Universidade Federal de São Paulo, São Paulo, SP, Brazil

Sandipan Bhattacharjee and Nina Vadiei
Department of Pharmacy Practice and Science, College of Pharmacy, The University of Arizona, Tucson, AZ, USA

Ziyad Alrabiah
Department of Pharmacy Practice and Science, College of Pharmacy, The University of Arizona, Tucson, AZ, USA

College of Pharmacy, King Saud University, Riyadh, Saudi Arabia

Lisa Goldstone
University of Southern California School of Pharmacy, Los Angeles, CA, USA

Scott J. Sherman
Department of Neurology, College of Medicine, The University of Arizona, Tucson, USA

Xi Wu, Yiqing Qiu, Keith Jiali Wang, Jianchun Chen and Xiaowu Hu
Department of Neurosurgery, Second Military Medical University, Changhai Hospital, No. 168 Changhai Road, Yangpu District, Shanghai, China

Simfukwe
Department of Neurosurgery, Changhai Hospital, Second Military Medical University, International College of Exchange, No. 800 Xiangyin Road, Shanghai 200433, China

Caroline Ran, Mehrafarin Ramezani, Anna Anvret, Dagmar Galter and Andrea Carmine Belin
Department of Neuroscience, Karolinska Institutet, 17177 Stockholm, Sweden

Lovisa Brodin, Thomas Willows, Olof Sydow, Anders Johansson and Per Svenningsson
Department of Clinical Neuroscience, Karolinska Institutet, 17177 Stockholm, Sweden

Karin Wirdefeldt
Department of Clinical Neuroscience, Karolinska Institutet, 17177 Stockholm, Sweden
Department of Medical Epidemiology and Biostatistics, Karolinska Institutet, 17177 Stockholm, Sweden

Marie Westerlund
Department of Neurobiology, Care Sciences and Society, Karolinska Institutet, 14183 Huddinge, Sweden

Fengqing Xiang
Department of Women's and Children's Health, Karolinska Institutet, 17176 Stockholm, Sweden

Luis I. G'omez-Jordana and C. (Lieke) E. Peper
Department of Human Movement Sciences, Faculty of Behavioural and Movement Sciences,
Vrije Universiteit Amsterdam, Amsterdam Movement Sciences, Amsterdam, Netherlands

James Stafford
School of Psychology, Queens University Belfast, David Kier Building, 18-30 Malone Road, Belfast BT7 1NN, UK

Cathy M. Craig
School of Psychology, Queens University Belfast, David Kier Building, 18-30 Malone Road, Belfast BT7 1NN, UK
INCISIV Ltd., Ormeu Avenue, Belfast, UK

Natalie Gasson, Andrew R. Johnson, Leon Booth and Andrea M. Loftus
Curtin Neuroscience Laboratory, School of Psychology and Speech Pathology, Curtin University, Bentley, WA 6102, Australia
ParkC Collaborative Research Group, Curtin University, Bentley, WA 6102, Australia

Blake J. Lawrence
Curtin Neuroscience Laboratory, School of Psychology and Speech Pathology, Curtin University, Bentley, WA 6102, Australia
ParkC Collaborative Research Group, Curtin University, Bentley, WA 6102, Australia
Ear Science Institute Australia, Subiaco, WA, Australia
Ear Sciences Centre, School of Surgery,)e University of Western Australia, Crawley, WA, Australia

Micaela Porta, Giuseppina Pilloni and Massimiliano Pau
Department of Mechanical, Chemical and Materials Engineering, University of Cagliari, Cagliari, Italy

Roberta Pili, Carlo Casula and Giovanni Cossu
A.O.B. "G. Brotzu" General Hospital, Cagliari, Italy

Mauro Murgia
Department of Life Sciences, University of Trieste, Trieste, Italy

Gencer Genc, Srivadee Oravivattanakul, Kathy Wilson, Russell Cerejo, Xin Xin Yu, Darlene Floden, Anwar Ahmed, Michal Gostkowski, Andre Machado and Hubert H. Fernandez
1Center for Neurological Restoration, Cleveland Clinic, 9500 Euclid Avenue, Mail Code U2, Cleveland, OH 44195, USA

Hesham Abboud
Center for Neurological Restoration, Cleveland Clinic, 9500 Euclid Avenue, Mail Code U2, Cleveland, OH 44195, USA
CaseWestern Reserve University, University Hospitals of Cleveland, 11100 Euclid Avenue, Cleveland, OH 44106, USA
Department of Neurology, Alexandria University, El Hadara University Hospital, El Hadara Kebly, Alexandria, Egypt

Faisal Alsallom
CaseWestern Reserve University, University Hospitals of Cleveland, 11100 Euclid Avenue, Cleveland, OH 44106, USA

Ayman Ezzeldin, Hazem Marouf and Ossama Y. Mansour
Department of Neurology, Alexandria University, El Hadara University Hospital, El Hadara Kebly, Alexandria, Egypt

Nicolas R. Thompson
Department of Quantitative Health Sciences, Cleveland Clinic, 9500 Euclid Avenue, Mail Code JJN3-01, Cleveland, OH 44195, USA
Neurological Institute, Center for Outcomes Research and Evaluation, Cleveland Clinic, 9500 Euclid Avenue, Cleveland, OH 44195, USA

Dennys Reyes
Department of Neurology, Cleveland Clinic Florida, 2950 Cleveland Clinic Blvd, Fl 3, Weston, FL 33331, USA

Timo Siepmann and Heinz Reichmann
Department of Neurology, University Hospital Carl Gustav Carus, Technische Universitaet Dresden, Dresden, Germany

Ana Isabel Penzlin
Department of Neurology and Rehabilitation, Klinik Bavaria Kreischa, Kreischa, Germany

Ben Min-Woo Illigens
Department of Neurology, Beth Israel Deaconess Medical Center, Harvard Medical School, Boston, MA, USA

Satoru Otsuki
Department of Rehabilitation, Juntendo University Nerima Hospital, 3-1-10 Takanodai, Nerima-ku, Tokyo 177-8521, Japan
Department of Rehabilitation Medicine, Juntendo University Graduate School, 2-1-1 Hongo, Bunkyo-ku, Tokyo 113-8421, Japan

Masanori Nagaoka
Department of Rehabilitation Medicine, Juntendo University Graduate School, 2-1-1 Hongo, Bunkyo-ku, Tokyo 113-8421, Japan

Jennifer A. Foley, Tom Foltynie and Patricia Limousin
National Hospital for Neurology and Neurosurgery, Queen Square, London, UK

UCL Institute of Neurology, Queen Square, London, UK

Lisa Cipolotti
National Hospital for Neurology and Neurosurgery, Queen Square, London, UK
Dipartimento di Scienze Psicologiche, Pedagogiche e della Formazione, Università degli Studi di Palermo, Palermo, Italy

Minrui Weng, Xiaoji Xie, Cheng-wu Zhang and Lin Li
Key Laboratory of Flexible Electronics (KLOFE) and Institute of Advanced Materials (IAM), Jiangsu National Synergetic Innovation Center for Advanced Materials (SICAM), Nanjing Tech University (Nanjing Tech), 30 South Puzhu Road, Nanjing 211816, China

Chao Liu and Kah-Leong Lim
Department of Physiology, Yong Loo Lin School of Medicine, National University of Singapore, Singapore,117593

Rita Moretti and Paola Caruso
Clinica Neurologica, Dipartimento Universitario Clinico di Scienze Mediche, Chirurgiche e della Salute, Università degli Studi di Trieste, Trieste, Italy

Matteo Dal Ben
FIF Science Park, University of Trieste, Trieste, Italy
Dipartimento Universitario Clinico di Scienze Mediche, Chirurgiche e della Salute, Università degli Studi di Trieste, Trieste, Italy

Wei Zhang, Hong He, Junjie Zhao, Tao Li, Leitao Wu and Jianzong Chen
Research Center of Traditional Chinese Medicine, Xijing Hospital, Fourth Military Medical University, Xi'an 710032, China

Hujie Song
Department of Encephalopathy, Xi'an Encephalopathy Hospital of Traditional Chinese Medicine, Xi'an 710032, China

Xiaojun Zhang
Department of Physics, Fourth Military Medical University, Xi'an 710032, China

Jing-ya Lin, Zhen-guo Liu, Cheng-long Xie, Lu Song and Ai-juan Yan
Department of Neurology, Xin Hua Hospital Affiliated to Shanghai Jiao Tong University School of Medicine, 1665 Kongjiang Road, Shanghai 200092, China

Alexandre Gironell, Berta Pascual-Sedano, Ignacio Aracil, Juan Mar´ın-Lahoz, Javier Pagonabarraga and Jaime Kulisevsky
Movement Disorders Unit, Department of Neurology, Hospital de la Santa Creu i Sant Pau, Autonomous University of Barcelona, Catalonia, Spain

Anson B. Rosenfeldt, Jay L. Alberts
Department of Biomedical Engineering, Cleveland Clinic, 9500 Euclid Ave., Cleveland, OH 44119, USA
Center for Neurological Restoration, Cleveland Clinic, 9500 Euclid Ave., Cleveland, OH 44119, USA
Cleveland FES Center, L. Stokes Cleveland VAMedical Center, 10701 East Blvd, Cleveland,OH 44106,USA

Tanujit Dey
Quantitative Health Sciences, Cleveland Clinic, 9500 Euclid Ave., Cleveland, OH 44119, USA

Jayakrishna Tippabathani, Jayshree Nellore, Vaishnavie Radhakrishnan, Somashree Banik and Sonia Kapoor
Department of Biotechnology, Sathyabama University, Chennai 600119, India

Louise Wiblin and Rory Durcan
Clinical Ageing Research Unit, Newcastle University, Newcastle upon Tyne NE4 5PL, UK

Mark Lee
2St Benedict's Hospice for Specialist Palliative Care, St. Benedict'sWay, Sunderland SR2 0NY, UK

Katie Brittain
Department of Nursing, Midwifery and Health, Northumbria University, Coach Lane Campus West, Room B128, Newcastle upon Tyne NE7 7XA, UK

Index

A

Action Tremor, 248-252

Activities of Daily Living, 20-22, 24-25, 80, 122, 125, 156, 159, 166, 179, 183, 212

Adl Disability, 20-24

Aerobic Exercise, 253-254, 256

Amyotrophic Lateral Sclerosis, 48, 54-55, 59, 67, 118, 142, 147, 275

Apathy, 48-49, 52, 54, 91, 100, 127, 137, 139, 183, 201, 203-205, 207-210, 212, 222-230

B

Basal Ganglia, 2-5, 10, 13-14, 16, 18, 29, 54, 100, 125, 148, 199, 218, 220, 240, 244, 246, 251-252

C

Cerebral Ischemia, 61, 66

Charles-bonnet Syndrome, 87, 89

Cognitive Decline, 34, 68, 72, 76, 82-83, 92-93, 99, 101, 107, 109, 164, 167, 200-201, 204, 206-208, 211, 229, 257, 272

Cognitive Training, 156-167

D

Dbs, 96, 102, 127-131, 137, 139, 157, 178-179, 181-183, 200-210, 212, 254

Deep Brain Stimulation Surgery, 178

Depression Treatment, 121-125

Differential Diagnosis, 47-48, 52-53, 89

Dopaminergic Neuron, 93, 213, 240

Dyskinesia, 1-2, 5-7, 9, 11, 13-16, 35, 38, 57, 178-185, 193, 201, 240-244, 246-247

E

Eeg, 68-70, 72, 74, 76-78, 104, 109

Endocannabinoid System, 2-5, 8-10, 12-13, 19

Event-related Potential, 103, 109

Executive Function, 48-49, 51-53, 73, 82, 103-104, 106-107, 156-159, 164-166, 200-208, 210-212

F

Foxa1, 259-260, 262-266

Freezing of Gait, 148-149, 154, 179, 183

G

Gait Patterns, 168-169, 175

Gait Variability, 148-149, 153

Globus Pallidus, 3-4, 139-140, 179, 184-185, 200

H

Hypomania, 127, 129, 133, 137, 139

I

Insomnia, 9, 79-84, 91

Iron Accumulation, 213-216

L

Lipid Peroxidation, 214, 216, 219

M

Marijuana, 1-4, 6-10, 16-19

Maximal Reach Distance, 192

Mild Cognitive Impairment, 26, 47-48, 54, 76, 78, 83, 103, 108, 156, 166-167, 230

Mitochondria Dysfunction, 214, 217-218

Mptp, 5-6, 13-15, 55, 64, 100, 113, 216, 219, 231-235, 239, 247

Mrna Expression, 63, 113, 116, 120, 141, 144-145, 241, 244-245, 259, 262, 264

Multiple System Atrophy, 53, 83, 118, 191, 267, 274-275

N

Neuroinflammation, 3, 8, 15, 17, 213-215, 217, 219

Nigrostriatal Dopamine, 1

Nrf2, 63, 141-147, 217, 221

Nurr1, 259-260, 262-266

O

Olfaction Function, 253-254, 256

Orthostatic Hypotension, 2, 11, 27-29, 32, 187-188

Oxidative Phosphorylation, 60, 63

Oxidative Stress, 3-4, 7, 56, 62, 66, 113, 141, 214, 216-220, 238-239, 254

P

Parkinson's Disease Therapy, 1, 4, 11

Parkinsonian Striatum, 240, 246-247

Peripheral Blood Lymphocytes, 259-260, 265

Physical Activity, 168-169, 172-177, 254

Phytocannabinoids, 1, 8, 18

Polymorphism, 9, 19, 32, 34, 39, 110-111, 114, 118-120, 256, 258, 260, 262

Postural Instability, 2, 27, 34, 36, 44, 47, 148, 178, 192, 199

Progressive Supranuclear Palsy, 47, 52-54, 229, 267, 274-275

Psychosis, 2, 7, 10-11, 85-102, 137, 227, 229-230

Psychotherapy, 121-125

Q

Quality of Life, 1, 8-9, 11, 18-20, 25-26, 68, 79, 83, 85, 98, 122, 126, 139, 154, 156, 159, 166-169, 176, 178-179, 183-184, 207-208, 210, 212, 229, 253, 256-257, 267, 270, 272, 274-275

R

Resting Tremor, 2, 6, 27, 43-44, 248-249, 251-252

Rivastigmine, 94-95, 101, 109, 222-224, 227-230

Ros, 56, 63, 213-217, 220, 232

S

Salidroside, 231-232, 238

Single Nucleotide Polymorphism, 110, 114, 118

Skin Biopsies, 186-189, 191

Sleep Disorders, 2, 9, 19, 79-83

Snca Gene, 110-111, 113, 117-118, 120

Social Isolation, 253, 267, 273, 275

Spatial Distance, 192-193, 195, 197

Substantia Nigra, 2-6, 8, 15, 55, 64, 116-117, 187, 213, 215, 220, 231, 238, 240, 247, 253, 259, 266

Subthalamic Nucleus, 6, 127, 139-140, 184-185, 200, 208-209, 212, 247, 257

Superoxide Dismutase, 7, 60, 216

T

Transcranial Direct Current Stimulation, 156-157, 160-163

V

Vascular Permeability, 55, 57, 60-61, 64

Vegf-a, 55-57, 59-61, 65-66

Vegf-b, 55-57, 59-67

Verbal Fluency, 47-49, 51-52, 54, 103-104, 106, 115, 200, 202, 204, 207-209

Visual Hallucination, 86, 103, 108

Visual Processing, 68, 72, 107, 207, 211

Visuospatial Ability, 68, 70, 72-73

www.ingramcontent.com/pod-product-compliance
Lightning Source LLC
Chambersburg PA
CBHW061330190326
41458CB00011B/3959

9 781632 427328